Anesthesia For Vascular Surgery

Anesthesia For Vascular Surgery

Edited by
Michael F. Roizen

Professor and Chairman
Department of Anesthesia and Critical Care
Professor
Department of Medicine
University of Chicago Pritzker School of Medicine
Chicago, Illinois

With contributions by

M. T. Bailin
D. J. Benefiel
D. J. Cullen
J. K. Davison
J. E. Ellis
P. J. Ford
M. A. Gettes
R. B. Glaser
D. D. Glass
I. J. Isaacson

J. A. Kaplan
G. H. Lampe
C. P. Larson, Jr.
J. J. Lunn
R. J. Lusby
D. T. Mangano
M. T. McCaffrey
J. D. Michenfelder
M. Nugent
M. F. O'Connor
F. K. Orkin

N. L. Pace
C. T. Petrovitch
T. L. K. Rao
N. B. Reddy
S. Roth
S. A. Shenaq
R. Teplick
J. P. Welch
M. P. Yeager
C. K. Zarins

Churchill Livingstone
New York, Edinburgh, London, Melbourne

Library of Congress Cataloging in Publication Data

Anesthesia for vascular surgery/edited by Michael F. Roizen
    p.   cm.
    Includes bibliographical references.
    ISBN 0-443-08567-6
    1. Blood-vessels—Surgery. 2. Anesthesia. I. Roizen, Michael F.
    [DNLM: 1. Anesthesia. 2. Vascular Surgery. WG 170 A579]
  RD598.5.A515 1990
  617.9'67413—dc20
  DNLM/DLC
  for Library of Congress   89-22134
                                        CIP

Distributed in the United Kingdom by Churchill Livingstone, Robert Stevenson House, 1–3 Baxter's Place, Leith Walk, Edinburgh EH1 3AF, and by associated companies, branches, and representatives throughout the world.

Accurate indications, adverse reactions, and dosage schedules for drugs are provided in this book, but it is possible that they may change. The reader is urged to review the package information data of the manufacturers of the medications mentioned.

The Publishers have made every effort to trace the copyright holders for borrowed material. If they have inadvertently overlooked any, they will be pleased to make the necessary arrangements at the first opportunity.

Copy Editor: *Kimberly Quinlan*
Production Designer: *Angela Cirnigliaro*
Production Supervisor: *Sharon Tuder*

Printed in the United States of America

First published in 1990

This volume is dedicated to vascular patients and surgeons everywhere who benefit from the care and devotion of their anesthesiologists; to my parents and Bill Hamilton, who taught me to do what is right and to say what is fact and what is bias; and to Nancy, Jeffrey, and Jennifer and the members of the Department of Anesthesia who allowed the time and sacrificed their own interests for the production of this work.

Contributors

Michael T. Bailin, MD
Instructor, Department of Anaesthesia, Harvard Medical School; Assistant Anesthetist, Department of Anesthesia, Massachusetts General Hospital, Boston, Massachusetts

David J. Benefiel, MD
Assistant Professor of Clinical Anesthesia, Department of Anesthesia, University of California, San Francisco, School of Medicine, San Francisco, California

David J. Cullen, MD
Professor, Department of Anaesthesia, Harvard Medical School; Director of Recovery Room, Department of Anesthesia, Massachusetts General Hospital, Boston, Massachusetts

J. Kenneth Davison, DDS, MD
Assistant Professor, Department of Anaesthesia, Harvard Medical School; Assistant Anesthetist, Department of Anesthesia, Massachusetts General Hospital, Boston, Massachusetts

John E. Ellis, MD
Assistant Professor, Department of Anesthesia and Critical Care, University of Chicago Pritzker School of Medicine, Chicago, Illinois

Penny J. Ford, MD
Instructor and Assistant Anesthetist, Department of Anesthesia, Massachusetts General Hospital, Boston, Massachusetts

Mark A. Gettes, MD
Assistant Professor, Department of Anesthesiology, Mount Sinai School of Medicine, New York, New York

Richard B. Glaser, MD
Assistant Professor, Department of Anesthesia, University of California, San Francisco, School of Medicine, San Francisco, California

D. David Glass, MD
Professor of Anesthesiology, Surgery, and Medicine, Department of Anesthesiology, Dartmouth Medical School, Hanover, New Hampshire

Ira J. Isaacson, MD
Associate Professor, Department of Anesthesiology, Emory University School of Medicine; Director of Anesthesia for Surgical Specialties, Emory University Hospital, Atlanta, Georgia

Joel A. Kaplan, MD
Horace W. Goldsmith Professor and Chairman, Department of Anesthesiology, Mount Sinai School of Medicine, New York, New York

George H. Lampe, MD
Assistant Professor, Department of Anesthesia, University of California, San Francisco, School of Medicine, San Francisco, California

C. Philip Larson, Jr, MD
Professor of Anesthesia and Surgery (Neurosurgery), Stanford University School of Medicine, Stanford, California

Jeffrey J. Lunn, MD
Assistant Professor, Department of Anesthesiology, Mayo Medical School and Mayo Foundation; Consultant, Anesthesiology and Critical Care, Mayo Clinic, Rochester, Minnesota

Robert J. Lusby, MD
Professor, Department of Surgery, University of Sydney School of Medicine, Sydney, Australia

Dennis T. Mangano, MD, PhD
Professor and Vice-Chairman, Department of Anesthesia, University of California, San Francisco, School of Medicine, San Francisco, California

Michael T. McCaffrey, MD
Assistant Professor, Departments of Neurology, Anesthesia, and Critical Care, University of Health Sciences/Chicago Medical School and the Brain Research Institute, Chicago, Illinois

John D. Michenfelder, MD
Professor, Department of Anesthesiology, Mayo Medical School and Mayo Foundation; Consultant, Department of Anesthesiology, Mayo Clinic, Rochester, Minnesota

Michael Nugent, MD
Professor and Chairman, Department of Anesthesiology, Medical College of Ohio, Toledo, Ohio

Michael F. O'Connor, MD
Fellow, Departments of Anesthesia and Critical Care, University of Chicago Pritzker School of Medicine, Chicago, Illinois

Fredrick K. Orkin, MD
Associate Professor, Department of Anesthesia, University of California, San Francisco, School of Medicine, San Francisco, California

Nathan L. Pace, MD
Professor, Department of Anesthesiology, University of Utah School of Medicine; Adjunct Professor, Department of Bioengineering, College of Engineering, University of Utah, Salt Lake City, Utah

Charise T. Petrovitch, MD
Chief, Department of Obstetric Anesthesia, Washington Hospital Center, Washington, DC

Tadikonda L. K. Rao, MD
Professor and Chairman, Department of Anesthesiology, Loyola University Stritch School of Medicine, Maywood, Illinois

Neeraja B. Reddy, MD
Assistant Professor, Department of Anesthesiology, Division of Cardiovascular Anesthesia and Division of the Pain Clinic, Loyola University of Chicago Stritch School of Medicine, Maywood, Illinois

Michael F. Roizen, MD
Professor and Chairman, Department of Anesthesia and Critical Care; Professor, Department of Medicine, University of Chicago Pritzker School of Medicine, Chicago, Illinois

Steven Roth, MD
Assistant Professor, Department of Anesthesia and Critical Care, University of Chicago Pritzker School of Medicine, Chicago, Illinois

Salwa A. Shenaq, MD
Associate Professor, Department of Anesthesiology, Baylor College of Medicine, Houston, Texas

Richard Teplick, MD
Associate Professor, Department of Anaesthesia, Harvard Medical School; Attending Anesthetist, Department of Anesthesia, Massachusetts General Hospital, Boston, Massachusetts

James P. Welch, MD
Instructor, Department of Anaesthesia, Harvard Medical School; Attending Anesthetist, Department of Anesthesia, Massachusetts General Hospital, Boston, Massachusetts

Mark P. Yeager, MD
Assistant Professor of Anesthesia and Medicine (Critical Care), Dartmouth Medical School, Hanover, New Hampshire

Christopher K. Zarins, MD
Professor, Department of Surgery; Chief, Section of Vascular Surgery, University of Chicago Pritzker School of Medicine, Chicago, Illinois

Preface

Despite the fact that practically all anesthesiologists provide anesthesia for vascular surgery, there has been a distinct lack of information published about the topic. This is unlike the situation in cardiac surgery, where a large body of knowledge has developed as a direct result of advances made in that field. For example, no major textbook has yet devoted itself to the science and clinical concerns of anesthesia for vascular surgery. This is unfortunate, as no other patient group needs attention so badly; in fact, the 30-day mortality rate is significantly higher for patients after vascular surgery than for those after cardiac surgery.

I believe there is no place in all of anesthesia in which the anesthetist can make as much of a difference to perioperative well-being as in vascular surgery. In vascular surgery, perioperative mortality is a direct result of the intra- and perioperative care rendered by the anesthetist. This is not to say that poor surgery cannot ruin a great anesthetic, much as poor anesthesia can certainly ruin great surgery. But good or great anesthesia can make great surgery even better and most vascular surgeons and patients realize this fact.

This book describes how anesthesia is provided for vascular surgery in various locales, supplying not only scientific foundations of practice, but also what I believe are clinical "pearls." Most of the sections are organized in the following general fashion. First, a surgeon describes a major vascular surgical procedure in terms of the cause, care, and treatment of an important vascular problem—the pertinent surgical issues, the underlying pathophysiologic changes, and the surgical approach. The section then continues with descriptions of the scientific basis of anesthesia care. Final chapters in each section describe how clinicians actually provide anesthesia at various institutions. At these institutions, anesthesia care for that particular vascular surgical procedure is considered among the very best. The inclusion of more than one of these "how-to" chapters in each section demonstrates that different techniques work equally well. This book hopes to show that a thorough understanding of underlying pathophysiologic principles is the most important factor determining superior anesthesia care for vascular surgery.

Although the book contains many discussions of surgical and theoretical approaches to many problems, plus controversial issues, it is not intended only for residents or other students of specific areas. The book was also written to help the practitioner, by describing what others have done, and are doing, with success. This "how-to" approach consists of different philosophies, manifested by different styles, and practiced at different institutions. Most of these practices and strategies do not conflict, but, in fact, complement each other. Some of them, such as Dr. Cullen's approach to prophylactic ventilation and Dr. Isaacson's preference for early extubation, clearly contrast. I believe such differences illustrate the art of anesthesia. In my view, it is not what clinicians actually do but, rather, the rationale for these preferences, plus the subsequent practices used to monitor the effectiveness of these techniques, that account for the success of such diverse strategies. The inclusion of these diverse points of view should strengthen the reader's understanding of not only how to monitor the patient but also their appreciation of what is truly important in monitoring. Readers can then select from among the several treatment strategies those most appropriate to their practice setting and their surgical colleagues.

The editor and contributors hope that knowledge gained from this book will increase the enjoyment and pride the reader takes in rendering excellent anesthesia care to vascular surgery patients.

Michael F. Roizen, MD

Acknowledgment

I would like to thank and acknowledge Pauline Snider for the excellent work she did in editing the manuscript so that all the chapters have uniform style and clarity in their presentation.

Contents

Section VI. CONTROVERSIES AND OTHER ISSUES

Section I

SCOPE OF THE PROBLEM

Morbidity and Mortality from Major Vascular Surgery

Richard B. Glaser

Several conditions produce the relatively high perioperative morbidity and mortality of major vascular surgery: interruption of normal blood flow, the stress of clamping and unclamping major vessels, blood and fluid shifts, and many morbid conditions that frequently coexist in these patients. Although physicians are greatly interested in identifying high-risk patients and modifying anesthesia and surgical techniques to minimize adverse outcomes, it is not yet possible to weigh accurately the risk of surgery against the benefits for all subsets of patients.

Measures of morbidity and mortality are not uniform or well defined. It is difficult to compare outcome from different centers and surgeons, much less the variation of outcome over time. Also, the definition of morbid states such as renal failure, congestive heart failure, stroke, and myocardial infarction vary from study to study. For example, mortality has been defined variously as resulting from surgery if death occurs within 24 hours of surgery, if it occurs anytime during hospitalization after surgery, or if it occurs within 6 months of surgery.

Clinical decision-making about surgical intervention should be based on information about outcome variables. Ideally, this information should be derived from well-designed, randomized clinical trials. In reality, data from poorly controlled retrospective studies (or worse yet, clinical impressions) are often the basis for decision-making. The popularity of certain surgical procedures that were initially well accepted (such as extracranial-intracranial bypass for the treatment of cerebral ischemia) often withers under the light of well-controlled outcome studies.[1] When interpreting studies on outcome for peripheral vascular procedures, one must remember that only a few of these study results have had, or are likely to have, validation by randomized clinical trials.

When a practitioner wants to weigh the risk of surgery against the expectation of benefit, information is needed about the likelihood of certain outcomes. What, for example, is the projected rate of myocardial infarction and death after repair of an abdominal aortic aneurysm in a 64-year-old patient who has hypertension and diabetes? When an anesthetist selects an anesthetic technique, information from outcome studies on similar patients should guide the choice. The more outcome information available, the easier it is to make an informed decision for a patient having a particular risk profile.

A complete assessment of risk must consider the natural course of the disease and the likelihood that surgery will alter that course. In the above example, one would need to know the natural course of an abdominal aortic aneurysm, both with and without surgical intervention. Moreover, the value of a procedure such as aortoiliac reconstruction is determined not only by knowing the possibility of limb salvage and favorable functional outcome, but also by considering the life expectancy in a population often having other potentially life-threatening degenerative disease. To the extent such information is available, it must then be modified to account for the continuing changes being made in surgical, medical, and anesthetic practices.

Taking these considerations into account, this chapter discusses morbidity and mortality in light of the following issues: the surgical procedure; the natural history of the disease and the effect of coexisting diseases; the risk according to underlying organ pathology; and the effect, if any, of specific types of anesthesia.

MORBIDITY AND MORTALITY AFTER SURGERY ON THE CAROTID ARTERY

The first carotid endarterectomies (CEAs) were performed in 1954 and 1955. Originally, only completed strokes and transient ischemic attacks (TIAs) were considered indications for CEA.[2] Later, the following were added: stroke in progress, asymptomatic carotid bruit, and occlusive carotid disease documented invasively and noninvasively. As a result, CEA has become increasingly popular in the United States. The number of CEAs performed in the United States increased from 15,000 in 1971[3] to over 100,000 in 1984.[4] Of the three prospective studies examining the effectiveness of CEA in treating TIAs or strokes, all have ultimately failed to show a statistically significant improvement in the surgically treated group.[5-7] Moreover, two of these studies predate the routine use of antiplatelet aggregation drugs for medically treated patients, a factor that may bias the outcome in favor of surgical intervention.

Several prospective randomized trials presently under way examine the usefulness of CEA for patients with asymptomatic carotid stenosis.[8] The Veterans Administration Cooperative Study expects to recruit 500 patients with angiographically proven occlusive carotid disease. The incidence of stroke, death, and TIAs in patients treated with CEA and aspirin will be compared with the incidence in patients given aspirin therapy alone. Data are not yet available.

Morbidity after Carotid Endarterectomy

Since 1968, the incidence of postoperative neurologic deficit after CEA has ranged from 45 to 3.6 percent.[9,10] Procedural morbidity and mortality improved from the introduction of CEA until about 1970. After 1970, variation in outcome correlated less well with time than with institution. No single variable seems to distinguish institutions with high morbidity and mortality from those with low rates, although, in general, larger centers—those more likely to tabulate and report results—have better outcome statistics than do smaller community hospitals.[11-13] Table 1-1 shows what some studies reported regarding the morbidity and mortality of CEA.

Table 1-1. Morbidity and Mortality from Carotid Endarerectomy

| Author(s) and Year | No. of Patients (n) | Neurologic Deficit | | Mortality (%) |
		Transient (%)	Permanent (%)	
DeWeese et al.[29] (1968)	205	7.9	18.9	11.2
Rainer et al.[110] (1968)	208	2.7	0.8	2.4
Fields et al.[7] (1970)	169	1.4	6.0	3.5
Thompson et al.[111] (1970)	592	0.5	2.7	3.4
Tytus et al.[9] (1970)	44	18.0	27.0	11.0
Howe and Kindt et al.[112] (1974)	62	0.0	1.4	0.0
Sundt et al.[10] (1975)	331	0.6	3.0	0.0
Toole et al.[113] (1975)	82	6.0	6.0	6.0
Baker et al.[114] (1977)	272	3.0	1.6	0.7
Prioleau et al.[115] (1977)	240		10.7	3.2
Fleming et al.[116] (1977)	189		2.1	1.6
Easton and Sherman [108] (1977)	194		14.5	6.6
Cornell[117] (1978)	100	3.0	2.0	4.0
Haynes and Dempsey[118] (1979)	232	2.5	0.4	1.1
Ennix et al.[12] (1979)	1,238		2.4	2.7
Brott and Thalinger[13] (1984)	371	1.6	6.3	2.8
Slavish et al.[109] (1984)	743	3.5	1.8	2.7
Fode et al.[33] (1986)	3,328	2.5	4.0	2.2
Graham et al.[119] (1986)	105	1.0	0.0	1.0
Smith et al.[17] (1988)	60	1.5	1.5	0.0

Asymptomatic Occlusive Carotid Artery Disease

The occurrence of asymptomatic carotid bruits constitutes one of the most problematic events with respect to analyzing the risks and benefits of surgical intervention. Observing for an average of 46 months 138 patients who had asymptomatic bruits, Thompson et al.[14] found a 27 percent incidence of TIAs and a 17 percent incidence of stroke. These patients were not chosen randomly, however, and the location of the stroke was not correlated with the site of the bruit. Evidence indicates that not all asymptomatic carotid bruits have the same prognosis.

Only one published report was a randomized trial to study CEA in patients with asymptomatic carotid bruits.[5] Of 19 patients who had abnormal results on ocular pneumoplethysmography, 15 had surgery and 14 were treated with aspirin. With these small numbers, no significant difference between treatment modalities was detected. When data for the 28 patients who refused random assignment of therapy and underwent CEA are included in the analysis, the surgically treated patients had a significantly poorer outcome. However, these patients may have had more serious symptoms and may have refused random assignment because they were not, in fact, asymptomatic.

Chambers and Norris[15] observed 500 patients with asymptomatic cervical bruits for up to 4 years. Thirty-six had cerebral ischemic events and 51 had cardiac events. Only eight had a frank stroke. Patients who had strokes were also much more likely to have coronary artery disease (CAD). This relationship suggests that heart disease contributes to stroke (by arrhythmias, hypotension, or embolism) or that patients likely to have a stroke also have more serious generalized atherosclerosis. Unfortunately, the presence of CAD makes these patients a greater surgical risk. The risk of an asymptomatic patient with a bruit having an unheralded stroke is less than 2 percent per year—a level clearly below the immediate serious morbidity associated with CEAs in most centers. Seventy-eight percent of the patients who had ischemic events presented with TIAs, suggesting that surgical intervention can usually be postponed until symptoms develop.

In another prospective study of carotid bruits, the severity of underlying carotid disease was determined by duplex scanning, an imaging technique that combines B-mode and Doppler ultrasonography. Of 167 patients observed for up to 3 years, 10 had either TIAs or stroke.[16] The annual rate of symptom occurrence (TIA or stroke) was calculated by life table analysis to be about 4 percent—a figure consistent with findings of Chambers and Norris.[15]

The degree of stenosis correlates with the likelihood that disease will progress and ischemic symptoms develop. Overall, carotid stenosis progresses in 30 to 40 percent of patients and even regresses in some.[17] In the Chambers and Norris study,[15] the incidence of stroke at 1 year was 1.7 percent for the entire group; however, when stenosis exceeded 75 percent (as determined by continuous Doppler ultrasonography), the 1-year incidence was 5 percent. A study by Javid et al.[18]

angiographically demonstrated that carotid atheromas increased in over 62 percent of patients. Atheromas increased in size by at least 25 percent per year in 34 percent of lesions. The presence on duplex scanning of stenosis greater than 80 percent correlated highly with either the occurrence of symptoms or progression to complete occlusion. A 1986 study by Hertzer et al.[19] also suggested that endarterectomy is more likely to prevent stroke if the stenosis is greater than 70 percent.

Duplex scanning is 84 percent as specific and 99 percent as sensitive as contrast angiography. The likelihood of discovering significant carotid occlusive disease is significantly less with only auscultation (i.e., discovery of a bruit) than with duplex scanning or other newer imaging techniques.[20,21] In patients with asymptomatic cervical bruits detected on physical examination in the Framingham study, the stroke rate was 12 percent in 171 patients observed for up to 8 years.[22] In a population-based study in rural Georgia, asymptomatic patients with a bruit had a stroke rate of 14 percent.[23]

Transient Ischemic Attacks

TIAs and stroke in evolution constitute the two most commonly accepted indications for the performance of CEA. Two randomized studies have compared the outcome of patients with TIAs treated either surgically or medically.[6,7] One study was terminated when three deaths and five strokes occurred in the first 20 surgical patients.[6] The second randomized study, a large multicenter trial, showed no difference in the two treatment modalities when in-hospital deaths and strokes were included in the comparison of long-term outcome.[7] This trial compared patients in the 1960s. It is difficult to interpret these findings in light of advances in both medical and surgical therapy for TIAs since that time. The impression persists in many centers, however, that patients fare better with surgery. This impression is supported by comparing morbidity and mortality rates at "better" institutions with rates for the natural course of untreated TIAs (see below).

TIAs are predictors of stroke. In one study, 46 percent of patients with stroke had had TIAs.[7] The risk of stroke in patients with TIAs ranges from 4 to 6 percent per year and from 24 to 37 percent overall.[24,25] Also, 15 percent of patients with TIAs have a stroke within 3 years.[26] Of patients who have a stroke after the onset of TIAs, approximately 21 percent have the stroke within the first month and 51 percent within a year of symptoms.[27] West et al.[28] calculated that the average combined stroke and mortality rates from published surgical series to 1979 was 9.1 percent. Comparing this figure with the estimated risk of stroke or death over 5 years in patients not having surgery (risk of 25 percent), these investigators suggested that the overall morbidity and mortality of TIAs or stroke would decrease with surgical intervention. At institutions having fewer adverse outcomes after surgery, the figures would favor surgical intervention even more.

Therefore, for surgery to be warranted, the surgery-induced decrease in morbidity and mortality of the untreated disease would have to exceed the adverse effects of surgery itself. Several studies examining the risk of stroke after CEA indicate that patients who survive the hospitalization for CEA without significant neurologic deficits have a better long-term prognosis than do patients undergoing the natural course of the disease.[7,9,29] Within 24 months of CEA, stenosis recurs in only 3.6 percent of patients.[30] Also, the fact that most of these strokes occur on the contralateral side suggests a protective ef-

fect of surgery. In one controlled study, the incidence of stroke in patients with unilateral carotid stenosis was lower in those who had had CEA than in similar nonsurgical patients.[7] However, when perioperative morbidity and mortality are factored in, it is not clear whether CEA provides a net benefit to the patient.

The rate of recurrent stroke in patients who have not undergone CEA ranges from 25 to 50 percent overall, with a yearly occurrence of 5 to 10 percent.[25,31,32]

These studies estimate that mortality from any stroke—initial or recurrent—ranges from 20 to 30 percent.

Risk Factors for Carotid Endarterectomy

Morbidity and mortality in patients undergoing CEA usually involve the heart or brain. Therefore, any attempt to limit the morbidity and mortality of CEA must not only decrease the risk factors for adverse cardiac and cerebrovascular effects but also modify surgical and anesthetic techniques to prevent their occurrence. The factors influencing the risk of CEA are as follows.

Severity of the Underlying Cerebrovascular Disease

Postoperative mortality and stroke depend greatly on the severity of the underlying disease.[14,28] Cerebrovascular disease in patients undergoing CEA ranges from unilateral asymptomatic partial occlusion to severe or complete occlusion of both carotid arteries. The following conditions that are considered indications for CEA are arranged in ascending order, according to the frequency of their association with postoperative mortality and neurologic deficit: asymptomatic carotid bruit, TIAs, history of prior cerebrovascular accident, and acute carotid occlusion with neurologic deficit. Table 1-2 shows the results of a retrospective analysis of CEA in 592 patients, in which Thompson et al.[14] relate outcome to three common indications for surgery.

In their retrospective analysis of 3,328 CEAs, Fode et al.[33] examined the combined rates for stroke and death by indication for surgery. Morbidity and mortality increased progressively as the presurgical neurologic status worsened (Table 1-3).

When acute carotid artery occlusion with profound neurologic deficit is the indication for surgery, morbidity and mortality are understandably high. However, because patency of blood vessels often is restored, neurologic outcome may improve. Meyer et al.[34] reported a 40 percent success rate in restoring patency in 34 such patients. Follow-up neurologic examinations produced normal results in 26.5 percent of patients, and an additional 31.2 percent had improved neurologic status. Seven patients (20.6 percent) died. These figures compare favorably with figures regarding the natural course of acute carotid occlusion: that is, 2 to 12 percent recover and 16 to 55 percent die.[35–37]

Age

The availability of large computerized databases enables estimates of mortality from CEA to be made for the entire country. Such estimates have greater external validity, that is, they are not biased by the attributes of a single surgeon, institution, or surgical technique. Large computerized databases also allow a more detailed analysis of the relationship between surgical mortality and demographic factors such as age, sex, and race. Information available on mortality rates for CEA from all nonfederal California hospitals in 1983 indicates that almost all mortality from CEA results from factors related to aging (Table 1-4).[38] The mortality data pertain only to deaths that occurred during the hospital admission for surgery. Thus, when estimating mortality, one must take into consideration the age of the patient.

For CEA, the relationship between surgical mortality and age is exponential. Figure 1-1A shows the percentage of people who died after CEA plotted against age. In Figure 1-1B, the y-axis has been converted to the logarithm of the percentage of patients who died. The regression line for the relationship of the variables is drawn through the data points. The plot of the natural logarithm (ln) of mortality against age is almost perfectly linear, the correlation coefficient (r^2) being 0.997. This high value means that essentially all of the variability in mortality experienced in this cohort is accounted for by increasing age and, by inference, the diseases associated with aging. To have an effect on mortality, the

Table 1-2. Surgical Mortality and Indication for Surgery, as Reported by Thompson et al.[111]

Indication for Surgery	No. of Patients $(n)^a$	Mortality (%)	
		Nonprocedural	Procedural
Asymptomatic bruit	51	0	0
TIAs	206	0.97	0.77
Frank stroke	112	4.5	3.7

^{a} Total number of patients = 592.
(Modified from Thompson et al.,[111] with permission.)

Table 1-3. Surgical Mortality and Indication for
Surgery, as Reported by Fode et al.[33]

Indication for Surgery	Combined Death and Stroke Rates from CEA (%)
Asymptomatic bruit	5.3
TIA	6.4
Minor stroke	7.7
Major stroke	9.8
Progressing stroke	21.1

(From Fode NC et al.,[33] with permission.)

different approaches to patient management (e.g., anesthetic technique, intraoperative carotid shunting, and postoperative care) would have to minimize the effect of the degenerative diseases of aging on surgical outcome. Therefore, to decrease the mortality and morbidity of CEA, medical personnel would have to direct their energy to limiting the ravages of cardiovascular, cerebrovascular, and renal disease in surgical patients and their susceptibility to infection.

The exponential relationship between age and mortality makes it possible to compare mortality from one decade to the next by using an odds ratio. The odds of dying from surgery at a particular age are equal to the number of patients who died divided by the number who underwent the procedure. The ratio of the odds rep-

Table 1-4. Relationship of Age and
Mortality from CEA[a]

Age (yrs)	No. of Patients	Deaths (%)
50 < 60	1,361	0.81
60 < 70	3,696	1.30
70 < 80	3,571	1.93
80 < 90	740	2.97
>90	24	4.17

[a] Data apply to all nonfederal hospitals in California in 1983.
(From Glaser and Feigal,[38] with permission.)

resents the increased likelihood of dying as age progresses from one decade to the next. For this data set, the odds ratio is 1.51 for CEA. If the projected mortality rate for a 40-year-old patient is 0.45 percent, the projected mortality rate for a 50-year-old would be 1.51 times 0.45 percent, or 0.68 percent. For a 60-year-old, the mortality rate would be 1.51 times 0.68 percent, or 1.03 percent; and so on.

Coronary Artery Disease

Patients undergoing CEA very often have other significant vascular disease. Of such diseases, CAD has the strongest correlation with late mortality after CEA. Among 335 patients observed for 6 to 11 years, 60 percent of the deaths within 60 days of CEA were caused by myocardial infarction.[39] This figure constituted 1.8 percent of the patients who had CEA. The overall mortality rate for survivors of the procedure was 27 percent at 5 years and 48 percent at 11 years. Regarding those who died within 11 years, myocardial infarction was the most common cause of death, significantly exceeding the proportion of deaths attributable to CAD in the general population (Table 1-5).

Reviewing 1,546 CEAs, Ennix et al.[12] divided patients into three groups on the basis of preexisting CAD. Group 1 had no

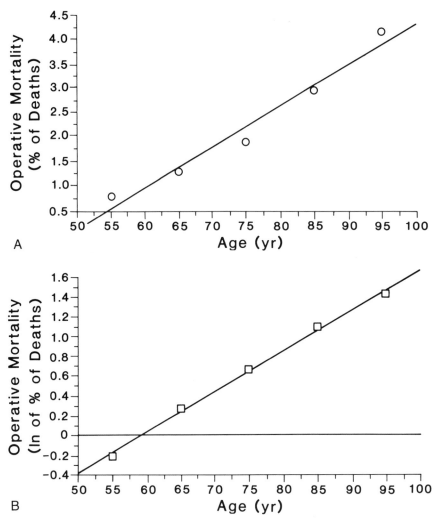

Fig. 1-1. Operative mortality from CEA increases exponentially with age. (**A**) Mortality is plotted against age. (**B**) The y-axis has been converted to the natural logarithm (ln) of the percentage of patients who died.

history or symptoms of CAD. Group 2 had symptomatic CAD (angina, congestive heart failure, or serious ventricular arrhythmias). Group 3 had histories of symptomatic CAD and had undergone coronary artery bypass before or with CEA. Table 1-6 shows that group 2 had significantly higher overall mortality rates than either group 1 or 2.

Patients with symptomatic CAD not only have greater cardiac mortality and morbidity but also greater cerebrovascular morbidity. If patients with CAD are generally older or sicker, they might be prone to greater neurologic morbidity after any surgical procedure. This assumption would be consistent with the fact that patients with asymptomatic

Table 1-5. Causes of Late Mortality (within 11 Years) after CEA[a]

Cause of Death	No.	% of Deaths
Myocardial infarction	59	37
Stroke	26	17
Neoplasm	15	10
Congestive heart failure	9	6
Pulmonary embolism	3	2

[a] A total of 335 patients having CEA were observed for 6 to 11 years.
(Modified from Hertzer and Lees,[39] with permission.)

bruits are much more likely to have a stroke if CAD is also present.[15] The assumption is less tenable in light of the outcome statistics for group 3, the patients who had coronary artery bypasses before or with CEA. This group not only had much lower rates for mortality and myocardial infarction than did patients with symptomatic CAD, but they also had a lower incidence of stroke and TIA. Perhaps those individuals who were likely to die or have myocardial or cerebral infarc-

tions did so at the time of coronary artery bypass grafting. Also, the patients selected to have coronary artery bypass grafting at that institution may have been healthier overall.

Although some physicians have stressed the potential benefit of coronary artery bypass prior to CEA or other vascular procedures,[37,39] to date these studies have not shown a significant difference in outcome when one takes into account the mortality associated with coronary artery bypass. An alternative explanation for the improved statistics on outcome after CEA in patients who have undergone coronary artery bypass is that those patients who are at greatest risk do not survive the bypass procedure. Although future studies may document an overall decrease in morbidity and mortality with the prophylactic use of coronary artery bypass, at present no scientific basis exists for this approach. Presumably, a subset of patients who have symptomatic CAD are at especially high risk. These might be patients with very advanced triple-vessel CAD, congestive heart failure, or left main coronary artery

Table 1-6. Percentages of 1,546 Patients with and without Preexisting CAD who Had Related Adverse Outcomes after CEA

Outcome	Group 1: No CAD Symptoms (n = 1,306)	Group 2: Symptomatic CAD (n = 85)	Group 3: Symptomatic CAD with Prior or Simultaneous CAB[a] (n = 155)
Myocardial infarction	0.8	12.9	2.6
TIA	1.0	2.4	0
Stroke (mild)	1.2	2.4	1.3
Stroke (severe)	1.1	2.4	0
Operative mortality	1.1	16.5	2.6

[a] CAB = coronary artery bypass.
(Modified from Ennix et al.,[12] with permission.)

disease. Identification of these high-risk patients by noninvasive techniques such as thallium scanning, Holter electrocardiographic monitoring, or echocardiography might allow for alternative management and a better overall prognosis.

Simultaneous or Staged Performance of Coronary Artery Bypass

Patients undergoing cardiopulmonary bypass for CAD are at especially high risk of stroke. In one prospective study, the rate of focal brain or ocular infarction after coronary artery bypass surgery was 5 percent; the rate of major stroke was 2 percent.[40] These adverse events were attributed to the flow characteristics of the bypass pump (nonpulsatile flow), embolization after dislodgement of atheromatous plaques or other material at the time of aortic cannulation, hypotension, or low cardiac output. Among patients whose carotid artery disease is detected noninvasively and whose disease is not pursued invasively, the incidence of stroke after coronary artery bypass may be much higher. A retrospective review of 234 patients with carotid artery disease found that the stroke rate after coronary artery bypass was 17 percent for patients who had abnormal results on oculoplethysmography and 1 percent for those who had normal results.[41]

One way of dealing with this problem is to submit the patient with both carotid artery and coronary artery disease to CEA and coronary artery bypass as either staged or simultaneous procedures.[42–45] This combined approach attempts to prevent both the cerebrovascular accidents that occur with relative frequency in patients undergoing coronary artery bypass and the myocardial infarctions that accompany CEA. Patients with unstable angina are at especially high risk of myocardial infarction in the perioperative period,[12] and patients with very advanced cerebrovascular disease seem to be at especially high risk of stroke during cardiopulmonary bypass.[42] Centers performing these two procedures simultaneously seem to produce morbidity and mortality rates that are either similar to or better than those occurring when either procedure is performed alone. For example, combined procedures in 331 patients at the Cleveland Clinic produced an operative mortality rate of 5.7 percent and a permanent perioperative stroke rate of 4.6 percent.[46] For the combined approach in 130 patients at the University of Cincinnati the operative mortality rate was 4.6 percent and the rate for additional stroke was 3.8 percent.[43]

Again, in the absence of a properly designed, randomized clinical trial, it is difficult to know whether or not this combined approach improves long-term survival rates. Although some studies purport to show a lower incidence of significant postoperative neurologic deficits when the two procedures are performed simultaneously, these studies do not correlate the severity of the underlying carotid disease with neurologic outcome. As has been shown, the severity of disease is an important determinant of outcome. If patients with asymptomatic carotid lesions undergo combined repair, their neurologic outcome cannot be compared with that of patients whose history may include stroke or TIAs. In a prospective study of patients undergoing cardiovascular surgery, the presence of asymptomatic carotid stenosis, as determined by duplex scanning, did not correlate with a higher rate of postoperative stroke.[47] Although overall mortality was higher if carotid obstruction was present, most of these deaths were caused by myocardial infarction. These data again point to the possibility that the coexistence of carotid obstruction or bruit with significant CAD indicates a sicker population—that is, patients who are, in general, at higher risk during surgical intervention. Available evidence does not support the assumption that patients undergoing coronary artery bypass who also have asymptomatic carotid lesions detected by angiography or noninvasive tests should undergo CEA and coronary artery bypass simultaneously.

Hypertension

Hypertension is common in patients with occlusive carotid disease. Postoperative hypertension occurs more commonly in patients with preexisting elevation in blood pressure and is associated with neurologic deficits after CEA.[48,49] Postoperative hypertension occurs in about 20 percent of patients who have had CEA, approximately 10 percent of whom also have postoperative neurologic deficit.[48,50] Towne and Bernhard[48] showed that neurologic deficit occurred in 3.4 percent of patients who had normal blood pressure after CEA and in 10.2 percent of patients who had elevated blood pressure. Similarly, Asiddao et al.[49] found neurologic deficit in 20 percent of patients with postoperative hypertension and in 6 percent of patients with normal blood pressure after CEA.

Hypertension is also associated with hemorrhagic cerebral infarction.[51,52] The removal of an occlusive carotid lesion may expose potentially fragile vessels to higher pressures.[51] These vessels may be more prone to rupture than vessels that have hypertrophied because of long exposure to hypertension. However, hypertension itself has not been shown to cause neurologic deficit after CEA. Hypertension may simply be a marker for patients who are at greater risk of neurologic complications for other reasons. Also, elevation in blood pressure may accompany a developing neurologic problem. The association of hypertension with neurologic deficit after CEA is frequently used as a rationale to treat hypertension if blood pressure exceeds 200 mmHg.

Diabetes

Although diabetic patients have impaired wound healing and immunocompetence,[53] the rate of complication after CEA is not much higher for diabetic than for nondiabetic patients. For example, of 156 patients undergoing CEA at New England Deaconess Hospital before 1980, two-thirds were diabetic and one-third were not.[54] The perioperative stroke rate for asymptomatic patients was 2.6 percent in the diabetic population and 0 percent in the nondiabetic population. Long-term follow-up showed that diabetic patients had significantly higher mortality rates than nondiabetics, primarily as a result of fatal myocardial infarction.

Type of Anesthesia

Either general or regional anesthesia may be used CEA. Advocates of regional anesthesia believe that it is easier to detect cerebral ischemia in awake patients and thereby prevent long-term neurologic deficit. In a 1985 review of CEA performed on awake patients, the need for placement of an intraluminal shunt was determined by evaluating the awake patient after a trial of carotid cross-clamping.[55] Only one death and one permanent neurologic deficit occurred among 100 consecutive patients. This figure is comparable to outcome statistics listed in Table 1-1 for recent series.

On the other hand, general anesthesia may offer a degree of protection against cerebral ischemia.[56,57] For example, isoflurane decreases cerebral metabolic oxygen requirements to a greater extent than other volatile anesthetic agents.[57] This property may explain why the incidence of electroencephalographic changes during clamping of the carotid artery is lower during isoflurane anesthesia than during anesthesia with other agents.[58] Nevertheless, no evidence shows that the choice of anesthetic affects outcome. Also, no convincing data have resolved the controversy as to whether placement of an intraluminal shunt protects against stroke during CEA.[59,60] Although electroencephalographic changes during CEA seem to correlate with postoperative neurologic deficit, intervention based on such changes appears not to affect outcome.[58,61]

MORBIDITY AND MORTALITY AFTER SURGERY ON THE ABDOMINAL AORTA AND MAJOR VESSELS OF THE EXTREMITIES

Patients with severe occlusive or aneurysmal disease of the aorta or with occlusive disease of the major vessels of the extremities are at especially high risk of death or morbidity from surgical attempts to correct these abnormalities. Two major reasons predominate. First, such patients often have significant coronary artery, cerebrovascular, and renal disease. Second, these pathologic conditions are often adversely affected by physiologic changes during surgery, for example, blood loss, volume shifts, and rapid changes in cardiac preload and afterload.

The major determinants of outcome for peripheral vascular surgery are the nature of the underlying disease and the type of surgery performed; the necessity of the surgery (emergency versus elective surgery); the presence of CAD; and age. Other factors that may affect outcome include anesthesia; renal disease; history of smoking and the presence of respiratory disease; and nutritional and metabolic status.

Nature of the Underlying Disease

There are several distinct patterns of peripheral vascular disease, each pattern having its own risk factors.[62] Type I pattern (isolated aortoiliac disease) is characterized by a relatively discrete area of disease involving the bifurcation of the aorta and the common iliac arteries. It occurs most commonly in smokers 40 to 55 years of age and is associated with claudication of the hip and thigh.

Type II pattern (diffuse aortoiliac disease) affects patients who are generally older and have more diffuse disease involving multiple levels of the vessels. In addition to being smokers, these patients are often hypertensive and have diabetes or lipid abnormalities that contribute to more widespread vascular disease. Severe claudication progressing to rest pain and ischemic ulcers is common. CAD and cerebrovascular disease are especially frequent in patients having the type II pattern of peripheral vascular disease.

Although the type III pattern (femoral-popliteal-tibial disease) most frequently affects elderly women with diabetes mellitus, men are certainly not spared. The disease is usually quite diffuse and involves smaller vessels as well. Foot ulcers and gangrene are common, and operative risk is often increased by coexisting illness.

Outcome is worse for patients with disease involving more distal vessels. The graft patency rate at 10 years is approximately 80 percent after correction of isolated aortoiliac disease but only 50 percent after correction of infrainguinal disease.[63] The 5-year survival rate after surgery is approximately 90 percent for type I disease, 80 percent for type II disease, and 65 percent for type III disease. A study at the Cleveland Clinic divided patients into three groups based on the distribution of disease.[64] Group A had isolated aortoiliofemoral disease (analogous to type I), group B had additional disease involving the femoropopliteal vessels (type II), and group C had femoropopliteal and tibioperoneal disease (type III). Late mortality was 28 percent for group A, 33 percent for group B, and 41 percent for group C. This increase in mortality is consistent with the increasing age and frequency of associated morbid conditions in type II and type III patients. Myocardial infarctions were responsible for much of the late mortality in all groups, occurring in 11, 15, and 20 percent of group A, B, and C patients, respectively.

Functional results also correlate with the extent of the disease at the time of surgery. About one-third of patients with infrainguinal disease, but only 13 percent of patients with limited disease, have incomplete relief of symptoms.[65] To improve functional outcome and decrease the incidence of postoperative graft occlusion by increasing distal runoff, one can now use balloon angioplasty for the major vessels of the extremities in conjunction with vascular reconstruction.

Type of Surgery

Surgery for Aneurysm versus Surgery for Occlusive Disease

Patients undergoing surgery for aortic aneurysm have higher rates of perioperative morbidity and mortality than do patients having surgery for aortic occlusion. Information regarding more than 2,000 aortic procedures by the Cleveland Vascular Society indicates mortality rates of approximately 4 percent for infrarenal aortoiliac revascularization and 8 percent for resection of abdominal aortic aneurysm (AAA).[66] The long-term survival rate is similarly worse after resection of an

Table 1-7. Median Survival Time of Caucasian Men after Peripheral Vascular Surgery

| Age (years) | Survival Time (years) after: | | |
	Surgery for Aneurysm	Aortic Bypass	Femoro-popliteal Bypass
<60	7.5	12.6	10.8
60–64	4.9	6.2	6.2
65–69	5.8	3.5	6.9
70–74	2.9	≤5.0	3.3
>75	6.7	0.9	6.7

(Modified from Burnham et al.,[67] with permission.)

AAA than after aortoiliac reconstruction. The lower long-term survival rate is largely due to the greater age of these patients. In a follow-up study, the median length of survival after hospital discharge was 5.8 years for AAA repair and 10.7 years for aortoiliac revascularization. Median age at the time of surgery was 66 and 57 years, respectively.[67] Table 1-7 shows that even after adjustment for age, survival time is usually shorter after surgery for aneurysm than after surgery for occlusive vascular disease.

Aortic Reconstruction versus Extraanatomic Bypass or Leg Revascularization

Procedures involving an aortic cross-clamp and aortic reconstruction carry a higher immediate operative mortality rate than extraanatomic bypass or more peripheral surgery involving the major vessels of the leg. Extraanatomic bypass and leg revascularization procedures, however, are generally associated with shorter periods of vascular patency and poorer long-term survival.[68] The shorter survival time relates more to the fact that such patients are older and sicker than to the surgical procedure itself.

Abdominal Aortic Aneurysmectomy

Treated versus Untreated Aneurysm. Since 1966, when Szilagyi et al.[69] compared the mortality of patients with untreated AAAs with that of patients who had undergone surgical repair, it has generally been accepted that the risk of dying from a large unresected aneurysm is greater than the risk of dying from an elective resection. In a retrospective review of 260 patients with ruptured AAAs, only 101 (39 percent) reached the hospital alive, and only 19.8 percent of the 260 survived hospitalization and surgery.[70] For patients with an aneurysm of 6 cm or larger, the most common cause of death is rupture of the aneurysm. For patients with aneurysms smaller than 6 cm, the most common cause of death is ischemic heart disease. Szilagyi and co-workers[69] determined that removal of an AAA would approximately double a patient's life expectancy. Aneurysms larger than 6 cm in diameter seemed to pose a significantly greater risk than smaller aneurysms. During a period of observation, 19 percent of aneurysms smaller than 6 cm ruptured. Overall, 34 percent of the nonsurgical patients died as the result of rupture of aneurysm.

As with CEA, both the severity of aneurysmal disease and the risk profile of an individual patient can vary widely. Little or no controversy exists about performing surgery on a patient who has a rapidly expanding or leaking aneurysm and who is a good candidate for surgery. However, controversy still exists regarding the other end of the spectrum—the patient who has a small aneurysm and is a poor surgical risk. A careful weighing of risk against potential benefit is most important for these patients.

Complications following abdominal aortic aneurysmectomy correlate closely with the severity and location of the aneu-

rysm. Surgery for asymptomatic aneurysm has the lowest mortality and morbidity. With rupture of an aneurysm, mortality increases dramatically, being highest for patients in shock.[68,70,71]

Emergency versus Elective Surgery. Surgery on ruptured AAAs incurs a much higher mortality rate than does elective repair of aneurysm.[72-75] Immediate perioperative mortality ranges from 3 to 6 percent for elective resection and from 25 to 70 percent for emergency repair after rupture. Patients in shock at the time of surgery have the highest mortality, the rate being approximately 80 percent. This difference in outcome for emergency versus elective surgery provides the rationale for early intervention once an aneurysm is discovered.

Emergency operations for revascularization of an occluded limb are similarly associated with as much as a 10-fold increase in perioperative mortality over elective procedures. In one series, mortality jumped from 3.3 percent for elective procedures to 37 percent for emergency surgery.[63]

Although morbidity and mortality for abdominal aortic aneurysmectomy have decreased significantly because of improvements in surgical and anesthetic care, outcome itself has not improved after repair of ruptured aneurysms.[70,74,75] A 1984 review of 898 aneurysmectomies at the University of Rochester showed how mortality from abdominal aortic aneurysmectomy had changed with time.[75] Mortality after elective surgery was 13 percent before 1965, 8.4 percent from 1966 to 1973, and 5.6 percent through 1981. However, for this same time period, mortality following resection of a ruptured aneurysm remained approximately 70 percent. Similarly, Crawford et al.[76] reported that mortality after operative repair of a ruptured aneurysm stayed approximately 23 percent for 25 years (1955 to 1980), whereas mortality from elective resection of aneurysm de-

Table 1-8. Age Distribution of Patients Undergoing Abdominal Aortic Aneurysmectomy[a]

Age (years)	1954 to 1968	1968 to 1976
40–49	1 (0.9%)	1 (0.7%)
50–59	21 (18.4%)	21 (14.6%)
60–69	55 (48.2%)	62 (43.1%)
70–79	29 (25.4%)	44 (30.6%)
80–89	8 (7.0%)	16 (11.1%)
Total	114	144

[a] Data pertain to patients at the Peter Bent Brigham Hospital in Boston.
(From Young et al.,[77] with permission.)

Table 1-9. Operative Mortality after Abdominal Aneurysmectomy

Authors and Years	No. of Patients	Operative Mortality (%)
Baird et al.[120] (1978)	160	5.6
Crawford et al.[121] (1979)	329	3.0
Whittemore et al.[122] (1980)	110	0
Diehl et al.[74] (1983)	350	5.1
Benefiel et al.[92] (submitted)	96	3.1*

* Mortality within 7 days of surgery; no operative mortality.

creased progressively to 2.5 percent in the last 5 years of the study.

Improvements in outcome with time are probably greater than these results indicate. Modern advances and increased experience in surgery and anesthesia have encouraged physicians to operate on older and sicker patients. This fact is illustrated by Table 1-8, which shows the age distribution for abdominal aortic aneurysmectomy at the Peter Bent Brigham Hospital in Boston over two decades.[77]

Although published reports tend to be biased in the direction of better outcome than might be expected in the general community (researchers tend not to publish results that are worse than the community average), it is clear that operative mortality for repair of intact aortic aneurysm has decreased to the point that such surgery can be advocated with confidence for all but the sickest of patients.[78] Table 1-9 provides statistics from several studies regarding operative mortality.

Long-term Outcome. Evaluation of risk versus benefit for abdominal aortic aneurysmectomy must take into account the long-term outcome after surgery. As with perioperative mortality, long-term survival is largely determined by the risk file of the patient. The most important fac-

tors determining long-term survival are age and the presence of cardiovascular disease. Crawford et al.[76] obtained long-term survival information on 816 patients who had surgical repair of AAA between 1955 and 1980 (representing follow-up on 99.6 percent of patients). Table 1-10 shows the relationship among age, cardiovascular disease, and long-term survival.

Table 1-10. Long-term Survival after Abdominal Aortic Aneurysmectomy[a]

	% of Patients Surviving at:		
	5 yrs	10 yrs	15 yrs
Cardiovascular status			
Without heart disease or hypertension	84	49	21
With heart disease or hypertension	54	34	17
Age			
<60 yr	71	53	24
60 to 71 yr	66	38	18
>71 yr	43	13	11

[a] Data pertain to 816 patients who had surgical repair of abdominal aneurysms between 1955 and 1980.
(Modified from Crawford et al.,[76] with permission.)

Close Observation and Nonresection of Abdominal Aortic Aneurysms. The advent of more reliable noninvasive techniques for closely monitoring the progress of an aortic aneurysm now makes it possible to intervene only if rupture of the aneurysm seems imminent. Using either computed tomography or ultrasonography, several groups have carefully measured the expansion rate of aortic aneurysms.[71,79,80] Good agreement exists among studies that the average aneurysm expands approximately 0.5 cm/year. Although larger aneurysms tend to expand more rapidly, the difference between their growth rate and that of small aneurysms is rather small. Variability is great, however, and for any particular aneurysm, the rate of expansion cannot be predicted with absolute certainty. For a high-risk patient, with a small aneurysm, careful observation with noninvasive imaging is a reasonable alternative. It should be noted, however, that in one autopsy series of 182 ruptured aneurysms, 18.1 percent were smaller than 5 cm in diameter.[81] Surgical intervention is indicated when the size of the aneurysm changes rapidly or when the diameter of the aneurysm exceeds 6 cm. Using these criteria produces long-term mortality rates from rupture of aneurysm that are similar to perioperative mortality from elective surgery, thus justifying a cautious "wait-and-see" approach. In centers having a low operative mortality, surgical intervention might be indicated for smaller aneurysms.

Cardiovascular Disease

Cardiovascular disease is the most common cause of both perioperative and late mortality in patients undergoing peripheral vascular surgery.[82–85] Asymptomatic CAD is present in a high percentage of such patients. Szilagyi et al.[69] reported that 71 percent of persons having an AAA would ultimately die of myocardial infarction or rupture of the aneurysm.

Among 557 patients who had abdominal aortic reconstruction at the Cleveland Clinic from 1974 to 1978, 210 had no clinical evidence of CAD.[74] Operative mortality was 2.9 percent, and postoperative myocardial infarction occurred in 1.4 percent. In patients with either angina or electrocardiographic evidence of ischemic heart disease preoperatively, mortality was 5.2 percent; the incidence of infarction was 6.2 percent.

The high incidence of symptomatic and asymptomatic ischemic heart disease has adversely affected both operative mortality and long-term survival following peripheral vascular surgery. The volume shifts and hemodynamic derangements that occur upon application of an aortic cross-clamp are particularly stressful to the patient with ischemic heart disease. To validate prospectively the risk index devised by Goldman et al.,[56] Jeffrey and colleagues[87] used the Goldman criteria to profile 99 patients undergoing abdominal aortic procedures. Eleven patients had life-threatening postoperative cardiac complications, five of which were myocardial infarctions and five, pulmonary edema. Thus, the cardiac risk index of Goldman significantly underestimated the likelihood of a postoperative cardiac event in patients undergoing abdominal aortic reconstruction. Given the prevalence of severe atherosclerotic heart disease in these patients, it is not surprising that myocardial infarction is responsible for approximately 40 percent of both early and late mortality after abdominal aneurysmectomy and for approximately 70 percent of operative mortality after aortic reconstruction for occlusive disease.[83,88] Late mortality after peripheral vascular surgery is 20.6 percent for patients with evidence of CAD and 3.8 percent for those without such evidence.[83]

The high late mortality rate from heart disease after aortic reconstruction clouds the overall risk-benefit analysis for many patients. It also provides the rationale for an aggressive simultaneous approach to both problems at some institutions but for a careful "wait-and-see" attitude at other centers.

Detecting Coronary Artery Disease

Newer diagnostic techniques enabling physicians to divide patient populations into subsets according to cardiac risk promise to decrease morbidity and mortality from peripheral vascular surgery. High-risk patients can undergo prophylactic coronary artery bypass or less invasive surgical procedures. They can also be monitored more closely in the perioperative period to reverse potentially damaging hemodynamic derangements.

Using exercise treadmill examinations given before vascular surgery, Cutler et al.[89] found that six postoperative myocardial infarctions occurred in 16 patients with abnormal results. No postoperative myocardial infarctions occurred in the 32 patients having normal results.

Exercise electrocardiography has several limitations. It cannot be used effectively in patients with certain preexisting electrocardiographic abnormalities, or in patients who are unable to exercise maximally (a frequent problem in those with peripheral vascular disease). Boucher et al.[90] attempted to overcome these limitations by using dipyridamole, a coronary vasodilator, instead of exercise to detect abnormalities in myocardial perfusion. Sixteen of 54 patients (30 percent) about to undergo peripheral vascular surgery had thallium redistribution, that is, evidence of impaired perfusion and myocardium vulnerable to ischemia. Fifty percent of these patients with evidence of significant CAD had perioperative cardiac events, three of which were myocardial infarctions. No such events occurred in patients without redistribution abnormalities. Significantly, patients with fixed perfusion abnormalities (suggestive of old myocardial infarction) but without evidence of jeopardized myocardium had no postoperative cardiac events. Although all of these patients had clinical evidence of CAD, on the basis of preoperative clinical signs, those who had postoperative cardiac events could not be distinguished from those who tolerated surgery without problems.

Coronary angiography performed before vascular surgery has shown that significant CAD exists in approximately 60 percent of patients undergoing such surgery and that only 8 percent of patients are completely free of CAD.[88] Among candidates for resection of aneurysm, severe, "correctable" CAD existed in 56 percent of patients having clinical evidence of ischemic heart disease and in 21 percent of patients having no signs of disease. Severe, potentially correctable CAD occurred in 31 percent of the entire group presenting for abdominal aortic aneurysmectomy and in 21 percent of patients undergoing lower extremity revascularization.

Prophylactic Coronary Artery Bypass

Many reports indicate that patients who have had coronary artery bypass can tolerate peripheral vascular surgery with approximately the same degree of success (i.e., morbidity and mortality) as those who do not have CAD. In one study, four patients with abnormal results on dipyridamole-thallium imaging studies had coronary arteriography and coronary artery bypass before vascular surgery.[90] All tolerated coronary artery bypass and vascular surgery without significant morbidity.

Ruel et al.[91] studied outcomes for 1,093 patients who had coronary artery bypass

Table 1-11. Outcome for 1,000 Patients Undergoing Peripheral Vascular Surgery after Routine Coronary Angiography

Patients[a]	No. of Patients	Mortality (%)
Those undergoing PVS	846	2.8
Those undergoing CAB	216	5.2
Those undergoing PVS after CAB	200	1.5[b]
Those with clinically suspected CAD who declined CAB and had PVS	35	12
Those with severe inoperable CAD who had PVS	28	14

[a] PVS = peripheral vascular surgery; CAB = coronary artery bypass.

[b] If mortality rate with CAB is included, figure becomes 7.0%.

(Data from Hertzer et al.[88])

before peripheral vascular surgery. Postoperative mortality was 2 percent overall, and none of the 120 patients undergoing abdominal aortic aneurysmectomy died. Among 559 patients who had coronary artery bypass during an earlier hospital admission, no deaths were related to cardiac events. For 534 patients who had both procedures during the same hospitalization because of severe or unstable coronary disease, mortality was 4 percent overall. This increase undoubtedly reflects the fact that patients who undergo these two procedures during one hospitalization tend to have more severe cardiac and aortic disease.

Table 1-11 lists the outcomes for 1,000 patients at the Cleveland Clinic who routinely had coronary angiography before peripheral vascular surgery (including CEA).[88] Statistical calculation of survival for this same group of patients after peripheral vascular surgery shows that patients with no CAD or only mild disease had the best survival rate after follow-up for 3 to 7 years. The next best statistical calculation of survival rate pertained to patients who had both coronary artery bypass and peripheral vascular surgery. Patients with advanced but compensated CAD had a 5-year survival rate of 63 percent, whereas patients who had clinically suspected but uncorrected CAD had a 5-year survival rate of 43 percent. With improvements in anesthesia and perioperative management, the incidence of postoperative myocardial infarction probably will continue to decline.[92,93] Therefore, it is hard to justify the routine use of coronary angiography unless it directly increases long-term survival.

Although accumulating evidence suggests that patients undergoing coronary artery bypass before peripheral vascular surgery do better in the long run than patients who have severe CAD but forego bypass surgery, no results from well-controlled, randomized studies support this hypothesis.

Age

A review of outcome in 557 patients undergoing abdominal aortic reconstruction showed that simply dividing patients by age (i.e., into groups of older or younger than 60 years) produced two groups having a markedly different risk of surgical mortality.[74] Mortality was 1 percent of patients under 60 years of age but 8.1 percent for those over 60. Age (i.e., older than 60 years) was associated with a greater increase in the relative risk of dying than was CAD, elevated serum creatinine levels, or even rupture of aneurysm.

In the California Health Facilities data set for the year 1983, 2,170 patients underwent aortoiliac reconstruction.[38] As with CEA, the relationship between increasing age and mortality from surgery for aortoiliac reconstruction was exponential. Figure 1-2A plots mortality against age and fits a least-squares regression line to the data. Figure 1-2B shows the same data with the y-axis converted to the natural logarithm of the mortality rate, again with the least-squares regression line. The almost-perfect fit of the data points to the regression line and the value of 0.98 for r^2 indicate that essen-

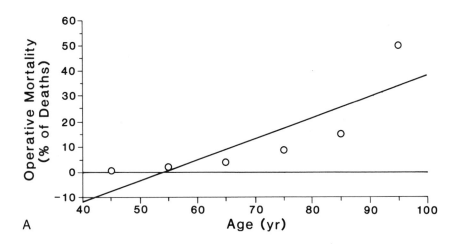

A

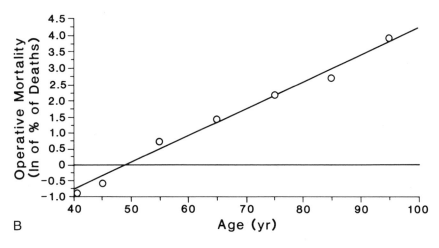

B

Fig. 1-2. Operative mortality from aortic reconstruction increases exponentially with age. (**A**) Mortality is plotted against age. (**B**) The y-axis has been converted to the natural logarithm (ln) of the mortality rate. Regression equation is: $y = 0.083x$; $r^2 = 0.981$.

tially all mortality from aortoiliac reconstruction is related in some way to aging. Using these data, one can see that with each decade, the risk of dying is 2.3 times higher. The expected mortality for an average 80-year-old patient after aortoiliac reconstruction would be $(2.3)^3$, or 12.2 times as high as that for a 50-year-old patient.

Despite the dramatic increase in operative mortality with aging, several investigators believe that careful patient selection and management still make surgical intervention appropriate even in the very elderly. In one report, patients over the age of 80 had a mortality rate of 3.3 percent for elective resection of an aortic aneurysm.[73] After repair of a ruptured aneurysm, mortality was 37 percent. In a study of 21 octagenarians who had AAAs (five of which ruptured), three deaths occurred after repair of the aneurysm.[94] Mortality after lower extremity revascularization was approximately 3 percent. The average life expectancy for an 80-year-old is 6.7 years for men and 7.8 years for women (National Center for Health Statistics). Approximately 50 percent of patients with an AAA will die within the first year of diagnosis.[95] In an elderly patient with life-threatening vascular disease, especially if coexisting disease is minimal, these statistics provide a rationale for elective surgical intervention.

Other Factors That May Affect Outcome

Anesthesia

Advances in anesthesia are responsible for much of the technical improvement in operative morbidity and mortality from vascular surgery. Improved management of patients undergoing coronary artery bypass, especially regarding manipulation of hemodynamic status and protection of the myocardium, has been extended to sick patients undergoing other major surgical procedures. As a result, the incidence of perioperative myocardial infarction has decreased.[90] In a 1985 analysis of perioperative ischemia in patients undergoing coronary artery bypass, Slogoff and Keats[96] implicated inappropriately treated intraoperative hemodynamic fluctuations as contributing to postoperative morbidity and mortality. For example, although application of an aortic cross-clamp induces myocardial ischemia[97] and wall motion abnormalities in susceptible individuals, appropriate anesthetic intervention seems to reverse these abnormalities.[98] Therefore, for patients undergoing major vascular surgery, the skill of the anesthetist and the effect of anesthetic interventions may greatly influence outcome and survival.

Several investigators also report that preoperative determination of myocardial performance curves and optimal preoperative volume loading may improve outcome (especially renal performance) after aortic cross-clamping procedures.[99,100]

Choice of anesthetic technique may also affect outcome. Benefiel et al.[92] compared isoflurane with sufentanil in patients undergoing reconstruction of the abdominal or thoracoabdominal aorta. Postoperative congestive heart failure or renal insufficiency occurred less frequently in patients given sufentanil than in patients given isoflurane. The only other difference in management was the postoperative epidural administration of opiates in some of the patients given isoflurane. The apparent differences between the two anesthetics, despite the small number of patients in the study (96), suggests a relatively powerful effect of anesthetic technique on outcome.

Renal Disease

The application of an aortic cross-clamp, underlying renal vascular disease, volume shifts, and perhaps choice of anesthetic all contribute to a significant incidence of postoperative renal dysfunction in vascular surgery patients. The development of postoperative renal failure requiring dialysis has a significant negative correlation with survival.[101] Preexisting renal disease contributes to impaired outcome. For example, operative mortality for aortic reconstruction is 19 percent when preoperative serum creatinine levels are higher than 2.0 mg/dl but only 4.6 percent when preoperative levels are lower.[74] Because intraoperative oliguria has many potential causes, the occurrence of oliguria by itself does not necessarily warrant aggressive hydration. For 137 patients undergoing abdominal aortic revascularization, intraoperative urinary output did not correlate with postoperative renal insufficiency.[102]

Smoking and Respiratory Disease

Because smoking is a significant risk factor for the development of peripheral vascular disease, discontinuation of smoking is one of the cornerstones of nonoperative management. Little information exists regarding the role of smoking and outcome after vascular surgery. Smokers have lower 2-year patency rates after femoral artery balloon angioplasty[103] and presumably have more rapid progression of atherosclerosis than do nonsmokers with an otherwise similar risk profile. The contribution of smoking to morbidity and mortality after vascular surgery procedures must be rather small, however, as smoking has not had an impact in studies of factors affecting outcome. On the other hand, cigarette smoking does correlate positively with respiratory complications after coronary artery bypass.[104] Discontinuation of smoking for at least 8 weeks decreases the rate of respiratory complications to a level one-third that of patients who have stopped smoking for less than 8 weeks. Although smoking may not strongly affect short-term survival, it does contribute to respiratory complications and probably decreases long-term vascular patency. Therefore, it seems prudent to advise discontinuation of smoking for as long as possible before elective vascular reconstruction.

Diabetes

Diabetic patients are prone to have vascular disease. They are also more likely to have more diffuse distal occlusive disease than nondiabetic patients. Despite this, the immediate effect of diabetes on outcome seems minimal. Diabetic patients have a higher incidence of wound complications after vascular surgery than do nondiabetic patients.[105] A retrospective review of 83 patients undergoing distal lower extremity bypass found no difference in operative morbidity or long-term patency rates between 24 diabetic and 59 nondiabetic patients.[106] However, two diabetic patients died of myocardial infarction.

Nutritional Status

Nutritional status affects outcome in two ways: directly, as a factor in wound healing; and indirectly, as a marker of general debility. One study reported that vascular patients who were malnourished (as evidenced by decreased serum albumin and transferrin levels) had impaired wound healing.[105] Specifically, 40 percent of patients having serum albumin levels below 3.0 g/dl (versus 12.5 percent of patients who had normal levels) had impaired wound healing. Sixty-four percent of patients having serum transferrin levels less than 150 mg/dl (versus 9 percent of patients with normal levels) had impaired wound healing. Similarly, in cancer patients undergoing vascular surgery and other major surgical procedures, complications occurred in 48 percent of malnourished patients and in 3 percent of patients without evidence of malnutrition.[107]

SUMMARY

There is no lack of information regarding morbidity and mortality after CEA. What is not available, however, is information collected in a rigorously scientific manner that can clarify which patients are likely to have a net benefit from CEA. Patients who have survived CEA without neurologic deficit seem to have better long-term morbidity and mortality than patients who have not undergone surgery. Although the weight of evidence supports CEA in patients having TIAs and high-grade stenosis, the issue has not been decided conclusively.

Difficulty in comparing outcome statistics is compounded by the enormous variability in morbidity and mortality from study to study and from institution to institution. At centers having very low morbidity and mortality rates, the argument for CEA for a broad range of indications is more convincing. Many CEAs, however, are still performed at institutions and community hospitals having generally higher morbidity and mortality rates.[11,13,108,109] With so many variables to consider, attempts are now being made to use outcome-based standards to justify or discourage CEA in specific subsets of patients.[2] The Rand Corporation has assembled a panel of experts from the fields of surgery, radiology, neurology, and medicine to evaluate the literature and establish standards for the advisability of CEA in 864 subgroups of patients. Use of their criteria assesses CEA to be inappropriate for all subgroups of patients if a hospital's perioperative death and stroke rate is 8 percent or more. When the institutional death and stroke rate is less than 5 percent, the relationship between risk and benefit becomes less clear, and surgery has an apparent benefit for some patients, especially those with symptomatic high-grade stenosis.

Because morbidity and mortality from resection of an abdominal aortic aneurysm and reconstruction for occlusive vascular disease have diminished with time, these surgical procedures are clearly capable of improving longevity and relieving symptoms in some subsets of patients. Large aneurysms in otherwise healthy patients provide the strongest rationale for surgical intervention. In centers having low surgical morbidity and mortality rates, even patients with significant systemic disease are likely to benefit from aneurysmectomy. Well-controlled studies have yet to be performed to support aggressive measures (i.e., angiography and coronary artery bypass) in patients scheduled for elective vascular surgery. Improvement in noninvasive diagnostic modalities and anesthesia care may obviate the need for such an aggressive approach. Advanced age, its attendant diseases, and the presence of CAD still constitute the greatest risk factors for patients undergoing vascular surgery.

REFERENCES

1. EC/IC Bypass Study Group: Failure of extracranial-intracranial arterial bypass to reduce the risk of ischemic stroke. Results of an international randomized trial. N Engl J Med 313:1191–1200, 1985
2. Eastcott HHG, Pickering GW, Rob CG: Reconstruction of internal carotid artery in a patient with intermittent attacks of hemiplegia. Lancet 2:994–996, 1954

3. Dyken ML, Pokras R: The performance of endarterectomy for disease of the extracranial arteries of the head. Stroke 15:948–950, 1984

4. Wennberg JE: Setting outcome-based standards for carotid endarterectomy (editorial). JAMA 256:2566–2567, 1986

5. Clagett GP, Youkey JR, Brigham RA et al: Asymptomatic cervical bruit and abnormal ocular pneumoplethysmography: a prospective study comparing two approaches to management. Surgery 96:823–830, 1984

6. Shaw DA, Venables GS, Cartildge NEF et al: Carotid endarterectomy in patients with transient cerebral ischaemia. J Neurol Sci 64:45–53, 1984

7. Fields WS, Maslenikov V, Meyer JS et al: Joint study of extracranial arterial occlusion. V. Progress report of prognosis following surgery or nonsurgical treatment for transient cerebral ischemic attacks and cervical carotid arterial lesions. JAMA 211:1993–2003, 1970

8. Veterans Administration Cooperative Study: Role of carotid endarterectomy in asymptomatic carotid stenosis. Stroke 17:534–539, 1986

9. Tytus JS, MacLean JB, Hill HD: Prognosis in patients with transient ischemic attacks after endarterectomy. Am Surg 36:623–626, 1970

10. Sundt TM, Sandok BA, Whisnant JP: Carotid endarterectomy. Complications and preoperative assessment of risk. Mayo Clin Proc 50:301–306, 1975

11. Modi JR, Finch WT, Sumner DS: Update of carotid endarterectomy in two community hospitals: Springfield revisited (abstract). Stroke 14:128, 1983

12. Ennix CL, Jr., Lawrie GM, Morris GC, Jr. et al: Improved results of carotid endarterectomy in patients with symptomatic coronary disease: an analysis of 1,546 consecutive carotid operations. Stroke 10:122–125, 1979

13. Brott T, Thalinger K: The practice of carotid endarterectomy in a large metropolitan area. Stroke 15:950–955, 1984

14. Thompson JE, Patman RD, Talkington CM: Asymptomatic carotid bruit: long-term outcome of patients having endarterectomy compared with unoperated controls. Ann Surg 188:308–316, 1978

15. Chambers BR, Norris JW: Outcome in patients with asymptomatic neck bruits. N Engl J Med 315:860–865, 1986

16. Roederer GO, Langlois YE, Jager KA et al: The natural history of carotid arterial disease in asymptomatic patients with cervical bruits. Stroke 15:605–613, 1984

17. Smith JS, Roizen MF, Cahalan MK et al: Does anesthetic technique make a difference? Augmentation of systolic blood pressure during carotid endarterectomy: effects of phenylephrine *versus* light anesthesia and of isoflurane *versus* halothane on the incidence of myocardial ischemia. Anesthesiology 69:846–853, 1988

18. Javid H, Ostermiller WE, Jr., Hengesh JW et al: Natural history of carotid bifurcation atheroma. Surgery 67:80–86, 1970

19. Hertzer NR, Flanagan RA, Jr., O'Hara PJ, Beven EG: Surgical *versus* nonoperative treatment of asymptomatic carotid stenosis. 290 patients documented by intravenous angiography. Ann Surg 204:163–171, 1986

20. Ziegler DK, Zileli T, Dick A, Sebaugh JL: Correlation of bruits over the carotid artery with angiographically demonstrated lesions. Neurology 21:860–865, 1971

21. Caplan LR: Carotid artery disease (editorial). N Engl J Med 315:886–888, 1986

22. Wolf PA, Kannel WB, Sorlie P, McNamara P: Asymptomatic carotid bruit and risk of stroke. JAMA 245:1442–1445, 1981

23. Heyman A, Wilkinson WE, Heyden S et al: Risk of stroke in asymptomatic persons with cervical arterial bruits. A population study in Evans County, Georgia. N Engl J Med 302:838–841, 1980

24. Goldner JD, Whisnant JP, Taylor WF: Long-term prognosis of transient cerebral ischemic attacks. Stroke 2:160–167, 1971

25. Bauer RB, Meyer JS, Fields WS et al: Joint study of extracranial arterial occlusion. III. Progress report of controlled study of long-term survival in patients with and without operation. JAMA 208:509–518, 1969

26. Ziegler DK, Hassanein RS: Prognosis in patients with transient ischemic attacks. Stroke 4:666–673, 1973

27. Whisnant JP: Epidemiology of stroke: emphasis on transient cerebral ischemic attacks and hypertension. Stroke 5:68–70, 1974

28. West H, Burton R, Roon AJ et al: Comparative risk of operation and expectant management for carotid artery disease. Stroke 10:117–121, 1979

29. DeWeese JA, Rob CG, Satran R et al: Surgical treatment for occlusive disease of the carotid artery. Ann Surg 168:85–94, 1968

30. Kistler JP, Ropper AH, Heros RC: Therapy of ischemic cerebral vascular disease due to atherothrombosis (first of two parts). N Engl J Med 311:27–34, 1984

31. Baker RN, Schwartz WS, Ramseyer JC: Prognosis among survivors of ischemic stroke. Neurology 18:933–941, 1968

32. Robinson RW, Demirel M, LeBeau RJ: Natural history of cerebral thrombosis. Nine to nineteen year follow-up. J Chronic Dis 21:221–230, 1968

33. Fode NC, Sundt TM, Jr., Robertson JT et al: Multicenter retrospective review of results and complications of carotid endarterectomy in 1981. Stroke 17:370–376, 1986

34. Meyer FB, Sundt TM, Jr., Piepgras DG et al: Emergency carotid endarterectomy for patients with acute carotid occlusion and profound neurological deficits. Ann Surg 203:82–89, 1986

35. Jones HR, Millikan CH: Temporal profile (clinical course) of acute carotid system cerebral infarction. Stroke 7:64–71, 1976

36. Grillo P, Patterson RH, Jr: Occlusion of the carotid artery: prognosis (natural history) and the possibilities of surgical revascularization. Stroke 6:17–20, 1975

37. Norrving B, Nilsson B: Carotid artery occlusion: acute symptoms and long-term prognosis. Neurol Res 3:229–236, 1981

38. Glaser RB, Feigal D: Age-specific surgical morbidity and mortality. An analysis of the California hospital discharge data tapes from the Office of Statewide Health Planning and Development. (Unpublished analysis, 1983).

39. Hertzer NR, Lees CD: Fatal myocardial infarction following carotid endarterectomy. Three hundred thirty-five patients followed 6–11 years after operation. Ann Surg 194:212–218, 1981

40. Breuer AC, Furlan AJ, Hanson MR et al: Central nervous system complications of coronary artery bypass graft surgery: prospective analysis of 421 patients. Stroke 14:682–687, 1983

41. Kartchner MM, McRae LP: Carotid occlusive disease as a risk factor in major cardiovascular surgery. Arch Surg 117:1086–1088, 1982

42. Furlan AJ, Craciun AR: Risk of stroke during coronary artery bypass graft surgery in patients with internal carotid artery disease documented by angiography. Stroke 16:797–799, 1985

43. Dunn EJ: Concomitant cerebral and myocardial revascularization. Surg Clin North Am 66:385–395, 1986

44. Matar AF: Concomitant coronary and cerebral revascularizlation under cardiopulmonary bypass. Ann Thorac Surg 41:431–435, 1986

45. Perler BA, Burdick JF, Williams GM: The safety of carotid endarterectomy at the time of coronary artery bypass surgery: analysis of results in a high-risk patient population. J Vasc Surg 2:558–563, 1985

46. Hertzer NR, Loop FD, Taylor PC, Beven EG: Combined myocardial revascularization and carotid endarterectomy. Operative and late results in 331 patients. J Thorac Cardiovasc Surg 85:577–589, 1983

47. Barnes RW, Marszalek PB: Asymptomatic carotid disease in the cardiovascular surgical patient: is prophylactic endarterectomy necessary? Stroke 12:497–500, 1981

48. Towne JB, Bernhard VM: The relationship of postoperative hypertension to complications following carotid endarterectomy. Surgery 88:575–580, 1980

49. Asiddao CB, Donegan JH, Whitesell RC, Kalbfleisch JH: Factors associated with perioperative complications during carotid endarterectomy. Anesth Analg 61:631–637, 1982

50. Bove EL, Fry WJ, Gross WS, Stanley JC: Hypotension and hypertension as consequences of baroreceptor dysfunction following endarterectomy. Surgery 85:633–637, 1979

51. Caplan LR, Skillman J, Ojemann R, Fields WS: Intracerebral hemorrhage following carotid endarterectomy: a hypertensive complication? Stroke 9:457–460, 1978

52. Lehv MS, Salzman EW, Silen W: Hypertension complicating carotid endarterectomy. Stroke 1:307–313, 1970

53. Goodson WH, III, Hunt TK: Wound healing and the diabetic patient. Surg Gynecol Obstet 149:600–608, 1979

54. Campbell DR, Hoar CS, Jr., Wheelock FC: Carotid artery surgery in diabetic patients. Arch Surg 119:1405–1407, 1984

55. Connolly JE: Carotid endarterectomy in the awake patient. Am J Surg 150:159–165, 1985

56. Newberg LA, Michenfelder JD: Cerebral protection by isoflurane during hypoxemia or ischemia. Anesthesiology 59:29–35, 1983

57. Casement B, Messick MD, Milde L et al: "Critical" rCBF during isoflurane anesthesia in man (abstract). Anesthesiology 63:A406, 1985

58. Blume WT, Ferguson GG, McNeil DK: Significance of EEG changes at carotid endarterectomy. Stroke 17:891–897, 1986

59. Ojemann RG, Heros RC: Carotid endarterectomy. To shunt or not to shunt? Arch Neurol 43:617–618, 1986

60. Ferguson GG: Carotid endarterectomy. To shunt or not to shunt? Arch Neurol 43:615–617, 1986

61. Rampil IJ, Holzer JA, Quest DO et al: Prognostic value of computerized EEG analysis during carotid endarterectomy. Anesth Analg 62:186–192, 1983

62. Hallett JW, Jr: Trends in revascularization of the lower extremity. Mayo Clin Proc 61:369–376, 1986

63. Nevelsteen A, Suy R, Daenen W et al: Aortofemoral grafting: factors influencing late results. Surgery 88:642–653, 1980

64. Martinez BD, Hertzer NR, Beven EG: Influence of distal arterial occlusive disease on prognosis following aortobifemoral bypass. Surgery 88:795–805, 1980

65. Mulcare RJ, Royster TS, Lynn RA, Conners RB: Long-term results of operative therapy for aortoiliac disease. Arch Surg 113:601–604, 1978

66. Plecha FR, Avellone JC, Beven EG, DePalma RG, Hertzer NR: A computerized vascular registry: experience of the Cleveland Vascular Society. Surgery 86:826–835, 1979

67. Burnham SJ, Johnson G, Jr., Gurri JA: Mortality risks for survivors of vascular reconstructive procedures. Surgery 92:1072–1076, 1982

68. Raviola CA, Nichter L, Baker JD et al: Femoropopliteal tibial bypass: what price failure? Am J Surg 144:115–123, 1982

69. Szilagyi DE, Smith RF, DeRusso FJ et al: Contribution of abdominal aortic aneurysmectomy to prolongation of life. Ann Surg 164:678–699, 1966

70. Ingoldby CJH, Wujanto R, Mitchell JE: Impact of vascular surgery on community mortality from ruptured aortic aneurysms. Br J Surg 73:551–553, 1986

71. Bernstein EF, Chan EL: Abdominal aortic aneurysm in high-risk patients. Outcome of selective management based on size and expansion rate. Ann Surg 200:255–263, 1984

72. Hicks GL, Eastland MW, DeWeese JA et al: Survival improvement following aortic aneurysm resection. Ann Surg 181:863–869, 1975

73. Harris KA, Ameli FM, Lally M et al: Abdominal aortic aneurysm resection in patients more than 80 years old. Surg Gynecol Obstet 162:536–538, 1986

74. Diehl JT, Cali RF, Hertzer NR, Beven EG: Complications of abdominal aortic reconstruction. An analysis of perioperative risk factors in 557 patients. Ann Surg 197:49–56, 1983

75. Pasch AR, Ricotta JJ, May AG et al: Abdominal aortic aneurysm: the case for elective resection. Circulation 70:suppl. I, I-1 to I-4, 1984

76. Crawford ES, Saleh SA, Babb JW, III, et al: Infrarenal abdominal aortic aneu-

rysm. Factors influencing survival after operation performed over a 25-year period. Ann Surg 193:699–709, 1981

77. Young AE, Sandberg GW, Couch NP: The reduction of mortality of abdominal aortic aneurysm resection. Am J Surg 134:585–590, 1977

78. Hollier LH: Surgical management of abdominal aortic aneurysm in the high-risk patient. Surg Clin North Am 66:269–279, 1986

79. Delin A, Ohlsén H, Swedenborg J: Growth rate of abdominal aortic aneurysms as measured by computed tomography. Br J Surg 72:530–532, 1985

80. Sterpetti AV, Schultz RD, Feldhaus RJ et al: Abdominal aortic aneurysm in elderly patients. Selective management based on clinical status and aneurysmal expansion rate. Am J Surg 150:772–776, 1985

81. Darling RC: Ruptured arteriosclerotic abdominal aortic aneurysms. A pathologic and clinical study. Am J Surg 119: 397–401, 1970

82. De Bakey ME, Crawford ES, Cooley DA et al: Aneurysm of abdominal aorta. Analysis of results of graft replacement therapy one to eleven years after operation. Ann Surg 160:622–639, 1964

83. Jamieson WRE, Janusz MT, Miyagishma RT, Green AN: Influence of ischemic heart disease on early and late mortality after surgery for peripheral occlusive vascular disease. Circulation, 66:suppl. I, I-92 to I-97, 1982

84. Hertzer NR: Fatal myocardial infarction following abdominal aortic aneurysm resection. Three hundred forty-three patients followed 6-11 years postoperatively. Ann Surg 192:667–673, 1980

85. Hertzer NR: Fatal myocardial infarction following lower extremity revascularization. Two hundred seventy-three patients followed six to eleven postoperative years. Ann Surg 193:492–498, 1981

86. Goldman L, Caldera DL, Nussbaum SR et al: Multifactorial index of cardiac risk in noncardiac surgical procedures. N Engl J Med 297:845–850, 1977

87. Jeffrey CC, Kunsman J, Cullen DJ, Brewster DC: A prospective evaluation of cardiac risk index. Anesthesiology 58:462–464, 1983

88. Hertzer NR, Beven EG, Young JR et al: Coronary artery disease in peripheral vascular patients. A classification of 1000 coronary angiograms and results of surgical management. Ann Surg 199:223–233, 1984

89. Cutler BS, Wheeler HB, Paraskos JA, Cardullo PA: Assessment of operative risk with electrocardiographic exercise testing in patients with peripheral vascular disease. Am J Surg 137:484–490, 1979

90. Boucher CA, Brewster DC, Darling RC et al: Determination of cardiac risk by dipyridamole-thallium imaging before peripheral vascular surgery. N Engl J Med 312:389–394, 1985

91. Reul GJ, Jr., Cooley DA, Duncan JM et al: The effect of coronary bypass on the outcome of peripheral vascular operations in 1093 patients. J Vasc Surg 3:788–798, 1986

92. Benefiel DJ, Roizen MF, Lampe GH et al: Does anesthetic choice make a difference? Morbidity after aortic surgery with sufentanil vs. isoflurane anesthesia. Anesthesiology (submitted)

93. Rao TLK, Jacobs KH, El-Etr AA: Reinfarction following anesthesia in patients with myocardial infarction. Anesthesiology 59:499–505, 1983

94. Edwards WH, Mulherin JL, Jr., Rogers DM: Vascular reconstruction in the octogenarian. South Med J 75:648–652, 1982

95. Thompson JE, Hollier LH, Patman RD, Persson AV: Surgical management of abdominal aortic aneurysms: factors influencing mortality and morbidity—a 20-year experience. Ann Surg 181:654–661, 1975

96. Slogoff S, Keats AS: Does perioperative myocardial ischemia lead to postoperative myocardial infarction? Anesthesiology 62:107–114, 1985

97. Attia RR, Murphy JD, Snider M et al: Infrarenal aortic cross-clamping during aortic surgery in patients with severe coronary artery disease. Circulation 53: 961–965, 1976

98. Roizen MF, Hamilton WK, Sohn YJ: Treatment of stress-induced increases in pulmonary capillary wedge pressure using volatile anesthetics. Anesthesiology 55:446–450, 1981

99. Bush HL, Jr., Huse JB, Johnson WC et al: Prevention of renal insufficiency after abdominal aortic aneurysm resection by optimal volume loading. Arch Surg 116:1517–1524, 1981

100. Grindlinger GA, Vegas AM, Manny J et al: Volume loading and vasodilators in abdominal aortic aneurysmectomy. Am J Surg 139:480–486, 1980

101. Bush HL, Jr: Renal failure following abdominal aortic reconstruction. Surgery 93:107–109, 1983

102. Alpert RA, Roizen MF, Hamilton WK et al: Intraoperative urinary output does not predict postoperative renal function in patients undergoing abdominal aortic revascularization. Surgery 95:707–711, 1984

103. Wilson AR, Fuchs JCA: Percutaneous transluminal angioplasty. The radiologist's contribution to the treatment of vascular disease. Surg Clin North Am 64:121–150, 1984

104. Warner MA, Divertie MB, Tinker JH: Preoperative cessation of smoking and pulmonary complications in coronary artery bypass patients. Anesthesiology 60:380–383, 1984

105. Casey J, Flinn WR, Yao JS et al: Correlation of immune and nutritional status with wound complications in patients undergoing vascular operations. Surgery 93:822–827, 1983

106. Gurri JA, Burnham SJ: Effect of diabetes mellitus on distal lower extremity bypass. Am Surg 48:75–76, 1982

107. Warnold I, Lundholm K: Clinical significance of preoperative nutritional status in 215 noncancer patients. Ann Surg 199:299–305, 1984

108. Easton JD, Sherman DG: Stroke and mortality rate in carotid endarterectomy: 228 consecutive operations. Stroke 8: 565–568, 1977

109. Slavish LG, Nicholas GG, Gee W: Review of a community hospital experience with carotid endarterectomy. Stroke 15:956–959, 1984

110. Rainer WG, Guillen J, Bloomquist CD, McCrory CB: Carotid artery surgery. Morbidity and mortality in 257 operations. Am J Surg 116:678–681, 1968

111. Thompson JE, Austin DJ, Patman RD: Carotid endarterectomy for cerebrovascular insufficiency: long-term results in 592 patients followed up to thirteen years. Ann Surg 172:663–679, 1970

112. Howe JR, Kindt GW: Cerebral protection during carotid endarterectomy. Stroke 5:340–343, 1974

113. Toole JF, Janeway R, Choi K et al: Transient ischemic attacks due to atherosclerosis. A prospective study of 160 patients. Arch Neurol 32:5–12, 1975

114. Baker WH, Dorner DB, Barnes RW: Carotid endarterectomy: is an indwelling shunt necessary? Surgery 82:321–326, 1977

115. Prioleau WH, Jr., Aiken AF, Hairston P: Carotid endarterectomy: neurologic complications as related to surgical techniques. Ann Surg 185:678–683, 1977

116. Fleming JFR, Griesdale DE, Schutz H, Hogan M: Carotid endarterectomy: changing morbidity and mortality (abstract). Stroke 8:14, 1977

117. Cornell WP: Carotid endarterectomy: Results in 100 patients. Ann Thorac Surg 25:122–126, 1978

118. Haynes CD, Dempsey RL: Carotid endarterectomy. Review of 276 cases in a community hospital. Ann Surg 189:758–762, 1979

119. Graham AM, Gewertz BL, Zarins CK: Predicting cerebral ischemia during carotid endarterectomy. Arch Surg 121:595–598, 1986

120. Baird RJ, Gurry JF, Kellam JF, Wilson DR: Abdominal aortic aneurysms: recent experience with 210 patients. Can Med Assoc J 118:1229–1235, 1978

121. Crawford ES, Palamara AE, Saleh SA, Roehm JOF, Jr: Aortic aneurysm: current status of surgical treatment. Surg Clin North Am 59:597–636, 1979

122. Whittemore AD, Clowes AW, Hechtman HB, Mannick JA: Aortic aneurysm repair. Reduced operative mortality associated with maintenance of optimal cardiac performance. Ann Surg 192:414–421, 1980

2

Morbidity Following Anesthetic Procedures in the Perioperative Period

Fredrick K. Orkin

Anesthesia care is rarely therapeutic by itself. Typically, anesthesia is therapeutic only in so far as it enables surgery to be performed. Thus, anesthesia per se offers no independent benefit, only risk of harm, which can be substantial. The spectrum of anesthetic-related morbidity is very broad, especially for patients having vascular surgery. This chapter captures the diversity by surveying some of the more salient anesthetic-related morbidity that may occur in the care of these patients who present with coexisting disease of multiple organ systems. Since space is limited and the selection is personal, the reader interested in greater detail or in additional topics should consult other sources.[1,2]

OVERVIEW

Morbidity is one form of patient outcome. Curiously, although we know a great deal about the risk of different events in association with anesthesia care, we know little about outcome, particularly socially meaningful outcome.[3,4]

In the absence of substantive information linking outcome with what we do, clinical decisions are often based on clinical experience, which may be biased by the worst or most recent cases encountered, and theoretic constructs, which may themselves be faulty owing to lack of knowledge.

Under these circumstances, coupled with what economists term a technologic imperative, new technology—whether a drug, device, surgical operation, treatment regimen, or practice pattern—is rapidly incorporated into clinical practice. In our zeal to improve care through adoption of new technology, we may worsen care.[4] This unexpected outcome may occur because all inputs to care have attendant risks and economic costs, as well as their intended benefits (Fig. 2-1, upper panel). Thus, we must focus on the *net benefit* of proposed changes in care as the difference between the benefit and the sum of the risks and costs involved (Fig. 2-1, lower panel). As additional resources, such as new technology, are committed to care, the resultant net benefits (ΔB_i) are smaller, because improvements in patient outcome are progres-

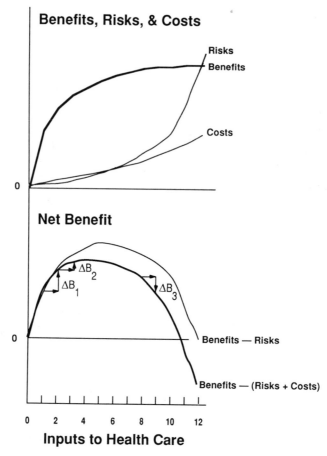

Fig. 2-1. Hypothetical relationships between health benefits and the risks and costs of health care as additional inputs are committed to health care. The segments ΔB_{1-3} denote the net benefits resulting from investing an additional input to care (see text). (Adapted from Donabedian A: The Definition of Quality and Approaches to Its Assessment. Vol 1. Explorations in Quality Assessment and Monitoring. p. 9. Health Administration Press, Ann Arbor, MI, 1980, with permission.)

sively smaller, while costs and risks continue to rise. A point is reached at which the net benefit of additional resources is negligible. Further investment beyond this point result in only *negative* net benefit (ΔB_3), which may be apparent as additional complications, deaths, and malpractice liability actions, as well as wasted dollars.

Health care in the United States is commonly viewed as being very high on the benefit curve in Figure 2.1, with the ex-

ception of situations in which access to care is restricted by lack of health insurance. Thus, there is a strong likelihood of wasting resources and even causing harm as we try to do better. A paradigm of this health care truism that is especially relevant to anesthesia care for the patient having vascular surgery is use of the pulmonary artery catheter: The availability of a flow-directed catheter that enables convenient pressure and cardiac output measurements and blood sampling on the right side of the heart was greeted with widespread adoption in many areas of anesthesia practice, as well as elsewhere throughout medicine. Clinical experience during the ensuing 15 years, however, has documented the substantial potential for serious complications and has caused many to question its benefit in many situations (see below). As a result, the use of this technology is attracting increasing circumspection, which probably would have been exhibited at its clinical introduction had the information been available. (Undoubtedly, many technologies are not even questioned because their associated problems are rarer, more subtle, or clinically less important.) Anesthesia care has many similar examples, as does medicine generally. Besides the medical and economic rationales for reducing the morbidity associated with the things that we do is the fact that much of this morbidity is preventable, especially with greater knowledge related to outcome. Obtaining greater knowledge of— and thus reducing—the morbidity associated with the things that we do requires additional objective studies especially clinical trials.[4] While all of the conditions and complications about to be discussed are not unique to vascular surgery patients, the perioperative conditions and treatments these patients often receive may make adverse drug interactions, complications of vascular access, pulmonary aspiration of gastric contents, dental injury, hemodynamic aberrations resulting from tracheal intubation, hypothermia, and awareness more common in this patient subset.

PREOPERATIVE CONSIDERATIONS

Drug Interactions

The patient presenting for vascular surgery typically has coexisting disease involving the cardiorespiratory and endocrine systems, including hypertension, coronary artery disease, chronic obstructive pulmonary disease, and diabetes mellitus, among other disorders. Not unexpectedly, the patient receives chronic medical therapy for each, with a variety of medications that pose the possibility of adverse drug interactions with one another and with drugs used as part of anesthesia care.

Etiology

Adverse drug interactions may be classified into two types: *Type A interactions* result from an exaggerated, but predictable, pharmacologic, often dose-dependent effect, whereas *type B interactions* are unexpected, unpredictable, and unrelated to the recognized pharmacologic effect.[5] Most of the interactions encountered in anesthesia care are classified as type A. These interactions may be differentiated further by noting that the exaggerated or diminished pharmacologic effect may be due to either pharmacokinetic interaction or pharmacodynamic interaction. In the former, the administration of one drug alters the disposition (absorption, distribution, metabolism, or elimination) of another drug; in the latter, one drug alters the response or "sensitivity" to another drug. Table 2-1 summarizes selected drug interactions associated with many of the medications administered to patients having vascular surgery. The spectrum of potential interactions is very broad, ranging from those of doubtful clinical importance to life-threatening reactions.

Incidence

Adverse drug interactions occur in 5 percent of those hospital inpatients who take 8 to 10 different medications; the incidence may rise to over 40 percent in patients receiving 10 to 20 drugs.[100–102] Although most drug interactions are transient and minor, about 3 percent of

Table 2-1. Selected Adverse Drug Interactions in the Patient having Vascular Surgery

Class of Drug and Prior Drug Therapy	Problem	Comments	References
Anticholinesterases			
Echothiophate eye drops	Inhibition of plasma pseudocholinesterase, causing prolonged apnea with succinylcholine.	Avoid succinylcholine. Change glaucoma therapy at least 4 weeks preoperatively.	6
Alkylating antineoplastic drugs (e.g., mechlorethamine, cyclophosphamide)	As above.	Avoid succinylcholine. Monitor neuromuscular function with nerve stimulator.	7–9
Antihypertensives			
Central α_2-adrenergic receptor agonist			
Clonidine	Decreased CNS sympathetic outflow. Withdrawal results in rebound hypertension. $MAC_{halothane}$ decreased.	Continue to time of surgery. Treat postoperative hypertension with sodium nitroprusside or clonidine patch or α-methyldopa.	10, 11
α-methyl-DOPA	$MAC_{halothane}$ decreased.		12
Peripheral α_1-adrenergic receptor antagonist			
Prazosin	Peripheral vasodilatation without tachycardia. Need higher dosage of vasopressor for given effect.		13
α_1- and α_2-adrenergic receptor antagonist			
Phenoxybenzamine	α-Adrenergic receptor blockade, with fall in peripheral resistance and tachycardia.	Tachycardia may be treated with β-adrenergic receptor antagonist.	
Adrenergic neuron blocker			
Guanethidine	No effect on $MAC_{halothane}$ (quaternary structure).		12, 14
Reserpine	Prevents norepinephrine reuptake at nerve terminal. $MAC_{halothane}$ decreased. Antagonizes indirectly acting and potentiates directly acting pressors.	Enhanced effect from direct sympathomimetic agents. Use infusions of direct acting agents, starting at lower doses than usual.	15–17
Diuretic			
Hydrochlorothiazide Furosemide	May enhance vasodilatation occurring with anesthetics. May cause hypovolemia with hypokalemia and dysrhythmias. May enhance neuromuscular blockade.	Continue drug but monitor intravascular volume and serum potassium.	18, 19
Vasodilators			
Hydralazine	Reflex tachycardia which may precipitate myocardial ischemia.	Combine with a β-adrenergic receptor-blocking drug (e.g., propranolol).	20
Minoxidil	Profound reflex sympathetic activity and sodium retention.	Give with diuretic and β-adrenergic receptor blocker. Monitor intravascular volume.	21

(continued)

Table 2-1. (*continued*)

Class of Drug and Prior Drug Therapy	Problem	Comments	References
Vasodilators (*continued*) Diazoxide	Profound reflex sympathetic activity. May precipitate myocardial ischemia.	As above.	22
Nitroglycerin	Potentiates nondepolarizing neuromuscular blockade.	Monitor neuromuscular function.	23
Sodium nitroprusside	Cyanide toxicity; metabolic acidosis.	Monitor dose and acid-base status. Hydroxycobalamin combines with cyanide ions to yield vitamin B_{12} and lower cyanide levels.	24
Ganglionic blocking agent Trimethaphan	Inhibits plasma cholinesterase, possibly producing prolonged apnea with succinylcholine.	Avoid succinylcholine. Monitor neuromuscular function.	25
Angiotensin-converting enzyme inhibitor Captopril Enalapril	Inhibits generation of angiotensin II. Enhanced hypotensive response to sodium nitroprusside. Intraoperative hypotension.	Give sodium nitroprusside especially cautiously.	26
β-Adrenergic receptor antagonists Propranolol Nadolol Timolol Metoprolol	Blunted sympathetic response to anesthesia and surgery. Potentiates inhalation agents in causing cardiovascular depression. Bradycardia. Bronchospasm. May aggravate congestive heart failure.	Continue through day of surgery; do not abruptly discontinue. Treat hypotension with calcium and inotrope (e.g., dopamine). Treat bradycardia with atropine, isoproterenol, or cardiac pacing. If respiratory disease present, use "cardioselective" β-adrenergic blocker.	27–36
Phosphodiesterase inhibitors Aminophylline	Increased levels of cyclic AMP. Dysrhythmias during halothane. Toxicity with overdosage (e.g., seizure, dysrhythmias, cardiorespiratory arrest, coma).	Monitor for dysrhythmias. Avoid halothane, reduce aminophylline infusion rate, or use isoflurane. Monitor theophylline levels (therapeutic range: 10–12 mg/L).	37, 38

(*continued*)

Table 2-1. *(continued)*

Class of Drug and Prior Drug Therapy	*Problem*	*Comments*	*References*
Calcium channel blocking agents			
Verapamil Nifedipine Diltiazem	Bradycardia; heart block; hypotension. Potentiates cardiovascular depression of inhalation agents. $MAC_{halothane}$ decreased. Interacts with β-adrenergic receptor antagonists.	Continue therapy. Monitor more closely when adding inhalation agents.	39–42 43
	Potentiates nondepolarizing neuromuscular blocking agents.	Monitor neuromuscular function.	44–46
Cardiac glycosides			
Digoxin	Diuretic interact to produce toxicity, hypokalemia, digitalis toxicity, and dysrhythmias. Leads to better cardiac function after surgery when begun prophylactically with patients who have borderline LV function.	Monitor serum potassium and correct hypokalemia, if time. Monitor especially closely when adding inhalation agent.	
Miscellaneous cardiotonic agents			
Amrinone	Hypotension. Higher dosage of this drug required during inhalation anesthesia.		
Antiarrhythmic agents			
Quinidine Phenytoin Disopyramide Lidocaine	Prolonged nondepolarizing neuromuscular blockade. Potentiates myocardial depression of inhalation anesthetics. Quinidine and procainamide can aggravate myasthenia gravis.	Monitor neuromuscular function.	48, 49
	Lidocaine decreases N_2O and halothane requirements.		50
	Lidocaine concentration higher during halothane anesthesia.	Monitor for lidocaine toxicity.	51
Bretylium	Blocks norepinephrine reuptake. Intraoperative hypotension. Exaggerated response to catecholamines owing to functional denervation hypersensitivity.	Treat hypotension with intravascular volume expansion. Avoid exogenous catecholamines, if possible.	52

(continued)

Table 2-1. (*continued*)

Class of Drug and Prior Drug Therapy	Problem	Comments	References
Antiarrhythmic agents (*continued*)			
Amiodarone	Bradycardia. Pulmonary fibrosis. Discontinuation leads to arrhythmia recurrence days or weeks later. Inhibits drug metabolism. Myocardial depression. Postoperative adult respiratory distress-like syndrome.	Check pulmonary function. Monitor especially closely when adding inhalation agents. Monitor respiratory function postoperatively.	53–55
Mexiletine Tocainide	Side effects: tremor, ataxia, nausea.		56
Histamine H_2-receptor antagonist			
Cimetidine	Inhibits drug metabolism, leading to increased concentrations of coadministered drugs, with possible toxicity (e.g., postoperative somnolence).	Drugs affected include lidocaine, diazepam, (other benzodiazepines), propanolol, meperidine, thiopental, warfarin.	57–61
Anticoagulants			
Heparin	Intraoperative bleeding. Contraindicates regional anesthesia.	Reverse heparin with protamine or delay surgery ($t_{1/2}$ = 1–3 h). Monitor partial thromboplastin time and whole blood clotting time.	62, 63
Warfarin	Intraoperative bleeding. Contraindicates regional anesthesia. Interacts with enzyme-inducing drugs (e.g., phenobarbital) to result in reduced anticoagulant effect; increased effect if inducer is discontinued, leading to hemorrhage. Cimetidine inhibits metabolism of warfarin to increase effect. Greater sensitivity to warfarin in elderly.	Reversed by vitamin K_1 but may take 24 h for prothrombin time to approach normal.	
Sedative-hypnotics			
Benzodiazepines (e.g., diazepam, midazolam)	$MAC_{halothane}$ reduced by diazepam. Enhances postoperative somnolence of inhalation anesthesia. Withdrawal syndrome after chronic use.		64, 65
Barbiturates	Chronic therapy causes enzyme induction, increasing metabolism of other drugs. Enhances postoperative somnolence of inhalation anesthesia.	Careful preoperative assessment of other drug therapy.	64

(continued)

Table 2-1.   *(continued)*

Class of Drug and Prior Drug Therapy	Problem	Comments	References
Antidepressants			
Tricyclic agent (e.g., amitriptyline, imipramine, nortriptyline)	Block re-uptake of norepinephrine. Cardiovascular instability; dysrhythmias. Enhanced sensitivity to sympathomimetic pressors, with tachycardia, and hypertension. Interact with pancuronium and halothane to produce tachyarrhythmias.	Monitor closely for dysrhythmias. Avoid sympathomimetics. Avoid halothane. Use muscle relaxant with minimal cardiovascular effects.	66–68
Monoamine oxidase inhibitor (MAOI) (e.g., phenelzine, pargyline, nialamide, iproniazid)	Interacts with sympathomimetic amine to produce hypertensive crisis; also, unpredictable response to pressor amines, with hypotension. Interacts with meperidine to produce syndrome of excitation, coma, sweating, rigidity, hyperpyrexia, and hyper- and hypotension.	Discontinue MAOI 2 weeks preoperatively, when need to treat pain postoperatively (judiciously balancing need for surgery and suicidal risk); substitute other drug. Treat hypertension with sodium nitroprusside, hypotension with IV fluids and direct-acting vasopressor. Avoid narcotics.	69–72 73
Major tranquilizers			
Phenothiazine (e.g., chlorpromazine)	Hypotension due to α-adrenergic receptor blockade. Heat loss due to vasodilatation and direct effect on central thermoregulating center.	Treat hypotension with α-adrenergic agonist. Monitor intravascular volume; add inhalation agent especially gradually.	74
Butyrophenone (e.g., haloperidol)	α-Adrenergic receptor blockade; anticholinergic effects. Hypotension with inhalation agents.	Treat hypotension with α-adrenergic agonist. Monitor intravascular volume; add inhalation agent especially gradually.	
Anticonvulsive drugs			
Phenytoin	See Antiarrhythmic agents, above.	Continue through time of surgery to minimize risk of withdrawal seizures.	
Phenobarbital	See Sedative-hypnotics, above.	Avoid enflurane.	
Miscellaneous CNS drugs			
Levodopa (L-DOPA)	Hypotension. Dysrhythmias. Large doses may cause hypertension. Interacts with inhalation agents to produce cardiovascular instability and dysrhythmias.	Discontinue day of surgery, but resume postoperatively as soon as possible. Avoid inhalation agents. Avoid droperidol (may worsen symptoms).	75, 76
Lithium	Potentiates nondepolarizing *and* depolarizing muscle relaxants. May reduce anesthetic requirement. Intraoperative hypotension; dysrhythmias.	Monitor neuromuscular function. Monitor serum lithium level. Monitor intravascular volume.	77 78, 79

(continued)

Table 2-1. *(continued)*

Class of Drug and Prior Drug Therapy	Problem	Comments	References
Endocrine drugs			
Adrenocorticosteroid (e.g., prednisone)	Chronic therapy may lead to suppression of pituitary-adrenal axis, with adreno-cortical insufficiency and resultant hypotension and respiratory insufficiency, if no "steroid cover" given. Sudden increase in dosage may lead to delayed wound healing, infection, exacerbation of hypertension, psychoses, and venous thrombosis.	Steroid cover not needed if therapy stopped 2 months preoperatively. Suggested steroid regimen: hydrocortisone, hemisuccinate or phosphate 100 mg IV or intramuscularly 1 h before anesthesia and q8–24 h for 36–48 h, and then taper to normal dosage over five to seven days. Monitor intravascular volume and cardiovascular system closely. Treat hypotension intra-operatively with hydrocortisone, IV fluids, and reduction of anesthetic dose.	80–88
Drugs for diabetes			
Insulin	Intraoperative hypo- and hyperglycemia; CNS manifestations of hypoglycemia often masked by general anesthesia and β-adrenergic receptor blockers. Antagonized by corticosteroids, thiazide and loop diuretics, and oral contraceptives.	Preoperative assessment and control of diabetes is important. Monitor blood glucose and urine ketones perioperatively.	76, 89, 90
Oral hypoglycemics (e.g., tolbutamide, chlorpropamide)	Hypoglycemia may occur up to 60 h after last dose. Interact with aspirin, phenylbutazone, sulfonamide to cause enhanced hypoglycemic effect (owing to displacement from binding sites). Interact with chloramphenicol, anticoagulants to cause enhanced hypoglycemic effect (owing to inhibition of metabolism).	Monitor blood glucose frequently.	91
Chemotherapeutic agents			
Aminoglycoside antibiotics (e.g., streptomycin, kanamycin, neomycin, gentamicin)	Cause neuromuscular block. Interact with nondepolarizing muscle relaxants to cause prolonged neuromuscular block.	Monitor neuromuscular function.	92–94
Alkylating agents (e.g., mechlorethamine cyclophosphamide)	See Anticholinesterases. May cause or potentiate nondepolarizing neuromuscular block.	Monitor neuromuscular function.	95, 96

(continued)

Table 2-1.   (continued)

Class of Drug and Prior Drug Therapy	Problem	Comments	References
Drugs of abuse			
Alcohol	Acute intoxication reduces anesthetic requirement; chronic use increases requirement. Interacts with most CNS depressants to produce enhanced sedation during acute intoxication. Acute intoxication is accompanied by larger volume of gastric acid. Chronic user has many coexisting disorders (e.g., cirrhosis, poor nutritional status, altered fluid and electrolyte status).	Administer anesthetics and sedative-hypnotics with greater caution. Give antacid and treat as "full stomach" before anesthetic induction? Monitor Mg^{++} and phosphate levels as low levels may be a cause of poor LV function. All drugs require cautious administration because of altered drug pharmacokinetics and pharmacodynamics. Beware of alcohol withdrawal? Treat with benzodiazepines.	97–99
Disulfiram	Blockade of acetaldehyde metabolism allows ethanol metabolites to accumulate in toxic amounts, leading to nausea and vomiting if ethanol is ingested.		

[Modified from Table 4-1 (Selected Drug Interactions) from Wood,[5] with permission.]

patients experience life-threatening problems.[101] Perhaps 90 percent of drug interactions are caused by a small group of drugs, including antihypertensives, diuretics, digoxin, anticoagulants, steroids, hypoglycemic agents, aspirin, and antibiotics, as suggested by Table 2-1.[102]

Treatment
Treatment must be directed to the underlying interaction and resultant pathophysiology, as indicated in Table 2-1.

Prevention
Prevention requires that one obtain a thorough drug history. In particular, this includes not only all medications that the patient is taking but also all those that the patient may have taken at any time during the past month. Especially problematic are eye drops, drugs affecting the autonomic nervous system, (e.g., α-adrenergic

receptor agonists, β-adrenergic antagonists, anticholinesterases) and some psychiatric drugs (e.g., monoamine oxidase inhibitors) (Table 2-1). It is also important to continue chronic medications through the time of surgery, with the exception of anticoagulants, cholinesterase inhibitors, and monoamine oxidase inhibitors, which often must be discontinued days to weeks before surgery.

IMMEDIATE PREOPERATIVE AND INTRAOPERATIVE PROBLEMS

Complications of Vascular Access

Cannulation of veins and arteries is undertaken to obtain a conduit for fluid therapy, pressure measurements, and blood sampling. Indeed, so commonplace is cannulation for vascular access that we rarely note its considerable potential for morbidity. Given the vast literature on this topic, only some of the more salient complications are surveyed here; for further detail, especially relating to specific access sites and devices, the reader should seek longer reviews.[103]

Infection

Infection is certainly an ever-present hazard whenever the skin, our protective covering, is trespassed with an indwelling foreign body. Typically, the organism is *Staphylococcus epidermidis* or perhaps *Staphylococcus aureus* that is present on the skin of the patient or the person performing the cannulation. Less common pathogens may be involved in patients with disorders of immune function (host defenses); the access device may also become colonized with bacteria or fungi originating in an infectious site in the patient; and occasionally the patient becomes infected with contaminated infusion fluid. The incidence of colonization varies with the duration and site of cannulation, the patient's host defenses, and the sterility with which the cannulation is performed and maintained. For example, 2 to 4 percent of central venous catheters are colonized after only 2 to 4 days in critically ill patients, whose host defenses are impaired; similarly, after a week, up to 14 percent of arterial catheters are colonized. Relative immobility appears important in maintaining sterility, for subclavian catheters have a lower incidence of colonization than jugular sites, which have a lower incidence than antecubital catheters. Although colonization of the catheter is relatively easy to document (e.g., culturing tip of catheter), the role of colonization in bacteremia and septicemia is considerably more difficult to determine. Typically, the incidence of blood-borne infection from vascular catheters is considerably lower than that of colonization.

If there is visible evidence of infection at a cannulation site, the catheter should be removed promptly and, only if bacteremia is suspected, cultures and Gram stains should be made from the catheter tip. Cultures of skin at the cannulation site correlate poorly with colonization of the catheter tip or the presence of bacteremia.

Minimizing the incidence of colonization and possible bacteremia requires undertaking the cannulation as a surgical procedure under sterile conditions, affixing the catheter so that it does not move in and out of the puncture site, applying a povidone antimicrobial ointment to the puncture site, affixing a sterile dressing that is changed every 2 days, or silver impregnated collar, minimizing the use of stopcocks and other potential breeches in the closed infusion system, changing the infusion set every 2 days, and, when possible, removing or changing the site of the cannulation every 2 to 4 days.[104]

Thrombus Formation

Thrombus formation is a natural response to the presence of foreign material in a vessel and begins within minutes of its insertion. Once formed, the thrombus propagates at a rate dependent on blood flow in the vessel (e.g., higher thrombus rate in low-flow states), size of the catheter in relation to vessel lumen, composition of the catheter (e.g., fewer thrombi with catheters made of Teflon), condition of the patient, and possibly whether the insertion was traumatic. Thrombus formation is problematic in so far as it results in vascular occlusion, thromboembolism, suppurative thrombophlebitis, and occlusion of the catheter. Finding a catheter thrombus-free at its removal can be misleading, because the thrombus may have slid off as the catheter was pulled through the vessel.

With regard to arterial cannulation, the principal concern is necrosis of the distal extremity resulting from occlusion of the vessel (typically the convenient, but small caliber, radial artery) or thromboembolism. Since cannulation results in an immediate decrease in distal blood flow, and often transient arterial spasm occurs at the time of insertion, confirming the presence of collateral circulation is widely recommended when choosing which extremity to cannulate. Among the methods are the Allen test, detecting retrograde distal flow with a Doppler probe when the radial artery is occluded, and use of a pressure transducer. None of these techniques, however, is documented to reduce risk. Although thrombus formation occurs probably in all cases with time, recannulation follows removal of the catheter, although the process may take months. Heparin flush solution not only maintains patency of the catheter but also reduces thrombus formation. However, continuous flushing is preferable to intermittent flushing, which, if not restricted to small volumes (e.g., 1 to 2 ml), is associated with embolization not only distally but also in a retrograde fashion to the cerebral circulation.[103]

Thrombus formation in relation to pulmonary artery catheterization carries not only the analogous risk of distal pulmonary artery obstruction with resultant pulmonary infarction, but also such extensive thrombus formation that there may be thrombocytopenia and venous obstruction to the head and upper extremities. Although current pulmonary artery catheters contain heparin bonded to their surface, the incidence of thromboembolic complications and the decrease in platelet count are unchanged, at least in patients having cardiac surgery; possibly the reversal of heparinization at the end of cardiopulmonary bypass also neutralizes the heparin bonded to the catheter.[103]

Hemorrhage

Hemorrhage, another of the diverse complications associated with vascular access, has itself diverse etiologies and presentations. Accidental disconnection or decannulation of an arterial catheter can result in substantial blood loss, especially if the catheter is concealed from view; thus, not only should the catheter be securely affixed, and connections have Luer-Loks if possible, but the catheter should remain in view whenever possible. Hemorrhage can also result when a large vein in the thorax or neck is sheared during attempted central venous cannulation, with the potential for considerable concealed bleeding leading to hemothorax.

A catastrophic variant of catheter-induced hemorrhage is perforation of the pulmonary artery, which occurs in about 0.2 percent of patients having cardiac surgery and is often lethal. It is usually heralded by hemoptysis following inflation of the pulmonary artery catheter's balloon or a change in catheter position. Typically, perforation occurs when the catheter is located too distal in the pulmonary vasculature in a patient with pulmonary hypertension. Also, since one-third of cases occur when cardiopulmonary bypass is ended, it is believed that distal migration of the catheter tip must occur during bypass. Too often, the catheter has been inserted too far or the balloon overinflated. Other risk factors include pulmonary hypertension (which distends distal pulmonary arteries, allowing distal catheter migration), advanced age (arteriosclerosis makes the vessel less distensible), female gender (shorter distance to migrate), and use of hypothermia (which stiffens the catheter). Prevention requires recognition of risk factors and scrupulous attention to detail. Treatment requires immediate administration of protamine (if heparin has been given and not reversed), institution of positive end-expiratory pressure (PEEP) at as high a level as can be tolerated to tamponade the rupture, identification of the bleeding site via fiberoptic bronchoscopy or pulmonary angiography, endobronchial intubation to isolate the bleeding lung, supportive cardiorespiratory care as needed, and evaluation for surgical resection of the affected pulmonary segment.

Misinterpretation of Data

Given the severity of illness experienced by the patient having vascular surgery, as well as the requirements of the planned surgical procedure, it is *expected* and entirely appropriate that the patient will be especially closely monitored with a wide variety of devices. However, there is an unfortunate temptation to ignore information obtained from other sources (e.g., one's five senses), rely exclusively on these devices, and, in particular, to regard the information displayed on meters and in blinking diodes as wholly valid. Recognition of the substantial opportunities for misinterpretation is necessary if mismanagement of the patient is to be avoided.

Partial obstruction of the tracheal tube, for example, may give rise to increasing peak inspiratory pressure and even wheezing. Unless patency of the breathing system is evaluated and remedied, therapy for bronchospasm may be instituted inappropriately, with resultant hypotension and arrhythmias. Similarly, gradual failure of the power supply in a multichannel monitor can simulate hypovolemia, with gradually falling arterial blood pressure, pulse pressure, and venous pressure. Vigorous treatment of the patient can give rise to fluid overload.

Especially prone to artifact are peripheral arterial waveforms. The shape and amplitude of the radial arterial waveform are determined by mechanical character-

istics of the myocardium, peripheral vascular tone, and compliance and length of catheter between the artery and pressure transducer (see Ch. 3).[103] Recognition of the potential for artifact in the pressure measured in the radial artery is important because this value is commonly considered a valid representation of central arterial pressure. A recent study from a large cardiothoracic center demonstrated that systolic blood pressures measured in the radial artery are about 10 percent higher than those in the subclavian artery during the prebypass period, are the same during bypass, and are about 10 percent below subclavian values postbypass.[105] Other measurement errors, of a nonsystematic nature, can arise from using an excessively long or compliance catheter or not purging all air bubbles from the catheter and transducer (see Chapter 3).

Monitoring devices can also mislead us by encouraging us to believe that all is well when such is not the case. A recent example is a series of six patients who had postoperative neurologic deficits after apparently "normal" intraoperative monitoring of somatosensory evoked potentials.[106]

Problems Related to Tracheal Intubation

Pulmonary Aspiration of Gastric Contents

Among the most feared anesthetic complications, pulmonary aspiration of gastric contents is more likely and poses a greater threat to the patient having vascular surgery. A chemical pneumonitis results, characterized by diffuse bronchospasm, interstitial and alveolar edema, hypoxemia, and hemorrhage into alveoli and bronchioles, which may progress to adult respiratory distress syndrome. Later, there may be destruction and sloughing of pneumocytes, decreased surfactant activity, hyaline membrane formation, accumulation of fibrin exudates, and destruction of pulmonary parenchyma, with resultant atelectasis or emphysema. The clinical as well as pathologic aspects are highly variable, depending on the volume and acidity of the material aspirated, as well as the amount of lung that is involved. Thus, symptoms very broadly range from coughing, through bronchospasm with tachycardia, tachypnea, and cyanosis (so-called Mendelson's triad), to respiratory failure. While many cases may be so mild that they are not recognized as aspiration, others may be fatal within minutes. As a result, the reported mortality of documented aspiration among surgical patients ranges from 0 to 100 percent.[107-112]

Etiology. Pulmonary aspiration, in its simplest form, requires an open glottis and foreign material, typically gastric contents. Normally, the glottic opening to the trachea forms an effective trap door, protecting the lungs from potentially noxious material. Respiratory gas exchange is so essential for life that the larynx is richly innervated by afferent nerves whose stimulation results in reflex closure of the glottis. However, this protective glottic reflex dulls progressively with advancing age,[113] accounting for the occasional aspiration in the awake patient.[114] Sedatives and narcotic analgesics dull the glottic reflex and thus also produce laryngeal incompetence, whereas general anesthesia blocks the reflex.[107]

Given laryngeal incompetence, the other requirement for pulmonary aspiration is foreign material, typically gastric contents, which consist of gastric fluid plus food. The acidity of the gastric fluid—at least 25 ml (0.4 ml/kg) at a pH below 2.5 in laboratory studies—is responsible for the chemical pneumonitis; food causes obstruction of airways. Gastric fluid volume increases with acute

ingestion of alcohol, duodenal ulcer, and morbid obesity. Although food is digested in a few hours, depending on the composition of the meal (longest with fats), gastric emptying time is prolonged by pain, anxiety, trauma, intra-abdominal masses, increased intracranial pressure, diabetic gastroparesis, and the administration of narcotic analgesics and parasympathomimetic drugs. Incompetence of the gastroesophageal sphincter facilitates passive regurgitation of stomach contents into the esophagus and posterior pharynx; among predisposing factors are a large meal, hiatus hernia, gastric suction tube, collagen vascular disease, pernicious anemia, abdominal mass, and advanced age.[107] Increased intragastric pressure, resulting from an intra-abdominal mass and acutely from the administration of succinylcholine, also facilitates regurgitation of gastric contents.

Table 2-2 summarizes many of the factors that predispose the patient having vascular surgery to suffer pulmonary aspiration.

Incidence. From the foregoing, it should be clear that pulmonary aspiration is a graded phenomenon, with the mildest cases escaping detection. Indeed, studies in which dye is introduced into the stomach preoperatively and then sought in the posterior pharynx, larynx, and trachea at the end of anesthesia have documented regurgitation in 14 to 26 percent of patients, with "silent" aspiration in at least 8 percent. The incidence of regurgitation is increased in the prone, lateral, and Trendelenburg positions, with the incidence of aspiration reaching 15 percent when general anesthesia is administered with a mask.

Until recently, our knowledge of pulmonary aspiration has been derived solely from the review of cases of documented aspiration. Although this would seem appropriate, retrospective case review provides an exaggerated view with

Table 2-2. Risk Factors for Pulmonary Aspiration in the Patient Having Vascular Surgery

Constitutional factors
    Advanced age
    Anxiety
    Difficult airway
    Gastric suction tube
    Recent meal (especially fats)
    Morbid obesity
    Pain
Disease-related factors
    Abdominal mass
    Collagen vascular diseases (e.g., scleroderma)
    Diabetes mellitus (e.g., peripheral neuropathy, gastroparesis)
    Duodenal ulcer
    Emergency surgery (e.g., rupturing abdominal aortic aneurysm)
    Hiatal hernia (especially with gastroesophageal reflux)
    Intestinal obstruction
    Metabolic disturbance
    Pernicious anemia
Pharmacologic factors
    Cigarette smoking
    Ethanol (acute ingestion)
    Methylxanthines (e.g., theophylline)
    Narcotic analgesics
    Parasympathomimetic agents
    Succinylcholine

regard to mortality and morbidity because it necessarily focuses on the more severe cases. Two recent studies focused instead on the population of patients presenting for surgery. A survey of ambulatory surgery centers, where 529,150 operations were performed during 1985, found 90 cases of suspected or definite aspiration, for an incidence of 1.7 cases per 10,000 anesthetics; there were no deaths.[111] An analysis of 12 years of computer-based anesthetic records at the Karolinska Hospital found an incidence of 4.7 aspirations per 10,000 anesthetics, with a death rate of 0.2 per 10,000 anesthetics.[112] The incidence of aspiration at night was more than sixfold higher than

that during the day. In 67 percent of cases, aspiration was preceded by difficulty involving the airway and/or tracheal intubation. In 83 percent, at least one risk factor for aspiration was present (see above list), including emergency surgery (43 percent), upper abdominal or emergency abdominal surgery (16 percent), and a history indicating delayed gastric emptying (61 percent). Thus, the investigators concluded, "Important causes of aspiration during anaesthesia are ignorance of risk factors and failure . . . to take the necessary measures to prevent the syndrome."

Treatment. Treatment, although limited in efficacy, must be instituted rapidly to relieve respiratory obstruction, thereby improving gas exchange and minimizing lung damage. As soon as aspiration is suspected, the upper airway should be suctioned. If aspiration appears to have occured, tracheal intubation should be undertaken in all but minor aspirations to facilitate clearing the airway, as well as administer oxygen in high concentration and implement controlled ventilation. Tracheal suctioning may stimulate coughing that helps clear airways; lavage with small volumes of saline may facilitate suctioning, although the mucosal damage occurs within seconds. Bronchoscopy should be undertaken promptly if solid material seems to have been aspirated.

Although administering oxygen by face mask or nasal cannula may be sufficient in minor cases, oxygen via tracheal intubation and controlled ventilation is required in severe cases, in which hypoxemia and carbon dioxide retention are present. Positive end-expiratory pressure improves oxygenation when large degrees of right-to-left shunt are present and allows the use of lower inspired oxygen concentrations. However, PEEP itself does not influence survival, which is dependent on the pre-existing severity of hypoxemia[115]; moreover, PEEP can aggravate pulmonary damage by causing increased transudation of fluid through injured capillary beds.[116,117] Pneumothorax is more common following aspiration, regardless whether PEEP is used.[118,119] Although controversial, the use of corticosteroids is not associated with improved outcome, except perhaps in those patients with severe bronchospasm. Similarly, because of the likelihood of selecting for infection with antibiotic-resistant bacteria, antibiotics should not be used prophylactically, except when feculent (or other grossly infected) material is aspirated. Once lung infection becomes manifest, cultures of tracheal aspirate should be obtained for both aerobic and anaerobic organisms, and antibiotic therapy begun, guided by Gram-stained smears. An important part of therapy is general supportive care, consisting of frequent tracheal suctioning, repositioning of the thorax, and chest physiotherapy.

Prevention.   Prevention is critically important, given that treatment efficacy is limited and largely supportive. Prevention begins with recognition of those patients and circumstances at increased risk for aspiration (see "Etiology"). In these situations, one must be especially cautious in using any drugs having sedative properties, so that protective reflexes are not impaired further. Gastric suction can substantially decrease the volume of fluid and air and, thereby, intragastric pressure; however, this maneuver does not ensure an empty stomach. Nasogastric tubes should not be left in place, if possible, at the time of anesthetic induction, because they impair the integrity of the gastroesophageal sphincter. Although a 6- to 8-hour period without oral intake is a time-honored requirement for elective surgery, there is support in the literature for a *variety* of fasting regimens. For example, the ingestion of 150 ml of water 2 to 3 hours preoperatively was associated

in one series with *decreased* residual gastric volume and acidity at the time of induction of anesthesia.[120,121]

For those patients especially at risk for aspiration, there are a variety of pharmacologic approaches to decreasing the volume and acidity of potential gastric aspirate: nonparticulate antacids (e.g., sodium citrate) raise the pH of gastric fluid without appreciable increase in gastric volume; H_2-histamine receptor-blocking agents (e.g., cimetidine, ranitidine) reduce the rate of acid production and also increase pH; and gastric stimulants (e.g., metoclopramide) increase gastroesophageal sphincter tone and decrease gastric emptying time.[107,122,123] Although these agents are effective in altering gastric volume and acidity, their influence, if any, on the incidence of aspiration is unknown. In part, their effect is extremely difficult to ascertain because the incidence of clinically important aspiration is itself so very low (e.g., 1.7 to 4.7 cases per 10,000 anesthetics), and aspiration is a graded response, with only the most severe cases being clinically apparent.[107,111,112] Given the high cost of some of these agents, their use may be cost-effective only for those patients at especially high risk for aspiration. These drug may also induce morbidity; cimetidine, for example, slows the metabolism of central nervous system depressant drugs administered at the same time, and may lead to postoperative somnolence.[57-61] Moreover, gastric volume and acidity may constitute necessary *but insufficient* conditions for aspiration; that is, an additional or concomitant factor, such as airway difficulties (e.g., difficult intubation) may be required for aspiration of a clinically important degree to occur. Because our clinical knowledge of aspiration is derived largely from patients who suffered the complication (especially the more serious cases), rather than the entire population at risk, we have a very incomplete view of the etiology and inadequate understanding upon which to base rational plans for prevention.

When faced with a patient at increased risk for aspiration, whose surgery cannot be postponed 8 to 12 hours to permit gastric emptying, anesthetic management can be designed to minimize the period during which the anesthetized patient's trachea (and lungs) are unprotected. The use of local or regional anesthesia does not obviate this concern, for aspiration may occur with heavy sedation, toxic reactions to local anesthetics, or when a high level of spinal or epidural anesthesia is obtained. If one opts for a nasotracheal (e.g., "blind" or with fiberoptic bronchoscope) or "awake" orotracheal intubation, great caution should be exercised in using sedatives and narcotics, lest unconsciousness or depression of protective airway reflexes ensue. Similarly, local anesthesia may be applied to the tongue and pharynx, but the vocal cords and trachea are best left unanesthetized if one's major concern is to prevent aspiration. When the foregoing alternatives are not appropriate, general anesthesia should be induced with intravenous agents, followed immediately by tracheal intubation, the so-called "rapid sequence induction." During the vulnerable period during which protective laryngeal reflexes are dulled, cricoid pressure is applied to compress the esophagus between the trachea and the vertebral column. If there is difficulty in accomplishing tracheal intubation and arterial desaturation begins, attempts at intubation can be abandoned temporarily and, with cricoid pressure maintained, ventilation with the mask begun; for patients die for lack of oxygen, not lack of intubation. Once the patient is again well-oxygenated and intubating conditions are improved (i.e., change in head position, different laryngoscope blade), tracheal intubation can be undertaken. Since the concern for aspiration persists at the end of the anesthesia and into the immediate postoperative period, tracheal extubation should be undertaken only when protective reflexes have returned.

Dental Injury

Although mundane, trauma to teeth and dental prostheses is both common and problematic in anesthetic practice.[124–128] The injuries include fracture, displacement, subluxation, and avulsion of teeth and restorations, such as fillings, crowns, caps, and bridge work; there may also be injury to the lips and tongue. In a large survey of anesthesiology residency programs, three-fourths of patients suffering dental injury required dental treatment which, on average, cost $2,800 (circa 1982) and 2 hours' administrative and legal time for each case.[124] Largely preventable, dental injury is disproportionately represented among malpractice claims (Fig. 2-2).

Etiology. The injury typically occurs during laryngoscopy for tracheal intubation but may also be related to the use of oropharyngeal airways, rigid suction devices, and surgical instruments used in the mouth at any time in the intraoperative and immediate postoperative periods. The emergence of a patient from general anesthesia may contribute to this complication by its association with forceful biting, especially if an oral airway or orotracheal tube is present. Underlying dental disease—including rampant caries, periodontal disease, and periodontosis—predisposes to dental damage during anesthesia care by weakening teeth and their supporting structures. Dental damage is also more likely during a "difficult intubation" or an intubation performed under emergent conditions.

Incidence. Most of the substantive information known about this complication arises from the responses of 81 percent of U.S. anesthesiology residency programs

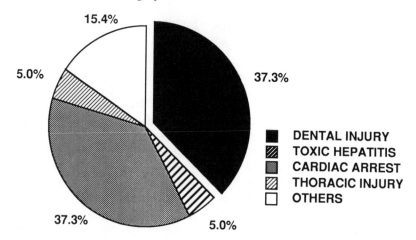

Fig. 2-2. Dental injury is over-represented among complications from general anesthesia cited in 541 closed malpractice liability claims during the 36-month period from 1978 to 1980. The number of claims related to dental injury is equal to that resulting from cardiac arrest (including brain damage). (National Association of Insurance Commissioners' data, modified from Lockhart, et al.[124] with permission.)

to a survey of specific dental trauma occurring in a 12-month period, in which there was 1 dental injury per 1,000 tracheal intubations.[124] The true incidence is undoubtedly higher, because some events probably escaped reporting. Almost half of the injuries involve dislodgement of loose teeth, 39 percent involve chipping or fracturing natural teeth, and 12 percent relate to damage to a dental prosthesis; the two central maxillary incisors are involved in 67 percent of cases. Three-fourths of the injuries occur during tracheal intubation in the operating room, with the others occurring at extubation (9 percent), in the postanesthetic care unit (9 percent), or at an unknown time (6 percent). Slightly over one-half of the injuries occur during difficult or emergency intubations.

Treatment.   When a dental complication occurs, the anesthesiologist can discuss it with the patient as soon as the patient is alert, as well as consider dental consultant. Displaced teeth should be placed in chilled saline for possible reimplantation later. Radiographs of the chest

and upper airway may be helpful in locating lost teeth and prostheses. One specific concern is pulmonary aspiration of teeth, which may give rise to bronchial obstruction, distal atelectasis, and lung abscess; thus, bronchoscopy may be indicated.

Prevention.   In each case of dental injury identified in the survey of anesthesiology residency programs, there was a readily identifiable oral condition that predisposed to dental trauma.[124] However, there was no documentation in the patient's medical record to suggest that the patient had been informed about the risk of dental injury or that measures were taken to prevent the injury. As is true for many other complications, prevention begins with awareness of the potential for the complication. As part of the preoperative interview, the anesthesiologist can note the condition of the patient's dentition: which teeth are loose, decayed, or heavily restored; whether oral disease has weakened dental support; where prosthetic devices are; whether direct laryngoscopy and tracheal intubation are likely to be difficult. When the likelihood of dental injury seems high, the anesthesiologist should inform the patient and take some specific steps to minimize the risk. These include avoiding tracheal intubation, when possible; resorting to nasotracheal intubation; or using the laryngeal mask, a recently developed airway that is passed blindly through the mouth to seat about the larynx.[129,130] When orotracheal intubation is necessary in a patient especially prone to suffering dental trauma, one can consider using custom rubber or plastic tooth protectors, which can be fabricated by the patient's dentist, and taping loose teeth to adjacent ones.

Cardiovascular Responses

For almost 20 years, it has been increasingly recognized that direct laryngoscopy and tracheal intubation may be associated with substantial increases in heart rate and arterial blood pressure, hemodynamic responses that are accompanied by increased myocardial oxygen demand.[131] Such responses in patients with normal coronary arteries and no other cardiac disease are usually of no greater clinical significance than as evidence of inadequate depth of anesthesia. However, an abrupt increase in myocardial oxygen demand in a patient with coronary artery disease and a resultant fixed coronary blood flow threatens myocardial ischemia that can lead to myocardial dysfunction or acute myocardial infarction.[131] Patients presenting for vascular surgery are at greatly increased risk for myocardial complications because of their underlying diffuse vascular disease (often involving coronary vessels) and the other aggravating diseases they usually have (e.g., hypertension, diabetes mellitus), as noted in Chapter 1 and elsewhere in this book.

Etiology. Perhaps not unexpected in an organ system that protects the lungs from noxious stimuli, the upper airway, larynx, trachea, and carina are richly innervated with sensory nerves. Direct laryngoscopy, with or without tracheal intubation, is associated with hypertension and elevation in circulating catecholamines, whereas intubation is associated also with increased heart rate.[132]

The cardiovascular responses to tracheal stimulation are mediated by both the sympathetic and parasympathetic nervous systems. Although parasympathetic stimulation can give rise to bradycardia that is mediated by a monosynaptic response involving increased vagal tone at the sinoatrial node, this reflex is much more common in infants and young children. The more common cardiostimulatory responses, hypertension and tachycardia, observed in adults consequent to laryngoscopy and tracheal intubation reflect the activity of sympathetic efferents via a polysynaptic pathway: impulses from vagal and glossopharyngeal afferents course to the brain stem, then to the sympathetic nervous system, which leads to a diffuse autonomic response that includes increased rate of firing of cardioaccelerator fibers, release of norepinephrine from adrenergic nerve terminals, secretion of epinephrine from the adrenal medulla, and probably even release of renin from the juxtaglomerular apparatus of the kidney.[133] Patients with poorly controlled hypertension preoperatively are especially prone to experience hypertension and tachycardia in response to tracheal intubation.[131,134]

These hemodynamic effector responses require yet another condition, an inadequate depth of anesthesia, or at least a relatively unimpaired sympathetic nervous system. This complication was never an important clinical problem before the introduction of neuromuscular blocking drugs into anesthetic practice. Before their use, tracheal intubation was generally attempted only when a sufficient depth of anesthesia had been obtained with inhalation anesthesia to produce muscle relaxation adequate for laryngoscopy; under these circumstances, the aforementioned cardiovascular reflexes were obtunded. Thus, this complication is truly a by-product of medical progress.

Treatment. The circulatory responses described above are typically short-lived. Nevertheless, given the inability of many patients undergoing vascular surgery (those with coronary artery disease) to meet the resultant increased myocardial oxygen demand, an attempt should be made to increase the depth of anesthesia and/or treat the sympathetic response more directly (e.g., sodium nitroprusside infusion or esmolol for hypertension, or propranolol or esmolol for tachycardia). Yet, none of these maneuvers has an immediate response, plus they pose additional complications (e.g., hypotension, bronchospasm), especially if implemented rapidly.

Prevention. Prevention, as with most other complications, is the best course. As with treatment, one may increase the depth of anesthesia or modify the sympathetic nervous system; however, the range of options is far broader.[133] Despite considerable interest in this complication, the depth of inhalation anesthesia required to avoid the hemodynamic stimulation associated with laryngoscopy and tracheal intubation is unknown. The dose of anesthetic required must be substantial, because the dose needed to prevent coughing during tracheal intubation is about 30 percent above that needed to block cardiovascular responses to skin incision,[135,136] the latter being 1.5 to 1.6 minimum alveolar concentration (MAC).[137]

An alternative approach is to supplement a more practical, lesser depth of inhalation anesthetic with adjuvant drugs. As might be expected, administering narcotic analgesics as preanesthetic medi-

cation is as ineffective as barbiturates.[138] Narcotic analgesics, administered in higher dosage as part of the anesthetic, offer dose-related protection against circulatory responses: whereas fentanyl citrate, 2 μg/kg intravenously (IV), is only partially effective, 6 μg/kg is often effective,[139] and 11 to 15 μg/kg offers almost complete protection.[140] Similarly, alfentanil in a dosage of 10 μg/kg or more prevents circulatory responses.[141]

Long recognized as an effective cough suppressant[142] and more recently noted to offer mild potentiation of inhalation anesthesia,[143] lidocaine is also effective in reducing the circulatory responses to laryngoscopy and intubation. However, lidocaine's efficacy for this application is influenced by dosage, route, and timing of administration: lidocaine, 1.5 mg/kg IV, attenuates circulatory responses when given 3 minutes before laryngoscopy,[144] but not when given earlier or later.[145] The efficacy of lidocaine administered topically (e.g., intratracheal aerosol) is more controversial: lidocaine, about 2.8 mg/kg intratracheally, attenuates circulatory responses when given 5 minutes before laryngoscopy[146,147] but is less effective than a lower dosage given intravenously.[147–149] Transtracheal administration of lidocaine, as well as specific nerve blocks of the upper airway, are more effective. Both may have cardiovascular effects of their own.

For patients at especially high risk of circulatory responses and their sequelae, one may attenuate the cardiovascular response by pretreating the patient with a variety of vasodilator and adrenergic antagonists—hydralazine,[150] sodium nitroprusside,[151] nitroglycerin,[152] labetalol,[153] and esmolol.[154]

Others have advocated the laryngeal mask for avoiding the problem. They maintain almost all of the advantages of tracheal intubation can be obtained with the laryngeal mask, whose blind insertion does not involve use of a laryngoscope, with resultant circulatory responses.[129,130] This mask has not been used for the prolonged situations of vascular surgery.

POSTOPERATIVE PROBLEMS

Unintended Hypothermia and Shivering

It is not uncommon for patients to be cold immediately after surgery; shivering (with resultant heat production) ensues as a thermoregulatory response.[155] Underlying the increased level of metabolism is a markedly increased utilization of oxygen (e.g., up to 500 percent normal). In turn, the increased oxygen use and carbon dioxide production place greater demands on the cardiopulmonary system. Elderly patients and others with limited cardiopulmonary reserve often cannot meet these demands and, thus, develop peripheral hypoxemia.[156] Especially vulnerable are patients rewarming from hypothermic extracorporeal circulation following coronary artery revascularization or rewarming after long periods where gut or other major areas are exposed in abdominal aortic surgery. A recent study documented that those who shiver have an oxygen consumption about twice that of patients who do not shiver and threefold that during anesthesia. Associated with the increased oxygen consumption are substantial increases in heart rate, cardiac index, and, thus, myocardial work.[157] As a result, the ideal physiologic balance between oxygen supply and demand is threatened when these patients emerge from anesthesia.

Etiology

In the awake human, body temperature is maintained at $37 \pm 0.5°C$ by a complex integration of multiple, redundant sensory inputs, each with different thermal sensitivities, from the brain (most notably the hypothalamus), spinal cord, and abdominal organs, among other tissues.[158] In a cold environment, two mechanisms for temperature regulation are invoked: behavioral (e.g., putting on warmer clothing) and physiologic (e.g., heat production via skeletal muscle shivering).[159] During anesthesia, however, the patient cannot invoke behavioral responses and most physiologic responses are progressively impaired with increasing depth of anesthesia and sympathetic block. General anesthesia (with or without muscle relaxants) and conduction anesthesia prevent shivering. The patient vasodilates, losing heat via radiation, convection, and conduction. On emergence from anesthesia, however, the thermoregulatory apparatus regains function, recognizes hypothermia, and responds, typically with shivering. Although some recent work suggests that the familiar postanesthetic muscular activity is actually a tremor resulting from failed inhibition of spinal reflex arcs,[160] the treatment is the same.

Treatment

Treatment of postoperative hypothermia is largely symptomatic, beginning with the application of warm blankets. However, the cold patient emerging from anesthesia responds with peripheral vasoconstriction, which limits the effectiveness of conductive heat transfer. Considerably more efficient is the use of radiant heat. Meperidine, in doses of 25 to 50 mg IV, has been found effective in controlling shivering following general anesthesia[161-163] and cardiopulmonary bypass.[164]

Prevention

The most important factor in avoiding intraoperative hypothermia is the operating room temperature. The critical ambient operating room temperature is 21°C, at or above which body temperature is maintained in the anesthetized patient, except for an initial mild temperature fall in the first 15 minutes owing to undraping, cool skin-cleaning solutions, and lack of patient movement.[165] The elderly patient awaiting vascular surgery in a colder operating room can become mildly hypothermic during induction of anesthesia and surgical preparation.[166] Radiant and convective heat loss can be reduced by covering the patient with plastic sheeting (e.g., garbage bags).[167] Given that much thermal energy is expended in humidifying dry anesthetic gases, there are a variety of methods of adding humidification: heated humidifier in anesthesia breathing system, artificial nose at the proximal end of the tracheal tube, and ultrasonic nebulizer. Warming transfused blood products, as well as all intravenous fluids in longer procedures, is also an important adjunct in avoiding hypothermia. Interestingly, the common practice of using a heating blanket beneath the patient is ineffective in prevention of conductive heat loss in patients with a surface area greater than 0.5 m², in short procedures[168] but a heating blanket combined with warming all fluids was the key to maintaining temperature in patients undergoing vascular surgery.[166]

Awareness During Anesthesia

Although the anesthesia may have been seemingly uncomplicated and the surgery successful, the patient may mention during the postoperative visit that he was awake during general anesthesia. Awareness, or unanticipated patient wakefulness, during anesthesia is often accompanied by great anxiety and pain.[169] More severe cases may give rise to a syndrome of "traumatic neurosis" consisting of repetitive nightmares, a preoccupation with death, and generalized irritability and anxiety.[170]

Etiology

Awareness is a complication of medical progress that has arisen in tandem with the use of long-acting muscle relaxants in 1942 and high-dose narcotic techniques in the late 1960s. These advances in anesthesia care have enabled avoiding the cardiovascular depressant effects of inhalation anesthetics. However, the muscle relaxants, in particular, also allow the dissociation of movement and muscular relaxation from analgesia and amnesia, giving rise to the possibility that an unmoving patient may be conscious and have full recall. Similarly, the recognition that high-dosage narcotic regimens do not produce "true anesthesia" was noted by one of its pioneers, when commenting on its rationale:

> Morphine produces profound analgesia without consistently causing loss of consciousness, in contrast to true "anesthesia." ... The priorities of anesthetic practice dictate that preservation of respiratory and circulatory integrity and provision of suitable conditions for operation take precedence over the provision of absolute patient comfort.[171]

Incidence

The published incidence of awareness during anesthesia depends on the anesthetic technique, strength of the stimulus, and the timing and persistence of attempts to elicit recall. Using a simple postoperative interview, an incidence of 0 to 8 percent is found, whereas an incidence as high as 44 percent may be obtained through hypnosis. Awareness is more likely during nitrous oxide-muscle relaxant techniques, depending on whether sedatives and narcotics are also given. The benzodiazepine sedatives are particularly effective in reducing the incidence of awareness during otherwise "light" anesthesia; the anticholinergic scopolamine is less reliable. The incidence is lowest with the use of potent inhalation agents, even in low concentration (e.g., 0.4 to 0.6 MAC); yet, cases of awareness have occurred during "true anesthesia."

Awareness is especially likely in certain types of surgery, of which two may involve the vascular patient: cardiac surgery and trauma surgery (e.g., rupturing abdominal aortic aneurysmectomy). Interestingly, a study of recall following trauma surgery noted that severity of injury is not a good predictor of recall.[172] A variety of mechanical and human errors also predispose to individual cases of awareness: ventilation with oxygen for a prolonged period after induction with an ultrashort-acting induction agent, beginning surgery before sufficient wash-in of inhalation anesthetic, failure of gas supply, admixture of air in the anesthesia breathing system, "syringe swap," among others.

Treatment
Intraoperatively, the presence of awareness should be considered and treated by increasing anesthetic depth when tachycardia, hypertension, and patient movement occur during "light" anesthesia. If awareness is discovered postoperatively, the patient must be given the opportunity to discuss and understand its occurrence. Psychiatric consultation should be obtained if discussion fails to allay the patient's anxiety and concerns.

Prevention
The incidence of awareness can be minimized, although not necessarily reduced to zero, by administering a surgical depth of inhalation anesthesia. During periods of cardiovascular instability, amnestic doses of inhalation anesthetic agents (e.g., 0.5 MAC) or benzodiazepine sedatives may be used to supplement nitrous oxide. In particular, the most valuable clinical method of avoiding (and detecting) intraoperative awareness is refraining from fully paralyzing the patient with muscle relaxant, thereby enabling movement in response to discomfort or awareness. Also, under these circumstances, one is able to have the patient respond to simple commands (e.g., "Open your eyes if you hurt"). The vigilant anesthesiologist may be warned of the potential for awareness during periods of "light" anesthesia, which may be accompanied by hypertension, tachycardia, sweating, and lacrimation, as well as movement. A variety of new technologies (e.g., cerebral function monitor, esophageal motility) have been proposed as adjuncts to assess depth of anesthesia but have little clinical utility or reliability at this time.

SUMMARY

Many things the anesthesiologist does that are not special or unique to anesthesia for vascular surgery can cause morbidity: drug interactions, complications of vascular access, pulmonary aspiration of gastric contents, dental injury, hemodynamic aberrations resulting from tracheal intubation, hypothermia, and awareness. However, their incidence may be higher because of the many drugs the vascular patient often chronically receives, the greater access number and more invasive nature of the vascular devices used for vascular patients, the prolonged exposure of the vascular patient to cool operating room air, and the instability of the vascular patient's cardiovascular system. As with many diseases, spending a few minutes paying attention to detail on preoperative evaluation and prevention may well reward the anesthetist and the patient.

REFERENCES

1. Taylor TH, Major E (eds): Hazards and Complications of Anaesthesia. Churchill Livingstone, New York, 1987
2. Orkin FK (ed): Complications in Anesthesiology, 2nd Ed. JB Lippincott, Philadelphia, (in press)
3. Brown DL (ed): Risk and Outcome in Anesthesia. JB Lippincott, Philadelphia, 1988
4. Orkin FK: Practice standards: the Midas touch or the emperor's new clothes? Anesthesiology 70:567, 1989
5. Wood M: Prior drug therapy. In Orkin FK (ed): Complications in Anesthesiology, 2nd Ed. JB Lippincott, Philadelphia, in press
6. Pantuck EJ: Echothiophate iodide eye drops and prolonged response to suxamethonium. BR J Anaesth 38:406, 1966
7. Gurman GM: Prolonged apnea after succinylcholine in a case treated with cytostatics for cancer. Anesth Analg 51:761, 1972
8. Zsigmond EK, Robins G: The effect of a series of anti-cancer drugs on plasma cholinesterase activity. Can Anaesth Soc J 19:75, 1972
9. Selvin BL: Cancer chemotherapy: implications for the anesthesiologist. Anesth Analg 60:425, 1981
10. Lowenstein J: Clonidine. Ann Intern Med 92:74, 1980
11. Kaukinen S, Pyykko K: The potentiation of halothane anesthesia by clonidine. Acta Anaesth Scand 23:107, 1979
12. Miller RD, Way WL, Eger EI II: The effects of alpha-methyldopa, reserpine, guanethidine and ipronizid on minimum alveolar anesthetic requirement (MAC). Anesthesiology 29:1153, 1968
13. Graham RM, Pettinger WA: Prazosin. N Eng J Med 300:232, 1979
14. Nielsen GD: Influence of various anaesthetics on the cardiovascular responses to noradrenaline in rats before and after guanethidine. Acta Pharmacol Toxicol 40:75, 1977
15. Alper MH, Flacke W, Krayer O: Pharmacology of reserpine and its implications for anesthesia. Anesthesiology 24:524, 1963
16. Katz RL, Weintraub HD, Papper EM: Anesthesia, surgery and rauwolfia. Anesthesiology 25:142, 1964
17. Ominsky AJ, Wollman H: Hazards of general anesthesia in the reserpinized patient. Anesthesiology 30:443, 1969
18. Miller RD, Yung JS, Matteo RS: Enhancement of d-tubocurarine neuromuscular blockade by diuretics in man. Anesthesiology 45:442, 1976
19. Oh TE: Furosemide and lithium toxicity. Anaesth Intensive Care 5:60, 1977
20. Koch-Waser J: Hydralazine. N Engl J Med 295:320, 1976
21. Mitchell HC, Pettinger WA: Longterm treatment of refractory hypertensive patients with minoxidil. JAMA 239:2131, 1978
22. McDonald AJ, Smith G, Woods JW, et al: Intravenous diazoxide therapy in hypertensive crisis. Am J Cardiol 40:409, 1977
23. Glissen SN, El-Etr AA, Lim R: Prolongation of pancuronium-induced neuromuscular blockade by intravenous infusion of nitroglycerin. Anesthesiology 51:47, 1979
24. Young M, Edwards MW: Complications of induced deliberate hypotension. In Orkin FK (ed): Complications in Anesthesiology. 2nd Ed. JB Lippincott, Philadelphia, (in press)
25. Wilson SL, Miller RN, Wright C, et al: Prolonged neuromuscular blockade associated with trimethaphan: a case report. Anesth Analg 55:353, 1976
26. Woodside J, Jr., Garner L, Bedford RF, et al: Captopril reduces the dose requirement for sodium nitroprusside induced hypotension. Anesthesiology 60:413, 1984
27. Horan BF, Prys-Roberts C, Hamilton WK, et al: Haemodynamic responses to

enflurane anaesthesia and hypovolaemia in the dog, and their modification by propranolol. Br J Anaesth 49:1189, 1977

28. Roberts JG, Foex P, Clarke TNS, et al: Haemodynamic interactions of high-dose propranolol pretreatment and anaesthesia in the dog. III. The effects of hemorrhage during halothane and trichloroethylene anaesthesia. Br J Anaesth 48:411, 1976

29. Roberts JG, Foex P, Clarke TNS, et al: Haemodynamic interactions of high-dose propranolol pretreatment and anaesthesia in the dog. I. Halothane dose-response studies. Br J Anaesth 48:315, 1976

30. Horan BF, Prys-Roberts C, Roberts JG, et al: Haemodynamic responses to isoflurane anaesthesia and hypovolaemia in the dog and their modification by propranolol. Br J Anaesth 49:1179, 1977

31. Chung DA: Anaesthetic problems associated with the treatment of cardiovascular disease. II. Beta-adrenergic antagonists. Can Anaesth Soc J 28:105, 1981

32. Wood AJJ: Beta-blocker withdrawal. Drugs 25:suppl. 2, 318, 1983

33. Slome R: Withdrawal of propranolol and myocardial infarction. Lancet 1:156, 1973

34. Roberts JG: Beta-adrenergic blockade and anaesthesia with reference to interactions with anaesthetic drugs and techniques. Anaesth Intensive Care 8:318, 1980

35. McCammon RL, Hilgenberg JC, Stoelting RK: Effect of propranolol on circulatory responses to induction of diazepam-nitrous oxide anesthesia and to endotracheal intubation. Anesth Analg 60:579, 1981

36. Hammon JW, Wood AJJ, Prager RL, et al: Perioperative beta-blockade with propranolol: reduction in myocardial oxygen demands and the incidence of atrial and ventricular arrhythmias. Ann Thorac Surg 38:363, 1984

37. Berger JM, Stirt JA, Sullivan SF: Enflurane, halothane and aminophylline: uptake and pharmacokinetics. Anesth Analg 62:733, 1983

38. Stirt JA, Berger JM, Sullivan SF: Lack of arrhythmogenicity of isoflurane following administration of aminophylline in dogs. Anesth Analg 62:568, 1983

39. Kapur PA, Bloor BC, Flacke WE, et al: Comparison of cardiovascular responses to verapamil during enflurane, isoflurane or halothane anesthesia in the dog. Anesthesiology 61:165, 1984

40. Tosone SR, Reves JG, Kissin I, et al: Hemodynamic responses to nifedipine in dogs anesthetized with halothane. Anesth Analg 62:903, 1983

41. Chelly JE, Rogers K, Hysing ES, et al: Cardiovascular effects of and interactions between calcium channel blocking drugs and anesthetics in chronically instrumented dogs. I. Verapamil and halothane. Anesthesiology 64:560, 1986

42. Kates RA, Zaggy AP, Norfleet EA, et al: Comparative cardiovascular effects of verapamil, nifedipine, and diltiazem during halothane anesthesia in swine. Anesthesiology 61:10, 1984

43. Maze M, Mason DM, Kates RE: Verapamil decreases MAC for halothane in dogs. Anesthesiology 59:327, 1983

44. Lawson NW, Kraynack BJ, Gintautas J: Neuromuscular and electrocardiographic responses to verapamil in dogs. Anesth Analg 62:50, 1983

45. Kraynack BJ, Lawson NW, Gintautas J, et al: Effects of verapamil on indirect muscle twitch responses. Anesth Analg 62:827, 1983

46. Durant NN, Nguyen N, Katz RL: Potentiation of neuromuscular blockade by verapamil. Anesthesiology 60:298, 1984

47. Makela VHM, Kapur PA: Dose-related cardiovascular effects of amrinone during enflurane anesthesia in the dog. Anesth Analg 65:S91, 1986

48. Harrah MD, Way WL, Katzung BG: The interaction of *d*-tubocurarine with antiarrhythmic drugs. Anesthesiology 33:406, 1970

49. Miller RD, Way WL, Katzung BG: The potentiation of neuromuscular blocking agents by quinidine. Anesthesiology 28:1036, 1967

50. Himes RS, DiFazio CA, Burney RG: Effects of lidocaine on the anesthetic requirements for nitrous oxide and halothane. Anesthesiology 47:437, 1977

51. Bentley JB, Glass S, Gandolfi AJ: The influence of halothane on lidocaine pharmacokinetics in man. Anesthesiology 59A:246, 1983

52. Koch-Waser J: Drug therapy: bretylium. N Engl J Med 300:473, 1979

53. Heger JJ, Prystowsky EN, Miles WM, et al: Clinical use and pharmacology of amiodarone. Med Clin North Am 68:1339, 1984

54. Latini R, Tognoni G, Kates RE: Clinical pharmacokinetics of amiodarone. Clin Pharmacokinet 9:136, 1984

55. Gallagher JD, Lieberman RW, Meranze J, et al: Amiodarone-induced complications during coronary artery surgery. Anesthesiology 55:186, 1981

56. Zipes DP, Troup PJ: New antiarrhythmic drugs: amiodarone, aprindine, disopyramide, ethmozin, mexiletine, tocainide, verapamil. Am J Cardiol 41:1005, 1978

57. Feely J, Wilkinson GR, McAllister CB, et al: Increased toxicity and reduced clearance of lidocaine by cimetidine. Ann Intern Med 96:592, 1982

58. Feely J, Wilkinson GR, Wood AJJ: Reduction of liver flow and propranolol metabolism by cimetidine. N Engl J Med 304:692, 1981

59. Gray DRP, Meatherall RC, Chalmers JL, et al: Cimetidine alters pethidine disposition in man. Br J Clin Pharmacol 18:907, 1984

60. Klotz U, Reimann I: Delayed clearance of diazepam due to cimetidine. N Engl J Med 302:1012, 1980

61. Lam AM, Parkin JA: Cimetidine and prolonged postoperative somnolence. Can Anaesth Soc J 28:450, 1981

62. Ellison N, Ominsky AJ: Clinical considerations for the anesthesiologist whose patient is on anticoagulant therapy. Anesthesiology 39:328, 1973

63. DeAngelis J: Hazards of subdural and epidural anesthesia during anticoagulant therapy. A case report and review. Anesth Analg 51:676, 1972

64. Chambers DM, Jefferson GC, Ruddick CA: Halothane-induced sleeping time in the mouse: its modification by benzodiazepines. Eur J Pharmacol 50:103, 1978

65. Perisho JA, Buechel DR, Miller RD: The effect of diazepam on minimal alveolar anesthetic requirements in man. Can Anaesth Soc J 18:536, 1971

66. Wong KC, Puerto AY, Puerto BA, et al: influence of imipramine and pargyline on the arrhythmogenicity of epinephrine during halothane, enflurane or methoxyflurane anesthesia in dogs. Life Sci 27:2675, 1980

67. Spiss CK, Smith CM, Maze M: Halothane-epinephrine arrhythmias and adrenergic responsiveness after chronic imipramine adminstration in dogs. Anesth Analg 63:825, 1984

68. Edwards RP, Miller RD, Roizen MF, et al: Cardiac response to imipramine and pancuronium during anesthesia with halothane or enflurane. Anesthesiology 50:421, 1979

69. Goldberg LI: Monoamine oxidase inhibitors: adverse reactions and possible mechanisms. JAMA 190:456, 1964

70. Vigran IM: Dangerous potentiation of meperidine hydrochloride by pargyline hydrochloride. JAMA 187:953, 1964

71. Clark B, Thompson JW: Analysis of the inhibition of pethidine N-demethylation by monoamine oxidase inhibitors and some other drugs with special reference to drug interactions in man. Br J Pharmacol 44:89, 1972

72. Rogers KJ, Thornton JA: The interactions between monoamine oxidase inhibitors and narcotic analgesics in mice. Br J Pharmacol 36:470, 1969

73. Evans-Prosser CD: The use of pethidine and morphine in the presence of monoamine oxidase inhibitors. Br J Anaesth 40:279, 1968

74. Gold MI: Profound hypotension associated with preoperative use of phenothiazines. Anesth Analg 53:844, 1974

75. Goldbert KL: Anesthetic management of patients treated with antihypertensive agents or levodopa. Anesth Analg 51:652, 1972

76. Stehling L: Hypoglycemic drugs. Clin Anesthesiol 10:233, 1973

77. Hill GE, Wong KC, Hodges MR: Lithium carbonate and neurmuscular blocking agents. Anesthesiology 46:122, 1977

78. Mannisto PT, Saarnivarra L: Effect of lithium and rubidium on the sleeping time caused by various intravenous anaesthetics in the mouse. Br J Anaesth 48:185, 1976

79. Jephcott G, Kerry RJ: Lithium: an anaesthetic risk. BR J Anaesth 46:389, 1974

80. Fraser CG, Preuss FS, Bigford WD: Adrenal atrophy and irreversible shock associated with cortisone therapy. JAMA 149:1542, 1952

81. Lewis L, Robinson RF, Tee J, et al: Fatal adrenocortical insufficiency precipitated by surgery during prolonged continuous cortisone treatment. Ann Intern Med 39:116, 1953

82. Salassa RM, Bennett WA, Keating FR, et al: Postoperative adrenal cortical insufficiency: occurrence in patients previously treated with cortisone. JAMA 152:1509, 1953

83. Winstone NE, Brooke BN: Effects of steroid treatment on patients undergoing operation. Lancet 1:937, 1961

84. Pooler HE: A planned approach to the surgical patient with iatrogenic adrenocortical insufficiency. Br J Anaesth 40:539, 1968

85. Plumpton S, Besser GM, Cole PV: Corticosteroid treatment and surgery. I. An investigation of the indications for steroid cover. Anaesthesia 24:3, 1969

86. Plumpton S, Besser GM, Cole PV: Corticosteroid treatment and surgery. II. The management of steroid cover. Anaesthesia 24:12, 1969

87. Symreng T, Karlberg BE, Kagedal B, et al: Physiological cortisol substitution of long-term steroid-treated patients undergoing major surgery. Br J Anaesth 53:949, 1981

88. Kehlet H, Binder C: Adrenocortical function and clinical course during and after surgery in unsupplemented glucocorticoid-treated patients. Br J Anaesth 45:1043, 1973

89. Rossini AA: Why control blood glucose levels? Arch Surg 111:229, 1976

90. Rossini AA, Hare JE: How to control the blood glucose in the surgical diabetic patient. Arch Surg 111:945, 1976

91. Schen RJ, Khazzam AS: Postoperative hypoglycemic coma associated with chlorpropamide. Br J Anaesth 47:899, 1975

92. Stanley VF, Giesecke AH, Jenkins MT: Neomycin-curare neuromuscular blockade and reversal in cats. Anesthesiology 31:228, 1969

93. Pittinger C, Adamson R: Antibiotic blockade of neuromuscular function. Ann Rev Pharmacol 12:169, 1972

94. Fogdall RP, Miller RD: Prolongation of a pancuronium-induced neuromuscular blockade by clindamycin. Anesthesiology 41:407, 1974

95. Bennett EJ, Schmidt GB, Patel KP, et al: Muscle relaxants, myasthenia and mustards? Anaesthesiology 46:220, 1977

96. Chung F: Cancer, chemotherapy and anaesthesia. Can Anaesth Soc J 29:364, 1982

97. Johnstone RE, Kulp RA, Smith TC: Effects of acute and chronic ethanol administration on isoflurane requirement of mice. Anesth Analg 54:277, 1975

98. Rubin E, Gang H, Misra PS, et al: Inhibition of drug metabolism by acute ethanol intoxication. Am J Med 49:801, 1970

99. Keity SR: Anesthesia for the alcoholic patient. Anesth Analg 48:659, 1969

100. Jick H, Miettinen OS, Shapiro S, et al: Comprehensive drug surveillance. JAMA 213:1455, 1970

101. Miller RR: Boston Collaborative Drug Surveillance Program: drug surveillance utilizing epidemiologic methods. Am J Hosp Pharm 30:584, 1973

102. May FE, Stewart RB, Cluff LE: Drug interactions and multiple drug administration. Clin Pharmacol Ther 22:322, 1977

103. Bedford RF: Complications of invasive cardiovascular monitoring. In Orkin FK (ed): Complications in Anesthesiology. 2nd Ed. JB Lippincott, Philadelphia, (in press)

104. Maki DG: Infections due to infusion therapy. p. 561–580. In Bennett JV, Brachman PS (eds): Hospital Infections. 2nd Ed. Little, Brown, Boston, 1986

105. Bazaral MG, Nacht A, Petre J, et al: Radial artery pressures compared with subclavian artery pressure during coronary

artery surgery. Cleve Clin J Med 55:448, 1988

106. Lesser RP, Raudzens P, Luders H, et al: Postoperative neurological deficits may occur despite unchanged intraoperative somatosensory evoked potentials. Ann Neurol 19:22, 1986

107. James CF, Modell JH: Pulmonary aspiration of gastric contents. In Orkin FK (ed): Complications in Anesthesiology. 2nd Ed. JB Lippincott, Philadelphia, (in press)

108. Awe WC, Fletcher WS, Jacob SW: The pathophysiology of aspiration pneumonitis. Surgery 60:232, 1966

109. Dines DE, Titus JL, Sessler AD: Aspiration pneumonitis. Mayo Clin Proc 45:347, 1970

110. Cameron JL, Mitchell WH, Zuidema GD: Aspiration pneumonia. Clinical outcome following documented aspiration. Arch Surg 106:49, 1973

111. Kallar SK: Aspiration pneumonitis: fact or fiction? Probl Anesth 2:29, 1988

112. Olsson GL, Hallen B, Hambraeus-Jonzon K: Aspiration during anaesthesia: a computer-aided study of 185,358 anaesthetics. Acta Anaesthesiol Scand 30:84, 1986

113. Pontoppidan H, Beecher HK: Progressive loss of protective reflexes in the airway with advance of age. JAMA 174:2209, 1960

114. Clark MM: Aspiration of stomach contents in a conscious patient: a case report. Br J Anaesth 35:133, 1963

115. Springer RR, Stevens PM: The influence of PEEP on survival of patients in respiratory failure: a retrospective analysis. Am J Med 66:196, 1979

116. Toung T, Saharia P, Permutt S, et al: Aspiration pneumonia: beneficial and harmful effects of positive end-expiratory pressure. Surgery 82:279, 1977

117. Kudsk KA, Pflug B, Lower BD: Value of positive end-expiratory pressure in aspiration pneumonia. J Surg Res 24:321, 1978

118. de Latorre FJ, Tomasa A, Klamburg J, et al: Incidence of pneumothorax and pneumomediastinum in patients with aspiration pneumonia requiring ventilatory support. Chest 72:141, 1977

119. Denlinger JK: Pneumothorax. In Orkin FK (ed): Complications in Anesthesiology. 2nd Ed. JB Lippincott, Philadelphia, (in press)

120. Maltby JR, Sutherland AD, Sale JP, et al: Preoperative oral fluids: is a five hour fast justified prior to elective surgery? Anesth Analg 65:1112, 1986

121. Sutherland AD, Maltby JF, Sale JP, et al: The effect of preoperative oral fluid and ranitidine on gastric fluid volume and pH. Can J Anaesth 34:117, 1987

122. Solanki DR, Suresh M, Ethridge HC: The effects of intravenous cimetidine and metochlorpropamide on gastric volume and pH. Anesth Analg 65:599, 1984

123. Manchikanti L, Colliver J, Marrero T, et al: Ranitidine and metochlorpropamide for prophylaxis of aspiration pneumonitis in elective surgery. Anesth Analg 63:903, 1984

124. Lockhart PB, Feldbau EV, Gabel RA, et al: Dental complications during and after tracheal intubation. JADA 112:480, 1986

125. Fisher TL: Teeth and the anaesthetist. Can Med Assoc J 106:602, 1972

126. Wright RB, Manfield FF: Damage to teeth during the administration of general anesthesia. Anesth Analg 53:405, 1974

127. Burton JF, Baker AB: Dental damage during anaesthesia and surgery. Anaesth Intensive Care 15:262, 1987

128. Garber JG, Herlich A, Orkin FK: Dental complications. In Orkin FK (ed): Complications in Anesthesiology. 2nd Ed. JB Lippincott, Philadelphia, (in press)

129. Brain AIJ: The laryngeal mask: a new concept in airway management. Br J Anaesth 55:801, 1983

130. Brain AIJ, McGhee TD, McAteer EJ, et al: The laryngeal mask airway: development and preliminary trials of a new type of airway. Anaesthesia 40:356, 1985

131. Prys-Roberts C, Greene LT, Meloche R, et al: Studies of anaesthesia in relation to hypertension. II. Haemodynamic consequences of induction and endotracheal intubation. Br J Anaesth 43:531, 1971

132. Shribman AJ, Smith G, Achola KJ: Car-

diovascular and catecholamine responses to laryngoscopy with and without tracheal intubation. Br J Anaesth 59:295, 1987

133. Bedford RF: Circulatory responses to tracheal intubation. Probl Anesth 2:201, 1988

134. Bedford RF, Feinstein B: Hospital admission blood pressure: a predictor for hypertension following endotracheal intubation. Anesth Analg 59:367, 1980

135. Yakaitis RW, Blitt CD, Angiulo JP: End-tidal halothane concentration for endotracheal intubation. Anesthesiology 47:386, 1977

136. Yakaitis RW, Blitt CD, Angiulo JP: End-tidal enflurane concentration for endotracheal intubation. Anesthesiology 50:59, 1979

137. Roizen MF, Horrigan RW, Frazer BM: Anesthetic doses that block adrenergic (stress) and cardiovascular responses to incision—MAC-BAR. Anesthesiology 54:390, 1981

138. Forbes AM, Dally FG: Acute hypertension during induction of anaesthesia and endotracheal intubation in normotensive man. Br J Anaesth 42:618, 1970

139. Kautto HM: Attenuation of the circulatory response to laryngoscopy and intubation by fentanyl. Acta Anaesthesiol Scand 26:217, 1982

140. Chen CT, Toung TJK, Donham RT, et al: Fentanyl dosage for suppression of circulatory response to laryngoscopy and endotracheal intubation. Anesthesiol Rev 13:37, 1986

141. Crawford DC, Fell D, Achola KJ, et al: Effects of alfentanil on the pressor and catecholamine responses to tracheal intubation. Br J Anaesth 59:707, 1987

142. Steinhaus JE, Gaskin L: A study of intravenous lidocaine as a suppressant of cough reflex. Anesthesiology 24:285, 1958

143. Himes RS Jr, DiFazio CA, Burney RG: Effects of lidocaine on the anesthetic requirements of nitrous oxide and halothane. Anesthesiology 47:437, 1977

144. Abou-Madi MN, Keszler H, Yacoub JM: Cardiovascular reactions to laryngoscopy and tracheal intubation following

small and large intravenous doses of lidocaine. Can Anaesth Soc J 24:12, 1977

145. Tam S, Chung F, Campbell M: Intravenous lidocaine: optimal time of injection before tracheal intubation. Anesth Analg 66:1036, 1987

146. Denlinger JK, Ellison N, Ominsky AJ: Effects of intratracheal lidocaine on circulatory responses to tracheal intubation. Anesthesiology 41:409, 1974

147. Stoelting RK: Circulatory changes during direct laryngoscopy and tracheal intubation: influence of duration of laryngoscopy with or without prior lidocaine. Anesthesiology 47:381, 1977

148. Youngberg JA, Graybar G, Hitchings D: Comparison of intravenous and topical lidocaine in attenuating the cardiovascular responses to endotracheal intubation. South Med J 76:1122, 1983

149. Hamill JF, Bedford RF, Weaver DC, et al: Lidocaine before endotracheal intubation: intravenous or laryngotracheal? Anesthesiology 55:578, 1981

150. Davids MJ, Cronin KD, Cowie RW: The prevention of hypertension at intubation: a controlled study of intravenous hydralazine on patients undergoing intracranial surgery. Anaesthesia 36:147, 1981

151. Stoelting RK: Attenuation of blood pressure response to laryngoscopy and tracheal intubation with sodium nitroprusside. Anesth Analg 58:116, 1979

152. Gallagher JD, Moore RA, Jose AB, et al: Prophylactic nitroglycerin infusions during coronary artery bypass surgery. Anesthesiology 64:785, 1986

153. Van Aken H, Puchstein C, Hidding J: The prevention of hypertension at intubation. Anaesthesia 37:82, 1982

154. Gold MI, Brown M, Coverman S, et al: Heart rate and blood pressure effects of esmolol after katamine induction and intubation. Anesthesiology 64:718, 1986

155. Ryan JF, Jones DE: Unintentional hypothermia. In Orkin FK (ed): Complications in Anesthesiology. 2nd Ed. JB Lippincott, Philadelphia, (in press)

156. Roe CF, Goldberg MJ, Blair CS, et al: The influence of body temperature on early postoperative oxygen consumption. Surgery 60:85, 1966

157. Ralley FE, Wynands JE, Ramsay JG, et al: The effects of shivering on oxygen consumption and carbon dioxide production in patients rewarming from hypothermic cardiopulmonary bypass. Can J Anaesth 35:332, 1988

158. Simon E, Pierau F-K, Taylor DCM: Central and peripheral thermal control of effectors in homeothermic temperature regulation. Physiol Rev 66:235, 1986

159. Chinyanga HM: Temperature regulation and anesthesia. Pharmacol Ther 26:147, 1984

160. Sessler DI, Israel D, Pozos RS, et al: Spontaneous post-anesthetic tremor does not resemble thermoregulatory shivering. Anesthesiology 68:843, 1988

161. Holdcroft A, Hall GM, Cooper GM: Redistribution of body heat during anaesthesia. Anaesthesia 34:758, 1979

162. Claybon LE, Hirsh RA: Meperidine arrests post-anesthesia shivering. Anesthesiology 53:S180, 1980

163. Pauca AL, Savage RT, Simpson S, et al: Effect of pethidine, fentanyl and morphine on post-operative shivering in man. Acta Anaesth Scand 28:138, 1982

164. Guffin A, Girard D, Kaplan JA: Shivering following cardiac surgery: hemodynamic changes and reversal. J Cardiothorac Anesth 1:24, 1987

165. Morris RH, Wilkey BR: The effects of ambient temperature on patient temperature during surgery not involving body cavities. Anesthesiology 32:102, 1970

166. Roizen MF, Sohn YJ, L'Hommedieu CS, et al: Operating room temperature prior to surgical draping: effect on patient temperature in recovery room. Anesthesiology 59:852, 1980

167. Telfer Brunton JLA, Thomas GMM, Blair I: Reduction of heat loss in neurosurgical patients using metallized plastic sheeting. Br J Anaesth 54:1201, 1982

168. Goudsouzian NG, Morris RH, Ryan JF: The effects of a warming blanket on the maintenance of body temperature in anesthetized infants and children. Anesthesiology 39:351, 1973

169. Goldberg M: Awareness during anesthesia. In Orkin FK (ed): Complications in Anesthesiology. 2nd Ed. JB Lippincott, Philadelphia, (in press)

170. Blacher RS: On awakening paralyzed during surgery: a syndrome of traumatic neurosis. JAMA 234:67, 1975

171. Lowenstein E: Morphine "anesthesia"—a perspective. Anesthesiology 35:563, 1971

172. Bogetz MS, Katz JA: Recall of surgery for major trauma. Anesthesiology 61:6, 1984

FURTHER READING

Taylor TH, Major E (eds): Hazards and Complications of Anaesthesia. Churchill Livingstone, New York, 1987

Orkin FK (ed): Complications in Anesthesiology. 2nd Ed. JB Lippincott, Philadelphia, (in press)

3

Monitoring Devices for Vascular Surgery: Basic Principles, Limitations, and Proper Functioning

Richard S. Teplick
James P. Welch
Penny J. Ford

Many therapeutic decisions regarding anesthesia for vascular surgery are based on information gathered from monitors, especially invasive pressure monitors and the electrocardiogram (ECG). However, such data are often inaccurate, imprecise, or misleading. For one thing, the limitations of monitoring equipment are not well understood. Also, data are not being collected to answer questions about the state of the patient. This chapter discusses the limitations of hemodynamic and electrocardiographic monitors by providing the background necessary for understanding how such devices obtain and process data. The chapter also discusses some basic principles of data interpretation.

THE ELECTROCARDIOGRAM

By using electronic filters to screen out certain frequencies, many electrocardiographic monitors provide a choice of di-

agnostic or monitoring frequency mode. The diagnostic electrocardiogram (the standard 12-lead ECG) has a larger bandwidth than the monitoring ECG, meaning that the range of frequencies effectively amplified is greater. However, monitoring ECGs (e.g., those displayed at bedside or in the operating room) can be interpreted as reliably and as meaningfully as diagnostic ECGs if correct calibration and mode are set properly. If these conditions are met, any differences between monitoring and diagnostic ECGs are caused by differences in lead placement and should not be considered artifactual.

Calibration of the ECG Electrocardiogram

Most diagnostic ECG machines and ECG monitors are equipped so that the electrical signal can be calibrated (standardized) before recording of ECGs. This process establishes a reference against which the amplitude of ECG waveforms can be measured. Many ECG machines place a calibration signal on the paper automatically. The standard used for diagnostic ECGs states that a 1-mV signal introduced into the circuit should produce a 1-mm deflection on the screen or paper. If not, the gain of the ECG should be adjusted so that application of the calibration signal does produce such a deflection, that is, a gain of 1 mm/mV. Otherwise, the magnitude of any changes in ST segment would be distorted and data possibly misinterpreted.

For example, if the ECG gain were set too high and the calibration were 4 mm/mV, a patient who would normally have a 0.5-mm depression of the ST segment (0.5 mV) on a correctly calibrated ECG machine would erroneously appear to have a 2-mm depression. This patient might be treated unnecessarily for ischemia. Often, the gain must be set too high so that the monitor can sense the QRS complex and thus determine and display heart rate. In this case, a separate screen or chart recorder gain should be adjusted to yield a gain of 1 mm/mV on the screen or recorder. This step would be taken after the amplifier gain has been set at a level sufficiently high to permit sensing of the QRS complex.

Unfortunately, many monitors do not have separate gain controls for the screen or recorder. The only solutions would be to decrease the gain periodically to achieve correct calibration or to ensure that the calibration mark is on all recorded ECGs and to adjust interpretation accordingly.

Electrocardiographic Mode

The difference in potentials generated by the heart between a typical pair of ECG limb leads is approximately 1 mV (0.001 V). However, the differences in potentials on the surface of the skin can be as high as 1 V. These differences may vary with time and are unrelated to the cardiac cycle. Therefore, to amplify the potential differences generated by the heart while lessening unwanted signals (noise), all ECGs are filtered to limit the range of frequencies amplified. The standard set by the American Heart Association defines diagnostic ECGs as having a bandwidth of 0.05 to 100 Hz.

The monitoring mode restricts bandwidth even further. In this mode, the frequency range effectively amplified is only approximately 0.5 to 40 Hz. Use of the monitoring mode improves immunity to 60-Hz interference (i.e., interference caused by the frequency of the alternating current line) and baseline variations such as those caused by ventilation. However, the monitoring mode can distort the ECG waveform, causing spurious elevation or depression in the ST segment (Fig. 3-1).[1,2]

Therefore, ST segments should only be analyzed in the diagnostic mode. The mode of an ECG monitor can be determined easily by pressing the calibration button and observing the rate of decay of the calibration signal and the degree of undershoot when the button is released. Figure 3-2 shows how calibration signals would look during these two modes.

Interpretation of the Electrocardiogram

If the gain and mode of the ECG monitor are set properly, deviations in ST segments from baseline are not artifacts. However, such changes may not show up on a standard 12-lead ECG because lead placement usually differs for a monitoring ECG and a diagnostic ECG. Also, as demonstrated by precordial mapping studies, the standard 12-lead configuration may miss changes in ST segment that non-

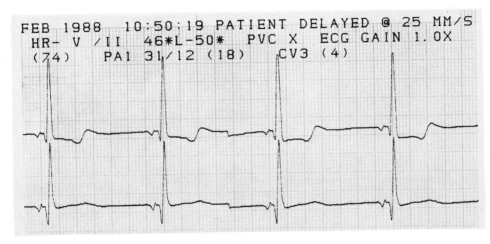

```
FEB 1988   10:50:19 PATIENT DELAYED @ 25 MM/S
HR- V /II   46*L-50*   PVC X   ECG GAIN 1.0X
(74)    PA1 31/12 (18)   CV3 (4)
```

Fig. 3-1. The top trace shows spurious depression in the ST segment owing to erroneous use of the monitoring mode. The first two QRS complexes on the left were obtained in the diagnostic mode. Note how the 1-mm depression in the ST segment in the diagnostic mode is converted into a 3-mm depression by switching to the monitoring mode. Therapy for ischemia would probably have been initiated if this error in mode setting had not been detected.

standard placement, such as that used with monitors, is able to detect. Conversely, for an individual without ST segment deviation, no changes would be detected by the monitor, regardless of lead configuration. Therefore, if changes in ST segment are detected on a properly calibrated monitor in the diagnostic mode, such changes should be considered to actually exist.

Although some of the newer monitors can display seven leads simultaneously (the limb leads plus one precordial lead), most monitors can display no more than two leads. In this case, it usually suffices to monitor the precordial lead (V_5) and

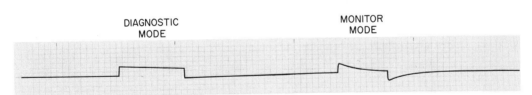

Fig. 3-2. One-millivolt electrocardiographic calibration signals applied in the diagnostic and monitoring modes produce characteristic forms. The paper speed is 25 mm/sec. The corners of the form are sharper in the diagnostic mode than in the monitoring mode. This characteristic, which is attributable to the greater high-frequency response, allows for better definition of abrupt changes in the waveform. Note also that amplitude decreases approximately 0.1 mV (1 small block) in 3 seconds (7.5 large blocks) in the diagnostic mode compared with 0.9 mV (9 small blocks) in the monitoring mode. When the calibration button is released, the signal becomes approximately 0.2 mV negative and slowly returns to baseline in the diagnostic mode. In the monitoring mode, the signal becomes almost 0.9 mV negative and rapidly returns to baseline. The more rapid voltage change in the monitoring mode and the overshoot when the calibration button is released tend to pull the origin of the ST segment away from the baseline and thus may produce spurious elevation or depression of this segment.

one inferior lead (e.g., lead II) continuously and to scan the remaining limb leads periodically. Obviously, if ischemia has been demonstrated previously on a particular lead, that lead should be monitored. Such information is often available preoperatively from referring physicians or from exercise or dipyridamole-thallium studies.

To have a reference point for changes, it is helpful to record the seven available leads and the calibration before surgery begins. In addition, it is helpful to record continuously at least two leads on paper at a slow speed (e.g., 10 mm/min) during the anesthetic. That is, changes in ST segments can often be detected by observing changes in the size of the very dark region of such a recording. Because the precordial electrode pad may be in the surgical field, it is sometimes necessary to replace it with a sterile needle electrode after skin preparation.

In summary, although clinicians sometimes are taught to regard acute changes in ST segments detected on monitors as artifactual, if the monitors are set in the proper mode and calibrated, it is impossible to produce spurious ST segment displacement, regardless of where the monitoring electrodes are placed on the patient. Thus, such changes should usually be regarded as indicating ischemia until proved otherwise and should be treated accordingly.

PRINCIPLES OF INVASIVE HEMODYNAMIC MONITORING

Invasive or direct measurement of pressures usually involves conversion of a mechanical signal, the pressure, into an electrical signal that can then be processed and displayed on a monitor. Early monitors simply amplified the electrical signal from the converting device (the transducer), displayed the signal on the monitor screen, and used the signal to deflect a voltmeter. Pressures could be read from the voltmeter, which was calibrated in pressures rather than volts, or directly from the display screen. However, the ability to read pressures directly from the display screen required the existence of horizontal markings on the screen. The markings had to correspond to the pressures in the range of interest (e.g., 25, 50, 75 mmHg, and so on, for systemic pressure). The amplifiers for the monitor would then have to be calibrated so that a given pressure applied to the transducer produced a deflection of the display trace to the corresponding line on the screen. The same signal also had to deflect the needle of the voltmeter to a value corresponding to the applied pressure. The calibration procedure was complex. The amplifiers first had to be adjusted to give the proper deflections on the meter and then the display amplifiers had to be adjusted to yield the proper deflections on the screen.

Over the past several decades, monitors have become much more complex electronically and simpler to calibrate. However, they are not necessarily simpler to operate. The most important change has been the incorporation of digital computer technology to produce the so-called "smart" monitors. In virtually all current-generation monitors, all input signals such as electrocardiographic signals and pressures are converted into digital data by sampling them rapidly. "Digitized" data are then stored and analyzed by computer algorithms. The incorporation of microcomputers permits selection of an enormous number of display options, plus generation of many derived variables. These impressive capabilities can mask major limitations.

The current generation of monitors have four characteristics in common.

First, they usually alter the electrical signal coming from the transducer in ways not clearly specified by the manufacturer. Second, the screens are not as tall as those on many older monitors, so that accurate calibration is difficult or impossible. This shortcoming is especially pertinent if several waveforms are displayed. Third, the monitors emphasize numerical pressure displays, which often take up one-third of the screen. These numerical values are derived by processing the data in a variety of ways, none of which is usually defined or characterized. Fourth, relatively simple knobs and buttons have given way to complex software requiring use of "soft keys" or a "touchscreen" to traverse a menu.

Soft keys are buttons, usually located just below the screen, that serve functions described on a small portion of the screen just above the buttons. These functions and descriptions change depending on which button has just been pushed. In this manner, a few buttons perform many different tasks. For example, a single soft key (button) may be labeled "setup." After the button is pressed, the screen label may change to "pressures" and the screen label over the adjacent key may change to "ECG." If the soft key is depressed a third time, the key functions may change to show pressure setup options.

A touchscreen operates in a similar manner. However, instead of having a fixed row of keys, regions of the screen are sensitive to touch or the proximity of a finger. In selecting a monitor, one simple criterion we apply is whether we can use the monitor without instruction. In our opinion, touchscreens are easier to use.

To understand how to use these monitors properly and the pros and cons of the technologic evolution just described, one must understand not only the basic principles governing transducers and monitors but also the purpose of measuring hemodynamic variables in the first place.

Transducers

Conversion of a mechanical pressure pulse into an electrical signal is accomplished by a diaphragm within a transducer. A difference in pressure across the diaphragm causes it to flex. The diaphragm is fixed within a chamber (the transducer), one side of which is exposed to intravascular pressure and the other to atmospheric pressure. In this way, changes in intravascular pressure cause the diaphragm to flex. Because the diaphragm is stiff (typically, 100 mmHg of pressure causes a volume displacement of 0.001 mm^3), its movement can track even the rapidly changing portions of pressure pulses.

The most common method of converting the motion of the diaphragm into an electrical signal is by having movement of the diaphragm change the length of a material. Resistance of the material varies with its length. These changes in resistance are measured by determining the change in a voltage (called the excitation voltage) that is applied to an electronic circuit incorporating this variable resistance. The relationship between applied pressure and changes in this measured voltage defines the sensitivity of the transducer. Most newer transducers used for hemodynamic monitoring are standardized to produce a change of 50 mV/mmHg of pressure if the excitation voltage is 1 V. That is, their sensitivity is 50 $\text{mV} \cdot \text{V}^{-1} \cdot \text{mmHg}^{-1}$.

The sensitivity of older transducers varied not only among manufacturers but also among transducers produced by the same manufacturer. Consequently, older monitoring equipment had to incorporate circuitry that the user then had to adjust to compensate for these differences (see below). Fortunately, the sensitivity of most newer transducers does not vary significantly from 50 mV·V^{-1}·mmHg^{-1}.

Static Calibration

Primarily because of variations in the sensitivities of transducers, calibration was more complicated for older monitors than it is for newer monitors. Functionally, almost all pressure monitors have three amplifiers. First, a preamplifier compensates for differences among transducers. The signal from the preamplifier is fed to a second amplifier that is adjusted to produce the proper deflections on a meter, digital display, or chart recorder. The output of the second amplifier goes to a third amplifier that is adjusted to produce the proper deflections on the screen. Newer monitors usually are designed assuming a transducer sensitivity of 50mV·V^{-1}·mmHg^{-1}, stable amplifiers, and fixed screen characteristics (i.e., no change in screen amplification). Consequently, some or all of their amplifiers cannot be adjusted. Nevertheless, it is instructive to review the steps in calibrating older monitors that permit adjustment of all three amplifiers.

The first step is to adjust the zero and gain of the main amplifier driving the meter, digital display, or chart recorder. (In a later step, the preamplifier will be adjusted to compensate for differences in transducers, so that it always produces the same voltage for a given pressure.) Adjustment of the main amplifier ensures that voltages from the preamplifier produce correct deflections on the meter, digital display, or chart recorder. This step is usually performed by ensuring that these devices show zero pressure when no signal is applied to the main amplifier (e.g., the "off" position on the slider switch of the Hewlett-Packard 8805 series amplifiers). Also, these devices

should show the correct pressures when a preset voltage (corresponding to that expected from the preamplifier for a given pressure) is applied. This preset voltage is usually provided by a front panel switch (e.g., the 100, 50, or 20 position on the Hewlett-Packard 8805 series amplifiers). For some monitors, these adjustments can be made with the transducer electrically disconnected from the amplifier. For others, the transducer must be connected, as this step incorporates a test of the resistance circuit within the transducer. However, in either case, such "internal" calibrations may be normal even if the transducer is totally dysfunctional, because there is no guarantee that the diaphragm moves appropriately or that the associated change in resistance is correct. Because the newer monitors have very stable amplifiers, this calibration is no longer necessary. However, some monitors still provide the ability to test, but not adjust, the main amplifier by applying a preset signal. If the monitor fails this test, it usually cannot be adjusted and must be serviced.

The next step is to adjust the transducer preamplifier (usually with the balance control) to show zero pressure when the transducer is open to air. This procedure subtracts out the weight of any water column on top of the transducer and compensates for any difference in baseline transducer voltage output. Therefore, this step ensures that zero pressure across the diaphragm yields a reading of zero. All monitors provide this adjustment, which should be performed routinely, as most transducers have some degree of zero drift owing to slight changes in the voltage generated when the transducer is opened to air.

Next, the preamplifier is adjusted to compensate for variations in the magnitude of the electrical signal produced by the transducer when the transducer is subjected to a given pressure, that is, differences in sensitivity. To do this, one applies a pressure in the midrange of the desired scale (for example, 100 mmHg for an arterial scale, or 20 mmHg for a central pressure scale), usually by using a mercury manometer attached to the transducer. The gain of the preamplifier (often a 10-turn dial) is then adjusted so that the meter, digital display, or chart deflects to the pressure applied to the transducer. *Newer monitors do not provide this adjustment because most transducers have a sensitivity of 50 mV·V^{-1}·mmHg^{-1}. Nonetheless, calibration to mercury should be routine unless a sufficient calibration history for the type of transducer being used has been established. Without this test, the entire system can appear to function normally even if the transducer is grossly inaccurate. If the monitor cannot be adjusted and an improper deflection is observed, the transducer must be replaced.*

The final step is to adjust the display amplifier so that the proper deflections occur on the screen. Specifically, the main amplifier is turned off or the transducer is opened to air and the display amplifier is adjusted to show zero on the screen. Then, one of the preset signals is applied to the main amplifier, and the gain of the display amplifier is adjusted to yield the proper deflection. Again, because of improvements in amplifier design and because the displays are designed to function with the amplifiers, this step is unnecessary for most newer monitors.

Despite these complexities and regardless of the monitor, accurate static calibration for a given scale is ensured if the screen and digital displays show zero pressure when the transducer is opened to air and when deflection is appropriate after a given amount of pressure is applied to the transducer. Calibration on other scales may be inaccurate if the proper procedure has not been followed.

Unfortunately, a successful static calibration, regardless of how it is performed, does not guarantee accurate transduction of pressure signals. The transducer may not be able to accurately reproduce the rapid pressure changes that occur in the systemic and pulmonary circulations. To ensure that these pressures are transduced with high fidelity, dynamic performance must be tested.

Signal Definition and Dynamic Performance

The shape of pressure waveforms can vary considerably, even within the same patient, over time. These shapes often do not conform to the expected or accustomed appearance. Although unusual waveforms may be caused by poor performance in the transducer and monitoring system, this is generally not true with newer systems that are set up properly. Fortunately, systems can be tested easily to determine whether they are introducing artifacts into displayed waveforms.

A system must be able to measure accurately not only static pressure applied to it but also dynamic pressure (as occurs in the cardiovascular system). Testing of this aspect of the system (called the *dynamic response*) is based on the principle that pressure waveforms can be described as a mixture of sine waves having different frequencies and amplitudes (heights). The lowest frequency of the sine waves is called the *fundamental frequency*, because it represents the heart rate. Fundamental frequency is expressed in cycles per second (Hz). If, for example, heart rate were 60 beats/min, a pulse would occur once a second, and the fundamental frequency would be 1 Hz. The additional sine waves required to describe the pressure waveform have frequencies that are multiples of the fundamental frequency. These multiples are called *harmonics*. A unique combination of such sine waves can reproduce the shape of any pressure waveform accurately. Generally, the amplitude of sine waves having high frequencies (high harmonics) becomes so small that such waves can be neglected. For most arterial pressure waveforms, this frequency occurs after the first six to eight harmonics (i.e., after a response that is six to eight times greater). Consequently, most arterial waveforms can be described accurately as a combination of sine waves spanning the fundamental frequency and including the first six harmonics. Additional harmonics may be required to describe arterial waveforms having unusual shapes, especially if their sharp corners have steep slopes.

To reproduce a pressure waveform accurately, the transducing system must be able to amplify all of these sine waves without distortion. This means that the size relationship between amplitudes of sine waves must be preserved. For example, if the pressure waveform is characterized by a first harmonic that has half the amplitude of the sine wave having the fundamental frequency, after conversion of pressure to an electrical signal by the transducer and amplification of the signal, the waveform must still have half the amplitude. For the patient whose heart rate is 120 beats/min, the fundamental frequency would be 120/60, or 2 Hz. Therefore, sine waves having frequencies of 2, 4, 6, 8, 10, and 12 Hz would be required to reproduce the shape of the pressure waveform. However, if rapid changes in the waveform occurred, frequencies as high as 20 Hz could be needed. Consequently, if the measurement system could transduce and display the mean pressure and sinusoidal pressure waves with frequencies up to 20 Hz without changing their relative amplitudes or the relative positions of their peaks (i.e., the phase differences), the

pressure waveform would be displayed on the screen without distortion. In this way, displayed pressures would accurately reflect the actual intraarterial pressures.

Although most amplifiers could easily meet this requirement, the transducer and tubing themselves may distort the size relationship of amplitudes of sine waves having even low frequencies. Distortion occurs because the combination of transducer and tubing tends to resonate (oscillate) at a certain frequency. Sine waves having frequencies near this resonant frequency (i.e., the natural frequency of the catheter-transducer system) are amplified to a greater degree than those having higher or lower frequencies (Fig. 3-3).

The tendency of these oscillating systems to return to rest is called *damping*. The speed with which the system comes to rest is expressed by the *damping coefficient*. Damping also determines how rapidly the rise in amplitude occurs as the resonant frequency is approached. Because the damping coefficient is usually 0.1 to 0.2 for most transducing systems, the rise in amplitude becomes significant at approximately one-half the resonant frequency. Thus, sine waves having frequencies below approximately one-half the resonant frequency of the transducer-catheter system are transformed into electrical signals without change in the size relationship of amplitudes.

Therefore, to avoid distortion, the system should resonate at a frequency that is at least twice the frequency of the highest harmonic necessary to reproduce the pressure waveform. For example, if the heart rate were 120 beats/min, the fundamental frequency would be 2 Hz and the highest harmonic needed for a normal waveform would be 12 Hz. The system should not resonate below 24 Hz. The frequency response of the system shown in Figure 3-3 resonates at 20 Hz; conse-

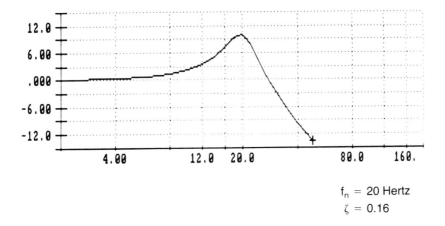

$$f_n = 20 \text{ Hertz}$$
$$\zeta = 0.16$$

$$H(s) = \frac{(2\pi f_n)^2}{s^2 + 4\pi\zeta f_n s + (2\pi f_n)^2}$$

Fig. 3-3. Frequency response of a transducer. The horizontal axis shows the frequency of a sine wave on a logarithmic scale. The vertical axis is amplification of the sine wave relative to amplitude of a sine wave having a frequency of 1 Hz. Note that all frequencies below approximately 10 Hz are amplified equally. However, from 10 Hz to the resonant frequency (natural frequency, f_n) of 20 Hz, there is progressive amplification of sine waves. Beyond the resonant frequency, the amplitude of the sine wave decreases rapidly. The amplitude of sine waves having frequencies beyond approximately 30 Hz are less than the amplitude of the sine wave having a frequency of 1 Hz. The width of the resonant peak is determined by the damping coefficient (ζ), which is 0.16 in this instance, and does not vary widely among transducers. In this example, if a patient had a heart rate of 120 beats/min, the arterial pressure waveform probably would be distorted because the amplitude of the sixth harmonic (12 Hz) is increased spuriously. This increase is caused by the inadequate frequency response of the transducing system.

quently, an arterial pressure waveform for a heart rate of 120 beats/min would be distorted. Distortion would probably manifest as a spurious increase in systolic pressure (Fig. 3-4) because of the amplification of relatively high frequency harmonics. If the resonant frequency were lower, the spurious increase in systolic pressure would probably disappear, the systolic upstroke would appear slowed, and sharp changes in pressure (such as the dicrotic notch) may disappear.

The most common cause of low resonant frequency is air in the tubing, es-

pecially near the transducer. This effect is magnified when the tubing between the cannula and transducer is long. With disposable dome transducers, resonant frequencies above 12 to 15 Hz may not be achievable, probably because of the compliance of the dome. In contrast, disposable systems may easily resonate above 40 Hz if carefully set up.

The dynamic performance of the combined tubing-transducer system can be determined easily by measuring the response to an abrupt change in pressure. This "pop test," shown in Figure 3-5, is

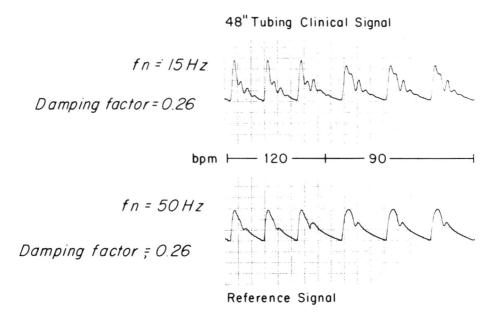

Fig. 3-4. Effects of a low resonant frequency of the transducing system on systemic arterial pressure at two different heart rates; fn is the resonant (natural) frequency of the system. Paper speed is 25 mm/sec, and each large division on the pressure scale (the vertical scale) is 25 mmHg. Although diastolic pressure and mean pressure (not shown) are virtually unaffected by the frequency response of the transducing system, the systolic pressure is artifactually increased by almost 25 mmHg at a heart rate of 120 beats/min (left half of top trace) but by only 15 mmHg at a heart rate of 90 beats/min. This distortion is accompanied by marked oscillations of the waveforms (called ringing). The improvement in accuracy at a rate of 90 beats/min is due to the lower frequency response required of the system at lower heart rates.

performed as follows. (1) The transducer-catheter system is closed to air and to the patient at the patient end by turning the stopcock to a 45-degree position. (2) The system is pressurized with the flushing solution to 150 mmHg or so. (3) The system is rapidly opened to air at the patient end, and oscillations in the subsequent waveform are observed. The resonant frequency of the system can be calculated by dividing the speed at which the waveform moves across the display screen (the sweep speed) by the distance between any two peaks of the oscillation. If the resonant frequency is low (less than approximately 15 times the fundamental frequency), the waveform may be distorted and the system should be checked for air.

Gardner[3] studied the transducer dynamic performance characteristics required for accurate measurement of blood pressure and described the pop test in greater detail.

Many newer monitors use filters to try to compensate for the frequency responses of transducing systems. Most of these filters prevent amplification of frequencies much above 12 Hz. It is hard to see how such filters could compensate for all systems, as resonant frequencies may vary widely. However, this issue has not been studied carefully, and the effects of such filters on displayed waveforms has not been well defined. The presence of such filters prevents high-frequency oscillations from occurring during pop tests.

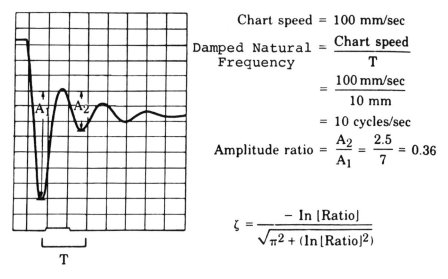

Chart speed = 100 mm/sec

$$\text{Damped Natural Frequency} = \frac{\text{Chart speed}}{T}$$

$$= \frac{100\,\text{mm/sec}}{10\,\text{mm}}$$

$$= 10\ \text{cycles/sec}$$

$$\text{Amplitude ratio} = \frac{A_2}{A_1} = \frac{2.5}{7} = 0.36$$

$$\zeta = \frac{-\ln\lfloor\text{Ratio}\rfloor}{\sqrt{\pi^2 + (\ln\lfloor\text{Ratio}\rfloor)^2}}$$

Fig. 3-5. A "pop test" can be used to determine the resonant frequency (also called the natural frequency) of a catheter-transducer system. In this example, paper speed is 100 mm/sec. The system is pressurized as described in the text and is then abruptly opened to air. This process, which is equivalent to striking a tuning fork, causes the system to oscillate at approximately its resonant frequency. Resonant frequency is determined by dividing the paper speed by the distance between peaks (in this instance, 10 mm). Also, in this example, the peaks recur 10 times per second, corresponding to a resonant frequency of 10 Hz. The damping coefficient, which describes how rapidly the oscillations die out, is calculated by determining the ratio of the amplitudes of two successive oscillations. However, because the damping ratio does not vary much among standard transducers, this calculation is usually not necessary.

Manufacturers might be queried about the presence and characteristics of such filters.

Digital Displays

With advances in technology, the original meters used to indicate beat-by-beat pressures were replaced with devices that displayed the desired pressures numerically. Current monitors usually dedicate part of the screen to the digital display of systolic, diastolic, and mean blood pressures. Because these displayed pressures would be distracting and difficult to read if they were updated with each beat, all monitors display pressures determined by some type of averaging scheme.

Older devices used a moving average. In effect, the pressures from each new beat are used to update the average pressures. Specifically, the new pressure is calculated as the old displayed value plus the difference between the old value and the new pressure divided by a weighting factor. For systemic blood pressure, the weighting factor is usually 2. As an example, assume that the displayed systolic pressure was 150 mmHg and that the new beat had a systolic pressure of 130 mmHg. The new displayed pressure would then be 150 + (130 − 150)/2, or 140 mmHg. If the pressure remained at 130 mmHg, the next displayed pressure would be 140 + (130 − 140)/2, or 135 mmHg. After approximately five beats, the digital display would show 130 mmHg. If the weighting factor were made larger (e.g., 5), the time until the display showed 130 mmHg would be considerably longer, but the display would flicker less with transient changes in pressure.

Most newer monitors use a weighting factor of 2 for peripheral arterial pressure but vary the factor for intrathoracic pressure according to how greatly the pressures in the new beat vary from the averages.[4] If these differences are great, a larger weighting factor is used so that the averages are affected to a lesser degree. The purpose of this variable weighting scheme is to detect the pressure at end-expiration, assuming that it is the most commonly occurring pressure. However, such systems seem no more accurate than those using fixed weighting factors.[5]

Thus, digital displays have two problems that render them basically uninterpretable. First, because of the averaging system, the numbers displayed may differ substantially from the actual pressures at the instant of measurement if the pressures are changing. The magnitude of this difference depends on the weighting scheme used and the true change in pressure. For example, the pressure displayed just before the onset of respiration may differ markedly from the actual pressure, because the displayed pressure incorporates pressures from a number of preceding beats. Second, the actual weights and the scheme for changing them for central vascular pressure measurements vary among manufacturers. The information about weighting algorithms is rarely available from the manufacturer; performance specifications are often not supplied. In fact, currently there is no standard set of waveforms against which the performance of different monitors may be compared. For these reasons, if accurate pressures are desired at a particular instant such as end-expiration or the onset of the QRS complex of the ECG (see below), the digital pressures might be disregarded and pressures could be determined from calibrated displays or paper recordings.

Auscultated versus Directly Measured Pressures

Systemic arterial pressure waveforms often take unusual shapes. For example, a radial arterial waveform may show a large spike indicating systolic pressure (Fig. 3-6). However, if auscultation indicates that systolic pressure occurs during the plateau of this waveform, a clinician might ignore the spike or call it overshoot. We believe that if the transducing system is calibrated accurately and the dynamic response is sufficiently high, the spike (and not auscultated pressure) would be the real indicator of systolic pressure.[6] The explanation is that auscultated pressure actually measures blood flow, not pressure. The Korotkoff sounds are caused by flow turbulence, or by "flapping" of the vessel wall with flow.

A simple hypothetical experiment illustrates the distinction between auscultated and directly measured pressures. Suppose all arteries leaving the left subclavian, axillary, brachial, and radial arteries were tied off, leaving a single path of flow from the aorta to the radial artery at the wrist. If a cannula were then inserted into the radial artery and the artery was tied off distally, the mean blood pressure measured from this cannula would be identical to that in the aorta. There would be no flow (the systolic and diastolic pressures would be unpredictable). Because of the lack of flow, no sounds would be heard by auscultation.

Thus, although usually related,[7] directly measured and auscultated pressures can be quite different. The failure to hear the pressure at the peak of the spike in Figure 3-6 is caused by insufficient flow or energy associated with the

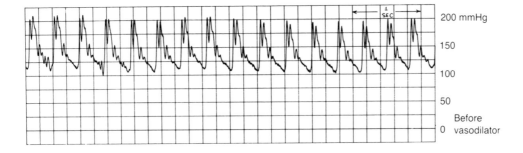

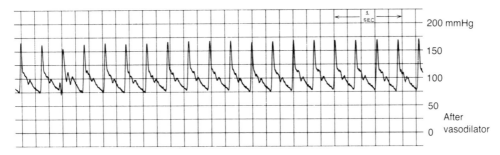

Fig. 3-6. Some unusual radial arterial waveforms have spikes (both the top and bottom arterial traces). The fact that the frequency response of the transducing system was adequate suggests that such peaks are not artifacts. The top trace was taken before (and the bottom trace, after) administration of a vasodilator. Pressures measured by cuff were approximately 30 mmHg lower than the systolic pressure transduced in the bottom trace. Because of the narrow width of the systolic peak in the bottom trace, the high systolic pressure has little effect on the mean pressure, and such high peaks may not be present elsewhere in the circulation.

spike. Nevertheless, the peak of this spike is systolic pressure at the point of measurement.

Consequently, rather than ignoring the spike or calling it overshoot, one should recognize the spike as real if the dynamic characteristics of the transducing system are adequate. The more important question is, Why is systolic pressure being measured?

MEASURING AND INTERPRETING PRESSURES

Issues of how or when to measure pressures usually can be resolved easily once the purpose for making the measure-

ments is defined clearly. Rather than trying to create hemodynamic profiles, it is more constructive to use the data to test hypotheses about the state of the cardiovascular system.

Systemic Arterial Pressures

The shape of the arterial pulse is determined by the properties of ventricular contraction and the characteristics of (and changes in) the vascular system as the pressure wave travels down the vascular tree (Fig. 3-7). These changes, caused by reflected waves within the vascular system,[8] generally decrease the width of pulse waves or pressure readings and increase systolic pressure as distance from

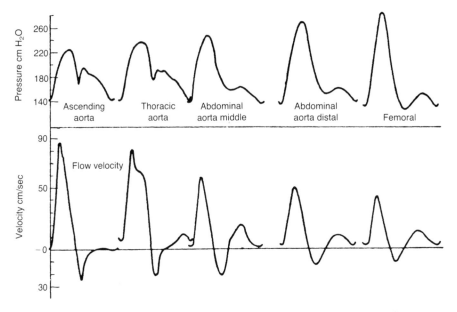

Fig. 3-7. This figure shows the changes in arterial pressure and flow waveforms at intervals between the aortic arch and femoral artery in a dog. Systolic pressure increases with distance from the arch, whereas diastolic pressure remains relatively constant. Also, the shape of the waveform changes, with transformation of the dicrotic notch into a dicrotic wave. The velocity profiles show that the relationship between pressure and flow at any instant varies with location, such that flow during diastole becomes more pronounced at more distal locations in the circulation. This effect occurs because of the compliance of large arteries. (From McDonald DA: Blood Flow in Arteries. 2nd Ed. p. 356. Williams & Wilkins, Baltimore, 1974, with permission.)

the aortic root increases. These effects become less marked with age, but in children they have been reported to increase systolic pressure between the aortic root and iliac artery more than 50 percent.[9] In contrast to systolic pressure, mean and diastolic pressures are less dependent on the physical characteristics of the vascular system and are therefore only slightly lower in peripheral arteries than in the root of the aorta. Changes in the characteristics of either the heart or the vascular system can produce changes in the features of the arterial pulse.

Mean Pressure

Mean arterial pressure is fortunately not only the easiest pressure to measure accurately but also the easiest to interpret physiologically. Mean pressure can be thought of as simply the average of blood pressures at many time points. In the past, the method used by clinicians to calculate mean pressure ($1 \times$ systolic $+ 2 \times$ diastolic $\div 3$) sometimes produced inaccurate results. Current machine averaging technology makes determination of an accurate mean pressure from an indwelling catheter an easy process.

The mean pressure is the average pressure during a period varying from one beat to many beats, depending on the monitor. Unless there is marked variation owing to respiration, the length of this period has little effect on the mean pressure. Mean pressure is of great physiologic significance because organ blood flow is largely determined by the difference between mean arterial blood pressure and venous blood pressure divided by the resistance of organ blood vessels. Cardiac output has no direct effect on organ blood flow. Instead, the effects of cardiac output occur indirectly through changes in mean blood pressure or through changes in vascular resistance mediated by baroreceptors. Changes in arterial and venous volumes that can increase cardiac output can also alter organ resistances by affecting such venous or atrial stretch receptors.

Although almost all organs maintain relatively constant blood flow during changes in blood pressure, the degree of autoregulation varies widely. One measure of an organ's ability to maintain blood flow as pressure decreases (that is, its autoregulatory reserve) is the degree to which blood flow through that organ can increase with maximum vasodilatation when the pressure difference across the organ is fixed (Fig. 3-8). It is important to recognize that there are enormous differences in the autoregulatory reserve of different organ beds[10] and that these differences reflect each organ's ability to maintain flow as mean blood pressure decreases. That is, organs having high reserve can maintain blood flow even when blood pressure is low, whereas organs having low reserve cannot. For example, the kidney can increase flow to approximately 1.25 times the basal flow, whereas muscle and skin can increase flow to almost 25 times the basal flow. Thus, the kidney has a very limited autoregulatory reserve and cannot maintain normal flow as mean pressure drops to relatively low values (e.g., 50 mmHg). Conversely, muscle and skin have an enormous reserve and thus can maintain blood flow even when mean blood pressures are very low.

The importance of these differences in reserve is that flow to various organs, such as the kidney, cannot be predicted by cardiac output. For example, if cardiac output is high and pressure low, most of the output would pass through organs having a large reserve, such as muscle and skin, whereas flow through the kidneys would probably decrease. This fact emphasizes the importance of maintaining adequate mean blood pressure, not cardiac output. This consideration is especially pertinent to vascular surgical patients because resistance through vital organ beds may be abnormally high owing to vascular disease. However, if blood pressure is maintained with administration of vasoconstricting drugs, blood flow to vital organs may still decrease, despite adequate pressures. For example, during strenuous exercise and despite very high cardiac output and normal or high blood pressure, renal blood flow decreases.

Because the arteries feeding the radial and pedal vessels are relatively large, their resistance is low. Therefore, even though flow through these vessels is relatively high, the decrease in mean pressure is small. Consequently, the mean pressure measured at an arterial cannula is usually close to the mean pressure in every organ system. However, because vascular surgical patients often have arterial stenoses, differences in pressures might be sought in the arms, and the cannula might preferentially be inserted in the side having the higher pressure.

Systolic Pressure

Although the most commonly measured pressure is systolic, it is also the most difficult to measure accurately and to interpret. As discussed above, if the transducer is properly calibrated and has a sufficiently high resonant frequency, the displayed systolic pressure will be accurate even though it may have a peculiar shape. Even assuming that the displayed systolic pressure is accurate, two additional problems in using systolic pressure would still exist. The first involves deciding why systolic pressure is being measured, that is, what is its physiologic significance. Although systolic pressure is believed to be an important determi-

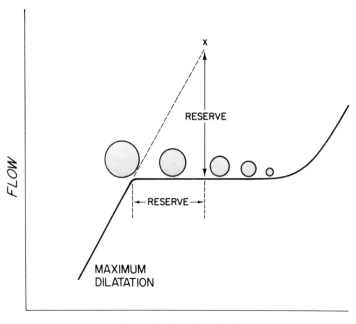

PRESSURE DIFFERENCE

Fig. 3-8. This schematic representation of the autoregulatory reserve of an organ shows the relationship among blood pressure, blood flow, and dilatation of blood vessels. The autoregulatory reserve is the maximum decrease in blood pressure that can occur before blood flow begins to decrease. The diameters of the circles show the increase in cross-sectional area that organ blood vessels must undergo to keep blood flow constant as pressure falls. If the pressure becomes low enough to cause maximal dilation of the vessels, further decreases in pressure will decrease flow, regardless of cardiac output. Autoregulatory reserve is often measured by keeping pressure constant and dilating the vessels maximally. This process increases blood flow, as shown by the vertical reserve line from the autoregulatory curve to point X. The autoregulatory reserve of different organs may be ranked by comparing the maximum flows achieved in this manner. The wide differences in reserve among organs permit normal flow at low pressures for organs having a large reserve, for example, muscle, whereas flow to organs with more limited reserve, such as the kidney, decreases. The oblique straight line from the lowest pressure to point X corresponds to the pressure-flow relationship that would occur if the vessels were maximally dilated.

nant of myocardial oxygen consumption, this assumption is incorrect unless the heart is markedly depressed. Even in this instance, it would be end-systolic pressure, not peak pressure, that would be important. And even then, end-systolic pressure would probably be important only insofar as it determines ventricular volume.[11] As discussed above and illustrated in Figure 3-7, systolic pressure does not directly relate to organ blood flow except through alterations in mean pressure. However, systolic pressure might be important in causing rupture of weakened areas in large vessels. This effect has not been established firmly.

Thus, it is often difficult to assign a physiologic significance to systolic pressure. The second problem involves the fact that even if the physiologic significance of systolic pressure were known with certainty, interpretation still would be difficult because, as discussed above, systolic pressure varies markedly throughout the vascular tree, generally increasing in more distal vessels. However, the magnitude of these changes varies among patients and also within a patient when conditions such as temperature or sympathetic tone are changing. Consequently, although a carefully set up system can measure systolic pressure accurately, it is difficult to interpret. Also, its value at other sites can differ substantially from that at the site of measurement.

Diastolic Pressure

Diastolic pressure is said to be the upstream pressure for coronary perfusion. No evidence supports this assertion, and much evidence even points to the contrary.[12] Although virtually all flow in the left ventricular muscle occurs during diastole, it does not necessarily all occur at the end of diastole. Furthermore, the substantial flow into the large epicardial arteries during systole may be important for diastolic perfusion. The coronary circulation is so complex that neither the upstream nor the downstream pressure is known, and both can vary as pressure changes. For these reasons, the pressures that make up coronary perfusion pressure are not known. In our view, these factors make the calculation of coronary vascular resistance meaningless and at time misleading. Although diastolic pressure varies only a small amount throughout the vascular tree and therefore can be estimated at any site using a peripheral arterial catheter, its physiologic significance is not well defined.

Variations in Pressure during Respiration

Many intravascular pressure tracings exhibit considerable variation, especially in systolic pressure, during the respiratory cycle. Usually, intravascular pressures decrease during spontaneous breaths. In contrast, during mechanical breaths, intravascular pressure increases initially, then decreases (the nadir occurring at about the time that airway pressure has returned to baseline), and gradually rises back to baseline. In our experience, the length of time required for this last phase varies considerably, ranging from a few beats to as many as 12 beats. If the ventilator rate is sufficiently high so that a breath occurs before pressure returns to baseline, pressure will decrease and hypotension may occur. The exact mechanisms for these variations in pressure are complex and depend on interaction with venous return, changes in pulmonary vascular blood volume, and left ventricular load. Because these pressure variations in the systemic arteries presumably affect tissue perfusion, systemic pressures probably should be averaged over the entire respiratory cycle if fluctuations in pressure are large. Unfortunately, it is difficult to determine the averaging period used by monitors. Such information might be sought from the manufacturer. Large respiratory variations in systolic blood pressure sometimes occur during hypovolemia.[13]

Central Pressures

To measure central vascular pressures (i.e., central venous or right atrial pressure, pulmonary artery pressure, pulmonary capillary wedge pressure [PCWP], and left atrial pressure) correctly, one must define the purpose for making such measurements. Unlike respiratory variations in peripheral arterial pressures, changes in central pressures resulting from respiration are artifactual. To solve this problem, many clinicians advocate measuring values that are averaged over respiratory cycles. However, such averages may be misleading if an estimate of ventricular end-diastolic pressure (EDP) is desired. In contrast, measurements of such pressures just before inspiration (called, for convenience, end-expiration) provide more accurate and precise estimates of EDP. To understand why, one must understand the difference between the measured central pressure and the transmural pressure.

For the reasons discussed earlier, digital displays on monitors generally cannot be used to obtain end-expiratory pressures. Instead, the pressures can be read accurately from a waveform displayed on a calibrated screen.

Relationship Between End-Diastolic Pressure and Volume

Probably the main reason for measuring left and right atrial pressures and PCWP is to estimate preload of the right and left ventricles. Although difficult to define precisely, preload is the ventricular end-diastolic volume (EDV). This is a useful definition because EDV is an important component of ventricular stroke volume. The relationship between volume and pressure in the ventricles at the end of diastole is represented by the ventricular compliance curve (Fig. 3-9). If this curve were the same for all individuals, EDV could always be determined by accurately measuring EDP. The substantial difference in compliance curves among patients (Fig. 3-9) means that EDV cannot be estimated accurately from EDP. Consequently, because changes in measurements govern therapeutic decisions, accuracy is not as important as precision when measuring EDP. For a given EDP, obtaining the correct value is less important than being able to obtain the same value (and the trend in values) on repeated measurements.[14]

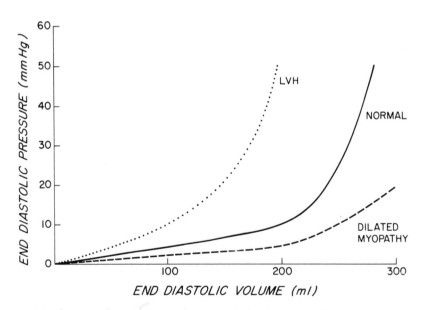

Fig. 3-9. Ventricular compliance curves for patients having normal hearts are contrasted with curves for patients having left ventricular hypertrophy (LVH) of dilated congestive cardiomyopathy. With LVH, the end-diastolic volume (EDV) at any end-diastolic pressure (EDP) is less than that of normal individuals. In contrast, with dilated congestive cardiomyopathy, EDV is always greater for a given EDP. Because the exact shape of the compliance curve for a given patient is usually unknown, even exact knowledge of EDP would not allow precise determination of EDV.

Transmural Pressure and End-Expiration

Although the exact relationship between EDP and EDV is usually not known, an increase in EDP is accompanied by some increase in EDV (Fig. 3-9). During a spontaneous breath, PCWP and right atrial pressure (which are assumed to reflect EDP of the left and right ventricles, respectively) decrease. However, EDV does not usually decrease and may actually increase. This seeming paradox can be explained as follows. The EDV of a ventricle depends on the pressure across its wall (i.e., the *transmural pressure—* the difference between the pressure in the ventricular cavity and that in the pericardium). The EDV does *not* relate to the difference between the pressure within the ventricle and atmospheric pressure. However, it is atmospheric pressure and not transmural pressure that is actually being measured.

Figure 3-10 illustrates these differences. During a spontaneous breath, intrathoracic pressure decreases. This decrease is transmitted to the pericardium so that pressure on the outer walls of the heart decreases. As a result, transmural pressure and EDV increase. However, the measured central pressures decrease because the pressure that the transducer is measuring is referenced to atmospheric rather than intrathoracic pressure. Consequently, the measured pressure equals the transmural pressure plus the intrathoracic pressure.

Because intrathoracic pressure decreases during a spontaneous breath, the intravascular pressure measured during such a breath will always be lower than the transmural pressure. Conversely, during positive-pressure ventilation, intrathoracic and pericardial pressures increase. These increases in pressure tend to compress the heart, making it smaller, while the measured intravascular pressures increase. Measured and transmural

pressures would be equal only if intrapericardial pressure, which is approximately the same as intrathoracic pressure, equals atmospheric pressure. Changes in pericardial pressure owing to respiratory variations in intrathoracic pressure will change transmural pressures in the direction opposite that of changes in measured pressures. Therefore, the point in the respiratory cycle at which pericardial pressure most closely approximates atmospheric pressure is at end-expiration.

The use of positive end-expiratory pressure (PEEP) introduces other considerations. During administration of PEEP, intrathoracic pressure is always greater than atmospheric pressure; therefore, measured central vascular pressures will always be greater than transmural pressures. The magnitude of this discrepancy depends on how much PEEP is transmitted to the intrathoracic cavity. In turn, transmission of PEEP depends on a number of variables, including chest wall and lung compliance. Although the use of PEEP precludes accurate measurement of transmural pressure without determination of intrathoracic pressure (which may be approximated by using an esophageal balloon), the error introduced is generally unimportant; even if transmural pressure were known, only an estimate of EDV could be obtained because of the variability in ventricular compliance curves.

The above argument suggests that the increase in accuracy gained by measuring central vascular pressure at end-expiration is not critical. However, the gain in precision is important in detecting changes in these pressures. For example, assume pressures were averaged over respiratory cycles in a mechanically ventilated patient and that the compliance of the thoracic cavity was suddenly reduced by surgical retraction. Reduction in compliance would increase intrathoracic pressure. This increase would in turn

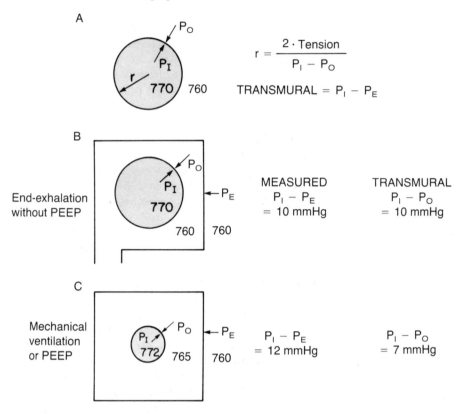

A

$$r = \frac{2 \cdot \text{Tension}}{P_I - P_O}$$

$$\text{TRANSMURAL} = P_I - P_E$$

B

End-exhalation
without PEEP

MEASURED	TRANSMURAL
$P_I - P_E$	$P_I - P_O$
= 10 mmHg	= 10 mmHg

C

Mechanical
ventilation
or PEEP

$P_I - P_E$
= 12 mmHg

$P_I - P_O$
= 7 mmHg

Fig. 3-10. This figure illustrates the difference between transmural pressure and the central pressure measured by a transducer. Paradoxically, the increase in central venous pressure or PCWP measured during a breath is usually accompanied by a decrease in ventricular volume. This decrease occurs because pressure in the cardiac chambers is measured relative to extrathoracic pressure (P_E) rather than intrathoracic pressure. The explanation for this seeming paradox is illustrated by imagining that the heart is an elastic balloon. As shown in panel **A**, the radius of the balloon (r) depends on the difference between the pressure inside (P_I) and outside (P_O) the balloon and the tension exerted by the balloon rubber. Panel **B** shows what happens when the balloon is placed in an open box. This situation represents, for example, the thoracic cavity at end-exhalation in patients not given PEEP. The pressure outside the balloon would remain atmospheric (in this instance, 760 mmHg), so that even though the transducer is outside the box, the pressure on the back of the transducer diaphragm (760 mmHg) would remain the same as that on the outside of the balloon. The pressure within the balloon would be 10 mmHg above atmospheric pressure (770 mmHg). The transducer would correctly show a transmural pressure difference of 10 mmHg. Panel **C** shows what would happen if the box were sealed and pressurized to an additional 5 mmHg by mechanical ventilation or the use of PEEP. The balloon would shrink because of the increased pressure outside the balloon. This decrease in balloon volume would be accompanied by a decrease in transmural pressure. That is, because P_O would now be 765 mmHg and P_I 772 mmHg, transmural pressure would be 7 mmHg. If the transducer still resides outside the box, the pressure difference across the diaphragm would be 12 mmHg. Consequently, pressure would appear to have increased while balloon volume decreased. This seeming paradox would not occur if the true transmural pressure were measured by placing the transducer within the box so that the pressures on the outside of the balloon and on the open side of the transducer diaphragm were the same.

magnify the increase in central pressures occurring during the respiratory cycle but would not directly affect end-expiratory pressures. An increase such as this in averaged pressures might be interpreted as an increase in EDV when, in fact, EDV had not changed or may have even decreased. Central pressures averaged over respiratory cycles can also change with alterations in tidal volume or respiratory rate while the end-expiratory values remain constant.

Thus, if central pressures are measured at a point in the respiratory cycle other than end-expiration (for example, at peak inspiration), the value will be affected by extracardiac factors, such as ventilatory pattern, that either do not change the EDV or transmural EDP or that change them in the direction opposite that of measured pressure changes. Because changes in central pressures coupled with changes in stroke volume can convey important information about cardiac function, the inaccuracy, and especially the imprecision, incurred by not measuring central pressures at end-expiration can lead to incorrect clinical decisions.

The simplest way of measuring end-expiratory pressure is to observe the chest wall or ventilator and to read the pressures directly from a calibrated screen. If screen calibrations are spaced too far apart to do this accurately, a chart recorder may be used. Because of small screen sizes and inadequate calibration marks, many newer monitors allow the user to move a horizontal cursor to any point in the waveform and to display the pressure corresponding to the cursor position. Although this procedure permits accurate measurement of end-expiratory pressures, it requires substantially more steps than reading a calibrated screen. Nevertheless, this step may be helpful in providing a marker to assess changes from baseline.

Waveform Features

The presence of atypical or abnormal configurations in central pressure waveforms can lead to errors in measurement. For example, the typical atrial waveform consists of an A wave, caused by right atrial contraction; a C wave, caused by bulging of the atrioventricular valve during isovolumic contraction; and a V wave that occurs during atrial filling and that peaks at the opening of the atrioventricular valves. Because these valves are closed from approximately the onset of systole until the peak of the V wave, atrial pressures during this time interval cannot reflect ventricular EDP. Also, because EDV, and thus EDP, increases with atrial contraction, the only time that atrial pressures can reflect EDP is after the A wave and before the onset of systole. Therefore, it is logical to measure atrial pressures at approximately the onset of the QRS complex of the ECG. However, because A, C, and V waves usually have amplitudes of only a few millimeters of mercury, atrial pressures can be averaged between respiratory cycles by, for example, transiently turning off the ventilator. (We do not recommend this because of the possibility of forgetting to turn the ventilator back on.) However, if the A, C, and V waves waves have large amplitudes, such averages can be misleading. For example, very large A waves can occur during a nodal rhythm when the atria and ventricles contract simultaneously (Fig. 3-11). Not only might the presence of such "cannon" waves be missed by displaying a mean central venous pressure, but the mean also could be markedly increased without a true change in EDP. Similar problems can occur if there are large V waves, as might occur with atrioventricular valvular regurgitation or volume overload.[15] In contrast, if fluid transudation in the lung is a concern, measuring mean left atrial pressures might be useful because pulmonary

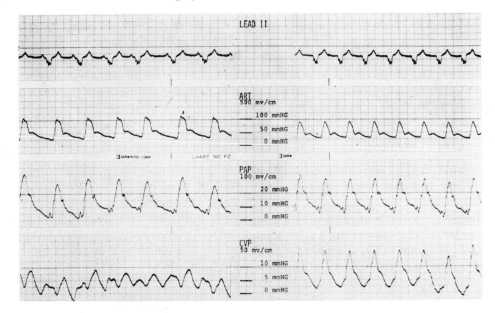

Fig. 3-11. Nodal rhythms of the heart produce cannon waves, very large A waves that occur when the atria contract against closed atrioventricular valves. The normal central venous pressure (CVP) trace is shown in the left side of the bottom panel. As seen in the right side of the same panel, the occurrence of a nodal rhythm is easily detected by the presence of large peaked cannon waves in the CVP trace. The presence of such waves is easier to detect than the absence of P waves in the ECG but might be missed if mean CVP were displayed. The figure also shows the drop in systemic pressure that usually occurs with nodal rhythm. Such abrupt changes in pressure are often caused by atrial dysrhythmias that can be detected easily from the CVP waveform.

edema might occur with high mean pressures even if the true EDP were normal.

Other Sources of Error in Measurement of Central Pressures

Occasionally, overinflation of the balloon in a pulmonary artery catheter can yield an erroneous value for pressure. This error probably results from transient obstruction of the catheter tip by the balloon or vascular wall, allowing pressure from the pressurized flushing system to build up within the transducer. Because correctly measured PCWP never exceeds pulmonary arterial disastolic pressure, this problem is readily detected by such a discrepancy. Balloon deflation, followed by slow reinflation, usually corrects this problem.

The term catheter whip is commonly used to describe pulmonary arterial waveforms having unusual spiking components of questionable origin. The term implies that these apparent waveform distortions are caused by mechanical motion of the catheter during the cardiac cycle. Given the fact that the catheter crosses through the right side of the heart into the pulmonary arterial inflow tract, this explanation seems plausible. However, the validity of this hypothesis has not been established; catheter whip may represent a true physiologic event.

Some believe that placement of the catheter tip in areas of the lungs having certain pressure-flow characteristics is also a potential source of overestimation of left atrial pressure from PCWP.[16] Specifically, these areas are the zones 1 and 2 of a model described by West et al.[17] when they divided lung vasculature into three functional categories. In zone 1, alveolar pressure is higher than both pulmonary arterial and venous pressures. As a consequence, there is no blood flow to these alveoli. In zone 2, pulmonary arterial pressure is greater than alveolar pressure, and pulmonary venous pressure is less than alveolar pressure. Therefore, flow is determined by the difference between pulmonary arterial and alveolar pressures. In zone 3, alveolar pressure is less than either pulmonary arterial or venous pressures, so that alveolar pressure does not affect flow.

We believe that placement of the catheter tip in areas having zone 1 or 2 characteristics is an unlikely source of error. First, placement of the catheter tip in a zone 1 region is unlikely because of the low blood flow. (However, changes in ventilation or position may convert other zones to zone 1 areas.) Regardless, although blood flow through alveoli may be absent in zone 1, flow to intraalveolar vessels should still exist,[18] thus providing the requisite continuity between the balloon and left atrium. If such continuity were lost, A, C, and V waves would not be observed on the PCWP trace, and PCWP should, by definition, be considerably higher than pulmonary artery diastolic pressure.

Second, placement of the catheter tip in a zone 2 region should not cause error because the pulmonary venous bed is open distal to the catheter tip unless inflation of the balloon causes all such venous channels to collapse (this is again unlikely because of the existence of extraalveolar vessels). As with a zone 1 region, A, C, and V waves would not be observed if such continuity were lost.

In our experience, the traces expected from these considerations do not occur. However, the possibility of their occurrence emphasizes the importance of examining the PCWP waveform for A, C, and V waves and of not displaying mean central pressures. We believe that the observed discrepancies between PCWP and left atrial pressure are more likely to result when relatively high flows or resistance in the vasculature between the balloon and left atrium cause a decrease in pressure. An additional source of error is the use of average values for PCWP and left atrial pressure. This practice occurs in many studies.

MEASUREMENT OF CARDIAC OUTPUT

Cardiac output is usually measured clinically by dilution of indicators. The principle involved is detection of changes in the concentration of an indicator, or in the temperature of blood, when the indicator is mixed with venous blood. Two indicators are commonly used. The first is indocyanine, a green dye, the concentration of which is measured at a site in the arterial circulation. The second indicator (a thermal indicator) is cold fluid, usually cold saline or dextrose in water. Changes in blood temperature are sensed in the pulmonary artery with a thermistor. Although other, noninvasive techniques based on Doppler flow or changes in impedance are becoming available, the validity of these methods is still controversial. Therefore, only the two dilution methods will be discussed.

Dilution methods for calculating cardiac output are based on the Stewart-Hamilton equation,[19] which is an expression of conservation of mass. That is, if no indicator is lost from the circulation, the amount recovered at the detection site must equal the amount injected. If blood flow is constant, the amount recovered is flow times the area under the concentration curve. Therefore, flow equals the amount injected divided by the area under the dilution curve.

The important assumptions in indicator dilution techniques are as follows.[20] (1) At some point distal to the injection site of the indicator and proximal to the measurement site, all blood passes through a single channel or at least intermixes. (2) Any alterations in flow, such as occur with each cardiac ejection, occur many times during the measurement period. This assumption may not be true because of respiration. (3) The indicator must remain in the vascular space, and large shifts of fluid to or from the vascular space cannot occur. If the third assumption were not true, the concentration of the indicator would change independent of blood flow. The two most commonly used indicator techniques are discussed below.

Dye Dilution Method

The dye dilution method consists of a bolus injection of a known quantity of dye into a central venous catheter. The change in concentration of the indicator resulting from mixing of the indicator in blood is detected by withdrawing blood from an arterial catheter and passing it through a densitometer. This device uses the optical density of the blood to determine the concentration of indicator. Such information is used to generate a curve showing the concentration of the dye over time. Because the blood is reinfused after the measurement, some of the indicator recirculates and mixes with the initial bolus, causing a bump in the last part of the curve. If this bump is not corrected for, the area under the curve would increase and produce an erroneously low cardiac output. To correct for recirculation of indicator, after the curve has de-

cayed to approximately 25 to 30 percent of the peak value, the rest of the curve is calculated by extrapolation, usually assuming a monoexponential decline. The validity of this assumption during respiration has not been established.[21] The shape of the dye curve also can yield valuable information on intracardiac shunting. For example, a right-to-left shunt might manifest as an early hump on the curve. Dye dilution is the standard against which most other techniques have been evaluated.

Thermodilution Technique

The thermodilution technique is similar to the dye dilution technique except that cold fluid is used as the indicator. A known volume of indicator, usually 5 percent dextrose in water at a known temperature below blood temperature (most often, 0°C or room temperature), is injected into the right atrium. The resulting change in temperature of pulmonary artery blood is measured by a calibrated thermistor on a pulmonary artery flotation catheter. These data are used to produce a thermodilution curve. The curve is similar to the dye dilution curve, except that no recirculation of indicator normally occurs. Cardiac output is proportional to the difference between the baseline and injectate temperatures divided by the area under the temperature change curve. The constant of proportionality depends on the volume, specific gravity, and specific heat of the injectate; the specific gravity and specific heat of the blood; and heat loss within the catheter.[22] These factors are accounted for in the calibration number set on the output computer.

As with the dye dilution method, the area under the temperature difference curve usually is calculated by terminating the measurement when the washout curve has decayed to approximately 25 to

30 percent of the peak value. Then, assuming exponential decay, the area of the remaining portion of the curve is extrapolated. However, this assumption has not been validated in vivo and is less likely to be correct than with the dye dilution method. A second assumption that is a source of error with thermodilution is that baseline blood temperature is constant during the measurement period. However, the temperature of central blood may vary with respiration, and such changes can produce errors in excess of 10 percent. In addition, because the changes in stroke volume with respiration occur rapidly with respect to the measurement period, thermodilution outputs may vary by 40 percent when injection is performed at different times during the respiratory cycle.[23] To solve this problem, one would inject the indicator at the end of expiration,[24] unless the average output is desired. In this case, multiple random injections should be used.

As is the case for pressure measurements, changes in stroke volume are more useful than the absolute number. Therefore, when measuring cardiac output, precision is once again more important than accuracy.

CONCLUSIONS

Because the equipment used to monitor the ECG and pressures for patients undergoing vascular surgery has many limitations, it is important to understand the principles governing such equipment. However, we believe that many of the potential ambiguities can be resolved by asking the proper questions rather than by making multiple measurements on a schedule and calculating hemodynamic profiles. In our view, such questions should be based on an understanding of the physiology and pathophysiology of the cardiovascular system.

REFERENCES

1. Stein RA, Seymour B-Z, LaBelle P: The modern monitor-defibrillator. A potential source of falsely abnormal ECG recordings. JAMA 246:1697–1698, 1981
2. Tayler D, Vincent R: Signal distortion in the electrocardiogram due to inadequate phase response. IEEE Trans Biomed Eng 30:352–356, 1983
3. Garnder RM: Direct blood pressure measurement—dynamic response requirements. Anesthesiology 54:227–236, 1981
4. Ellis DM: Interpretation of beat-to-beat blood pressure values in the presence of ventilatory changes. J Clin Monit 1:65–70, 1985
5. Fish DJ, Teplick R: Clinical value of variable weight filter algorithm equipped monitors for invasive pressure measurement (abstract). Anesthesiology 65:A156, 1986
6. Ladin Z, Trautman E, Teplick R: Contribution of measurement system artifacts to systolic spikes. Med Instrum 17:110–112, 1983
7. Bruner JMR, Krenis LJ, Kunsman JM, Sherman AP: Comparison of direct and indirect methods of measuring arterial blood pressure. Med Instrum 15:11–21, 1981
8. O'Rourke MF: Arterial Function in Health and Disease. Churchill Livingstone, New York, 1982
9. O'Rourke MF, Blazek JV, Morreels CL, Jr., Krovetz LJ: Pressure wave transmission along the human aorta. Changes with age and in arterial degenerative disease. Circ Res 23:567–579, 1968
10. Zelis R: Mechanisms of vasodilation. Am J Med 74(6B):3–12, 1983
11. Suga H, Hayashi T, Shirahata M: Ventricular systolic pressure-volume area as predictor of cardiac oxygen consumption. Am J Physiol 240:H39–H44, 1981
12. Olsson RA, Bungi WJ: Coronary circula-

tion. p. 987–1037. In Fozzard HA, Haber E, Jennings RB et al (eds): The Heart and Cardiovascular System: Scientific Foundations. Raven Press, New York, 1986

13. Perel A, Pizov R, Cotev S: Systolic blood pressure variation is a sensitive indicator of hypovolemia in ventilated dogs subjected to graded hemorrhage. Anesthesiology 67:498–502, 1987

14. Teplick RS: Measuring central vascular pressures: a surprisingly complex problem (editorial). Anesthesiology 67:289–291, 1987

15. Haskell RJ, French WJ: Accuracy of left atrial and pulmonary artery wedge pressure in pure mitral regurgitation in predicting left ventricular end-diastolic pressure. Am J Cardiol 61:136–141, 1988

16. Nadeau S, Noble WH: Misinterpretation of pressure measurements from the pulmonary artery catheter. Can Anaesth Soc J 33:352–363, 1986

17. West JB, Dollery CT, Naimark A: Distribution of blood flow in isolated lung; relation to vascular and alveolar pressures. J Appl Physiol 19:713–724, 1964

18. Permutt S, Howell JBL, Proctor DF, Riley RL: Effect of lung inflation on static pressure-volume characteristics of pulmonary vessels. J Appl Physiol 16:64–70, 1961

19. Hamilton WF: Measurement of the cardiac output. p. 551–584. In Handbook of Physiology. Section 2: Circulation. Vol. 1. American Physiological Society. Washington, DC, 1962

20. Zierler KL: Circulation times and the theory of indicator-dilution methods for determining blood flow and volume. p. 585–615. In Handbook of Physiology. Section 2: Circulation. Vol. 1. American Physiological Society, Washington, DC, 1962

21. Howard AR, Hamilton WF, Dow P: Limitations of the continuous infusion method for measuring cardiac output by dye dilution. Am J Physiol 175:173–177, 1953

22. Yang SS, Bentivogolio LG, Maranhão V, Goldberg H: From Cardiac Catheterization Data to Hemodynamic Parameters. 2nd Ed. p. 77–88. FA Davis, Philadelphia, 1978

23. Jansen JRC, Schreuder JJ et al: Thermodilution technique for measurement of cardiac output during artificial ventilation. J Appl Physiol 51:584–591, 1981

24. Stevens JH, Raffin TA, Mihm FG et al: Thermodilution cardiac output measurement. Effects of the respiratory cycle on its reproducibility. JAMA 253:2240–2242, 1985

Section II

ANESTHESIA AND SURGERY FOR CEREBROVASCULAR INSUFFICIENCY

4

Surgery for Cerebrovascular Disease: Surgical Goals and Methods

Robert J. Lusby

Carotid artery surgery has developed rapidly since the first successful procedures for symptomatic extracranial cerebrovascular disease in the early 1950s.[1,2] The enthusiasm associated with the rapid advancement of vascular surgery as a specialty has seen carotid endarterectomy become the third most common operation in the United States: approximately 100,000 procedures are performed annually, 40 percent of which involve asymptomatic disease.[3,4] However, recent criticism of the criteria for surgery has prompted several large prospective studies to examine closely the arguments for and against carotid endarterectomy.

The rationale for surgery has been based on information from a limited number of prospective and retrospective studies. Unfortunately, the retrospective reviews have not clearly documented the natural history of carotid disease and have lacked proper control groups. Although the role of surgery in preventing stroke in *symptomatic* carotid disease is generally accepted, the effectiveness of prophylactic carotid endarterectomy in *asymptomatic* patients is controversial.[5,6] The presence of a cervical bruit or an asymp-

tomatic lesion of greater than 50 percent stenosis also carries a high risk of myocardial infarction, the leading cause of morbidity in this patient population. Therefore, these conditions may be more worthy of investigation and treatment than carotid lesions.[5,6] Because progression of an asymptomatic lesion to greater than 80 percent stenosis carries a higher risk of significant cerebral events (stroke, transient ischemic attack, or asymptomatic occlusion), surgical correction of this type of lesion appears justified.[7,8]

Other important pathologic conditions of the extracranial vessels include vertebrobasilar disease, aneurysmal disease of both carotid and vertebrobasilar systems, acute arterial dissection, fibromuscular dysplasia, and postoperative recurrent stenoses.

CAUSES AND NATURE OF CAROTID DISEASE

Occlusive carotid disease is usually caused by atherosclerosis at the bifurcation of the common carotid artery and in-

85

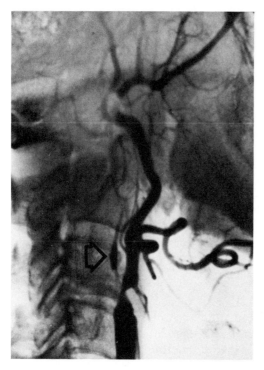

Fig. 4-1. Angiogram showing the carotid bifurcation with moderate stenosis of external carotid origin and severe stenosis of the internal carotid origin with "string" sign (arrow).

volves the origins of both the internal and external carotid arteries[9-13] (Fig. 4-1). Atherosclerotic lesions occur more frequently in the extracranial arterial system than in the intracranial system. Although the origin of the vertebral artery is the site next most likely to be affected, minor diffuse involvement tends to occur throughout the entire vessel. Cerebrovascular disease is also often accompanied by atherosclerosis of the coronary arteries. In all areas, atherosclerosis is more marked in hypertensive patients and increases in severity and frequency with age.[13-16]

Atheromatous plaque tends to form at the carotid bifurcation, possibly because of the impedance mismatch or altered hemodynamic conditions associated with the division of the vessel into a large in-

ternal and relatively small external carotid artery.[17] The flow pattern differs in each vessel, flow being continuous and forward in the internal carotid artery and forward and reverse in the external carotid artery. The plaque that forms may produce symptoms either by reducing flow to the brain or by undergoing degenerative changes that lead to atheroemboli or thromboemboli. Intraplaque hemorrhage (Fig. 4-2), luminal thrombus formation, and ulcerative breakdown at this site have all been associated with the onset of ischemic cerebral symptoms.[9-12] The size and composition of the embolus, the adequacy of collateral blood flow, the presence or absence of a complete circle of Willis, and the ability of the embolus to disaggregate are all factors that affect the severity of the ischemic cerebral event. Carotid endarterectomy removes the friable, degenerative stenotic lesions found at the carotid bifurcation, and the vessel heals with scar formation. Because the resulting fibrous scar tissue is stable and no longer a source of emboli, the risk of stroke from this lesion is removed.

Atheroembolism also causes cerebral dysfunction in other diseases of the extracranial arterial system, including aneurysmal disease and fibromuscular dysplasia. Acute arterial dissection, an uncommon occurrence, may cause embolic problems but is more likely to lead to acute occlusion of the vessel and circulatory insufficiency owing to poorly developed collateral anastomoses. Although these diseases occur only infrequently, the variety of surgical approaches required makes knowledge of these processes and their management important.[18-20]

Occasionally, early acute thrombotic occlusion and symptoms occur after successful carotid endarterectomy. In this situation, immediate reoperation and thrombectomy provide the best results.[21-24] Symptomatic restenosis occurs

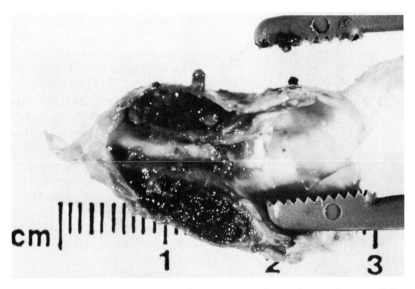

Fig. 4-2. Carotid endarterectomy specimen showing intraplaque hemorrhage and degenerative atheroma.

in as many as 1.5 percent of patients. The cause of this lesion is usually neointimal hyperplasia if the lesion occurs within 12 months of endarterectomy, or recurrent atherosclerosis if it occurs later. Occasionally, both conditions occur together. Reoperation with repeated endarterectomy and patch angioplasty usually prevent further cerebral attacks.[25,26]

INDICATIONS FOR CAROTID SURGERY

Symptomatic Stenosis

Surgical intervention for patients with hemispheric symptoms and carotid atheromatous plaques is considered the best way of preventing further ipsilateral ischemic symptoms, particularly stroke. The 1970 report of the Joint Study of Extracranial Arterial Occlusion documented a significantly lower incidence of transient ischemic attacks and stroke after car-

otid endarterectomy for symptomatic lesions, noting that most of the long-term mortality for these patients was attributable to cardiac disease.[27] Early in this study, surgical mortality and perioperative stroke were relatively high. In the last 5 years of the study, however, improvements in technique, patient selection, and perioperative management reduced perioperative mortality to 1.5 percent.

Approximately 25 to 60 percent of patients having transient ischemic attacks will progress to a completed stroke.[28] The risk of stroke is highest in the months after the initial symptoms: up to 21 percent of strokes occur within 1 month of onset of symptoms, and 51 percent occur within the first year.[29,30] However, fewer than 10 percent of patients with cerebral infarction have preceding transient ischemic attacks.[30] These facts emphasize the dilemma of treating asymptomatic stenosis and of deciding the usefulness of prophylactic surgery. Among those presenting with stroke, recurrent stroke occurs at

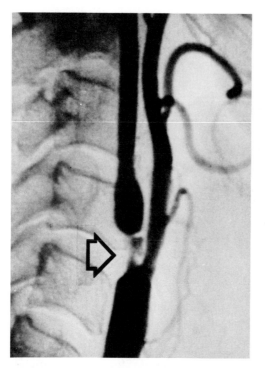

Fig. 4-3. Angiogram showing localized stenosis of the internal carotid artery, with ulceration (arrow), associated with ipsilateral cerebral ischemic symptoms.

the rate of 10 percent in the first year and then approximately 4 percent per year.[31] Thus, with transient ischemic attacks or stroke, untreated carotid lesions incur an annual incidence of stroke of approximately 5 percent, with the maximum risk in the first year approaching 15 percent[32] (Fig. 4-3).

Surgery at any particular institution can be justified for symptomatic disease if the overall rate for surgical morbidity and mortality for that hospital or particular surgeon is less than 5 percent. Most recent assessments from major institutions satisfy this criterion. However, because expertise comes from continuing practice, carotid endarterectomy is not a procedure for the surgeon who performs vascular surgery only occasionally.

Antiplatelet Agents

The benefit of administering antiplatelet agents for symptomatic cerebrovascular disease is another area of uncertainty. The Canadian Cooperative Study Group reported that the incidence of stroke or death was lower for male patients given regular aspirin (325 mg daily) after transient cerebral events than in a similar group given only placebo.[33] However, another study showed that aspirin decreased the incidence of transient cerebral events but not stroke.[34] Therefore, by masking the progression of atheromatous disease, aspirin may be deleterious: fewer patients would be offered surgery before the onset of stroke.

Antiplatelet agents are commonly used postoperatively to protect against platelet aggregation, thrombus formation, and neointimal hyperplasia at the site of endarterectomy.[35]

Timing of Surgery

An important lesson learned in the early years of carotid surgery was that mortality and morbidity decreased if surgical intervention was timed appropriately. Specifically, surgical mortality was unacceptably high (approximately 42 percent) if surgery was performed within 2 weeks of the onset of an acute stroke having moderate or severe deficit. If surgery was delayed at least 2 weeks, surgical mortality decreased to approximately 17 percent.[36] Surgical mortality for patients presenting with transient ischemic attack was 1.3 percent.[36]

As a result, patients with clinical evidence of stroke who had residual deficit lasting more than 24 hours usually were not considered for surgery for at least 30 days.[37] This clinical guideline has become less certain because of the advent of computed tomographic scanning. Cerebral infarction occurs in as many as 46 percent of patients who have clinically evident transient ischemic attacks.[38–41] Patients with large infarcts on computed tomographic scanning have a higher incidence of perioperative deficit.[42] Therefore, computed tomographic evidence of large infarction should be considered an indication for surgical delay, despite a benign presentation.

Neurologically Unstable Patients

Although it is well accepted that acute stroke patients should not have early surgery, the place of surgery is less well defined for patients who have crescendo transient ischemic attacks, fluctuating deficits ("stuttering stroke"), and acute deficit soon after an initially successful carotid endarterectomy. Aggressive surgical approach to the stroke occurring after endarterectomy has shown a high association with thrombotic occlusion of the internal carotid artery at the site of surgery, with good success rates following early reoperation. Best results occur with reoperation within 2 hours, with most investigators recommending no angiographic evaluation because of the delay involved.[21–24] Similar results could be expected for hospitalized patients who have had full preoperative evaluation but have a stroke while awaiting surgery, and in patients who have a stroke after diagnostic angiography demonstrating acute occlusion. Again, speed of action is paramount.

Experience in other neurologically unstable patients with demonstrated carotid bifurcation disease has been limited but encouraging.[43,44] However, a major deficit or altered state of consciousness is still a definite contraindication to surgery, and controlled prospective studies documenting the advantage of surgical intervention do not yet exist.

Occlusion of the Internal Carotid Artery

The usefulness of surgery for occlusion of the internal carotid artery remains controversial. Although many patients tolerate occlusion of this artery without major deficit, the incidence of new ipsilateral cerebral symptoms following occlusion is significant.[45] Benefit has been documented for surgical procedures on both ipsilateral and contralateral carotid bifurcations. Stenotic lesions of the carotid bifurcation involving the origin of the external carotid on the side of the occlusion may contribute to ipsilateral symptoms because of reduction in flow or the passage of atheroemboli through the external carotid-ophthalmic artery anastomoses. Endarterectomy of the external carotid lesion, with exclusion of the confirmed occlusion of the internal carotid artery, reduces the incidence of new symptoms.[46] Embolization of material across the circle of Willis is theoretically possible and probably likely with major occlusive disease of the contralateral carotid bifurcation. This possibility is confirmed if endarterectomy of the contralateral carotid bifurcation significantly reduces symptoms ipsilateral to the occluded internal carotid artery[47] (Fig. 4-4).

Extracranial-to-Intracranial Bypass

Extracranial-to-intracranial (EC-IC) bypass does not decrease the risk of subsequent cerebral events in the presence of internal carotid artery occlusion.[48] This procedure endeavors to correct the problem of low cerebral blood flow but does not prevent atheroembolism from the extracranial carotid artery. The failure of EC-IC bypass to benefit these patients lends support to the atheroembolic theory of cerebral ischemic syndromes.

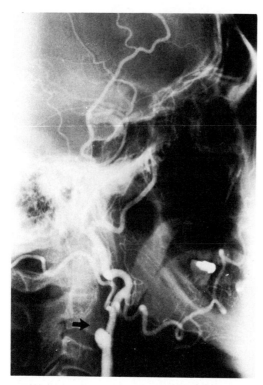

Fig. 4-4. Angiogram showing occluded internal carotid artery.

Asymptomatic Stenosis or Bruit

The ability of surgery to prevent stroke when asymptomatic stenosis of the internal carotid artery exists is a controversial issue. The argument against surgery contends that the risk of unheralded stroke ipsilateral to a noncritical carotid stenosis or bruit is relatively low (1 to 2 percent annually). This risk is less than the risk of stroke during surgery for such lesions.[7,8,49,50]

The argument in favor of surgery asserts that the risk of perioperative stroke for asymptomatic lesions is very low.[51,52] Also, at least one-third of strokes are not preceded by warning symptoms such as transient ischemic attacks.[7,8,53] The dilemma in managing asymptomatic carotid disease is that physicians still do not

know which patients and which lesions warrant therapy, which tests should be given to detect such lesions, and which therapies should be attempted.[54] Current efforts are directed at identifying the asymptomatic patient at high risk of stroke who may benefit from surgery before the onset of symptoms.

Central to the management dilemma is poor understanding of the natural history of atherosclerosis of the carotid bifurcation.[53–55] Although early studies used the presence of a cervical bruit as an indicator of disease of the carotid bifurcation, later work showed poor correlation between cervical bruit and ipsilateral stenosis of the internal carotid artery. These earlier studies were likely to underestimate the risk of carotid lesions.[55] More accurate assessment of stenosis of the carotid bifurcation is now available by the noninvasive techniques of ocular plethysmography and duplex scanning. Also, intravenous digital subtraction angiography produces good arterial imaging with minimal risk and discomfort. Using these techniques, recent studies have shown that atherosclerosis of the internal carotid artery progresses at a relatively low rate, approaching 26 percent at 12 months; the progression to stenosis greater than 50 percent occurs at a rate of approximately 8 percent a year. In 2 percent of cases, the disease had regressed at 12 months.[53] In follow-up outcome studies of patients with asymptomatic cervical bruits, more cardiac ischemic events (10 percent) occurred than cerebral ischemic events (7 percent).[7]

Patients likely to be at high risk of stroke are those with asymptomatic tight stenosis of the internal carotid artery.[7,8, 50,55] Progression of a lesion to more than 80 percent stenosis (Fig. 4-5) carries a 35 percent risk of cerebral ischemia or internal carotid occlusion within 6 months and a 46 percent risk at 12 months.[53] Controversy still exists, however, regarding

ploying noninvasive duplex imaging to document disease at the carotid bifurcation found no increased risk of stroke during surgery at a remote site.[50] On the other hand, these patients do have a higher incidence of cerebral ischemic events on follow-up than patients without carotid disease. Close follow-up and patient awareness of transient ischemic symptoms may enable appropriate surgical intervention before the occurrence of stroke.[50] This risk, however, is that the first attack may be a completed stroke.

Our current knowledge provides little justification for prophylactic carotid surgery in any patient having asymptomatic stenosis of less than 80 percent.[49] This group should undergo duplex scanning and ocular plethysmography at regular 6- or 12-month intervals. If stenosis progresses to more than 80 percent or if ipsilateral cerebral symptoms develop, surgical removal of the carotid lesion should be considered. Surgery would be justified if the expected patient survival was at least 5 years, and if the combined surgical mortality and serious morbidity was less than 3 percent. Attention must be paid to the modification of risk factors and a careful cardiac evaluation sought.

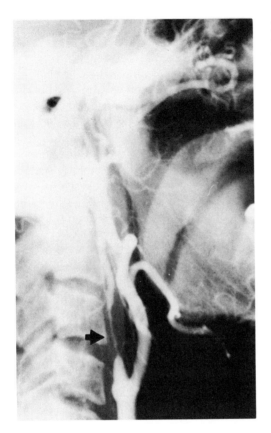

Fig. 4-5. Angiogram showing greater than 80 percent stenosis of the proximal internal carotid artery (arrow).

the usefulness of prophylactic surgery for such patients.[8] Because the benefits of surgery are not apparent for approximately 5 years, the life expectancy of the individual must be assessed prior to surgical intervention. In addition, the surgeon should be able to perform the procedure with minimal risk to the patient. The combined perioperative mortality and morbidity should be no more than 3 percent in order to obtain an advantage from surgery in this asymptomatic group.[55]

The place of prophylactic carotid surgery in patients with asymptomatic stenosis having major surgery in other areas is also controversial. Recent studies em-

SURGICAL PROCEDURE

Surgeons operating on the extracranial vessels endeavor to remove stenotic and degenerative atheromatous lesions from the mainstream blood supply to the brain and thus reduce the incidence of stroke, monocular blindness, and transient ischemic attacks.

Carotid Endarterectomy

Endarterectomy of the carotid bifurcation has become the preferred surgical technique for stenotic disease of the carotid artery, owing mostly to the limited nature of the atherosclerotic process in this position and the relatively large size of the vessels. The details of the surgery are fairly standardized.[52,56]

Surgeons usually perform this operation using general anesthesia, endotracheal intubation, and controlled ventilation.[52] However, some surgeons prefer local anesthesia, either regional nerve block of the cervical plexus or infiltration of the operative area.[57,58] Although this approach may be stressful for the patient, surgeon, and anesthetist, the patient becomes the monitor of cerebral perfusion. If the need for increased cerebral perfusion arises at any time during surgery, a shunt may be inserted.

Use of Intraluminal Shunts

The need for intraluminal shunts in carotid surgery is a controversial issue. Some surgeons use shunts routinely, some never use them, and others use them selectively.[59–62] Advocates maintain that the technique is relatively easy and that the shunt is not intrusive to the operation itself. Maintenance of normal or near normal blood flow patterns by this method is thought to protect against ischemic events. Those who do not use shunts point out that placement of the shunt may dislodge particulate atheroma and cause embolic events. Technical problems with air embolization, kinking of the shunt, and shunt occlusion against the side wall of the vessel are to be avoided.

Selective use of shunts may reduce some of the problems while providing cerebral protection for patients at high risk. The measurement of internal carotid stump pressure is a guide to the adequacy of collateral vessels and their ability to maintain cerebral circulation.[63] In general, surgeons who use this monitoring technique will shunt carotid blood if back pressure is less than 50 mmHg; some surgeons use a figure of 25 mmHg.[64] In ad-

dition, neurologically unstable patients, or those who have had a prior stroke, may also benefit from selective shunting.

Of major importance is the fact that perioperative neurologic events are not totally eliminated by use of a shunt. Recent work with electroencephalographic monitoring has indicated that a combination of embolic problems and reduced blood flow probably causes such perioperative events.[63,65] Hypotensive events during induction of anesthesia are thought to be the cause of operative stroke in some cases.

Emboli dislodged at the time of surgery are likely to cause a large percentage of operative deficits that shunting would not prevent. Particular care in manipulating the neck during induction of anesthesia and extreme caution in dissecting out the carotid artery will lessen the risk of such emboli. Once emboli have been dislodged, of course, insertion of a shunt does not prevent a deficit. Also, whether insertion of a shunt helps reduce a deficit has not been proven.

Operative Technique

During general anesthesia, the patient is gently positioned to avoid overextension or extreme lateral rotation of the neck. These maneuvers can occlude the vertebral artery and contribute to perioperative deficits.[66] The patient is placed in the supine position with a soft liter pack or sandbag between the shoulders. The incision used to approach the carotid bifurcation is usually a curved skin crease incision 2 to 3 cm below the angle of the mandible, or along the anterior border of the sternocleidomastoid muscle.[56]

After division of the platysma muscle, the artery is approached by first mobilizing the internal jugular vein. The carotid bifurcation lies under the junction of the common facial vein and the internal jugular vein. Several cranial nerves are identified during dissection. The ansa cervicalis lying anterior to the artery may be divided to expose the vessel fully. The vagus nerve usually lies lateral to the artery and deep to the bulb but may meander anteriorly to lie over the more proximal common carotid artery. In this position, the vagus nerve is vulnerable to injury.

Changes in voice, usually temporary, are quite common after carotid endarterectomy and are presumed to be caused by neurapraxia secondary to handling of either the vagus nerve or the external branch of the superior laryngeal nerve. However, permanent deficits have occurred from damage to the superior laryngeal nerve and recurrent laryngeal nerve.[67] At the upper limits of the dissection of the internal carotid artery lies the hypoglossal nerve, which is held close to the internal carotid artery by the occipital branch of the external carotid artery. Division of this small vessel and its accompanying vein greatly facilitates full mobilization of the internal carotid artery.[67] Other neural damage can occur—specifically, to the greater auricular nerve, the mandibular branch of the facial nerve, the glossopharyngeal nerve, and the accessory cranial nerves.[67]

Once adequate exposure is obtained, systemic heparinization is used to reduce the risk of thrombotic occlusion during clamping of the artery. The usual dose of heparin given intravenously is 5,000 to 7,500 units. Distal clamps and then proximal clamps are applied to reduce the risk of emboli. Should final mobilization of the bifurcation area be needed, it is done once clamps are on. Arteriotomy is then performed from the common carotid artery and is extended into the internal carotid artery beyond the obvious limits of the disease. At this point, a shunt is inserted, if indicated. I believe that careful maintenance of blood pressure is important is ensuring cerebral perfusion during endarterectomy.[59]

Performance of the endarterectomy is the most critical step in the operation. Endarterectomy can be done properly and without hurry in approximately 20 minutes.[68] The plane of cleavage is important, with special attention being directed to feathering the distal intima to a clean and complete endpoint. It is most unusual to have the plaque of atheroma extend more than 5 cm distal to the bifurcation, and inadequate removal of the atheroma can lead to early recurrence of stenosis.[69] In an exceptional case, it may be necessary to secure the distal edge of the intima by suture. Although prolonged clamping of the carotid appears to increase operative morbidity, inadequate endarterectomy almost certainly leads to postoperative deficit. Therefore, every effort must be made to remove the atheroma completely.

Closure of the arteriotomy is usually performed with direct approximation by running suture. A small internal carotid artery may require patch angioplasty with either autogenous vein or synthetic material.[59] When suturing is almost complete, the internal and common carotids are flushed by brief release of clamps to remove any thrombus or particulate matter, and the lumen is washed with heparinized saline. The suture line is then completed and flow is reestablished, first into the external carotid artery and then into the internal carotid artery. The distal internal carotid artery is then inspected for a pulse and gently palpated to detect any thrill. Some centers assess the final result by ultrasonography, duplex imaging, or contrast radiography. Evidence of loose fragments, intimal flaps, or stenosis requires immediate reexploration.

Postoperative management is vitally important to the successful outcome of carotid endarterectomy. Until an intimal layer reforms, the large area of media now in contact with the blood is quite thrombogenic. To avoid thrombus formation and platelet aggregation in the early post-operative period, we usually do not reverse intraoperative heparin but, instead, administer antiplatelet agents. Aspirin, dipyridamole, and Rheomacrodex (low-molecular-weight dextran) in various combinations are commonly used immediately after surgery. The unwanted side effect of antiplatelet therapy is oozing of the wound, hematoma being the most common wound complication.[59] The need for careful hemostasis is obvious.

The other important variable to be controlled postoperatively is blood pressure. Hypotension must be avoided, as this condition aggravates the thrombotic tendency at the site of endarterectomy. Hypertension may also cause or aggravate neurologic deficit.[70] Deficit is particularly evident as the patient is waking and may require aggressive intervention with short-acting antihypertensive agents. Postoperatively, patients are usually cared for in an intensive care unit, or in an intensive care-like postanesthesia care unit (recovery room), using the arterial line to monitor blood pressure accurately.

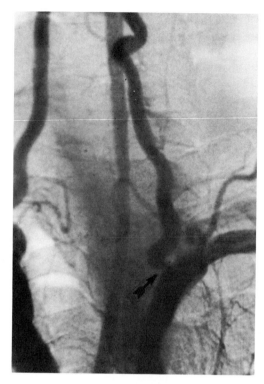

Fig. 4-6. Angiogram showing stenosis of the origin of the vertebral artery (arrow).

Surgical Procedures for Vertebrobasilar Insufficiency

Disease of the vertebrobasilar system is less well understood than disease of the carotid arteries. Symptoms, which are bilateral or nonlocalizing and imprecise, include vertigo, ataxia, blurred vision, dizziness, syncope, "drop attacks," bilateral paresthesia or paresis, dysarthria, headache, and confusion. Symptoms sometimes relate to exercise, posture, or position.[71]

Again, atherosclerosis-induced stenosis is the most common pathologic process affecting the vertebrobasilar arteries. Disease most commonly affects the origins of the verebral arteries, usually in association with disease of the subclavian vessels from which they arise (Fig. 4-6). Plaque rarely extends more than 2 to 3 mm beyond their origins and infrequently shows evidence of subintimal hemorrhage similar to that occurring at the carotid bifurcation.

Redundancy of these vessels can cause kinking that reduces blood flow on assumption of certain head positions.[72] Because the usual cause of vertebrobasilar symptoms is flow reduction and not atheroembolism, unilateral vertebral stenosis is not an indication for surgery if angiography demonstrates normal confluence to a basilar artery. It is important to remember that the posterior communicating vessels in the circle of Willis may be deficient in 25 percent of people.[73] However, as many as 52 percent of patients with vertebrobasilar symptoms have normal vertebrobasilar and subclavian vessels with significant stenotic disease at the carotid bifurcations.[74] For these reasons, the relative importance of various lesions in both carotid and vertebral systems, as well as in the circle of Willis, is difficult to determine when nonspecific symptoms of the posterior fossa occur. Although numerous reports have documented improvement in vertebrobasilar symptoms after endarterectomy of the carotid bifurcation alone, surgeons do not universally agree that this is the most appropriate way to treat the disease.[75-78]

Surgery performed directly on the vertebral arteries is rare, constituting only 5.6 percent of all procedures for extracranial cerebral vessels. This procedure is reserved for patients with bilateral vertebral lesions and ischemic symptoms.[79]

Surgical techniques for improving blood flow in the vertebral artery are numerous, reflecting the general lack of experience with this vessel. Major aortic branches from which the vertebral arteries arise may be diseased and thus require endarterectomy, bypass, or direct reimplantation procedures. These procedures often require thoracotomy for adequate control of proximal blood vessels. Extraanatomic bypasses or anastomoses may be performed in suitable circumstances; bypasses that are entirely extrathoracic have a lower reported morbidity. Such procedures include carotid-subclavian artery bypass, subclavian-subclavian bypass, and side-to-side subclavian-to-carotid anastomosis.[80]

Procedures specifically directed to the lesion at the origin of the vertebral artery include internal plication with vein patch angioplasty,[81] autogenous vein bypass,[82] simple patch angioplasty of the origin,[83] transposition of the vertebral origin to other sites,[84,85] and local endarterectomy of the origin through a subclavian arteriotomy.[86] All procedures seem to be successful in relieving symptoms and incur low morbidity. Surgical repair is possible at all levels, including intracranial anastomoses to posterior cerebral artery branches; however, higher levels of vertebral artery disease occur only infrequently.[87-89]

As with carotid artery disease, technical expertise in dealing with lesions at various sites on the vertebral arteries has developed quickly. Unfortunately, our basic knowledge of the natural history of vertebrobasilar arterial disease is poor, and justification of surgical risk for unquantified benefit is not available.[90,91] Specific studies of these syndromes seem to be many years behind those being developed for carotid artery disease. Until we acquire a more precise understanding of vertebrobasilar symptoms and their relationship to varous anatomic lesions, we will remain unable to adequately justify many surgical endeavors into the vertebrobasilar arterial system.

Surgery for Other Lesions

Although extracranial carotid aneurysms are rare, embolism or thrombosis may cause cerebrovascular symptoms. These aneurysms very rarely rupture and hemorrhage but can be sites for generation of thromboemboli.[18] The lesion is usually caused by atherosclerosis or trauma or follows surgery (false aneurysm) (Fig. 4-7). Although most of these lesions occur at the carotid bifurcation, the distal internal carotid artery may also be affected. Aneurysms at other sites are common. Treatment depends on the location and extent of the aneurysm and the presence of infection. Locally accessible lesions are best managed by excision and replacement with autogenous or synthetic material. A saccular defect not involving the entire vessel may be treated by aneurysmorrhaphy and patch repair.

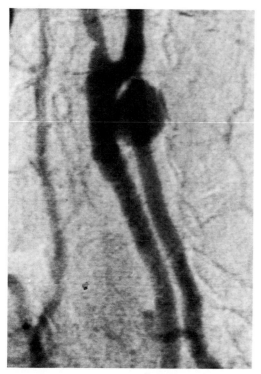

Fig. 4-7. Digital subtraction angiogram showing false aneurysm after carotid endarterectomy.

Inaccessible high cervical aneurysms are often related to trauma. If they remain asymptomatic, a nonsurgical approach may be most appropriate. Symptomatic lesions in this position need exclusion from the circulation. Although proximal ligation has a high rate of neurologic deficit, measuring collateral blood pressure with ocular pneumoplethysmography and compression of the common carotid artery in the root of the neck may predict this complication.[92] Alternatively, EC-IC bypass may be required prior to ligation to ensure adequate cerebral perfusion.[18]

Fibromuscular dysplasia has been reported to affect many vessels, including the extracranial carotid and vertebral arteries.[19] This disease of unknown origin usually occurs in women approximately 50 to 55 years of age. Although more car-

otid than vertebral lesions have been reported, both are rare. The carotid lesion normally involves only the extracranial internal carotid artery; lesions on the vertebral artery are seen at any level in its extracranial course. Symptoms can be caused by embolism, dissection, or occlusion of the vessel. Currently, the preferred treatment for symptomatic lesions is sequential dilation of the involved segment to a maximum of 3.5 to 4 mm by using a series of rigid dilators. Surgical exposure of the involved segment during dilation ensures visualization of the dilators when the stenotic lesions are traversed. Several studies report favorable results, a perioperative stroke rate of 3 percent, and no mortality.[19,93] Long-term follow-up shows long-lasting results from this technique and a low incidence of new cerebral symptoms.[93]

Spontaneous dissection of the internal carotid and vertebral arteries is also rare. Spontaneous dissection of the carotid artery is not associated with atherosclerosis, and most patients present with neurologic deficit.[20] Acute dissection is usually treated conservatively with heparin infusion to reduce thrombotic complications. Surgical options, though rarely indicated, include resection of the affected vessels with graft interposition, thrombectomy and removal of the involved intima, and ligation of the affected vessel with or without EC-IC bypass. Dissection also sometimes occurs with traumatic hyperextension of the neck, again commonly presenting with neurologic deficit. These lesions usually extend to the base of the skull, making control of blood flow during surgical procedures very difficult.

CONCLUSIONS

Most surgeons would agree that the goal of surgery for cerebrovascular disease is to prevent stroke, monocular blindness, and transient ischemic attacks. However, very few other statements about this field of surgery would obtain consensus. Nevertheless, several important concepts are widely accepted in the literature. Carotid endarterectomy decreases morbidity and increases survival under certain circumstances. Specifically, patients who have either angiographically demonstrated ipsilateral tight stenosis or transient ischemic attacks from ulcerative ipsilateral plaques appear to benefit from carotid encarterectomy. However, for this statement to be true, the combined perioperative mortality and morbidity associated with the operative team (surgeon, anesthetist, nurses, and others) must be less than 3 percent. Surgery on the patient who has similar lesions but is asymptomatic is controversial. Drugs that prevent platelet aggregation may also prevent the warning symptoms of stroke but not the stroke itself. Surgery on acute stroke not related to extracranial carotid thrombosis is probably not indicated. In contrast, surgery to remove an acute extracranial thrombosis, as after carotid endarterectomy, appears beneficial within the first 2 hours of thrombosis. The role of tissue plasminogen activator in these situations remains to be determined.

The surgical approach to the carotid artery is relatively simple and straightforward, requiring a smooth endpoint and careful dissection. Controversy exists over the benefit and risk associated with use of shunts, neurologic-monitoring modalities, choice of anesthesia, and radiographic imaging at the completion of surgery. Morbid outcomes have been attributed to hypotension, hypertension, and vessel manipulation with subsequent embolization.

Fibromuscular dysplasia is often treated with dilation under direct visualization. Inoperably placed aneurysms associated with embolization may be one of the indications for EC-IC bypass surgery prior to ligation of the aneurysm. Vertebrobasilar artery surgery and symptoms are additional areas for which consensus does not exist regarding indications for surgery and the most effective surgical approach. Use of consensus panels, chart review, and almost all indications supported by data in the literature reveal that almost one-third of the 100,000 carotid endarterectomies performed in the United States were inappropriate.[94] However, when appropriate indications are used, these operations can meet their goals of reducing the incidence of stroke, monocular blindness, and transient neurologic deficit. One should remember that atherosclerosis is a systemic disease and that the leading cause of death among individuals who either have asymptomatic carotid bruits or are undergoing carotid endarterectomy is myocardial dysfunction.

ACKNOWLEDGMENT

I thank G. Hayman for dedicated secretarial work.

REFERENCES

1. Eastcott HHG, Pickering GW, Rob CG: Reconstruction of internal carotid artery in a patient with intermittent attacks of hemiplegia. Lancet 2:994–996, 1954
2. DeBakey ME: Successful carotid endarterectomy for cerebro-vascular insufficiency. Nineteen-year follow-up. JAMA 233:1083–1085, 1975
3. Moore DJ, Miles RD, Gooley NA, Sumner DS: Noninvasive assessment of stroke risk in asymptomatic and nonhemispheric patients with suspected carotid disease. Five-year follow-up of 294 unoperated

and 81 operated patients. Ann Surg 202:491–504, 1985

4. Thompson JE: Don't throw out the baby with the bath water. A perspective on carotid endarterectomy. J Vasc Surg 4:543–545, 1986

5. Colgan MP, Kingston W, Shanik DG: Asymptomatic carotid stenosis: is prophylactic endarterectomy justifiable? Br J Surg 72:313–314, 1985

6. Barnes RW, Nix ML, Sansonetti D et al: Late outcome of untreated asymptomatic carotid disease following cardiovascular operations. J Vasc Surg 2:843–849, 1985

7. Chambers BR, Norris JW: Outcome in patients with asymptomatic neck bruits. N Engl J Med 315:860–865, 1986

8. Bogousslavsky J, Despland P-A, Regli F: Asymptomatic tight stenosis of the internal carotid artery: long-term prognosis. Neurology 36:861–863, 1986

9. Lusby RJ, Ferrell LD, Ehrenfeld WK et al: Carotid plaque hemorrhage. Its role in production of cerebral ischemia. Arch Surg 117:1479–1488, 1982

10. Edwards JH, Kricheff II, Gorstein F et al: Atherosclerotic subintimal hematoma of the carotid artery. Radiology 133:123–129, 1979

11. Imparato AM, Riles TS, Mintzer R, Baumann FG: The importance of hemorrhage in the relationship between gross morphologic characteristics and cerebral symptoms in 376 carotid artery plaques. Ann Surg 197:195–203, 1983

12. Imparato AM, Riles TS, Gorstein F: The carotid bifurcation plaque: pathologic findings associated with cerebral ischemia. Stroke 10:238–245, 1979

13. Fisher CM, Gore I, Okabe N et al: Atherosclerosis of the carotid and vertebral arteries—extracranial and intracranial. Neuropathol Exp Neurol 24:455–476, 1965

14. Battacharji SK, Hutchinson EC, McCall AJ: Stenosis and occlusion of vessels in cerebral infarction. Br Med J 3:270–274, 1967

15. Cole FM, Yates PO: Comparative incidence of cerebrovascular lesions in normotensive and hypertensive patients. Neurology 18:255–259, 1968

16. Kannel WB, Wolf PA, Verter J, McNamara PM: Epidemiologic assessment of the role of blood pressure in stroke. The Framingham Study. JAMA 214:301–310, 1970

17. Ross R: The pathogenesis of atherosclerosis—an update. N Engl J Med 314:488–500, 1986

18. Busuttil RW, Davidson RK, Foley KT, Livesay JT, Barker WF: Selective management of extracranial carotid artery aneurysms. Am J Surg 140:85–91, 1980

19. Stanley JC, Fry WJ, Seeger JF et al: Extracranial internal carotid and vertebral artery fibrodysplasia. Arch Surg 109:215–222, 1974

20. Ehrenfeld WK, Wylie EJ: Spontaneous dissection of the internal carotid artery. Arch Surg 111:1294–1301, 1976

21. Kwaan JHM, Connolly JE, Sharefkin JB: Successful management of early stroke after carotid endarterectomy. Ann Surg 190:676–678, 1979

22. Najafi H, Javid H, Dye WS et al: Emergency carotid thromboendarterectomy. Surgical indications and results. Arch Surg 103:610–614, 1971

23. Treiman RL, Cossman DV, Cohen JL et al: Management of postoperative stroke after carotid endarterectomy. Am J Surg 142:236–238, 1981

24. Takolander R, Bergentz S-E, Bergqvist D et al: Management of early neurologic deficits after carotid thromboendarterectomy. Eur J Vasc Surg 1:67–71, 1987

25. French BN, Rencastle NB: Recurrent stenosis at site of carotid endarterectomy. Stroke 8:597–605, 1977

26. Stoney RJ, String ST: recurrent carotid stenosis. Surgery 80:705–710, 1976

27. Fields WS, Maslenikov V, Meyer JS et al: Joint Study of Extracranial Arterial Occlusion. V. Progress report of prognosis following surgical or nonsurgical treatment for transient cerebral ischemic attacks and cervical carotid artery lesions. JAMA 211:1993–2003, 1970

28. Acheson J, Hutchinson EC: Observations on the natural history of transient cerebral ischemia. Lancet 2:871–874, 1964

29. Goldner JC, Whisnant JP, Taylor WF: Long-term prognosis of transient cerebral ischemic attacks. Stroke 2:160–167, 1971

30. Whisnant JP: Epidemiology of stroke: emphasis on transient cerebral ischemic attacks and hypertension. Stroke 5:68–70, 1974

31. Matsumoto N, Whisnant JP, Kurland LT, Okazaki H: Natural history of stroke in Rochester, Minnesota, 1955 through 1969: an extension of a previous study, 1945 through 1954. Stroke 4:20–29, 1973

32. West H, Burton R, Roon AJ et al: Comparative risk of operation and expectant management of carotid artery disease. Stroke 10:117–121, 1979

33. The Canadian Cooperative Study Group: A randomized trial of aspirin and sulfinpyrazone in threatened stroke. N Engl J Med 299:53–59, 1978

34. Fields WS, Lemak NA, Frankowski RF, Hardy RJ: Controlled trial of aspirin in cerebral ischemia. Stroke 8:301–315, 1977

35. Edwards WH, Edwards WH, Jr., Mulherin JL, Jr., Jenkins JM: The role of antiplatelet drugs in carotid reconstructive surgery. Ann Surg 201:765–770, 1985

36. Bauer RB, Meyer JS, Fields WS et al: Joint Study of Extracranial Arterial Occlusion. III. Progress report of controlled study of long-term survival in patients with and without operation. JAMA 208:509–518, 1969

37. Fields WS: Selection of stroke patients for arterial reconstructive surgery (editorial). Am J Surg 125:527–529, 1973

38. Berguer R, Sieggreen MY, Lazo A, Hodakowski GT: The silent brain infarct in carotid surgery. J Vasc Surg 3:442–447, 1986

39. Perrone P, Candelise L, Scotti G et al: CT evaluation in patients with transient ischemic attack. Correlation between clinical and angiographic findings. Eur Neurol 18:217–221, 1979

40. Waxman SG, Toole JF: Temporal profile resembling TIA in the setting of cerebral infarction. Stroke 14:433–437, 1983

41. Bogousslavsky J, Regli F: Cerebral infarction with transient signs (CITS): do TKAs correspond to small deep infarcts in internal carotid artery occlusion? Stroke 15:536–539, 1984

42. Graber JN, Vollman RW, Johnson WC et al: Stroke after carotid endarterectomy: risk as predicted by preoperative computerized tomography. Am J Surg 147:492–497, 1984

43. Bourke BM, McCollum CN, Greenhalgh RM: Carotid endarterectomy in patients with actively changing neurological deficits—correlations with CT brain scans. Aust NZ J Surg 55:335–340, 1985

44. Goldstone J, Moore WS: Emergency carotid artery surgery in neurologically unstable patients. Arch Surg 111:1284–1291, 1976

45. Burnett JR, Lusby RJ: Surgery for the occluded carotid artery. p. 41–50. In Greenhalgh R (ed): Indications in Vascular Surgery. W B Saunders, Philadelphia, PA, 1988

46. O'Hara PJ, Hertzer NR, Beven EG: External carotid revascularization: review of a ten-year experience. J Vasc Surg 2:709–714, 1985

47. Nordhus O, Ekeström S, Liljeqvist L: Unusual indications for carotid artery surgery. Acta Chir Scand 146:5–8, 1980

48. EC-IC Bypass Study Group: Failure of extracranial-intracranial arterial bypass to reduce the risk of ischemic stroke. N Engl J Med 313:1191–1200, 1985

49. Chambers BR, Norris JW: The case against surgery for asymptomatic carotid stenosis. Stroke 15:964–967, 1984

50. Barnes RW: Asymptomatic carotid stenosis: the argument against prophylactic carotid endarterectomy. p. 599–605. In Moore WS (ed): Surgery for Cerebrovascular Disease. Churchill Livingstone, New York, 1987

51. Thompson JE, Patman RD, Talkington CM: Asymptomatic carotid bruit: long term outcome of patients having endarterectomy compared with unoperated controls. Ann Surg 188:308–316, 1978

52. Thompson JE, Talkington CM: Carotid endarterectomy. Ann Surg 184:1–15, 1976

53. Roederer GO, Langlois YE, Jager KA et al: The natural history of carotid arterial disease in asymptomatic patients with cervical bruits. Stroke 15:605–613, 1984

54. Caplan LR: Carotid-artery disease (editorial). N Engl J Med 315:886–888, 1986

55. Quinones-Baldrich WJ, Moore WS:

Asymptomatic carotid stenosis: the argument in favour of carotid endarterectomy. p. 589–598. In Moore WS (ed): Surgery for Cerebrovascular Disease. Churchill Livingstone, New York, 1987

56. Wylie EJ, Stoney RJ, Ehrenfeld WK: Carotid atherosclerosis. p. 49–84. In Egdahl RH (ed): Manual of Vascular Surgery. Part 1. (Comprehensive Manuals of Surgical Specialties Series.) Springer-Verlag, New York, 1980

57. Riles TS, Imparato AM, Kopelman I: Carotid artery stenosis with contralateral internal carotid occlusion: long-term results in fifty-four patients. Surgery 87:363–368, 1980

58. Hobson RW, II, Wright CB, Sublett JW et al: Carotid artery back pressure and endarterectomy under regional anesthesia. Arch Surg 109:682–687, 1974

59. Thompson JE: Complications of carotid endarterectomy and their prevention. World J Surg 3:155–165, 1979

60. Whitney DG, Kahn EM, Estes JW, Jones CE: Carotid artery surgery without a temporary indwelling shunt. 1,917 consecutive procedures. Arch Surg 115:1393–1399, 1980

61. Hertzer NR, Beven EG, Greenstreet RL, Humphries AW: Internal carotid back pressure, intraoperative shunting, ulcerated atheromata, and the incidence of stroke during carotid endarterectomy. Surgery 83:306–312, 1978

62. Baker WH, Littooy FN, Hayes AC et al: Carotid endarterectomy without a shunt: the control series. J Vasc Surg 1:50–56, 1984

63. String ST, Callahan A: The critical manipulable variables of hemispheric low flow during carotid surgery. Surgery 93:46–49, 1983

64. Moore WS, Yee JM, Hall AD: Collateral cerebral blood pressure. An index of tolerance to temporary carotid occlusion. Arch Surg 106:520–523, 1973

65. Sundt TM, Jr., Sharbrough FW, Piepgras DG et al: Correlation of cerebral blood flow and electroencephalographic changes during carotid endarterectomy: with results of surgery and hemodynamics of cerebral ischaemia. Mayo Clin Proc 56:533–543, 1981

66. Sherman DG, Hart RG, Easton JD: Abrupt change in head position and cerebral infarction. Stroke 12:2–6, 1981

67. Lusby RJ, Wylie EJ: Complications of carotid endarterectomy. Surg Clin North Am 63:1293–1302, 1983

68. Littooy FN, Halstuk KS, Mamdani M et al: Factors influencing morbidity of carotid endarterectomy without a shunt. Am Surg 50:350–353, 1984

69. Javid H, Dye WS, Hunter JA et al: Surgical treatment of cerebral ischemia. Surg Clin North Am 54:239–255, 1974

70. Towne JB, Bernhard VM: The relationship of postoperative hypertension to complications following carotid endarterectomy. Surgery 88:575–580, 1980

71. Imparato AM, Riles TS: Surgery for vertebral and subclavian artery occlusions. p. 521–542. In Bergan JJ, Yao JS (eds): Cerebrovascular Insufficiency. Grune & Stratton, Orlando, FL, 1983

72. Hardin CA, Poser CM: Rotational obstruction of the vertebral artery due to redundancy and extraluminal cervical fascial bands. Ann Surg 158:133–137, 1963

73. Battacharji SK, Hutchinson EC, McCall AJ: The circle of Willis—the incidence of developmental abnormalities in normal and infarcted brains. Brain 90:747–758, 1967

74. Ueda K, Toole JF, McHenry LC, Jr: Carotid and vertebrobasilar transient ischemic attacks: clinical and angiographic correlation. Neurology 29:1094–1101, 1979

75. Ford JJ, Jr., Baker WH, Ehrenhaft JL: Carotid endarterectomy for nonhemispheric transient ischemic attacks. Arch Surg 110:1314–1317, 1975

76. Rosenthal D, Cossman D, Ledig CB, Callow AD: Results of carotid endarterectomy for vertebrobasilar insufficiency. An evaluation over ten years. Arch Surg 113:1361–1364, 1978

77. Dye WS, Brown CM: Surgical correction of carotid and vertebral artery stenosis. Surg Clin North Am 53:241–251, 1973

78. McNamara JO, Heyman A, Silver D, Mandel ME: The value of carotid endarterectomy in treating transient cerebral ischemia of the posterior circulation. Neurology 27:682–684, 1977

79. Imparato AM: Vertebral arterial reconstruction: a nineteen-year experience. J Vasc Surg 2:626–634, 1985

80. Edwards WH, Mulherin JL, Jr: The surgical reconstruction of the proximal subclavian and vertebral artery. J Vasc Surg 2:634–642, 1985

81. Imparato AM, Lin JP-T: Vertebral arterial reconstruction: internal plication and vein patch angioplasty. Ann Surg 166:213–221, 1967

82. Berguer R, Andaya LV, Bauer RB: Vertebral artery bypass. Arch Surg 111:976–979, 1976

83. Myers KA: Reconstruction of vertebral artery stenosis. Aust NZ J Surg 47:41–48, 1977

84. Diaz FG, Ausman JI, de los Reyes RA et al: Surgical reconstruction of the proximal vertebral artery. J Neurosurg 61:874–881, 1984

85. Edwards WH, Mulherin JL, Jr: The surgical approach to significant stenosis of vertebral and subclavian arteries. Surgery 87:20–28, 1980

86. Thevenet A, Ruotolo C: Surgical repair of vertebral artery stenoses. J Cardiovasc Surg 25:101–110, 1984

87. Berguer R: Distal vertebral artery bypass: technique, the "occipital connection," and potential uses. J Vasc Surg 2:621–626, 1985

88. Senter HJ, Bittar SM, Long ET: Revascularization of the extracranial vertebral artery at any level without cross-clamping. J Neurosurg 62:334–339, 1985

89. Sundt TM, Jr., Whisnant JP, Piepgras DC et al: Intracranial bypass grafts for vertebral-basilar ischemia. Mayo Clin Proc 53:12–18, 1978

90. Caplan LR: Occlusion of the vertebral or basilar artery. Follow up analysis of some patients with benign outcome. Stroke 10:277–282, 1979

91. Caplan LR: Vertebrobasilar disease. Time for a new strategy. Stroke 12:111–114, 1981

92. Gee W, Mehigan JT, Wylie EJ: Measurement of collateral cerebral hemispheric blood pressure by ocular pneumoplethysmography. Am J Surg 130:121–127, 1975

93. Effeney DJ, Krupski WC, Stoney RJ, Ehrenfeld WK: Fibromuscular dysplasia of the carotid artery. Aust NZ J Surg 53:527–531, 1983

94. Chassin MR, Kosecoff J, Park RE et al: Does inappropriate use explain geographic variations in the use of health care services? A study of three procedures. JAMA 258:2533–2537, 1987

5

Anesthesia Goals for Operations to Relieve or Prevent Cerebrovascular Insufficiency

Michael F. Roizen

The primary goals of anesthesia for vascular surgery are to minimize patient morbidity and maximize surgical benefit. I believe that understanding the major types of morbidity and their causes facilitates meeting these goals.

The two most frequently performed operations for cerebral vascular insufficiency in the United States are carotid endarterectomy and extracranial-to-intracranial (EC-IC) bypass. Approximately 100,000 (± 30 percent) carotid endarterectomies are performed yearly in the United States[1]; EC-IC bypass is not performed even $\frac{1}{100}$th as frequently as is carotid endarterectomy (see Ch. 7). Thus, information regarding morbidity is much better defined for carotid endarterectomy than for EC-IC bypass.

MORBIDITY AND MORTALITY AFTER CAROTID ENDARTERECTOMY

Surgical success, morbidity, and mortality after carotid endarterectomy vary directly with neurologic and cardiac status of the patient before surgery. Of surgical patients in a large Mayo Clinic series who had strokes in progress or unstable neurologic status, 2.5 percent died of postoperative neurologic deficits and 1 percent died of cardiovascular complications.[2] Of patients with coronary artery disease (CAD), 1.9 percent died from myocardial ischemia. Because more patients in this series had CAD than unstable neurologic status, the primary cause of morbidity and mortality after carotid endarterectomy was myocardial dysfunction (Table 5-1). Two other surgical series performing routine neurologic and cardiologic examinations described morbidity and mortality after carotid endarterectomy. Hertzer and Lees[3] reported that myocardial dysfunction accounted for 60 percent of deaths within 60 days of carotid endarterectomy. Table 5-2 shows results by Ennix et al.[4] regarding myocardial infarction and severe stroke after carotid endarterectomy in patients having various degrees of CAD.

Ennix et al.[4] and Hertzer et al.[5] have stressed the potential benefits of performing coronary artery bypass graft (CABG)

Table 5-1   Morbidity and Mortality after Carotid Endarterectomy

Reference	No. of Patients Studied	Percentage of Patients Who Died or Had Serious Morbidity from:	
		Cardiac Causes	CNS Causes
Ennix et al.[4] (1979)	1,546	60	30
Sundt et al.[2] (1981)	1,145	50	31
Hertzer and Lees[3] (1981)	335	60	17
Burke et al.[11] (1982)	1,141	67	33
Graham et al.[12] (1986)	105	100	0
Smith et al.[10] (1988)	60	0	100

procedures prior to carotid endarterectomy or other surgical procedures. That is, the morbidity and mortality associated with carotid endarterectomy are lower in patients who have first undergone CABG procedures. However, this reduction may be attributable to the fact that the patients at greatest risk may die or have myocardial or central nervous system (CNS) morbidity after the CABG procedure. The studies by Ennix et al.[4] and Hertzer et al.[5] in fact show no significant reduction in mortality when mortality owing to the CABG procedure is included in the over-

Table 5-2. Myocardial Infarction and Severe Stroke after Carotid Endarterectomy in Patients Having Various Degrees of CAD

Cardiac Status	Percentage of Patients Having:	
	Myocardial Infarction	Severe Stroke
No symptoms of CAD	0.8	1.1
Symptoms of CAD	12.9	2.4
History of CAD plus prior or current CABG procedure	2.6	1.3

(Data from Ennix et al.[4])

all mortality rate. Identification of high-risk patients by noninvasive tests, or better intraoperative monitoring and management of myocardial ischemia, may be able to alter these results.

Patients with *symptomatic* carotid artery disease appear to be as much as 17 times more likely to have a stroke during CABG procedures than are patients who have no carotid artery disease.[6] Such statistics have led to simultaneous performance of carotid and coronary vascular procedures; however, even in the best series, the rate of mortality and serious morbidity is approximately 10 percent.[7,8] In contrast, patients with *asymptomatic* carotid stenosis do not have a higher stroke rate following coronary artery surgery than do patients who have no carotid stenosis; the mortality rate is higher, however, owing mostly to myocardial infarction.[9]

Age also undoubtedly affects morbidity. Chapter 1 discusses the strong correlation between age and both myocardial and CNS morbidity after carotid endarterectomy.

Thus, morbidity and mortality statistics from virtually all series but our own (Smith et al.,[10] Table 5-1) show, surprisingly, that even when a vessel to the brain is occluded, the major cause of morbidity and mortality after carotid endarterectomy is myocardial dysfunction (Table 5-1).[2–4,9–12] Even in our own series, 34 percent of patients had myocardial ischemia intraoperatively; however, none of these patients had myocardial infarcts or died from myocardial events during the rest of their hospital stay.[10] Perhaps our results and those of other published series differ because we so heavily emphasize the goals of decreasing myocardial stress and maintaining myocardial well-being perioperatively.

THE SURGICAL PROCEDURE

Extracranial-to-Intracranial Bypass

As mentioned above, two general surgical approaches are available for treating and preventing cerebrovascular insufficiency: EC-IC bypass and carotid endarterectomy. Randomized studies (see Ch. 7) indicate that the EC-IC bypass has limited indications. One might be to prevent a stroke when transient ischemic attacks (TIAs) believed to be related to flow and not embolus occur in a patient who has bilateral carotid occlusions or lesions located so high in the carotid as to preclude extracranial carotid surgery. In EC-IC bypass, blood flow to the brain should be interrupted only during the short period of EC-IC anastomosis to the recipient vessel, and shunting of the flow during such time is usually not an option. Therefore, the monitors one would use for making judgments about the need for shunting, the adequacy of the shunt, and the adequacy of repair would not be necessary. Otherwise, the basic surgical and anesthetic goals, monitoring strategies, and anesthetic techniques are quite similar to those for carotid endarterectomy. The patients in both groups have similar

medical and surgical problems and present similar challenges.

Carotid Endarterectomy

In carotid endarterectomy, surgical approaches vary by surgical group, but the general aim is to gain a "smooth" ulcer- and plaque-free vessel with "smooth" endpoints and to avoid emboli and intraoperative neurologic ischemia (see Ch. 4). To reach these goals, most surgeons would like to have some measure of cerebral blood flow or neurologic function. Some rely solely on shunting of carotid blood flow and use a shunt in all applicable patients. Others rely on skillful general anesthesia and a short occlusion time. Each technique has been used successfully by surgeons experienced in that particular method.[1,3,10–16]

The first step in the surgical plan is to isolate the internal carotid artery at the location of the plaque or ulcerative lesion (this is determined radiographically and usually starts near the bifurcation). Heparin is given in a dose of 2,000 to 20,000 units per 70 kg of body weight. The dose varies according to the surgical group and is based, in my best estimate, on custom. The surgeon then isolates the diseased segment of the carotid by placing clamps or ties on the proximal and distal internal carotid artery and on the external carotid. A period of test occlusion follows, during which time personnel may evaluate regional cerebral blood flow, neurologic function, the electroencephalogram (EEG), the processed EEG, somatosensory evoked potentials, carotid artery stump pressure, or none of these. Next, an incision is made into the artery, a shunt is inserted (usually first into the proximal vessel and then into the distal vessel; often with clamps but sometimes with ties; and often with a pressure-measuring side arm to ensure that one or more ends are not crimped or occluded). Because insertion of a shunt incurs an embolism-associated stroke rate of at least 0.7 percent,[17] not all surgeons advocate routine shunting.

The next step is to remove the ulcerated or plaque-containing area, leaving a smooth intimal surface joining the endarterectomized vessel and native vessel. Occasionally, a long or tortuous region is shortened by resection and reanastomosis. In some instances, the remaining portion of the intima is too thin, in which case a vein or synthetic textile (Dacron) patch is employed. Because suturing the patch requires more time than suturing the native vessel, an internal shunt is frequently used during these procedures. Time is of the essence: at a carotid artery stump pressure of 40 mmHg, neurologic dysfunction can occur in 40 minutes and is common when occlusion time exceeds 60 minutes[18] (see below, "Carotid Artery Stump Pressure").

If a shunt has been used, it is now removed; in all cases, the arteriotomy is closed, usually with a running suture. Placement and removal of the shunt rarely take less than 1 minute or more than 4 minutes. In my fortunate experience with eight technically outstanding surgeons, total occlusion time has rarely exceeded 40 minutes.

Most surgeons wish to have their patients awaken soon after skin closure, as some surgeons treat a new neurologic deficit with immediate reexploration, or at least arteriography. Although a few surgeons request routine arteriography after restoration of blood flow, most believe that the complications of routine arteriography (formation of emboli, allergic reactions, vasospasm, bleeding from the puncture wound, and stroke) are greater than its benefits (the rare detection of inadequate repair, suture lines, or blood flow).

ANESTHESIA GOALS

For minimal morbidity and mortality, I believe the goals of anesthesia should be, first, to protect the heart from ischemia; and second, to protect the brain from ischemia. Some prominent anesthesiologists believe that this priority should be reversed (see Chs. 6 and 7). However, in my view, two considerations strongly argue for protection of the heart as the higher priority: (1) myocardial ischemia is the leading cause of morbidity in carotid endarterectomy; and (2) protection of the heart is the area in which anesthesiologists can exert, I believe, the greatest effect. Unfortunately, these two goals are often at odds with each other.

To decrease myocardial oxygen requirements, one tries to decrease heart rate, blood pressure, and myocardial contractility.[19] One also tries to maintain oxygen delivery to the brain, to increase cerebral perfusion pressure, and to decrease cerebral metabolic requirements. To increase cerebral perfusion pressure, one tries to increase arterial blood pressure to above the threshold required for normal brain autogregulation.[12,17,19–21] This activity usually involves avoiding severe bradycardia or decreasing central venous pressure.

Not only do reduction in blood pressure and augmentation of cerebral perfusion pressure lead to conflict in managing the priorities of the heart and those of the brain, but changes in heart rate can also cause conflict. Nevertheless, I believe there are compromise solutions that allow both goals to be met. To decrease myocardial work, one tries to decrease heart rate. However, sudden bradycardia can occur when the surgeon stretches the baroreceptor nerve endings directly. (Because of atherosclerosis, these nerve endings are supersensitive, as they usually have not been stretched easily by changes in blood pressure for many years.) Bradycardia can decrease arterial pressure substantially, an event that could compromise collateral cerebral perfusion. In my practice, the compromise solution allowing or facilitating a stable heart rate of approximately 70 beats/min has been injection of 1 percent lidocaine into the area of the bifurcation 10 to 15 minutes before occlusion of the carotid artery. In addition, the goals of decreasing myocardial contractility and cerebral metabolic rate are consonant, regardless of whether thiopental or isoflurane is used as the major anesthetic.

To maintain blood pressure, I usually employ light anesthesia (without paralysis, so that inadequate anesthesia can be detected), allowing endogenous vasopressor substances to maintain blood pressure. The incidence of myocardial ischemia has been substantially lower with this light-anesthesia technique than with deeper anesthesia and administration of phenylephrine.[12] In fact, I believe one of the major benefits of monitoring the EEG or processed EEG is that a normal or unchanged EEG after clamping of the carotid artery allows one to decrease blood pressure to facilitate protection of the heart.

MONITORING

These hemodynamic and metabolic methods of protecting the heart and brain from ischemia described in theory should work in practice. It would be reassuring, however, to have monitors confirm that these goals are actually being met. Unfortunately, the detection of both myocardial and cerebral ischemia by monitors during general or regional anesthesia is imperfect at present, and both false-negative and false-positive results confuse monitoring personnel. I will review the

monitoring techniques that are available and commonly used for myocardial and cerebral ischemia, giving my views on the benefits and problems of each.

Monitoring for Myocardial Ischemia

Electrocardiographic Changes in the ST Segment

When monitoring the electrocardiogram (ECG), one usually selects lead V_5. However, we have found that monitoring even seven electrocardiographic leads did not allow us to detect 75 percent of the instances of myocardial ischemia detected by changes in regional wall motion and by wall-thickening defects on a two-dimensional transesophageal echocardiogram (2D TEE).[22–24] In other vascular surgery employing segmental wall motion abnormalities and wall-thickening abnormalities as the ultimate standard, the sensitivity of the ECG in detecting myocardial ischemia was 40 to 80 percent. In addition, compared with other leads (notably lead II), lead V_5 was insensitive in detecting myocardial ischemia during cartotid endarterectomy. For our discussion, a monitoring technique is said to be sensitive if it detects myocardial ischemia when myocardial ischemia does, in fact, exist. For example, if the 2D TEE contained wall motion and wall-thickening abnormalities indicating myocardial ischemia in 10 subjects and the ECG had changes in ST segment in only 6, the ECG would said to be 60 percent as sensitive to myocardial ischemia as the 2D TEE.

Automated Electrocardiographic ST-Segment Trend Analysis

Two or three leads are usually used for electrocardiographic monitoring with automated ST-segment trend analysis.

Some devices available for this purpose claim to make detection of myocardial ischemia an easier process than it would be with simple oscilloscopic electrocardiographic traces. Although these devices might meet this goal,[23-25] they should not be expected to be as sensitive as a 2D TEE or a printout of a 12-lead ECG. In our studies, ST-segment trend analysis devices were approximately 40 to 90 percent as sensitive in detecting myocardial ischemia as were printouts of ECGs.[23-25]

Changes in Wedge Pressure, or the Appearance of V Waves on Pulmonary Capillary Wedge Pressure Tracings

Although changes in wedge pressure in the absence of fluid administration or changes in systemic pressure may be a sensitive indicator of myocardial ischemia, such changes are not specific. A monitoring technique is said to be specific if it is normal when myocardial ischemia has not occurred. For example, if the ECG and 2D TEE readings are normal, pulmonary capillary wedge pressure (PCWP) tracings should not indicate myocardial ischemia. On the other hand, V waves on PCWP tracings may not occur very often when myocardial ischemia is, in fact, occurring. Therefore, the appearance of V waves on PCWP tracings may be a specific indicator but is not a sensitive detector of myocardial ischemia.[26] In addition, the reported 2 percent carotid puncture rate on cannulation of the internal jugular vein makes it difficult to justify that route during this operation. Most surgeons would postpone carotid endarterectomy to another day after disturbing the contralateral carotid. I believe that the risk of inserting a pulmonary artery catheter from subclavian, external jugular, arm, or femoral sites does not justify the benefit. The rare exception might be the patient about to

undergo general anesthesia whose only signs or symptoms of myocardial ischemia are changes on the PCWP tracing but no changes in the ST segment. The other exception might be the instance in which a 2D TEE is not available, or when pictures from it cannot be obtained.

Angina in Patients Undergoing Regional Anesthesia

No reports are available regarding the usefulness of angina in detecting myocardial ischemia. The incidences of myocardial ischemia and death from myocardial causes after carotid endarterectomy are similar for both regional and general anesthesia.[27]

Monitoring for Cerebral Ischemia

Repeated Neurologic Evaluation of the Conscious Patient

Chapter 6 discusses this topic in detail. A brief synopsis of the statements in that chapter regarding the use of regional anesthesia for carotid endarterectomy follows. Usually, the carotid artery is occluded for a 1- to 4-minute trial period; if neurologic examination reveals no new deficit, the surgeon proceeds with endarterectomy. If a new neurologic deficit occurs, the surgeon releases the clamp and allows reperfusion to occur and neurologic function to return. At this point, some surgeons immediately reocclude the vessels, rapidly insert a shunt, and complete the procedure. However, most of the surgeons in my experience have preferred to cancel surgery and return on another day to perform the procedure under general anesthesia with a shunt. Still other surgeons apparently consider the lack of tolerance for carotid occlusion to be a contraindication to any further carotid surgery in such patients.[18] The disadvantages of using regional anesthesia include the following: the need for patient cooperation; the possible loss of patient cooperation (because of confusion, panic, or seizures) with the onset of a new neurologic deficit; the possibility that an unexpected delayed deficit will occur some time after the test period; the inability to administer drugs such as thiopental that might protect the brain against ischemia; and the inability to secure the airway if panic, seizure, or oversedation occurs. Those surgeons who revert to general anesthesia in the event of a new neurologic deficit in response to test occlusion seem to perceive general anesthesia as being the "best" technique for the "worst" cases. If this is so, then, as Dr. Michenfelder reasons in Chapter 6, general anesthesia should be considered the best technique for most cases.

Evaluation of Neurologic Function during General Anesthesia

The more frequently used indicators of neurologic function during general anesthesia consist of the EEG, somatosensory evoked potentials, regional cerebral blood flow, and carotid artery stump pressure.

The Electroencephalogram.

The scalp-recorded EEG reflects the electrical activity of the underlying cortical tissue. Conventional recording methods provide vast amounts of information, including a voltage value at each instant in time for each pair (16 or more) of electrodes. However, interpretation of this type of information is unwieldy in the operating room. Therefore, currently available data reduction methods now describe the EEG in terms of several calculated variables, and changes in these variables are charted over time.

Various physiologic and anesthetic manipulations affect the EEG. Reductions in cerebral blood flow, changes in temperature, the occurrence of hypotension, and administration of anesthetic agents all produce characteristic changes on the EEG. The proper interpretation of such changes during surgery depends on familiarity with the effects of the commonly used anesthetic agents, and of temperature, on the EEG. It should be remembered, however, that the blood flow threshold for electrical failure (approximately 18 ml/min per 100 g of brain) is higher than the blood flow threshold for metabolic failure (approximately 10 to 12 ml/min per 100 g of brain) (see Ch. 25).

The EEG can be viewed in its raw form or after undergoing various transformations. For example, the development of rapid computer analysis of the EEG by Fourier transformation into spectral arrays of power and frequency has simplified on-line assessment of the brain's electrical activity. Generally, if focal ischemia occurs, the usual change is a localized decrease in frequency or amplitude, or both.

How good is the EEG as an early warning signal of ischemia, and how effective is it in improving outcome after carotid endarterectomy? These are two quite different questions. It is my impression that the EEG is a sensitive early warning device but that it is not very specific (too many false-positive results occur); moreover, we have no idea whether its use improves outcome. However, the EEG may be more effective in improving myocardial well-being than in improving cerebral well-being. Results from several studies provide the basis for this conclusion.

In the Mayo Clinic series of 1,145 carotid endarterectomies monitored with EEG and measurements of blood flow (as determined by clearance of xenon), no patient awoke from anesthesia with a new neurologic deficit not predicted by EEG.[2] Another report described a series of 111 carotid endarterectomies monitored with a single channel of the EEG analyzed in "real time" to produce a density spectral array.[28] Among patients with no preoperative neurologic deficit, new postoperative deficits appeared in only the five patients having ischemic electroencephalographic events lasting 5 or more minutes. However, the EEG was not as predictive of outcome in patients who had a neurologic deficit before surgery. One such patient who had no changes on EEG during surgery had a new deficit after surgery, and one patient with changes on EEG lasting 13 minutes had no demonstrable new deficit after surgery.

The need for caution when monitoring patients with preexisting neurologic deficits was emphasized in a report describing 125 patients who had strokes or reversible ischemic neurologic deficits before undergoing carotid endarterectomy.[29] Four patients awoke with new deficits, despite unchanged EEGs.

In one series, only the last 93 of 172 carotid endarterectomies were monitored by EEG.[30] Monitoring of the EEG was associated with a reduction in the use of indwelling shunts (from 49 to 12 percent) and with a reduction in the combined major neurologic morbidity and mortality (from 2.3 to 1.1 percent). However, this study suffers from the use of historic controls and lack of randomization. Other investigators have shown a lower sensitivity (55 percent) for the EEG (Table 5-3).[31]

Another criticism is that monitoring of the EEG may have, at best, limited use, as 65 to 95 percent of neurologic deficits after carotid endarterectomy are caused by thromboembolic and not flow-related events. Although both conditions can be detected easily with the EEG, no major benefit accrues from any therapeutic maneuver in response to detection of such problems. In fact, if afterload or the use of shunts increases, the number of emboli

Table 5-3. Sensitivity,[a] Specificity,[b] and Predictive Positive[c] and Negative[d] Rates for the EEG in One Recent Study

EEG	New Postoperative Neurologic Problem	
	+	−
+	6	45
−	5	330

[a] Sensitivity = 6/11 = 55% at worst. Sensitivity is positivity (abnormality) of the EEG if the patient has a neurologic deficit.

[b] Specificity = 330/335 = 98.5% at worst. Specificity is negativity (normality) of the EEG when the patient remains neurologically intact.

[c] Predictive positive rate = 6/56 = 10.8% at worst. Predictive positive rate is the percentage of times an abnormal EEG successfully predicts a new neurologic deficit.

[d] Predictive negative rate = 330/380 = 87% at worst. Predictive negative rate is the percentage of times a normal EEG successfully predicts a neurologically intact patient.

(From McFarland et al.,[31] with permission.)

could increase and myocardial oxygen balance could become worse. Description of one group's experience with 176 consecutive patients undergoing carotid endarterectomy without shunts but with monitoring of the EEG provides an example.[32] Although most of the clamp-associated changes on EEG were related to decreased regional cerebral blood flow, postoperative deficits were usually caused by embolism. Other studies have yielded similar results.[33]

Other considerations in evaluating the appropriateness of electroencephalographic monitoring for carotid endarterectomy include false-positive and false-negative results and cost-effectiveness. Several factors can account for the occurrence of intraoperative false-positive results (i.e., changes on the EEG not accompanied by demonstrable deficits). First, the brain can tolerate brief periods of ischemia without infarction. Thus, one should not expect temporary, reversible changes on the EEG to necessarily indicate postoperative deficits. Second, the EEG must be viewed as a sensitive but nonspecific indicator of ischemia, as the EEG responds not only to cerebral ischemia but also to administration of anesthesia and changes in temperature and blood pressure. Third, as stated earlier, the blood flow threshold for electrical failure is higher than the threshold for metabolic failure. This means that even though the EEG may be an early warning system for cerebral ischemia, not all changes on the EEG indicate that ischemia is taking place. Fourth, the EEG may not detect focal embolic events.

Except as noted above (i.e., in patients with preexisting neurologic deficits, strokes in evolution, or recent reversible ischemic neurologic deficits), there are relatively few reports of false-negative results on EEG.

In general, patients who do not have intraoperative changes in EEG do not awaken with new neurologic deficits. Because most neurologic deficits after carotid endarterectomy are not caused by flow-related ischemia, detection of changes on EEG does not guarantee that placement of a shunt will reverse the deficit. In fact, the use of shunts is associated with a low but definite risk of causing emboli.

Chapter 25 provides a detailed discussion of the cost-effectiveness of monitoring the EEG. I believe a slightly different view results if one assumes that monitoring involves not only costs and benefits but also risks. Thus, monitoring should perhaps be evaluated in terms of risks versus benefits rather than cost versus benefits.

Using annual figures, let us assume that 100,000 carotid endarterectomies are performed each year; that 3,000 new deficits occur (making the deficit rate 3 percent); and that monitoring might prevent one-sixth of these new deficits (500 deficits;

these are related to blood flow and not emboli[31–33]). Let us also assume that an additional 15 percent of patients would undergo temporary shunting of carotid blood flow because of monitoring of the EEG and that 2 percent of these would have neurologic deficits associated with insertion of the shunt. Therefore, monitoring would be responsible for an additional 300 deficits. The *net* number of deficits preventable by monitoring would be 200 per year.

However, let us now assume that the annual deficit rate is 1 percent (1,000 new deficits per year) and that monitoring might prevent one-sixth of these deficits (160 deficits). Furthermore, if one assumes, as in the previous example, that an additional 15 percent of patients would undergo shunting because of monitoring of the EEG and that 2 percent would have neurologic deficits related to insertion of the shunt, then, once again, 300 new deficits would be attributable to monitoring. When one then subtracts the number of deficits caused by monitoring (300) from the number of deficits preventable by monitoring (160), one sees that monitoring of the EEG would prevent no deficits and would, in fact, cause 140 additional deficits.

Thus, monitoring of the EEG might either benefit or harm the neurologic status of the patient, depending on the deficit rate the anesthetist and the surgeons normally incur with that type of patient. Of course, variation in the values for the percentage of deficits preventable by monitoring, the deficit rate, and the rate of deficits related to insertion of the shunt changes the point at which benefits and risks are even. Nevertheless, this "break-even" point can be calculated if one has determined the rates in question.

However, it is entirely possible that monitoring of the EEG allows maintenance of a lower blood pressure during temporary carotid occlusion than would be feasible if only assessment of carotid artery stump pressure were used. Therefore, monitoring of the EEG may provide the benefit of allowing one to decrease afterload in the patient at risk of myocardial ischemia. Electroencephalographic monitoring may also permit an unhurried and technically superior endarterectomy, may identify delayed ischemia, and may aid in the detection of other problems such as shunt malfunction.

Unfortunately, no data yet demonstrate that this method of detection of neurologic dysfunction during carotid endarterectomy results in better patient outcome than does any other method of detection.

Somatosensory Evoked Potentials. Monitoring of evoked potentials relies on the fact that neural activity occurs after application of a stimulus. The resulting electrical activity that is related to the stimulus (the signal) must be separated from the activity that is not related to the stimulus (the noise). The primary problem with evoked potentials is that the signal-to-noise ratio is unfavorable. This issue and the effectiveness of using somatosensory or motor evoked potentials in carotid endarterectomy are reviewed in Chapter 26. To summarize, the benefit of using somatosensory evoked potentials to monitor neurologic function during carotid endarterectomy is even more conjectural than is the role of monitoring the EEG.

Regional Cerebral Blood Flow. Measurement of regional cerebral blood flow usually involves washout of a radioisotope such as xenon 133 after its injection into a surgically occluded carotid artery.[1] Flows above 24 ml/min per 100 g of brain are regarded as satisfactory, and those below 18 ml/min per 100 g of brain are believed to indicate the potential for cerebral ischemia. Obtaining such measurements requires expensive and highly technical equipment in the operating room. Of the few centers having such equipment, one has reported excellent correlation between cerebral blood flow and outcome; however, flow differences representing ischemia did depend on the anesthetic agents used.[1,34] Questions about this method of monitoring involve both its sensitivity and its specificity. As with all of the other monitors of neurologic function during carotid endarterectomy, no benefit has yet been shown.

Carotid Artery Stump Pressure. Stump pressure (mean blood pressure distal to the carotid clamp; also sometimes called back pressure) is widely used for evaluating the adequacy of cerebral perfusion during carotid surgery. During halothane anesthesia, cerebral ischemia rarely occurs at stump pressures above 60 mmHg, presumably because of the excellent collateral circulation required for maintaining that pressure[18,35] and the autoregulation present at this level. If stump pressure decreases below 60 mmHg, the likelihood of ischemia increases. However, since pressure is not identical to flow, stump pressures may be less than 60 mmHg while blood flow is perfectly adequate.

The major criticism of using stump pressure to monitor cerebral perfusion concerns the large number of false-positive results that occur, that is, a stump pressure of less than 60 mmHg when regional cerebral blood flow is actually more than 24 ml/min per 100 g of brain. Such results occur in about 30 percent of patients.[35] Thus, a shunt may be placed when none is needed. However, the simplicity of the measurement and its validity when pressure exceeds 60 mmHg during anesthesia with volatile anesthetics make it still the most useful clinical method for ensuring adequate perfusion during carotid endarterectomy. During narcotic-based anesthesia, stump pressure must be higher for blood flow to be adequate.[35]

As with all other measures, no clear benefit has been demonstrated for the use of stump pressure. However, logic dictates that monitoring techniques ensuring adequate cerebral function at the lowest myocardial work (such as the EEG, somatosensory evoked potentials, and stump pressure) would have a place in carotid endarterectomy.

CONCURRENT DISEASE IN THE PATIENT UNDERGOING CAROTID ENDARTERECTOMY

Many disorders are associated with vascular disease; diabetes, smoking and its sequelae, chronic pulmonary disease, hypertension, and ischemic heart disease are the most common. Management of anesthesia for concurrent diseases is reviewed elsewhere.[36] Perhaps the most important considerations when planning the perioperative management of concurrent diseases is to understand and search for the end-organ effects of such conditions and to understand the appropriate drug therapy. Although one usually does not anesthetize patients who have uncontrolled hypertension, uncontrolled metabolic disease, untreated pulmonary infections, or recent (within 3 to 6 months) myocardial infarction if other portions of the myocardium are still at risk,[36,37] crescendo TIAs can force one's hand. Attempts at rapid control of blood pressure or electrolytes may be more hazardous than leaving the condition untreated and trying to control the abnormality slowly. For example, rapidly reducing blood pressure in a patient with TIAs may precipitate cerebral ischemia and should be postponed until after surgery (assuming that surgery cannot be delayed to permit gradual preoperative control of blood pressure). Similarly, discontinuing a drug may be more hazardous than continuing drug therapy and being cognizant of its effects.

Specific attempts have been made to identify, prior to surgical operations, patients at risk of myocardial injury.[5,37] However, until these procedures gain widespread acceptance and extensive trials demonstrate reduced overall mortality, the goal of optimizing care—specifically, minimizing myocardial morbidity—seems logical. Two facts support this goal: (1) patients who have carotid artery disease are also likely to have CAD; and (2) the primary case of morbidity and mortality after carotid artery surgery is cardiac in nature.

ANESTHESIA FOR SURGERY FOR CEREBROVASCULAR INSUFFICIENCY: ONE APPROACH

Preoperative Assessment and the Anesthesia Plan

Our surgeons prefer general anesthesia for cerebrovascular insufficiency. If the patient has no medical problem that needs optimization before surgery, my preoperative interview focuses on reducing anxiety, obtaining informed consent, and determining the status of end organs likely to be affected by atherosclerosis, hypertension, or other diseases. In addition, multiple blood pressure and heart rate readings are obtained while the patient is in various positions, and the nurses are asked to obtain at least four more such readings before surgery (one every 2 hours while the patient is awake, and one during the night).

These preoperative values are important when formulating the range of acceptable intraoperative values. Specifically, preoperative data are used to determine the individualized range of values this particular patient can tolerate during and after surgery. For example, if blood pressure is 180 mmHg systolic and 100 mmHg diastolic, heart rate is 96 beats/min on admission, and no signs or symptoms of myocardial ischemia are present, my belief is that the patient can tolerate these levels during surgery. If blood pressure decreases during the night to 80 mmHg systolic and 50 mmHg diastolic and heart rate to 48 beats/min and the patient does not awaken with signs of a new cerebral deficit, I believe that the patient can safely tolerate such levels during anesthesia. Thus, from preoperative data, an individualized set of values is derived for each patient. I then try to keep the cardiovascular variables within that range and, in fact, plan prior to induction of anesthesia what therapies to use to accomplish that goal (e.g. administration of more or less anesthesia; nitroglycerin; nitroprusside-dopamine; dobutamine; phenylephrine; or propranolol-esmolol-isoproterenol or atropine).

I believe that this type of planning is relatively unimportant for the totally healthy patient but is especially important for the patient suspected of having cardiovascular disease, such as patients undergoing carotid endarterectomy. Although I am not certain that keeping cardiovascular variables within an individualized range of acceptable values improves outcome, I do believe that using such a plan reduces morbidity. For example, several studies have shown that major intraoperative deviations in blood pressure from the preoperative level correlate with the occurrence of myocardial ischemia.[10,38,39]

The acceptable values are kept in mind during surgery by listing them at the top of the anesthesia record before induction. Prior to working with surgeons who routinely use the EEG, I worked with surgeons who wanted the patient's blood pressure to be at the upper end of ward pressure. This desire arose from data indicating that a higher systemic blood pressure would increase collateral cerebral blood flow distal to a carotid occlusion.[20] On the other hand, such an increase in blood pressure increases myocardial work and thus the likelihood of myocardial ischemia.[10,19] At our institution, if the surgeons want the anesthesiologists to increase blood pressure to above the upper limits of the patient's normal ward pressure, as they sometimes do for a patient whose carotid blood flow cannot be shunted because of the anatomy of the lesion, we do so in a preoperative test period. At that time, we ask about angina and examine seven electrocardiographic leads for evidence of ischemia. Only in rare patients having changes in PCWP indicating myocardial ischemia but no changes on ECG would we use a pulmonary artery catheter during carotid surgery. (In my practice, this has occurred only twice in approximately 1,500 anesthetics for carotid endarterectomy.) I avoid inserting pulmonary artery catheters during carotid surgery for two reasons: (1) little fluid shift occurs during these operations; and (2) at our institution, the rate of complications from using a pulmonary artery catheter exceeds that of carotid surgery itself.

Other information I try to determine during the preoperative visit and assessment are the electrocardiographic lead most likely to reveal ischemia (often found on an exercise electrocardiographic study, or from the best guess on a thallium redistribution study), and the value of the patient's normal carbon dioxide level. The latter usually can be assumed to be normal if the bicarbonate level is normal or if the patient does not have a history suggestive of chronic obstructive pulmonary disease.

Anesthesiologists at the two institutions I have been associated with (the University of California, San Francisco, and the University of Chicago) do not premedicate patients about to undergo carotid surgery, as their surgeons believe that premedication delays awakening and my confuse preoperative tests of mental function. My own initial reaction was concern that lack of premedication might increase anxiety[40] and cause myocardial ischemia. However, in my practice, only one patient of the 1,500 "premedicated" for carotid endarterectomy with only an interview has arrived in the preoperative holding area or operating room with angina or electrocardiographic evidence of myocardial ischemia. Either the preoperative interview is very effective[40] or patients in my practice in San Francisco and Chicago differ substantially from those of Slogoff and Keats[39] in Houston. These investigators reported a high incidence of preinduction ischemia in approximately 1,500 patients undergoing CABG procedures.

Thus, local custom and logical considerations have both contributed to formulation of the following goals and techniques I use for patients undergoing carotid endarterectomy.

(1) Avoid myocardial ischemia by keeping hemodynamic variables (especially heart rate) at normal levels. For this purpose, I usually monitor lead V_5 and lead II of the ECG for changes in the ST segment and heart rate and the transesophageal echocardiogram for abnormal wall motion or thickening.

(2) Avoid cerebral ischemia by maintaining normal or high-normal blood pressure and by shunting carotid blood flow if an abnormal EEG occurs. Keep the patient in a slightly hypocarbic state.

(3) Use general anesthesia, but have the patient awake at the end of the operation. To accomplish this, I avoid drug premedication and "premedicate" only by interview. For general anesthesia, light levels of volatile agents are used.

(4) Unless crescendo TIAs are present, delay surgery in patients who have uncontrolled hypertension, untreated pulmonary disease, myocardial infarction less than 3 months old if areas of myocardium are still at risk, or uncontrolled metabolic diseases.

Some of these goals are in conflict and have been modified by study results. For example, one could provide deeper anesthesia while maintaining blood pressure by means of an α_1-adrenergic drug such as phenylephrine. However, I found that the incidence of myocardial ischemia was three times greater with deep anesthesia and the use of vasopressors to maintain blood pressure than with light anesthesia at the same systolic pressure.[10] My usual procedure for administering light anesthesia is as follows.

Preparation of the Patient

After the preoperative interview, all oral intake is restricted after midnight, and an intravenous infusion of 5 percent dextrose in half-normal saline is begun through an 18-gauge plastic cannula at a maintenance rate of 100 ml/h per 70 kg of body weight. Administration of fluids ensures that the patient is not hypovolemic and thus subject to a large decrease in blood pressure during induction of anesthesia. When the patient arrives in the preoperative holding area, the intravenous solution is changed to normal saline. After skin preparation with iodine and raising of a lidocaine skin wheal, an 18-gauge arterial line is inserted into the radial artery contralateral to the planned carotid surgery. In my opinion, 18-gauge lines are preferable to 20-gauge lines because no greater morbidity ensues with the larger catheter[41] and because the 20-gauge line tends to incur a 5 to 10 percent incidence of kinking when our surgeons push on the arm with their bellies during carotid dissection. Normal saline is used rather than dextrose or lactated Ringer's solution because lactate is metabolized to dextrose. Also, recent animal studies indicate that increasing blood glucose may increase neurologic damage after global ischemia.[42] Although at least one laboratory has reported different results for focal CNS ischemia,[43] and some investigators believe that survival is better with fructose than with saline,[44] my view is that the most prudent approach at this time seems to be maintenance of normoglycemia.

The patient is then brought to the operating room and transferred to an operating table having an already warmed heating mattress. I believe that the heating mattress is important for maintaining normothermia and thus helps in reducing postoperative circulatory instability.[45] Standard monitoring devices and techniques (e.g., the EEG, ECG, measurement of blood pressure, and pulse oximeter) are then applied and the data examined prior to induction of anesthesia.

Induction of Anesthesia

Anesthesia is induced with a barbiturate. At this time and during carotid occlusion, some anesthesiologists titrate the dose to achieve burst suppression on the EEG (see Ch. 7). Electrical suppression not only reduces cerebral metabolism to as little as 40 to 50 percent of awake levels but also decreases cerebral blood flow and intracranial pressure. Once burst suppression occurs, barbiturates have no further cerebral metabolic effect, or any effect in protecting the brain from ischemia.[46] One hundred percent oxygen, thiopental (1 to 2 mg/kg), and 3 mg of *d*-tubocurarine are then administered, followed by thiopental (25 to 50 mg/min

per 70 kg of body weight intravenously), along with increasing concentrations of isoflurane in oxygen by mask. When systolic blood pressure has decreased by 20 to 30 percent, succinylcholine (1.5 mg/kg), atracurium besylate, or vecuronium bromide is given. No muscle relaxants are given if muscle or lower motor neuron dysfunction is present (see Ch. 16). It is also my practice to administer 100 mg of either lidocaine or thiopental intravenously to blunt the cardiovascular response (i.e., in blood pressure and heart rate) to laryngoscopy and tracheal intubation. After routine checks and verification of endotracheal intubation by endtidal capnography, a transesophageal echocardiographic probe is inserted to obtain cross-sectional views of the left ventricle at the level of the papillary muscles.

Controlled ventilation is then begun, often with 50 percent nitrous oxide in oxygen, and sometimes with oxygen alone, titrating the concentration of isoflurane or enflurane and adjusting the table position to achieve the desired blood pressure. My tendency is to avoid administering more than 10 ml of crystalloid (or other fluids) per kg of body weight in this 2-hour operation, for I suspect (but have not confirmed) that a greater administration of fluids would contribute to postoperative hypertension. This effect may result from the absence of baroreceptor function so common in patients undergoing carotid endarterectomy.[47] The lack of baroreceptor function may also account for the stable intraoperative heart rate of these patients.[10]

Controversy exists concerning the optimum intraoperative carbon dioxide level for patients undergoing carotid endarterectomy.[21] Most practitioners now prefer a slightly hypocarbic state or normocarbia[21] (see Chs. 6 and 7). Maintenance of a slightly hypocarbic state has the possible advantage of preferentially diverting cerebral blood flow to potentially ischemic areas of the brain by constricting the nonischemic, normally reactive vessels.

Intraoperative Considerations

During the operation, light anesthesia is usually employed, using patient movement and hemodynamic changes to signal inadequate anesthesia. If anesthetization sufficient to inhibit movement during temporary occlusion of the carotid cannot be ensured, a muscle relaxant is added. The desired heart rate response determines the choice of muscle relaxant.

Although the effects of anesthetics on normal cerebral blood flow are known, the preference for one anesthetic over another for carotid endarterectomy appears to have no scientific basis. Perhaps the only information suggesting that one should choose isoflurane over other inhalational agents or narcotics is that from a nonrandomized study at the Mayo Clinic.[34] In that study, the "critical regional cerebral blood flow" (the blood flow below which electroencephalographic signs of ischemia occur) was 10 ml/min per 100 g of brain during isoflurane anesthesia, as opposed to approximately 20 ml/min per 100 g of brain during halothane anesthesia. Also, the need to shunt was less frequent during isoflurane anesthesia than during halothane anesthesia.

My tendency to avoid narcotics in these operations is based on the desire to have patients awaken shortly after the last stitch is placed (although this may now be possible with alfentanil) and on the desire to avoid the hemodynamic effects of naloxone and of muscle relaxant reversal. Avoidance of narcotics is not based on published anecdotal reports that narcotics worsen neurologic outcome after focal or global cerebral ischemia.[48]

Before beginning carotid occlusion, the surgeon infiltrates the carotid artery at the bifurcation with 1 percent lidocaine, with the hope of preventing the sudden onset of bradycardia during stretching of the baroreceptor itself or of the nerve coming from the baroreceptor(see above, "Anesthesia Goals"). Anesthetic depth is kept at a minimum, so that blood pressure increases to the upper end of the ward value. If no evidence of ischemia is found on EEG, or if carotid artery stump pressure is comfortably above 50 mmHg, depth of anesthesia would be increased somewhat and systemic blood pressure would decrease slightly. If monitoring indicates myocardial ischemia, the hemodynamic cause, if any would be reversed. When no obvious hemodynamic cause exists, nitroglycerin is given. Our studies found that 8 to 35 percent of the instances of myocardial ischemia occurred at this point in surgery.[10] Why this should be so is not known, as the hemodynamic state did not differ substantially from that just prior to cross-clamping of the carotid artery.

After completion of carotid repair and restoration of blood flow, the focus shifts completely to myocardial well-being. During repair of the muscle layer, the patient is allowed to resume spontaneous ventilation. Normally, our surgeons identify the recurrent laryngeal nerve. This identification prevents worry about vocal cord paresis, which allows the anesthesiologist to extubate the trachea with as light a plane of anesthesia as possible, but before the gag reflex is restored. Usually within 2 to 3 minutes after the last stitch, the patient will respond to pain; before leaving the operating room (i.e., within 4 to 6 minutes after the last stitch), the patient is able to follow simple commands.

Postoperative Complications

The four problems feared most in the recovery room are hemodynamic instability, respiratory insufficiency (most frequently caused by vocal cord paresis), formation of hematomas, and onset of new neurologic dysfunction.

Although, in my experience, circulatory instability has usually manifested as hypertension, reports in the literature also describe the occurrence of hypotension. Since inception of my current regimen, the incidence of postoperative hypotension has dropped to zero, and the incidence of postoperative hypertension has decreased from 35 to approximately 10 percent. This regimen consists of hydrating patients starting the night before surgery; giving antihypertensive drugs, including diuretics, on the morning of surgery; using a heating blanket to help maintain temperature; and limiting intraoperative administration of crystalloid to 10 ml/kg. Although these decreases in hemodynamic instability are based on historic controls and are anecdotal, I believe that any instance of hypertension needs vigorous treatment to reduce myocardial work. I often titrate combinations of either nitroprusside or hydralazine with propranolol, esmolol, or labetalol to achieve normotension. An elegant study by Stinson et al.[49] on post-CABG patients found such therapies superior to administration of nitroglycerin or trimethaphan camsylate in reducing blood pressure. Of course, other causes of hypertension are sought (e.g., pain, a full bladder, myocardial ischemia, hypoxia, hypercarbia). However, the association of hypertension with postoperative neurologic deficit is too strong to allow hypertension to persist.[50]

Although some investigators believe that hypotension after carotid endarterectomy is caused by hypersensitivity of the carotid sinus nerve,[51] in my experience, significant hypotension (systolic blood pressure of less than 80 mmHg) has often accompanied myocardial ischemia. My practice is to routinely obtain a 12-lead ECG shortly after the patient's arrival in the recovery room and monitor the lead(s) most likely to detect ischemia. After carotid surgery, this often proves to be lead II and not lead V_5.[22]

Ventilatory insufficiency has three chief sources. It can appear as stridor caused by unilateral or, more often, bilateral vocal cord paresis after the second of bilateral carotid operations, or after carotid endarterectomy preceded by thyroidectomy. Ventilatory insufficiency can also be caused by hematoma or deficient carotid body function (these patients are chronic carbon dioxide retainers). In the case of stridor, immediate securing of the airway is necessary. Treatment of hematomas often consists of opening the suture line and applying external drainage (this may need to be done even in the recovery room). (In my practice, each of the two above-described procedures has occurred only once in approximately 1,500 anesthetics given for carotid surgery.) The chemoreceptor function of the carotid body is predictably damaged for up to 10 months after carotid endarterectomy; complete loss of the ventilatory and circulatory response to hypoxia occurs after bilateral endarterectomy.[47] Because such loss increases carbon dioxide tension by 6 mmHg at rest, the routine use of supplemental oxygen is justified, at least until the patient ambulates.

Although wound hematoma from venous oozing usually accumulates slowly, this postoperative complication and arterial hemorrhage can both threaten the airway. Wound hematoma probably constitutes the most painful part of most carotid operations; most patients do not require more pain relief than that provided by acetaminophen. On occasion, reexploration in the operating room is necessary; in an emergency, rapid opening of the wound in the recovery room can be lifesaving.

Neurologic dysfunction after carotid endarterectomy is discussed in Chapter 8.[52,53]

CONCLUSIONS

Taking into consideration the most common causes of morbidity following carotid endarterectomy, I believe that the goals of anesthesia management for these patients should be as follows: (1) protecting the heart from ischemia; (2) protecting the brain from ischemia; and (3) having the patient awaken soon after surgery. These seemingly diverse goals can be accommodated by use of carefully selected techniques and therapies. For example, monitoring of the EEG aids both the heart and the CNS if observation of normal CNS electrical activity on the EEG then allows the anesthesiologist to reduce afterload. In a second example, injection of local anesthetic around the carotid sinus nerve not only prevents increases in myocardial oxygen demand but also decreases the likelihood of sudden bradycardia and hypotension. As in most aspects of anesthesia, meticulous attention to details such as overnight hydration and intraoperative use of warming mattresses may be as important as the choice of anesthetic agents or even of monitoring techniques.

Although my biases regarding both monitoring and anesthetic techniques are evident, it should be clear that many other techniques can be used for avoiding postoperative myocardial and cerebral dysfunction. Four important postoperative complications can lead to adverse sequelae. Circulatory instability can be caused by either myocardial or cerebral ischemia, inadequate or too vigorous hydration, or inadequate prevention of hypothermia. Respiratory insufficiency results from edema or laryngeal nerve trauma or from deficit carotid chemoreceptor function. Wound hematoma is a serious complication because it may compromise the airway. Finally, new neurologic deficits sometimes occur postoperatively. Each of these complications may require emergency treatment.

REFERENCES

1. Winslow CM, Solomon DH, Chassin MR et al: The appropriateness of carotid endarterectomy. N Engl J Med 318:721–727, 1988
2. Sundt TM, Jr., Sharbrough FW, Piepgras DG et al: Correlation of cerebral blood flow and electroencephalographic changes during carotid endarterectomy. With results of surgery and hemodynamics of cerebral ischemia. Mayo Clin Proc 56:533–543, 1981
3. Hertzer NR, Lees CD: Fatal myocardial infarction following carotid endarterectomy. Three hundred thirty-five patients followed 6–11 years after operation. Ann Surg 194:212–218, 1981
4. Ennix CL, Jr., Lawrie GM, Morris GC, Jr. et al: Improved results of carotid endarterectomy in patients with symptomatic coronary disease: an analysis of 1,546 consecutive carotid operations. Stroke 10:122–125, 1979
5. Hertzer NR, Beven EG, Young JR et al: Coronary artery disease in peripheral vascular patients: a classification of 1000 coronary angiograms and results of surgical management. Ann Surg 199:223–233, 1984
6. Kartchner MM, McRae LP: Carotid occlusive disease as a risk factor in major cardiovascular surgery. Arch Surg 117:1086–1088, 1982
7. Dunn EJ: Concomitant cerebral and myocardial revascularization. Surg Clin North Am 66:385–395, 1986

8. Hertzer NR, Loop FD, Taylor PC, Beven EG: Combined myocardial revascularization and carotid endarterectomy. Operative and late results in 331 patients. J Thorac Cardiovasc Surg 85:577–589, 1983

9. Barnes RW, Marzalek PB: Asymptomatic carotid disease in the cardiovascular surgical patient: is prophylactic endarterectomy necessary? Stroke 12:497–500, 1981

10. Smith JS, Roizen MF, Cahalan MK et al: Does anesthetic technique make a difference? Augmentation of systolic blood pressure during carotid endarterectomy: effects of phenylephrine *versus* light anesthesia and of isoflurane *versus* halothane on the incidence of myocardial ischemia. Anesthesiology 69:846–853, 1988

11. Burke PA, Callow AD, O'Donnell TF, Jr et al: Prophylactic carotid endarterectomy for asymptomatic bruit. Arch Surg 117:1222–1227, 1982

12. Graham AM, Gewertz BL, Zarins CK: Predicting cerebral ischemia during carotid endarterectomy. Arch Surg 121:595–598, 1986

13. Roizen MF, Ellis JE, Smith JS et al: Anesthesia for major vascular surgery, p. 183–186. In Estafanous FG (ed): Anesthesia and the Heart. Butterworth, Stoneham, MA, 1988

14. Baker WH, Dorner DB, Barnes RW: Carotid endarterectomy: is an indwelling shunt necessary? Surgery 82:321–326, 1977

15. Ferguson GG: Intra-operative monitoring and internal shunts: are they necessary in carotid endarterectomy (editorial)? Stroke 13:287–289, 1982

16. West H, Burton R, Roon AJ et al: Comparative risk of operation and expectant management for carotid artery disease. Stroke 10:117–121, 1979

17. Sundt TM, Houser OW, Sharbrough FW, Messick JM, Jr: Carotid endarterectomy: results, complications, and monitoring techniques. Adv Neurol 16:97–119, 1977

18. Wylie EJ: Is an asymptomatic carotid stenosis a surgical lesion? Presidential Address, Society of Cardiovascular Surgeons, 1982

19. Hamilton WK: Do let the blood pressure drop and do use myocardial depressants! Anesthesiology 45:273–274, 1976

20. Boysen G, Engell HC, Henriksen H: The effect of induced hypertension on internal carotid artery pressure and regional cerebral blood flow during temporary carotid clamping for endarterectomy. Neurology 22:1133–1144, 1972

21. Ehrenfeld WK, Hamilton FN, Larson CP, Jr et al: Effect of CO_2 and systemic hypertension on downstream cerebral arterial pressure during carotid endarterectomy. Surgery 67:87–96, 1970

22. Smith JS, Cahalan MK, Benefiel DJ et al: Intraoperative detection of myocardial ischemia in high-risk patients: electrocardiography versus two-dimensional transesophageal echocardiography. Circulation 872:1015–1021, 1985

23. Ellis JE, Roizen MF, Aronson S et al: Frequency with which ST segment trends predict intraoperative myocardial ischemia (abstract). Anesthesiology 67:A2, 1987

24. Ellis JE, Roizen MF, Aronson S et al: Comparison of two automated ST-segment analysis systems, EKG (including T wave inversion analysis), and transesophageal echocardiography for the diagnosis of intraoperative myocardial ischemia (abstract). Anesthesiology 69:A5, 1988

25. Kotrly KJ, Kotter GS, Mortara D, Kampine JP: Intraoperative detection of myocardial ischemia with an ST segment trend monitoring system. Anesth Analg 63:343–345, 1984

26. Pichard AD, Diaz R, Marchant E, Casanegra P: Large V waves in the pulmonary capillary wedge pressure tracing without mitral regurgitation; influence of pressure/volume relationship on the V wave size. Clin Cardiol 6:534–541, 1983

27. Riles TS, Kopelman I, Imparato AM: Myocardial infarction following carotid endarterectomy: a review of 683 operations. Surgery 85:249–252, 1979

28. Rampil IJ, Holzer JA, Quest DO et al: Prognostic value of computerized EEG analysis during carotid endarterectomy. Anesth Analg 62:186–192, 1983

29. Rosenthal D, Stanton PE, Jr., Lamis PA:

Carotid endarterectomy. The unreliability of intraoperative monitoring in patients having had stroke or reversible ischemic neurological deficit. Arch Surg 116:1569–1575, 1981

30. Cho I, Smullens SN, Streletz LJ, Fariello RG: The value of intraoperative EEG monitoring during carotid endarterectomy. Ann Neurol 20:508–512, 1986

31. McFarland HR, Pinkerton JA, Jr., Frye D: Continuous electroencephalographic monitoring during carotid endarterectomy. J Cardiovasc Surg 29:12–18, 1988

32. Blume WT, Ferguson GG, McNeil DK: Significance of EEG changes at carotid endarterectomy. Stroke 17:891–897, 1986

33. Morawetz RB, Zeiger HE, McDowell HA, Jr et al: Correlation of cerebral blood flow and EEG during carotid occlusion for endarterectomy (without shunting) and neurologic outcome. Surgery 96:184–189, 1984

34. Messick JM, Jr., Casement B, Sharbrough FW et al: Correlation of regional cerebral blood flow (rCBF) with EEG changes during isoflurane anesthesia for carotid endarterectomy: critical rCBF. Anesthesiology 66:344–349, 1987

35. McKay RD, Sundt TM, Michenfelder JD et al: Internal carotid artery stump pressure and cerebral blood flow during carotid endarterectomy: modification by halothane, enflurane, and Innovar. Anesthesiology 45:390–399, 1976

36. Roizen MF: Anesthetic implications of concurrent diseases. p. 255–357. In Miller RD (ed): Anesthesia. 2nd Ed. Vol. 1. Churchill Livingstone, New York, 1986

37. Boucher CA, Brewster DC, Darling RC et al: Determination of cardiac risk by dipyridamole-thallium imaging before peripheral vascular surgery. N Engl J Med 312:389–394, 1985

38. Roizen MF, Beaupre PN, Alpert RA et al: Monitoring with two-dimensional transesophageal echocardiography. Comparison of myocardial function in patients undergoing supraceliac, suprarenal-infraceliac, or infrarenal aortic occlusion. J Vasc Surg 1:300–305, 1984

39. Slogoff S, Keats AS: Further observations on perioperative myocardial ischemia. Anesthesiology 65:539–542, 1986

40. Egbert LD, Battit GE, Turndorf H, Beecher HK: The value of the preoperative visit by an anesthetist. A study of doctor-patient rapport. JAMA 185:553–555, 1963

41. Bedford RF: Radial arterial function following percutaneous cannulation with 18- and 20-gauge catheters. Anesthesiology 47:37–39, 1977

42. Lanier WL, Stangland KJ, Scheithauer BW et al: The effects of dextrose infusion and head position on neurologic outcome after complete cerebral ischemia in primates: examination of a model. Anesthesiology 66:39–48, 1987

43. Pearl RG, Larson CP: Effect of hyperglycemia on neurologic outcome after focal ischemia. Stroke (in press)

44. Farias LA, Willis M, Gregory GA: Effects of fructose-1,6-diphosphate, glucose, and saline on cardiac resuscitation. Anesthesiology 65:595–601, 1986

45. Roizen MF, Sohn YJ, L'Hommedieu CS et al: Operating room temperature prior to surgical draping: effect on patient temperature in recovery room. Anesth Analg 59:852–855, 1980

46. Nehls DG, Todd MM, Spetzler RF et al: A comparison of the cerebral protective effects of isoflurane and barbiturates during temporary focal ischemia in primates. Anesthesiology 66:453–464, 1987

47. Wade JG, Larson CP, Jr., Hickey RF et al: Effect of carotid endarterectomy on carotid chemoreceptor and baroreceptor function in man. N Engl J Med 282:823–829, 1970

48. Hosobuchi Y, Baskin DS, Woo SK: Reversal of induced ischemic neurologic deficit in gerbils by the opiate antagonist naloxone. Science 215:69–71, 1982

49. Stinson EB, Holloway EL, Derby G et al: Comparative hemodynamic responses to chlorpromazine, nitroprusside, nitroglycerin, and trimethaphan immediately after open-heart operations. Circulation, 51/52: suppl. I, I-26 to I-33, 1975

50. Asiddao CB, Donegan JH, Whitesell RC, Kalbfleisch JH: Factors associated with perioperative complications during carotid endarterectomy. Anesth Analg 61:631–637, 1982

51. Tarlov E, Schmidek H, Scott RM et al: Reflex hypotension following carotid endarterectomy: mechanism and management. J Neurosurg 39:323–327, 1973

52. Goldstone J, Effeney DJ: The role of carotid endarterectomy in the treatment of acute neurologic deficits. Prog Cardiovasc Dis 22:415–422, 1980

53. Mentzer RM, Jr., Finkelmeier BA, Crosby IK, Wellons HA, Jr: Emergency carotid endarterectomy for fluctuating neurologic deficits. Surgery 89:60–66, 1981

6

Anesthesia and Surgery for Cerebrovascular Insufficiency: One Approach at the Mayo Clinic

John D. Michenfelder

Patients who require surgery for cerebrovascular insufficiency present a particular challenge to the anesthetist, not only because they have or may have cerebral ischemia but also because such patients frequently have multisystem disease. The major goals of management are (1) to avoid drugs and techniques that might initiate or aggravate cerebral ischemia; (2) to avoid drugs and techniques that might aggravate pathologic conditions in areas other than the brain (although avoidance of cerebral ischemia always takes precedence); (3) to select drugs and techniques that might protect the brain or minimize cerebral ischemia (note that protection against ischemia is not the same as avoidance of ischemia); and (4) to monitor the brain for ischemia. The basic principles involved in the anesthetic management of patients undergoing surgery for occlusive vascular disease are similar regardless of procedure, that is, carotid endarterectomy or bypass. Accordingly, I first describe management of the patient undergoing carotid endarterectomy at the Mayo Clinic

and then identify the important differences in anesthetic management that apply to other surgical procedures for cerebrovascular occlusive disease.

REGIONAL VERSUS GENERAL ANESTHESIA

As judged by the number of reports published in the past 10 to 15 years, interest in the use of regional anesthesia for carotid surgery appears to be growing.[1-10] From a technical standpoint, regional anesthesia (deep cervical block) is simple, reliable, and virtually free of complications when performed by an experienced anesthetist. Alternative choices not generally recommended for carotid surgery include superficial cervical block with deep surgical infiltration of local anesthetic or cervical epidural anesthesia.

The major advantage of regional anesthesia is that the conscious patient can undergo repeated neurologic evaluation. Thus, an accurate and sensitive assessment of cerebral function can be made during occlusion of the carotid. To achieve this goal, the patient cannot be heavily sedated. Regional anesthesia thus requires a cooperative patient, a completely successful block, and a sugeon accustomed to working with regional anesthesia.

In the usual technique, the surgeon exposes the carotid artery and carries out a trial occlusion for 1 to 4 minutes. Endarterectomy proceeds if the patient has no new neurologic deficit. If a deficit occurs, the clamps are released. At this point, some surgeons cancel surgery, scheduling it for another day, at which time they give general anesthesia and use a shunt.[1,2] Still others believe that further carotid surgery is contraindicated for such patients.[3] Most surgeons, however, wait for reperfusion and return of normal neurologic function. They then reocclude the vessels, rapidly (within 2 minutes) insert a shunt, and complete the surgical procedure.

The disadvantages of regional anesthesia include patient discomfort and, as a result, loss of cooperation; the perceived need for hasty surgery while inserting and removing the shunt; the possible loss of patient cooperation (because of confusion, panic, or seizures) with the onset of a neurologic deficit; the possible occurrence of a neurologic deficit after the test period; the inability to administer drugs that might protect the brain (e.g., thiopental); and the inability to "fine tune" blood gases and blood pressure. We believe that if general anesthesia is perceived to be the safest choice for the riskiest cases (as evidenced by its use on development of a new neurologic deficit), it seems reasonable to assume that general anesthesia would be the safest choice for all cases.

We have opted for general anesthesia based on the above considerations. However, we believe this decision imposes an obligation to provide cerebral monitoring that is as sensitive and reliable as its alternative (repeated neurologic assessment of possible cerebral ischemia in the awake patient). As described in this text, we believe such monitoring is available. We reject the two other approaches used with general anesthesia: to use a shunt in all instances (and monitor nothing), or to perform the surgery as fast as possible without a shunt (and monitor nothing). The former practice incorrectly suggests that use of shunts is without risk and that shunts guarantee adequate blood flow. The latter practice, in our opinion, invites inadequate surgical repair.

PREOPERATIVE ASSESSMENT

If the patient is neurologically stable, it is important to determine the range of blood pressures normal for that patient, as this dictates to us the range of values we will permit during general anesthesia. In all instances, a minimum permissible blood pressure should be established to determine at what point immediate treatment would be initiated. If the patient is not stable and demonstrates a progressing deficit, consideration should be given to preoperative interventions such as pharmacologically increasing blood pressure, blood transfusion, and administration of heparin. In rapidly deteriorating patients requiring emergency surgery (e.g., middle cerebral artery embolectomy), premature induction of anesthesia with thiopental may protect the brain—that is, prolong its tolerance for the existing ischemia by reducing its need for oxygen.

If the patient has no history or physical findings suggesting pulmonary dysfunction, it is reasonable to assume that blood gas values will be normal. If, however, pulmonary disease is suspected or demonstrable, I believe preoperative determination of blood gas values is imperative. Only this practice establishes the normal carbon dioxide level, which dictates the arterial carbon dioxide partial pressure ($PaCO_2$) to be set during general anesthesia. Thus, if a patient has chronic obstructive pulmonary disease and a preoperative $PaCO_2$ of 50 mmHg, it must be assumed (regarding the reactivity of that patient's cerebrovasculature) that 50 mmHg represents normocarbia. Induction of true normocarbia ($PaCO_2$ of 35 to 40 mmHg) during anesthesia in such a patient would produce relative hypocarbia, a reduction in total cerebral blood flow (CBF), and a possible redistribution of blood flow that might be either favorable or unfavorable (see below).

The most common coexisting problems in patients with occlusive cerebrovascular disease are hypertension and ischemic heart disease. If hypertension is not well controlled, it is probably a mistake to attempt acute preoperative reduction and control of blood pressure. Such actions are likely to precipitate cerebral ischemic episodes and should be postponed until after surgery (assuming that surgery cannot be delayed to permit gradual preoperative control of blood pressure).

The hazards of general anesthesia in patients who have had a previous myocardial infarction are well known (see Ch. 1). The risk of a second infarction following anesthesia is particularly great in the 3 to 6 months after the first infarction. Accordingly, the cerebral risk of delaying surgery must be weighed carefully against the cardiac risk of proceeding without delay. When the patient is not neurologically stable, there is no choice but to proceed.

The many systemic disorders that may exist in these patients must be dealt with individually in the preoperative period. However, common problems such as obesity, diabetes, arthritis, and abnormal hepatic or renal function rarely directly affect pathologic conditions of the brain and therefore do not require special consideration here.

INDUCTION OF ANESTHESIA

As already indicated, a major goal of anesthesia is to keep hemodynamic function and gas exchange within a normal range. By necessity, anesthesia alters cerebral function. This alteration may be beneficial, in that most anesthetics reduce cerebral oxygen demand. The effects of anesthesia on CBF are variable and of unknown importance in patients with regional cerebral ischemia. Induction with a barbiturate (usually thiopental) briefly reduces cerebral metabolism to as little as 40 to 50 percent of control and at the same time decreases CBF and intracranial pressure. The combined effect is demonstrably protective in experimental animals given incomplete global or regional cerebral ischemia, and in humans as well.[11] The mechanism by which such protection occurs is probably reduction in oxygen demand to a level that matches reduced oxygen delivery. This reduced oxygen demand occurs primarily as the result of inhibition of functioning neurons. However, in the absence of functional neurons, as manifested by an isoelectric electroencephalogram (EEG), barbiturates have no cerebral metabolic effect and no protective effect. Therefore, if the barbiturate is being administered for the dual purposes of producing anesthesia and protecting the brain, the EEG should be monitored and the anesthetic depth set and maintained (with additional barbiturates) to produce a burst suppression pattern on the EEG.

With induction of anesthesia, control of the airway is paramount to avoid both hypoxia and abrupt changes in carbon dioxide levels. Muscle relaxation may be obtained with any of several drugs, the choice being determined by possible side effects. Succinylcholine might be avoided in patients with muscle dysfunction secondary to neurologic disease; in such patients, potassium release from skeletal muscle and abrupt hyperkalemia may follow intravenous succinylcholine and lead to cardiac arrest. Both *d*-tubocurarine and atracurium besylate (the latter in large doses only) can cause histamine release and significant hypotension, whereas pancuronium bromide can cause hypertension and tachycardia. Vecuronium bromide has the least potential for any of these side effects and may be the drug of choice in these patients.

MAINTENANCE OF ANESTHESIA

Although the effects of individual anesthetics on normal CBF are known, no scientific data provide a rational basis for preferring either a cerebral vasodilating or vasoconstricting drug for maintenance of anesthesia in patients with occlusive vascular disease. All of the volatile agents are cerebral vasodilators, halothane being the most potent and isoflurane the least. All of the intravenously administered anesthetics except ketamine are cerebral vasoconstrictors, thiopental being the most potent; narcotics appear to be only weak vasoconstrictors. Intuitively, one might select a vasodilator for patients with cerebral ischemia. However, as is the case with carbon dioxide, anesthetics probably affect cerebral vascular resistance only through action on normal cerebral vasculature. If so, cerebral vasodilating anesthetics might have the potential, like hypercarbia, of stealing blood flow from ischemic regions. Conversely, vasocon-

stricting anesthetics might have the potential, like hypocarbia, of increasing blood flow to ischemic regions. No convincing data are available to resolve these apparent contradictions.

We compared 11 patients who were anesthetized with nitrous oxide, fentanyl citrate (a narcotic), and droperidol (a neuroleptic drug and potent cerebral vasoconstrictor) with 19 patients given halothane and 30 patients given enflurane.[12] Values for CBF before and after occlusion were significantly lower in patients given narcotics than in those given halothane or enflurane (Table 6-1). However, during occlusion, mean CBF for the three groups did not differ significantly; the patients given narcotic had numerically the lowest mean CBF. These results suggest that the choice of anesthetic is not a critical factor in terms of aggravating cerebral ischemia during occlusion, as long as hemodynamic values are kept adequate. Table 6-1 also shows that back pressure of the internal carotid artery (stump pressure) was highest in patients given narcotics and lowest in those given halothane, reflecting the differing cerebrovascular effects of these agents.

From a metabolic standpoint, arguments could be made for using either isoflurane anesthesia or an anesthetic composed primarily of barbiturate, as both techniques are protective in experimental animals subjected to incomplete ischemia. However, such protection has been shown only at depths of anesthesia associated with varying degrees of hemodynamic depression and hypotension. Furthermore, unlike thiopental, isoflurane may not offer protection when ischemia is regional rather than global. This impression results from a primate study of temporary occlusion of the middle carotid artery.[13] Those results require confirmation, however, because of differences in blood pressures and drug therapies used in the study. It seems more

Table 6-1. Effect of Halothane, Enflurane, and Innovar[a] on regional CBF and Stump Pressure in Patients Undergoing Carotid Endarterectomy[b] (Mean ± SE)[c]

| | Halothane (n = 19) | Enflurane (n = 30) | Innovar (n = 11) | Comparisons Between Anesthetics | | |
				Halothane vs. Enflurane	Halothane vs. Innovar	Enflurane vs. Innovar
Before occlusion rCBF (ml·100 g^{-1}·min^{-1})	66 ± 9	59 ± 4	34 ± 3	NS	$P < 0.05$	$P < 0.05$
During occlusion rCBF (ml·100 g^{-1}·min^{-1})	42 ± 3	37 ± 2	31 ± 3	NS	$0.05 < P < 0.10$	NS
Stump pressure (mmHg)	49 ± 4	55 ± 4	76 ± 8	NS	$P < 0.05$	$P < 0.05$
MAP (mmHg)	112 ± 4	110 ± 2	112 ± 5	NS	NS	NS
After occlusion rCB (ml·100 g^{-1}·min^{-1})	92 ± 7	64 ± 4	41 ± 5	$P < 0.05$	$P < 0.05$	$P < 0.05$

[a] Innovar = trademark combination of droperidol (a neuroleptic) and fentanyl citrate (a narcotic) in a 50:1 ratio.
[b] These patients had regional rCBF of greater than 18 ml·100 g^{-1}·min^{-1}.
[c] rCBF = regional cerebral blood flow; stump pressure = back pressure in the internal carotid artery; NS = not significant; and MAP = mean arterial blood pressure.

appropriate to try to prevent ischemia than to prolong the brain's tolerance for ischemia. We thus recommend light levels of anesthesia and maintenance of blood pressure at the high end of the normal range. Furthermore, if the EEG is used to detect the onset of ischemia (as is our practice), light levels of anesthesia are mandatory to recognize the characteristic changes of ischemia on EEG.

We currently prefer to maintain anesthesia in these patients by giving a combination of nitrous oxide, isoflurane, and small doses of fentanyl citrate. The rationale is twofold. First, this combination of a weak vasodilator and a weak vasoconstrictor should result in minimal effect on normal cerebral vessels and, hence, CBF; undesirable shifts in regional blood flow should not occur. Second, modest concentrations of isoflurane *might* offer a degree of protection on a metabolic basis. We have shown that the "critical" CBF (that is, the flow associated with ischemic changes on EEG) is significantly lower with isoflurane than with halothane (10 versus 20 ml·100 g^{-1}·min^{-1}).[14] Although this reduction in critical CBF is not direct evidence of a protective effect on the brain, it is certainly strong indirect evidence of such. Furthermore, in a retrospective analysis of over 2,000 carotid endarterectomies, we determined that the incidence of ischemic changes on EEG after surgical occlusion of the carotid artery was significantly ($P < 0.001$) lower with isoflurane anesthesia (19 percent) than with either enflurane or halothane anesthesia (25 and 26 percent, respectively). These data are direct evidence that isoflurane is the most protective of the volatile anesthetics, but still fail to address the critical question: Is isoflurane as protective as thiopental?

CONTROL OF BLOOD PRESSURE

Control and maintenance of blood pressure are critical in these patients. One must assume that autoregulation has been lost in areas of the brain threatened by ischemia. Accordingly, blood flow would passively follow systemic blood pressure in these regions. Therefore, blood pressure should be increased 15 to 25 percent during carotid occlusion so as to increase perfusion pressure and hence blood flow to the affected hemisphere. Some patients having surgery under regional anesthesia have been reported to tolerate occlusion when their blood pressure was elevated but not when it was normal. However, Boysen et al.[15] did not find this to be true. Cerebral blood flow did not increase significantly after eight of their patients had induced hypertension because of potentially ischemic blood flows during occlusion. A 20 percent increase in blood pressure increased mean CBF from 17 to only 19 ml·100 g^{-1}·min^{-1}.

One effective way of increasing blood pressure when a volatile anesthetic is given is by infusing phenylephrine. Some physicians are rightly concerned that deliberately increasing afterload on the heart with an α-agonist could be particularly dangerous because of the tendency of this patient group to have underlying heart disease. Such an increase in cardiac workload could precipitate cardiac failure, ischemia, or both. We believe that these concerns are appropriate; in our experience, the second most common cause of morbidity and mortality in these patients is cardiac in origin.

In practice, we do not deliberately elevate blood pressure in patients with known cardiac disease. Furthermore, we always monitor the V$_5$ chest lead on the electrocardiogram (ECG) and avoid deliberate increases in blood pressure if ST-segment depression occurs at any time. These precautions should greatly lessen the risk associated with induced hypertension.

Another routine precaution is the injection of a local anesthetic into the carotid sinus by the surgeon after exposure of the carotid bifurcation. Clinical experience suggests that these patients vary widely in their response to surgical manipulation of the carotid sinus and that sudden bradycardia and hypotension are possible. Injection of a local anesthetic abolishes this unpredictable variable during surgical manipulation. If variability in carotid sinus pressure extends into the postoperative period, this condition might contribute to the transient postoperative hypertension that frequently occurs in these patients (see below).

CONTROL OF CARBON DIOXIDE LEVELS

The controversy concerning optimum carbon dioxide levels in patients undergoing carotid surgery is largely a historical one, with most practitioners now opting for normocarbia as the best compromise. In certain experimental animal models, paradoxical response to carbon dioxide can be demonstrated such that hypercarbia produces a "steal" effect and hypocarbia improves ischemic regional blood flow. However, in patients undergoing carotid surgery, the response of CBF to changes in carbon dioxide is unpredictable (Fig. 6-1). We believe that if the response is unpredictable and if the patient is stable at normal carbon dioxide levels, these levels should be maintained.

There is one exception in our current practice. If marked reactive hyperemia (CBF exceeding 80 to 100 ml·100 g^{-1}·min^{-1}) occurs after repair of a severely stenotic carotid artery, we may attempt to reduce blood flow by inducing hypocarbia and modest hypotension. These maneuvers are usually reserved for patients who have had a previous stroke on the operated side and who are therefore at risk of intracerebral bleeding after repair.

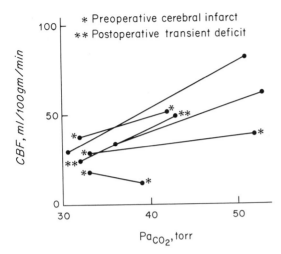

* Preoperative cerebral infarct
** Postoperative transient deficit

Fig. 6-1. Effects of change of $PaCO_2$ on cerebral blood flow before carotid endarterectomy. In six patients, cerebral blood flow changed variably and unpredictably in response to changes in $PaCO_2$—either no response or a paradoxical response.

MONITORING

We believe that the use of general anesthesia in patients undergoing carotid surgery imposes the obligation of monitoring brain function as reliably as one would monitor the awake patient having surgery under regional anesthesia. We monitor both the EEG and regional CBF. We currently rely on the standard 16-lead EEG using conventional electrode placements.[16] A trained technician assigned exclusively to the task continuously monitors the EEG from before induction of anesthesia until emergence from anesthesia. Any ischemic changes on the EEG that are concomitant with carotid occlusion are considered absolute indications for placement of a shunt if technically feasible. We determine CBF from the washout of xenon 133 that is injected intermittently into the common carotid artery by the surgeon (after occlusion of the external carotid artery). The calculation of CBF is based on the half-time washout of

xenon 133 and provides information primarily about the fast-flow compartment. We routinely measure blood flow just prior to occlusion of the carotid, immediately after occlusion (xenon 133 being injected immediately before occlusion), and after repair of the carotid. If a shunt is placed, we measure flow after placement. Whenever preocclusion CBF is considered near the critical level (defined earlier), a shunt is placed even if no changes have occurred on EEG. When these criteria for the EEG and CBF were used, approximately one-third of our patients had temporary shunts inserted during carotid repair.

The other monitoring devices and techniques used routinely for patients undergoing carotid endarterectomy include the ECG (lead V_5), direct measurement of arterial blood pressure (via radial or dorsalis pedis artery), determination of inspired and expired gas concentrations by mass spectroscopy, esophageal stethoscope, temperature determination, and intermittent determinations of blood gases. The mass spectrometer permits accurate control of the concentrations of anesthetics, oxygen, and carbon dioxide and thereby aids in maintaining a stable baseline pattern on EEG. This pattern is critical in recognizing subtle changes on EEG caused by marginal ischemia. Similarly, to interpret changes in CBF, we attempt to keep both carbon dioxide levels and blood pressure with a narrow range from just before carotid occlusion until the carotid has been reopened and the final determination of CBF has been made.

In the event of ischemic changes on EEG or CBF within the critical range during occlusion, the insertion of a shunt does not greatly alter anesthetic management. Patients have already been given heparin (5,000 to 7,000 units just prior to carotid occlusion), and no pharmacologic "protection" is given to permit continued meaningful monitoring of the EEG. Assuming that blood flow through the shunt is demonstrated to be adequate, we normally would *not* continue to induce hypertension.

We do not monitor stump pressure routinely because we believe it correlates only crudely with CBF.[12] In a study of 91 patients, CBF and stump pressure did not correlate in 42 percent when the critical (minimally acceptable) stump pressure was assumed to be 50 mmHg and the critical CBF was 18 to 24 ml·100 g^{-1}·min^{-1} (Fig. 6-2). Among these were 12 patients with stump pressures greater than 50 mmHg and CBF values within the critical range or lower. Of these, four patients had changes on EEG indicating ischemia. Had the critical stump pressure been taken to be 60 mmHg, these four patients would have been identified as having ischemia; however, a number of unnecessary shunts would have been inserted in

patients who had adequate CBF but stump pressures below 60 mmHg.

We have also evaluated how well other monitoring devices correlate with the standard EEG and measurements of CBF. A nasal plethysmograph was said to estimate "cerebral perfusion" by measuring pulsations originating from branches of the anterior ethmoidal artery. However, measurements of CBF did not correlate with pulse height before, during, or after carotid occlusion.[17] Similarly, a device for measuring conjunctival oxygen partial pressure was said to reflect the adequacy of CBF. Our group (B. Gibson, R. Cucchiara, J. McMichan, unpublished data) found no correlation between these two variables. On the other hand, a processed electroencephalographic signal was found to correlate reasonably well with the standard EEG in terms of recognizing major ischemic changes.[18] This processed EEG device (the Cerebral

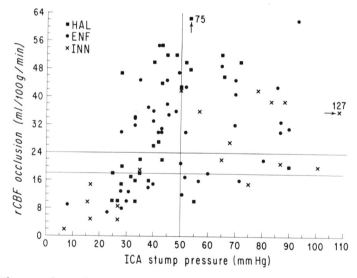

Fig. 6-2. The correlation between stump pressure (back pressure in the internal carotid artery) and occlusion cerebral blood flow during carotid endarterectomy is crude at best. The lower right-hand quadrant represents those patients at risk who had marginal or ischemic blood flows despite stump pressures higher than 50 mmHg. HAL = halothane; ENF = enflurane; and INN = Innovar (a combination of fentanyl citrate and droperidol).

Function Monitor, Devices Limited, New Brunswick, NJ) is one of several available and is among the least expensive. In the case of the Cerebral Function Monitor, which converts frequency and amplitude to "power," the cost of simplification includes loss of sensitivity. Two of our study patients who had subtle changes on EEG were not identified by Cerebral Function Monitor output; however, major changes on EEG were always recognized. Whether other devices that depend on averaging and that provide a compressed spectral array or a similar processed signal also sacrifice sensitivity remains to be determined.

POSTOPERATIVE MANAGEMENT

The most common immediate postoperative problem in patients undergoing carotid surgery is blood pressure lability. In our experience, this most commonly presents as transient hypertension, although occasional hypotension also occurs. Carotid sinus dysfunction can cause either abnormality. Tarlov et al.[19] reported a high incidence of hypotension, which was prevented by surgical denervation of the carotid sinus. They reasoned that the sinus was hypersensitive postoperatively because the covering plaque that had dampened the pressure signals had been removed. The more common ocurrence is hypertension, which may be attributable to carotid sinus insensitivity caused by surgical trauma. However, Wade et al.[20] found that carotid sinus function was blunted in these patients preoperatively and did not change within 1 to 4 weeks of carotid endarterectomy, even when performed bilaterally. It thus seems unlikely that acute loss of sinus sensitivity would be responsible for postoperative hypertension.

Regardless of cause, treatment of hypertension in many of these patients is desirable, and is attainable in a variety of ways. Successful control of blood pressure can be achieved variably with intravenously administered hydralazine (10 to 20 mg), chlorpromazine (1 to 3 mg), propranolol (1 to 5 mg), or labetalol (20 to 80 mg); or with infusion of a potent vasodilator such as nitroprusside. The last approach requires more intense monitoring and introduces the possibility of rebound hypertension on discontinuation of the drug.

Carotid endarterectomy causes damage to the carotid body that is irreversible for up to 10 months; complete loss of the ventilatory and circulatory responses to hypoxia occurs after bilateral endarterectomy.[20] Patients who have lost the ventilatory response to hypoxia also have a resting $PaCO_2$ that is 6 mmHg higher than preoperative resting levels. These patients must not be exposed to circumstances that could cause hypoxemia, because compensatory mechanisms would not be in force. Rather, high inspired concentrations of oxygen should be administered, and drugs that might depress ventilation (such as opiates) should be avoided or monitored closely.

The most dreaded postoperative complication in patients undergoing carotid surgery is probably spontaneous hemorrhage into the wound, with compromise of the patency of the upper airway. Abrupt, life-threatening arterial bleeding requires rapid reopening of the wound and establishment of an airway. The latter is usually not possible until the wound has been evacuated. If venous oozing is the cause of hemorrhage, the event is considerably less dramatic and can usually be managed in a more controlled (and sterile) fashion without complete loss of the airway.

ANESTHETIC CONSIDERATIONS FOR BYPASS PROCEDURES

A major difference in our management of patients undergoing bypass procedures is the lack of special monitoring, that is, the EEG and measurement of CBF. We believe neither is necessary. These monitoring techniques are used primarily to make judgments regarding the need for shunting, the adequacy of the shunt, and the adequacy of repair in carotid endarterectomy. Such considerations are not applicable to bypass surgery. In other respects, our basic anesthetic and monitoring approach to these patients is quite similar to that for carotid endarterectomy; both groups present similar problems and challenges to anesthetic management. These two groups do not differ regarding preoperative assessment, induction and maintenance of anesthesia, control of blood pressure and carbon dioxide levels, and routine monitoring.

The only major intraoperative difference in anesthetic management relates to the use of barbiturates to minimize the possibility of ischemic effects. Because bypass requires temporary occlusion of the recipient vessel, ischemia may increase during this period. Therefore, we give a "sleep dose" of thiopental (3 to 5 mg/kg) just before occlusion. The rationale is as follows. A sleep dose produces a transient burst-suppression pattern on the EEG that is associated with near maximal suppression of oxygen metabolism. If at that point the recipient vessel is occluded, any region made ischemic by occlusion would retain a near-maximal concentration of barbiturate with continued metabolic suppression. If the barbiturate washes out from the region normally supplied by the recipient vessel, protection will be short-lived but not needed. By the same reasoning, successive doses of barbiturate are not given during occlusion; presumably, a significant concentration could not be delivered to any regions of existing ischemia.

Whether such barbiturate therapy affects outcome in terms of postoperative neurologic deficits is unknown; settling this issue would require a blind, randomized prospective study. We do not plan to pursue such a study for several reasons. The treatment itself is relatively innocuous and has been shown to be effective in humans[11] and in animal models of incomplete regional ischemia.[21–23] Thus, it would be difficult to deny patients whatever benefit might accrue in order to carry out a scientifically valid study. Indeed, these circumstances seem to represent the perfect application of such barbiturate therapy: the patient is already anesthetized and adequately monitored, any ischemia induced by occlusion would be transient, and the dose of barbiturate is modest and associated with only mild side effects.

REFERENCES

1. Hobson RW, II, Wright CB, Sublett JW et al: Carotid artery back pressure and endarterectomy under regional anesthesia. Arch Surg 109:682–687, 1974
2. Rich NM, Hobson RW, II: Carotid endarterectomy under regional anesthesia. Am Surg 41:253–259, 1975
3. Yared I, Martinis AJ, Mack RM: Carotid endarterectomy under local anesthesia: a retrospective study. Am Surg 45:709–714, 1979
4. Imparato AM, Ramirez A, Riles T, Mintzer R: Cerebral protection in carotid surgery. Arch Surg 117:1073–1078, 1982
5. Bosiljevac JE, Farha SJ: Carotid endarterectomy: results using regional anesthesia. Am Surg 46:403–408, 1980
6. Gabelman CG, Gann DS, Ashworth CJ, Jr., Carney WI, Jr: One hundred consec-

utive carotid reconstructions: local versus general anesthesia. Am J Surg 145:477–482, 1983

7. Kwaan JHM, Peterson GJ, Connolly JE: Stump pressure. An unreliable guide for shunting during carotid endarterectomy. Arch Surg 115:1083–1085, 1980

8. Whittemore AD: Carotid endarterectomy. An alternative approach. Arch Surg 115:940–942, 1980

9. Levin BH, Schanno JF: Local anesthesia: serious consideration for extracranial carotid artery surgery. Am Surg 46:174–179, 1980

10. Peitzman AB, Webster MW, Loubeau J-M et al: Carotid endarterectomy under regional (conductive) anesthesia. Ann Surg 196:59–64, 1982

11. Nussmeier NA, Arlund C, Slogoff S: Neuropsychiatric complications after cardiopulmonary bypass: cerebral protection by a barbiturate. Anesthesiology 64:165–170, 1986

12. McKay RD, Sundt TM, Michenfelder JD et al: Internal carotid artery stump pressure and cerebral blood flow during carotid endarterectomy: modification by halothane, enflurane, and Innovar. Anesthesiology 45:390–399, 1976

13. Nehls DG, Todd MM, Spetzler RF et al: A comparison of the cerebral protective effects of isoflurane and barbiturates during temporary focal ischemia in primates. Anesthesiology 66:453–464, 1987

14. Messick JM, Jr., Casement B, Sharbrough FW et al: Correlation of regional cerebral blood flow (rCBF) with EEG changes during isoflurane anesthesia for carotid endarterectomy: critical rCBF. Anesthesiology 66:344–349, 1987

15. Boysen G, Engell HC, Henriksen H: The effect of induced hypertension on internal carotid artery pressure and regional cerebral blood flow during temporary carotid clamping for endarterectomy. Neurology 22:1133–1144, 1972

16. Sharbrough FW, Messick JM, Jr., Sundt TM, Jr: Correlation of continuous electroencephalograms with cerebral blood flow measurements during carotid endarterectomy. Stroke 4:674–683, 1973

17. Cucchiara RF, Messick JM: The failure of nasal plethysmography to estimate cerebral blood flow during carotid occlusion. Anesthesiology 55:585–586, 1981

18. Cucchiara RF, Sharbrough FW, Messick JM, Tinker JH: An electroencephalographic filter-processor as an indicator of cerebral ischemia during carotid endarterectomy. Anesthesiology 51:77–79, 1979

19. Tarlov E, Schmidek H, Scott RM et al: Reflex hypotension following carotid endarterectomy: mechanism and management. J Neurosurg 39:323–327, 1973

20. Wade JC, Larson CP, Jr., Hickey RF et al: Effect of carotid endarterectomy on carotid chemoreceptor and baroreceptor function in man. N Engl J Med 282:823–829, 1970

21. Michenfelder JD, Milde JH, Sundt TM, Jr: Cerebral protection by barbiturate anesthesia. Use after middle cerebral artery occlusion in Java monkeys. Arch Neurol 33:345–350, 1976

22. Michenfelder JD, Milde JH: Cerebral protection by anaesthetics during ischaemia (a review). Resuscitation 4:219–233, 1975

23. Michenfelder JD, Theye RA: Cerebral protection by thiopental during hypoxia. Anesthesiology 39:510–517, 1973

7

Anesthesia and Surgery for Cerebrovascular Insufficiency: One Approach at Stanford

C. Philip Larson, Jr

SURGICAL OPTIONS FOR CEREBROVASCULAR INSUFFICIENCY

Extracranial-to-Intracranial Bypass Surgery versus Carotid Endarterectomy

There are basically two types of operations for correction of cerebrovascular insufficiency: extracranial-to-intracranial (EC-IC) bypass surgery and carotid endarterectomy. The purpose of EC-IC bypass is augmentation of collateral circulation to a presumably ischemic focal area of the brain. However, indications for the use of EC-IC bypass remain unclear and controversial.[1] Current evidence suggests that this procedure does not lessen the severity of a stroke in evolution and does not significantly improve neurologic deficits from a completed stroke by enhancing flow to "border zones of ischemia."[1,2] Furthermore, a recent study did not describe favorable results with EC-IC bypass surgery.[3] Specifically, 1,377 patients with symptomatic atherosclerosis of the internal carotid or middle cerebral arteries were randomly assigned to receive either medical treatment or EC-IC bypass. Disability (in vision, speaking, toileting, and walking) was greater in the surgical group for the first 6 months after treatment. Also, at 6 months after operation, functional status was no better than for patients given medical treatment. Clearly, patients who had EC-IC bypass surgery had greater disability and long-term benefits that were no better than those achieved by medical therapy alone.

If EC-IC bypass has any application, it may be to prevent strokes in patients having transient ischemic attacks (TIAs) plus either bilateral carotid occlusion or severely stenotic lesions well above the carotid bifurcation. These conditions would not be amenable to extracranial surgery. However, before surgical anastomosis is undertaken, TIAs must be shown to be caused by inadequate blood flow and not embolism.

Because of these limitations, EC-IC bypass surgery is rarely performed at Stanford. For the occasional procedure that is performed, however, the principles of anesthetic management are the same as for carotid endarterectomy.

In contrast, carotid endarterectomy is a common operation at Stanford. Three distinct surgical groups perform this procedure: neurosurgeons, vascular surgeons, and cardiac surgeons. In general, their criteria for operation, the surgical techniques used, and patient outcome are similar. No doubt, subtle differences exist among surgical groups and individual surgeons in all three categories. Some of these differences may be important to outcome. However, of greater importance to the anesthetist is the fact that anesthetic management does not differ appreciably when working with any of these three surgical groups. Although an anesthetist may work with a variety of surgeons performing the same surgical procedure, the principles important to good anesthetic care remain the same.

The three surgical groups have a similar criterion for surgery, namely, the occurrence of TIAs caused by a stenotic or ulcerative lesion in the carotid system. In general, patients with asymptomatic carotid bruits are treated conservatively and are given medical therapy. Such therapy includes administration of drugs for hypertension; elimination of smoking; regulation of diet to lower serum triglyceride levels; and administration of drugs that impair platelet aggregation, such as aspirin. This conservative approach is supported by several studies demonstrating that the risk of stroke unheralded by a TIA is less than 2 percent in patients with asymptomatic carotid bruits.[4–6] Because the risk of a serious complication from carotid endarterectomy is at least 2 percent, our surgeons do not perform carotid endarterectomy for asymptomatic carotid bruits. Instead, they educate their patients regarding the symptoms of cerebral ischemia and observe those patients regularly for worsening of the disease. Then,

if TIAs occur, full evaluation and surgery are considered.

Before coming to operation, all patients undergo angiography to identify the type of lesion (ulcerative or stenotic), its exact location, and the extent of the collateral circulation. To circumvent the need for arterial catheterization, some surgeons use digital subtraction angiography (DSA) and resort to conventional angiography only if DSA images are unsatisfactory.

Concomitant Symptomatic Heart Disease

The one major difference among surgical groups relates to surgical management of the patient who has both cerebrovascular insufficiency and symptomatic coronary artery disease. Some cardiac surgeons perform carotid endarterectomy followed immediately by coronary artery bypass grafting. Others believe that the two procedures should be performed on separate occasions, thereby providing time for the patient to recover from endarterectomy before being subjected to cardiac surgery. I prefer the latter approach. I am primarily concerned that unknown and undiagnosed cerebral ischemia may develop during endarterectomy and that the periods of low blood pressure or flow at the beginning and end of cardiopulmonary bypass would then worsen such ischemia. Because no rigorous studies have compared these two surgical approaches, the issue remains unresolved.

Most surgeons performing carotid endarterectomies at Stanford routinely use an internal shunt during temporary occlusion of the carotid artery. Although use of a shunt certainly decreases the potential time for cerebral ischemia, it does not guarantee that focal ischemia will not occur from hypoperfusion or inadvertent embolization during surgery. Therefore, from the standpoint of anesthetic management, I believe the same precautions should be taken whether or not a shunt is used.

ANESTHETIC APPROACH TO CAROTID ENDARTERECTOMY

Preanesthetic Preparation

In addition to the usual measures taken in preoperative evaluation of any patient undergoing anesthesia and surgery, special considerations apply to patients having carotid endarterectomy. Most important among these is careful evaluation of cardiovascular status. Such evaluation includes a detailed history of cardiovascular function and serial determinations of blood pressure in both arms to establish the range of normal pressures and the possible existence of regional differences. If blood pressure differs in the two arms, I measure it during and after surgery in the arm having the higher values. I believe these higher values are better reflections of the pressures transmitted to the brain by unobstructed vessels before surgery and by the repaired vessel after surgery. I also consider a preoperative electrocardiogram (ECG) mandatory.

This concern about cardiovascular function relates to the need to regulate blood pressure artificially during endarterectomy. Often one must increase blood pressure as much as 20 percent above the highest resting pressure to maintain optimal collateral circulation during surgical occlusion of the carotid.[7] In addition, regulation of blood pressure is often necessary in the early postoperative period. Because the incidence of perioperative myocardial infarction is at least 1 percent in this surgical population, it seems only

prudent to be familiar with the patient's cardiovascular status when called on to regulate blood pressure.

Except in emergencies, we delay anesthesia and surgery if the patient has severe, uncontrolled hypertension, uncontrolled diabetes, or recent (within the last 3 months) myocardial infarction. We give antihypertensive medications up to the time of anesthesia.

The use of premedication in patients undergoing carotid endarterectomy is controversial. Some anesthetists believe that rather heavy premedication is mandatory to minimize the hypertensive response to anxiety and stress that may accompany preparation for and induction of anesthesia. In my opinion, premedication is unnecessary in most endarterectomy patients and may even be harmful. If a patient has a new TIA or stroke immediately before surgery, its signs may be difficult to distinguish from those associated with excessive responses to premediation. I have found that detailed discussion about the anesthetic and surgical plan, with appropriate reassurance, is usually enough to allay anxiety in patients of this age group.

If medication is desired, small doses of sedative-hypnotics such as flurazepam (15 to 30 mg) or diazepam (5 to 10 mg) are preferable to opiates, because the former depress the central nervous system to a lesser degree. If one desires to give glycopyrrolate, this agent may be given as premedication or administered just before the start of anesthesia.

Propranolol (1 to 2 mg/kg, given orally in divided doses in the 12-hour period before anesthesia) may enhance cardiovascular stability during induction of anesthesia and placement of the endotracheal tube.[8] Presumably, propranolol also lessens reflex tachycardia, should it become necessary to administer vasodilating drugs during or after operation. In my experience, tachycardia does not necessarily develop during induction, intubation, or administration of a vasodilating drug. Therefore, I generally do not administer propranolol or any other β-adrenergic receptor-blocking drug preoperatively but, instead, wait until the need is clear. The rapid action of intravenously administered propranolol makes it a good drug for quick control of heart rate if tachycardia occurs.[9]

Management in the Operating Room

Monitors

In my view, monitoring of arterial blood pressure directly from a cannula placed in a radial or other convenient artery is essential for detecting sudden and marked fluctuations in blood pressure that necessitate hypertensive or hypotensive drug therapy, as well as for analysis of blood gas levels. If surgery is performed with the patient in the semiseated position, the transducer should be placed at the level of the head rather than the heart. This level is used because cerebral perfusion pressure, which is of primary concern during this operation, is estimated by subtracting intracranial pressure from arterial blood pressure at the level of the brain.

A central venous pressure catheter is very useful in virtually all patients undergoing carotid endarterectomy, both for monitoring the adequacy of fluid therapy and for administering vasoactive drugs quickly and safely. Although several sites for insertion are available in the arm and groin, I strongly prefer either the internal or external jugular or subclavian approaches. The main reason for this preference is that these sites permit insertion of a short catheter with minimal dead space. The longer arm or leg catheters act as a reservoir for whatever is being infused through the catheter, thereby making it more difficult to effect

rapid changes in the actions of vasoactive drugs. Of course, if a neck site is chosen, the catheter should be placed on the side opposite the operative field. Efforts should be made to avoid puncture of the nonoperative carotid artery during identification of the internal jugular vein. If inadvertent puncture does occur, I believe that several minutes of light pressure at the puncture site while the patient is still awake would be a safe procedure.

Additional monitoring aids used routinely for carotid endarterectomy include an ECG (preferably using the modified V_5 precordial lead so that potential myocardial ischemia during and after operation can be detected more readily), an esophageal stethoscope, and body temperature. Two additional monitors that are extremely valuable in patients undergoing carotid endarterectomy are a pulse oximeter and an infrared carbon dioxide analyzer. The pulse oximeter gives a continuous readout of peripheral oxygen saturation (and pulse rate), data that help ensure adequate oxygenation during anesthesia. Once correlated with a simultaneously drawn arterial blood gas sample, the end-tidal carbon dioxide analyzer provides a continuous determination of arterial carbon dioxide levels. In addition, we commonly monitor the electroencephalogram (EEG) during anesthesia and surgery (see below).

Choice of Anesthetic Drugs

In my view, there are three special objectives of anesthesia for carotid endarterectomy: to maintain optimal cerebral perfusion pressure during and after surgery; to minimize the metabolic rate of cerebral oxygen consumption in potentially ischemic areas of the brain during temporary occlusion of the carotid artery; and to render the patient responsive to gross evaluation of neurologic function soon after surgery. A combination of anesthetic drugs is needed to accomplish these goals, as no one agent has all of the desired properties. I believe the two key anesthetic drugs are thiopental and a low-dose volatile anesthetic (either isoflurane or halothane). Additional anesthetic drugs that are useful in most of these patients include an opiate and a muscle relaxant of moderate duration of action.

The principal advantage of thiopental is its demonstrated ability to protect the brain from focal ischemia.[10-13] These studies and others confirm that thiopental lessens the severity of brain damage when focal areas of the brain are subjected to ischemia from either embolism or hypoperfusion. Because either of these conditions may occur without warning during carotid endarterectomy, I believe it is highly desirable to incorporate thiopental into the anesthetic management. How thiopental protects the brain from focal ischemia is not entirely clear, but at least two mechanisms are likely. First, thiopental decreases cerebral metabolic oxygen consumption; it is the most potent of all anesthetic drugs in this regard. Decreasing cerebral oxygen requirement at a time when cerebral flow may be impaired (either from temporary occlusion of the carotid artery or from embolization of plaque material during endarterectomy) may prevent or limit the severity of ischemic damage. Second, thiopental is a potent cerebral vasoconstrictor, a pharmacologic property that is often forgotten. The vasoconstrictive action of thiopental affects only normally reactive cerebral vessels. Therefore, if focal cerebral ischemia occurs, cerebral blood flow would be preferentially diverted from normal areas of brain (in which thiopental vasoconstriction would be occurring) to potentially ischemic areas of the brain (in which vasodilation from focal acidosis would be overriding the effect of thiopental). In essence, thiopental and hypocarbia produce similar results: they both cause a preferential diversion of blood flow from areas of normal blood flow to areas of potential ischemia.

The use of low-dose (1 MAC (minimum anesthetic concentration of anesthesia at 1 atm that keeps 50% of patients from moving when exposed to a noxious stimuli) or less) isoflurane or halothane provides adequate but rapidly reversible surgical anesthesia that permits early postoperative neurologic evaluation. When halothane or isoflurane is used in low doses and in combination with thiopental and hypocarbia, the potential deleterious effects of these drugs—namely, cerebral vasodilation and loss of cerebral autoregulation—are minimized.[14,15] Whether either agent is preferable is uncertain. Unlike thiopental, halothane does not protect the brain from focal cerebral ischemia.[10] Whether isoflurane protects the brain from focal cerebral ischemia during carotid occlusion remains in doubt.[16] However, Messick and colleagues[17] report that the regional cerebral blood flow associated with abnormalities on EEG (what they call "critical rCBF") is lower with isoflurane than with halothane in patients undergoing carotid endarterectomy. Critical rCBF was less than 10 ml/min per 100 g of brain tissue in patients anesthetized with isoflurane. In contrast, an earlier study had reported critical rCBF of 18 to 20 ml/min per 100 g of brain tissue in patients anesthetized with halothane.[18] These results suggest that isoflurane is preferable to halothane for patients undergoing carotid endarterectomy. However, at an inspired concentration of 0.6 percent or less, the choice may be immaterial.

My typical routine for induction and maintenance of anesthesia in elderly patients undergoing carotid endarterectomy is as follows. After placement of the appropriate arterial and venous catheters and monitors, and after preoxygenation, I induce anesthesia with meperidine (1.0 to 1.5 mg/kg) and thiopental (5 to 10 mg/kg), in divided doses, to allow for assessment of cardiovascular responses. In my view, meperidine is preferable to fentanyl citrate because the duration of action of meperidine matches the length of operation to a better degree, and because it costs less. The use of meperidine in this dose range smoothes both induction of anesthesia and, more important, recovery from anesthesia. When the patient loses consciousness, I administer a combination of muscle relaxants, which is called, for want of a better name, "Curalon." This 10-ml mixture consists of 7 ml of d-tubocurarine (2.1 mg/ml) and 3 ml of pancuronium bromide (0.3 mg/ml) and is usually given in doses of 6 to 10 ml. "Curalon" produces neuromuscular blockade as quickly, and perhaps even more quickly, than does either drug alone. More important, it does not cause hypotension or tachycardia, which either muscle relaxant may do when used alone in equipotent doses. Generally, no additional dose of muscle relaxant is needed.

After endotracheal intubation, I add isoflurane or halothane, at a concentration of approximately 1 MAC, to the inspired gas mixture. Sixty percent nitrous oxide may or may not be used, depending on cardiovascular and pulmonary function. Several minutes before occlusion of the carotid artery, I gradually administer an additional dose of thiopental, 5 to 10 mg/kg, the total dose generally not exceeding 15 mg/kg.

Control of Ventilation

Ventilation is controlled with a mechanical ventilator from the end of induction until the wound is closed. Tidal volume and frequency are adjusted so that arterial carbon dioxide partial pressure ($PaCO_2$) ranges from 25 to 30 mmHg. Although some authorities advocate that $PaCO_2$ be kept at the normal value,[19] I believe there is no real basis for that view. In contrast, maintenance of hypocarbia has two potential advantages: it causes a preferential diversion of cerebral blood flow to potentially ischemic areas of the brain by constriction of nonischemic, normally reactive vessels, and it may decrease anesthetic requirement. In my opinion, any possible hazards of this level of hypocarbia are either managed easily or strictly theoretical in nature. For example, the decrease in cardiac output that may occur is managed readily by fluid therapy or administration of a lower dose of volatile anesthetic. The leftward shift in the oxyhemoglobin dissociation curve and the increase in ventilation-perfusion abnormality are of theoretical but not clinical interest. Last, there is no evidence that this level of hypocarbia exacerbates the adverse metabolic effects of cerebral ischemia.

Control of Blood Pressure

Regulation of blood pressure is one of the most critical processes controlled by the anesthetist during carotid endarterectomy. It is highly desirable to keep systemic blood pressure at, or up to, 20 percent above the patient's highest recorded resting pressure while awake. The reason for this is that temporary occlusion of the carotid system during surgery often decreases distal perfusion pressure (stump pressure) below that required for maintenance of autoregulation (60 mmHg). Also, the use of volatile agents such as halothane may impair autoregulation to some degree. The consequences of these effects are that cerebral blood flow distal to the surgical clamp or via collateral channels may be pressure dependent. Therefore, the higher the pressure, the more likely it is that cerebral perfusion will be adequate during surgical occlusion. I prefer administering an agent that stimulates only α-adrenergic receptors (e.g., phenylephrine) to support blood pressure because such drugs have minimal potential for producing dysrhythmias. A dilution of 10 mg in 250 ml of 5 percent dextrose in water is infused as needed with a microdrip infusion set and flow regulator. Monitoring of the modified V_5 lead of the ECG usually can help indicate whether the increase in blood pressure is causing myocardial ischemia.

If hypertension occurs during operation and the dose of anesthetic is deemed adequate (as judged from the quantities administered and the clinical response of the patient), I administer sodium nitroprusside by microdrip infusion. I prefer this hypotensive agent to trimethaphan camsylate or nitroglycerin because of its prompt and controllable action. Also, sodium nitroprusside does not cause tachyphylaxis.

Fluid Therapy

In general, I try to limit the total volume of crystalloid fluid administered throughout surgery to 10 to 15 ml/kg. The choice of crystalloid probably does not matter as long as it does not contain dextrose. Recent studies in animals indicate that increased blood glucose levels may decrease the tolerance of the brain to global ischemia.[20] However, a recent study on cats in our laboratory indicates that glucose may have the opposite effect in focal cerebral ischemia.[21] That is, it may protect ischemic brain from injury. Because glucose may have different effects on focal and global cerebral ischemia, the most prudent approach would be to limit the quantity of dextrose-containing solutions until more evidence is forthcoming. To maintain adequate circulating blood volume and urinary output, I give 6 percent hetastarch and blood replacement as needed. Because of its large molecular size, hetastarch remains in the vascular compartment longer than crystalloid fluids and can be administered in doses up to 20 ml/kg. I would not exceed this dose, because larger doses of hetastarch appear to cause a clotting disorder.[22]

Monitoring of the Adequacy of Cerebral Perfusion

Even if a shunt is used, monitoring of the adequacy of cerebral perfusion is desirable because periods of temporary occlusion of a major cerebral vessel are always necessary. In addition, sometimes a shunt cannot be used because of the location of the stenotic or ulcerative lesion. The most informative data are measurements of regional cerebral blood flow by using the washout of a radioisotope such as xenon 133 after its injection into a surgically occluded carotid artery. Flows above 24 ml/min per 100 g of brain tissue are regarded as satisfactory, whereas those below 18 ml/min indicate the potential for cerebral ischemia. Although it would be ideal to measure regional cerebral blood flow in the operating room, we do not have the expensive and highly technical equipment necessary to do so.

A more widely used method is measurement of responses on the EEG. The development of spectral-compression electroencephalographic techniques has made on-line assessment of cerebral perfusion possible. Various new instruments permit computerized analysis of the EEG in the operating room by the anesthetist. If focal ischemia were to occur, the expected changes on the EEG would be a decrease in frequency or amplitude, or both, of the waveform. However, it is important to recognize that electroencephalographic monitoring is not a perfect process and that it may give false-positive or false-negative results. For example, because the EEG usually does not change until severe cerebral ischemia occurs, changes on EEG are not good prodromal indicators of ischemia. Also, the EEG may not identify small focal areas of ischemia, the most likely event during carotid endarterectomy. Finally, a "worsening" of the EEG during operation, with no change in anesthetic state, does not necessarily mean that neurologic injury has occurred. Despite its shortcomings, we use the EEG routinely during carotid endarterectomy.

Stump pressure (mean blood pressure distal to the carotid clamp; also sometimes called back pressure) is used by many to evaluate the adequacy of cerebral perfusion during carotid surgery. Cerebral ischemia rarely occurs at stump pressures above 60 mmHg because of the excellent collateral circulation required to maintain that pressure. As stump pressure decreases below that value, the risk of ischemia increases. However, because pressure is not identical to flow, it is possible for stump pressure to be less than 60 mmHg while blood flow is perfectly adequate. The major criticism of using stump pressure as an indicator of cerebral perfusion is that it is not always accurate. Stump pressure may be less than 60 mmHg while regional cerebral blood flow is more than 24 ml/min per 100 g of brain tissue. Because this situation occurs in approximately 30 percent of patients,[23] judging cerebral perfusion by stump pressure alone would often result in placement of a shunt when none is needed. However, the simplicity of the measurement and its validity when pressure exceeds 60 mmHg make stump pressure still the most useful clinical method for ensuring adequate perfusion during carotid endarterectomy.

Most of our surgeons have little interest in any form of monitoring of cerebral perfusion during endarterectomy, relying entirely on a surgical shunt or skillful general anesthesia and short occlusion times. Review of the literature indicates that this is not an unreasonable or cavalier approach.[24]

Management of Anticoagulation

When the carotid vessels have been exposed and the surgeons are ready to occlude the carotid artery, the anesthetist administers 10 mg of heparin (1,000 units/

mg) intravenously. After endarterectomy is completed and before the wound is closed, 50 mg of protamine sulfate is administered slowly over 10 minutes to partially reverse the effect of heparin. Complete reversal is not generally desired, as our surgeons believe that partial anticoagulation in the postoperative period lessens the chance of thrombus formation at the surgical site.

POSTOPERATIVE COMPLICATIONS

The most important postoperative complications after carotid endarterectomy are circulatory instability with or without myocardial infarction, loss of carotid body function, respiratory insufficiency, and stroke. Circulatory instability in the form of either hypotension or hypertension is common after this operation. We found that hypotension or hypertension (defined as a change in systolic blood pressure of more than 40 mmHg from the patient's resting pressure) occurred in 47 of 100 patients after endarterectomy.[25] Although the mechanism for hypotension is not known, a variety of factors may contribute to its occurrence: hypovolemia, depression of circulation by anesthetics or other drugs, dysrhthmias, or excessive reflex response after exposure of the baroreceptor mechanism to a new, higher pressure.

The most convincing hypothesis regarding the cause of hypertension is loss of the normal carotid baroreceptor mechanism as a result of the operation. The carotid sinus is an integral part of the anatomy of the carotid bifurcation. In the dog, clamping above and below the sinus or denervation of the sinus causes persistent, fluctuant hypertension. Using the standard Valsalva test to evaluate the baroreceptor reflex in patients before and after carotid endarterectomy, we found that the reflex was outside the normal range before surgery and that it was further depressed by the operation.[25] It is well known from animal studies that the carotid baroreceptor is a fragile structure easily damaged by surgery in the area.

Potential complications from failure to control hypertension include excessive bleeding at the operative site, increased myocardial oxygen consumption or arrhythmias and myocardial infarction, intracerebral hemorrhage, and increased intracranial pressure from cerebral edema. We commonly find it necessary to administer sodium nitroprusside, often in combination with propranolol, to control heart rate postoperatively and to keep blood pressure in the desired range. Much less often, but on occasion, mild blood pressure support with phenylephrine is needed. However, before resorting to vasoconstrictive therapy, the anesthetist must make certain that intravascular volume is adequate.

Of equal importance to the loss of carotid baroreceptor function is the loss of carotid body function after carotid endarterectomy. We demonstrated that chemoreceptor function ceases in most patients after this operation, as evidenced by loss of ventilatory and circulatory responses to hypoxia and a modest increase in resting $PaCO_2$.[25] The loss may be temporary or permanent and represents a potentially serious hazard to the patient. Anesthetists must be aware of this and avoid or obviate situations known to provoke hypoxemia. I recommend that these patients be given augmented concentrations of oxygen to breathe postoperatively until they are fully conscious. Furthermore, special attention must be directed toward preventing serious atelectasis or other pulmonary or circulatory abnormalities that might cause arterial hypoxemia. The response to these adverse conditions would be further respiratory and circulatory depression, loss of consciousness, and death.

Acute respiratory insufficiency may occur soon after surgery because of hematoma formation with tracheal deviation, vocal cord paralysis from surgical traction on laryngeal nerves, or tension pneumothorax from dissection of air through the wound into the mediastinum and pleural space. Unexpected respiratory distress should bring these three possibilities immediately to mind. In general, a hematoma that causes respiratory distress should be evacuated before endotracheal intubation is attempted. Likewise, tension pneumothorax should be relieved immediately by needle evacuation if there is evidence of circulatory insufficiency.

At centers where carotid endarterectomy is commonly performed, the incidence of perioperative stroke is 3 percent or less.[24] If a patient emerges from anesthesia for carotid endarterectomy with a new neurologic deficit, immediate cerebral angiography should be performed to determine whether an intimal flap has formed at the site of operation. This flap is a surgically correctable lesion if operated upon immediately, and the severity of the subsequent neurologic deficit from the flap may be lessened. Postoperative myocardial infarction occurs in about 1 percent of patients. This figure is not surprising, considering that atherosclerosis is a generalized vascular disease involving the coronary as well as the cerebral circulation. The overall mortality from carotid endarterectomy, including angiography, is less than 3 percent at centers where this operation is commonplace.[24]

SUMMARY

Because carotid stenosis and ulceration are primarily diseases of the elderly, carotid endarterectomy will be performed with increasing frequency in the coming years. The routine use of an internal shunt by the surgeon does not obviate the need for the type of anesthetic management that maximizes protection from cerebral ischemia. I believe that the goals of anesthetic management should be to optimize cerebral perfusion pressure, to minimize cerebral oxygen requirement during temporary occlusion of the carotid artery, and to render the patient responsive to neurologic evaluation at the end of surgery. The anesthetics most effective in accomplishing these goals are thiopental, because of its ability to protect the brain from focal ischemia, and low-dose isoflurane or halothane, because of their ability to provide reversible surgical anesthesia. In may view, the critical variables to monitor during carotid endarterectomy are arterial blood pressure and end-tidal carbon dioxide tension. The EEG, while interesting, is not essential to anesthetic management. Both during and after surgery, I keep blood pressure at, or up to, 20 percent above the patient's usual pressure. I do so by administering phenylephrine or sodium nitroprusside and light anesthesia as needed. The most important complications after carotid endarterectomy are circulatory instability with or without myocardial infarction, loss of carotid chemoreceptor and baroreceptor function, respiratory insufficiency, and stroke.

REFERENCES

1. EC-IC Bypass Study Group: Failure of extracranial-intracranial arterial bypass to reduce the risk of ischemic stroke. Results of an international randomized trial. N Engl J Med 313:1191–1200, 1985

2. Samson DS, Boone S: Extracranial-intracranial (EC-IC) arterial bypass. Past performance and current concepts. Neurosurgery 3:79–86, 1978

3. Haynes RB, Mukherjee J, Sackett DL et al: Functional status changes following medical or surgical treatment for cerebral ischemia. Results of the Extracranial-Intracranial Bypass Study. JAMA 257:2043–2046, 1987

4. Chamber BR, Norris JW: Outcome in patients with asymptomatic neck bruits. N Engl J Med 315:860–865, 1986

5. Hennerici M, Rautenberg W, Mohr S: Stroke risk from symptomless extracranial arterial disease. Lancet 2:1180–1183, 1982

6. Ford CS, Frye JL, Toole JF, Lefkowitz D: Asymptomatic carotid bruit and stenosis. A prospective follow-up study. Arch Neurol 43:219–222, 1986

7. Ehrenfeld WK, Hamilton FN, Larson CP et al: Effect of CO_2 and systemic hypertension on downstream cerebral arterial pressure during carotid endarterectomy. Surgery 67:87–96, 1970

8. Prys-Roberts C, Foëx P, Biro GP, Roberts JG: Studies of anaesthesia in relation to hypertension. V. Adrenergic beta-receptor blockade. Br J Anaesth 45:671–681, 1973

9. Safwat AM, Reitan JA, Misle GR, Hurley EJ: Use of propranolol to control rate-pressure product during cardiac anesthesia. Anesth Analg 60:732–735, 1981

10. Smith AL, Hoff JT, Nielsen SL, Larson CP: Barbiturate protection in acute focal cerebral ischemia. Stroke 5:1–7, 1974

11. Hoff JT, Smith AL, Hankinson HL, Nielsen SL: Barbiturate protection from cerebral infarction in primates. Stroke 6:28–33, 1975

12. Michenfelder JD, Milde JH, Sundt TM, Jr: Cerebral protection by barbiturate anesthesia. Use of middle cerebral artery occlusion in Java monkeys. Arch Neurol 33:345–350, 1976

13. Nussmeier NA, Arlund C, Slogoff S: Neuropsychiatric complications after cardiopulmonary bypass: cerebral protection by a barbiturate. Anesthesiology 64:165–170, 1986

14. Adams RW, Gronert GA, Sundt TM, Jr., Michenfelder JD: Halothane, hypocapnia, and cerebrospinal fluid pressure in neurosurgery. Anesthesiology 37:510–517, 1972

15. Adams RW, Cucchiara RF, Gronert GA, Messick JM, Michenfelder JD: Isoflurane and cerebrospinal fluid pressure in neurosurgical patients. Anesthesiology 54:97–99, 1981

16. Nehls DG, Todd MM, Spetzler RF et al: A comparison of the cerebral protective effects of isoflurane and barbiturates during temporary focal ischemia in primates. Anesthesiology 66:453–464, 1987

17. Messick JM, Jr., Casement B, Sharbrough FW et al: Correlation of regional cerebral blood flow (rCBF) with EEG changes during isoflurane anesthesia for carotid endarterectomy: critical rCBF. Anesthesiology 66:344–349, 1987

18. Sharbrough FE, Messick JM, Jr., Sundt TM, Jr: Correlation of continuous electroencephalograms with cerebral blood flow measurements during carotid endarterectomy. Stroke 4:674–683, 1973

19. Marshall K: Carotid artery surgery: perioperative considerations. p. 1–6. 1985 ASA Refresher Course Lectures, no. 113. American Society of Anesthesiologists, Park Ridge, IL, 1985

20. Lanier WL, Stangland KJ, Scheithauer BW et al: The effects of dextrose infusion and head position on neurologic outcome after complete cerebral ischemia in primates: examination of a model. Anesthesiology 66:39–48, 1987

21. Zasslow MA, Pearl RG, Shuer LM, Steinberg GK, Lieberson RE, Larson CP: Hyperglycemia decreases acute neuronal ischemic changed after middle cerebral artery occlusion in cats. Stroke 20:519–523, 1989

22. Cully MD, Larson CP, Jr., Silverberg GD: Hetastarch coagulopathy in a neurosurgical patient (correspondence). Anesthesiology 66:706–707, 1987

23. McKay RD, Sundt TM, Michenfelder JD et al: Internal carotid artery stump pressure and cerebral blood flow during carotid endarterectomy: modification by halothane, enflurane, and Innovar. Anesthesiology 45:390–399, 1976

24. Ferguson GG: Intra-operative monitoring and internal shunts: are they necessary in carotid enderterectomy [sic] (editorial)? Stroke 13:287–289, 1982

25. Wade JG, Larson CP, Jr., Hickey RF et al: Effect of carotid endarterectomy on carotid chemoreceptor and baroreceptor function in man. N Engl J Med 282:823–829, 1970

8

Anesthesia for Emergency Surgery for Cerebrovascular Insufficiency

Michael F. Roizen

Recent data indicate that the reluctance to perform emergency carotid endarterectomy on patients who have fluctuating neurologic deficits may be unwarranted.[1,2] Therefore, in the future, anesthetists may be seeing more patients who have crescendo transient ischemic attacks or strokes in evolution and who are therefore candidates for emergency carotid revascularization. A full explication of the risk-benefit ratio for such emergency carotid revascularizations can be found in Chapter 1. Conditions indicating the need for emergency surgery include tight (greater than 95 percent) stenosis with or without symptoms, symptomatic occlusion within 6 to 10 hours of the onset of occlusion, and recent carotid endarterectomy that has either bled or produced new neurologic symptoms.

PREOPERATIVE PREPARATION

Because a patient undergoing emergency carotid endarterectomy may have a full stomach and thus require protection against aspiration of gastric contents, rapid-sequence induction of anesthesia is used. My main goal is to minimize the hemodynamic stress of rapid-sequence induction while maintaining adequate perfusion pressure across the stenotic lesion. Because patients undergoing emergency carotid endarterectomy have medical problems similar to those of patients undergoing elective carotid revascularizations, much of the following text repeats material discussed in Chapter 5. Such material is presented here, however, for the sake of completeness, and to spare the reader the inconvenience of having to refer frequently to Chapter 5.

At our institution, surgeons prefer general anesthesia for emergency surgery for cerebrovascular insufficiency. Therefore, the preoperative visit does not need to concern itself with choice of general versus regional anesthesia. If the patient has no medical problem needing optimization before surgery, my preoperative interview focuses on reducing anxiety and determining the status of end organs likely to be affected by atherosclerosis, hypertension, and other diseases. Clearly, in emergency circumstances, this process can take only 90 seconds rather than the usual 10 to 15 minutes. At this time, I also obtain informed consent.

147

In addition, I examine the range of readings on the multiple blood pressure and heart rate determinations that the patient has undergone. If surgery has not been scheduled for 4 or more hours (as is sometimes the case in tight carotid stenosis without current symptoms), I ask the nurses to obtain a least four more readings of blood pressure and heart rate before surgery. From this preoperative information, I derive an individualized set of values for each patient. I then try to keep cardiovascular variables within that range during surgery. Prior to induction of anesthesia, I plan what therapies to use to accomplish that goal (e.g., administration of more or less anesthesia; nitroglycerin; nitroprusside/dopamine; dobutamine; phenylephrine; or propranolol/esmolol/isoproterenol or atropine). Clearly, in the patient with fluctuating neurologic symptoms or with tight stenosis, the lore and practice is to keep blood pressure at the upper end of ward pressure, or slightly above. My practice is to obtain this level of blood pressure (or allow it to occur) but to avoid increasing heart rate, as I believed aggressive control of heart rate is important in preventing myocardial ischemia.[3]

In my view, this type of planning is especially important for the patient who has suspected cardiovascular disease (which is usual in patients undergoing carotid endarterectomy) but relatively unimportant for the totally healthy patient. I do not know for certain that keeping cardiovascular variables within an individualized range of acceptable values improves surgical outcome, but I do believe that using such a plan reduces morbidity. I keep the acceptable values in mind during surgery by listing them at the top of my anesthesia record before induction.

The desire to keep blood pressure elevated in patients who have fluctuating neurologic symptoms is based on data indicating that collateral cerebral blood flow distal to a carotid occlusion is greater if systemic blood pressure is higher.[4] On the other hand, an increase in blood pressure increases the work of the heart and, thus, the likelihood of myocardial ischemia.[5,6]

I tend to avoid using pulmonary artery catheters for carotid surgery for several reasons. First, there are few fluid shifts during these operations. Also, at our institution, the rate of complications from pulmonary artery lines exceeds the rate from carotid surgery. In addition, taking the 10 to 15 minutes that insertion of a pulmonary artery line requires is often not feasible in an emergency situation. Only when myocardial ischemia has been indicated by changes in pulmonary capillary wedge pressure without accompanying changes on the electrocardiogram (ECG) have I used a pulmonary artery catheter during carotid surgery. In my practice, this has happened only twice among approximately 1,500 patients anesthetized for carotid surgery.

During the preoperative assessment, I also try to ascertain which electrocardiographic lead is most likely to reveal ischemia (often found on an exercise ECG study or from a "best guess" on a thallium redistribution study) and the value of the patient's normal carbon dioxide level. Usually, the latter can be assumed to be normal if the patient's bicarbonate level on an electrolyte panel is normal or if the patient does not have a history suggestive of chronic obstructive pulmonary disease.

Anesthetists at our institution traditionally have not premedicated patients about to undergo carotid surgery, as our surgeons believe premedication delays awakening and may confuse preoperative tests of mental function (see Ch. 5). These concerns are even more applicable regarding patients scheduled for emergency carotid revascularization.

Thus, local custom and logical considerations have persuaded me to set the following goals and to use the following techniques goals when treating patients undergoing emergency cerebrovascular surgery.

(1) Avoid cerebral ischemia by maintaining high-normal or slightly elevated blood pressure and by shunting carotid flow if abnormalities on the electroencephalogram (EEG) occur. I also keep the patient in a slightly hypocarbic state.

(2) Avoid myocardial ischemia by maintaining normal heart rates. For this purpose, I usually monitor lead V_5 and lead II of the ECG for changes in heart rate and in the ST segment. I monitor the transesophageal echocardiogram for abnormalities in wall motion and thickening.

(3) Use general anesthesia but have the patient awake at the end of the operation. To accomplish this, I avoid premedication with drugs and "premedicate" (allay anxiety) only by interview. I use light levels of volatile agents for general anesthesia.

When these goals are at odds with one another, study results can guide effective modification of goals and methods. For example, I could provide deeper levels of anesthesia and mantain blood pressure with an α-adrenergic drug such as phenylephrine. However, I have found that light anesthesia at a particular systolic pressure incurs only one-third the incidence of myocardial ischemia as that incurred with deep levels of anesthesia and the use of vasopressors to attain that same blood pressure.[5] The usual procedure for providing light general anesthesia is as follows.

As soon as possible, I begin an intravenous infusion of normal saline through an 18-gauge plastic cannula. If the operation is not to be performed immediately, infusion is begun before the patient is transported to the operating room. Fluid administration helps ensure that the patient is not hypovolemic and thus subject to large decreases in blood pressure dur-

ing induction of anesthesia. I use an 18-gauge arterial line rather than a 20-gauge line because no greater morbidity ensues with the larger catheter[7]; also, the smaller 20-gauge line tends to incur a 5 to 10 percent incidence of kinking when our surgeons push on the arm with their bellies during carotid dissection. I use normal saline rather than dextrose or lactated Ringer's solution because lactate is metabolized to dextrose. In addition, animal studies indicate that increasing blood glucose may increase neurologic damage after global ischemia.[8] Although at least one laboratory has reported different results regarding focal central nervous system ischemia,[9] and some investigators report that survival is better with fructose than with saline,[10] I believe that the most prudent approach at this time is to maintain normoglycemia.

As in elective situations, I like to transfer the patient to an operating table covered by a heating blanket that has been warmed prior to induction of anesthesia. The heating mattress, I believe (with some evidence),[11] is important for maintaining normothermia, which probably helps to reduce circulatory instability after surgery.

INDUCTION OF ANESTHESIA

Patients who are brought immediately to the operating room are allowed to breathe 100 percent oxygen. Venous access is secured, and peripheral arterial cannulation is performed for direct monitoring of systemic blood pressure and obtaining of blood samples for determination of gas tensions. I then proceed with a rapid-sequence intravenous induction using a short-acting barbiturate, a muscle relaxant, and endotracheal intubation. Before intubation, a bolus of lidocaine

(1.5 mg/kg) or sodium nitroprusside (1 to 2 μg/kg) may be administered intravenously for attenuation of the hypertensive response to visualization of the larynx and tracheal intubation. Hypotension is treated by tilting the table or with intravenous infusion of phenylephrine or methoxamine (direct α-adrenergic agonists). If a pulmonary artery catheter is desired, a peripheral brachial or subclavian vein contralateral to the operative side can be used as the site of insertion. However, few circumstances appear to warrant use of a pulmonary artery catheter in the patient undergoing emergency exploration of the carotid artery.

When the patient is believed to have an empty stomach, gentle titration of anesthesia with a barbiturate, followed by inhalation of increasing concentrations of volatile anesthetic, is often used to induce anesthesia.

If a hematoma is noted near the operative site and surgical exploration is anticipated, oxygen is given at high concentration by face mask with a reservoir bag or Ayre's T-piece. A tracheostomy or cricothyrotomy tray should be immediately available. Visualization of the trachea may be difficult because of edema or because pressure of the hematoma has caused deviation of the trachea away from the hematoma. In the event of acute airway obstruction, a high concentration of oxygen in the functional residual volume of the lung may provide additional protection against hypoxemia until the airway has been secured by intubation or the hematoma has been evacuated surgically.

If the hematoma does not obstruct the airway and the patient is not having difficulty breathing spontaneously, induction may be accomplished as in an elective procedure. If the airway appears obstructed, topical anesthesia for the lips, tongue, posterior pharynx, and epiglottis is provided. The larynx is then visualized.

If no difficulty with endotracheal intubation is anticipated, induction is performed as described above. However, if difficulty is expected, the wound is opened and drained externally, and endotracheal intubation is performed before general anesthesia is induced.

The role of nonparticulate antacids, histamine receptor-blocking drugs, and metoclopramide in preventing acid aspiration in patients with full stomachs remains controversial.

Why is induction usually begun with a barbiturate? Barbiturate-induced electrical burst suppression on the EEG is associated with reduction in cerebral metabolism to as little as 40 to 50 percent of awake levels and with a simultaneous decrease in cerebral blood flow and intracranial pressure. Once burst suppression occurs, barbiturates have no further effect on cerebral metabolism, or any effect in protecting the brain from ischemia.[12] Specifically, in the patient with an empty stomach I give 100 percent oxygen, thiopental (1 to 2 mg/kg), and 3 mg of d-tubocurarine. This is following by intravenous administration of thiopental (25 to 50 mg·min^{-1}·70 kg^{-1}), along with increasing concentrations of isoflurane in oxygen by mask. When systolic blood pressure has decreased 20 to 30 percent, and assuming the patient has no muscle or lower motor neuron dysfunction, I administer 1.5 mg/kg of succinylcholine or appropriate doses of atracurium or vecuronium. No muscle relaxants are given if muscle or lower motor neuron dysfunction exists. Either 100 mg of lidocaine or 100 mg of thiopental is given intravenously to blunt blood pressure and heart rate responses to laryngoscopy and tracheal intubation. After routine checks and verification of endotracheal intubation by end-tidal capnography, I insert a transesophageal echocardiographic probe to obtain cross-sectional images of the left ventricle at the level of the papillary muscles.

At this time, I institute controlled ventilation, often with 50 percent nitrous oxide in oxygen, and at other times with oxygen alone, titrating the concentration of isoflurane or enflurane and adjusting the table position to achieve the desired blood pressure. I usually avoid giving more than 10 ml of crystalloid or other fluid per kg of body weight in this 2-hour operation, as I believe (without good evidence) that increasing fluid administration to these patients contributes to postoperative hypertension. This effect may result from the absence of baroreceptor function such patients usually exhibit.[13] Lack of baroreceptor function may also account for the stability in heart rate we find in these patients during surgery.[5]

Controversy exists concerning the optimum intraoperative carbon dioxide level in patients undergoing carotid endarterectomy.[4] Most practitioners now opt for slight hypocarbia or normocarbia (see Chs. 6 & 7). Maintenance of a slightly hypocarbic state has the possible advantage of preferentially diverting cerebral blood flow to potentially ischemic areas of the brain by constricting the nonischemic, normally reactive vessels.

MAINTENANCE OF ANESTHESIA

During surgery, I usually employ light anesthesia, using patient movement and hemodynamic changes as indicators of inadequate anesthesia. If I cannot ensure that the patient will be anesthetized sufficiently to prevent movement during temporary occlusion of the carotid, I add a muscle relaxant, the choice of which would depend on the heart rate response I wish to obtain.

Although the effects of anesthetics on normal cerebral blood flow are known, no sound scientific basis appears to exist for choosing one anesthetic over another for cerebrovascular surgery. Perhaps the only information suggesting that one should select isoflurane over other inhalational agents or narcotics originates from a nonrandomized study at the Mayo Clinic.[14] In that study, the cerebral blood flow at which ischemic changes occurred on the EEG was only $10\,\mathrm{ml\cdot100\,g^{-1}\cdot min^{-1}}$ during isoflurane anesthesia but approximately $20\,\mathrm{ml\cdot100\,g^{-1}\cdot min^{-1}}$ with other agents. Also, the need to shunt was less frequent with isoflurane than with other agents.

My tendency to avoid narcotics in these operations is based on my desire to have patients awaken shortly after the last stitch is placed (although this may now be possible with alfentanil), and on the wish to avoid the hemodynamic effects of naloxone and muscle relaxant reversal. Avoidance of narcotics is not based on anecdotal reports that narcotics worsen neurologic outcome after focal or global cerebral ischemia.[15]

Before occluding the carotid, the surgeon infiltrates the carotid at the bifurcation with 1 percent lidocaine to prevent the sudden onset of bradycardia during stretching of the baroreceptor or of the nerve coming from the baroreceptor. Then, depth of anesthesia is kept at a minimum, so that blood pressure increases to the upper end of the ward level. If no evidence of ischemia occurs on the EEG, or if stump pressure (blood pressure in the carotid artery distal to the clamp) is comfortably above 50 mmHg, depth of anesthesia is increased somewhat, and systemic blood pressure falls slightly. If monitoring indicates the occurrence of myocardial ischemia, I treat the hemodynamic cause, if known, or administer nitroglycerin, if no obvious hemodynamic cause exists. In studies at our institution, 8 to 35 percent of the instances of myocardial ischemia occurred at this point in the operation.[5] I do not know why this event occurred at this particular time, as hemodynamic status did not differ substantially from that existing just before cross-clamping of the carotid.

After carotid repair has been completed and blood flow restored, the focus again shifts totally to the patient's myocardial well-being. When the muscle layer is being repaired, I allow the patient to resume spontaneous ventilation. Our surgeons usually identify the recurrent laryngeal nerve, which enables me to extubate the trachea in as light a plane of anesthesia as possible but before the gag reflex is restored (this point pertains to patients who have been judged to have an empty stomach). Usually within 2 to 3 minutes after the last stitch, the patient will respond to pain; before leaving the operating room (and generally within 4 to 6 minutes after the last stitch), the patient is able to follow simple commands. If the patient has been judged not to have an empty stomach preoperatively, I suction the stomach with a nasogastric tube, begin a titration of metoprolol or infusions of nitroprusside and esmolol, and wait until the patient is awake before extubating the trachea.

POSTOPERATIVE COMPLICATIONS

The four problems feared most in the recovery room are hemodynamic instability, respiratory insufficiency (usually caused by vocal cord paresis), hematoma formation, and onset of new neurologic dysfunction. These potential problems are discussed in detail in Chapter 5.

CONCLUSION

The most common causes of morbidity after emergency operations for cerebrovascular insufficiency probably differ from those after elective carotid endarterectomy. However, no large series has quantitated the relative risks of cerebrovascular versus myocardial ischemia in emergency operations. Nevertheless, logic plus data from the Mayo Clinic regarding surgery on patients with fluctuating neurologic deficit[16] dictate that, in emergency cerebrovascular surgery, preserving brain function is more important than protecting the heart from ischemia. As Chapter 5 explains, these priorities are reversed when carotid endarterectomy is performed on an elective basis. In addition, in emergency surgery, securing the airway rapidly and preventing aspiration must also be considered.

REFERENCES

1. Goldstone, J, Effeney DJ: The role of carotid endarterectomy in the treatment of acute neurologic deficits. Prog Cardiovasc Dis 22:415–422, 1980
2. Mentzer RM, Jr., Finkelmeier BA, Crosby IK, Wellons HA, Jr: Emergency carotid endarterectomy for fluctuating neurologic deficits. Surgery 89:60–66, 1981
3. Slogoff S, Keats AS: Further observations on perioperative myocardial ischemia. Anesthesiology 65:539–542, 1986
4. Ehrenfeld WK, Hamilton FN, Larson CP, Jr et al: Effect of CO_2 and systemic hypertension on downstream cerebral arterial pressure during carotid endarterectomy. Surgery 67:87–96, 1970
5. Smith JS, Roizen MF, Cahalan MK et al: Does anesthetic technique make a difference? Augmentation of systolic blood pressure during carotid endarterectomy: effects of phenylephrine *versus* light anesthesia and of isoflurane *versus* halothane on the incidence of myocardial ischemia. Anesthesiology 69:846–853, 1988
6. Hamilton WK: Do let the blood pressure drop and do use myocardial depressants! Anesthesiology 45:273–274, 1976

7. Bedford RF: Radial arterial function following percutaneous cannulation with 18- and 20-gauge catheters. Anesthesiology 47:37–39, 1977
8. Lanier WL, Stangland KJ, Scheithauer BW et al: The effects of dextrose infusion and head position on neurologic outcome after complete cerebral ischemia in primates: examination of a model. Anesthesiology 66:39–48, 1987
9. Pearl RG, Larson CP: Effect of hyperglycemia on neurologic outcome after focal ischemia. Stroke (in press)
10. Farias LA, Willis M, Gregory GA: Effects of fructose-1,6-diphosphate, glucose, and saline on cardiac resuscitation. Anesthesiology 65:595–601, 1986
11. Roizen MF, Sohn YJ, L'Hommedieu CS et al: Operating room temperature prior to surgical draping: effect on patient temperature in recovery room. Anesth Analg 59:852–855, 1980
12. Nehls DG, Todd MM, Spetzler RF et al: A comparison of the cerebral protective effects of isoflurane and barbiturates during temporary focal ischemia in primates. Anesthesiology 66:453–464, 1987
13. Wade JG, Larson CP, Jr., Hickey RF et al: Effect of carotid endarterectomy on carotid chemoreceptor and baroreceptor function in man. N Engl J Med 282:823–829, 1970
14. Messick JM, Jr., Casement B, Sharbrough FW et al: Correlation of regional cerebral blood flow (rCBF) with EEG changes during isoflurane anesthesia for carotid endarterectomy: critical rCBF. Anesthesiology 66:344–349, 1987
15. Hosobuchi Y, Baskin DS, Woo SK: Reversal of induced ischemic neurologic deficit in gerbils by the opiate antagonist naloxone. Science 215:69–71, 1981
16. Sundt TM, Jr., Sharbrough FW, Piepgras DG et al: Correlation of cerebral blood flow and electroencephalographic changes during carotid endarterectomy. With results of surgery and hemodynamics of cerebral ischemia. Mayo Clin Proc 56:533–543, 1981

Section III

SURGERY FOR VISCERAL ISCHEMIA AND SUPRARENAL AORTIC RECONSTRUCTION

9

Visceral Ischemia: Surgical Goals and Methods

Robert J. Lusby

CHARACTERISTICS OF VISCERAL ISCHEMIA

Visceral ischemia presents to the surgeon as gangrenous or pregangrenous bowel urgently requiring surgery, or as a syndrome characterized by chronic abdominal pain and weight loss.

Acute Mesenteric Occlusion

Patients with acute mesenteric occlusion present with severe abdominal pain but few other abdominal signs until infarction and peritonitis develop 4 to 6 hours later. Early diagnosis is often missed unless high clinical suspicion prompts immediate arteriography. Once massive bowel infarction occurs, the mortality rate soars to 85 to 100 percent.[1] If revascularization can be achieved early, the pregangrenous bowel may be saved and mortality rates reduced dramatically.[1] Even when overt intestinal gangrene is present in some areas, marginally ischemic bowel may still be salvageable in other areas and revascularization may be beneficial in limiting the extent of needed gut resection.

Chronic Visceral Ischemia

The recognition of chronic visceral ischemia as a cause of abdominal pain is credited to Dunphy,[2] who first described the condition in 1936. In 1957, Mikkelsen[3] applied the term intestinal angina to the dominant symptom. The syndrome consists of abdominal pain, frequently dull and aching, situated in the periumbilical and epigastric area. Pain usually starts 15 to 60 minutes after ingestion of food and lasts 1 to 4 hours. The resulting fear of eating leads to very restricted oral intake and often ingestion of only liquids. Weight loss, a product of poor intake rather than malabsorption, is usually marked, sometimes exceeding 15 percent of ideal body weight.[4] Nausea, vomiting, and changed of bowel habit may, but do not always, occur.[5]

Chronic visceral ischemia is four times more common in women than men, the mean age being 57 years.[6,7] Excessive cigarette smoking is a well-recognized risk factor.[4,8] No specific signs on physical examination distinguish patients with chronic visceral ischemia, and no single test is diagnostic. Inanition and malnutrition frequently produce malignant cachexia. Although signs of generalized

155

atherosclerosis with symptomatic cere-brovascular, cardiovascular, and periph-eral vascular disease are common, these conditions are not evident in young pa-tients who have arcuate ligament con-striction. An abdominal bruit is audible in approximately 87 percent of all pa-tients who have chronic visceral is-chemia.[4]

These patients are often symptomatic for extended periods, having extensive investigations of the upper and lower gas-trointestinal tract with normal findings before vascular disease is considered as a possible cause.[8,9] Although these tests are helpful in excluding other causes of abdominal pain and weight loss, diag-nosis depends on recognition of the spe-cific symptom complex and arterio-graphic demonstration of advanced splanchnic occlusive disease.

Most *symptomatic* visceral vascular disease involves narrowing of the origins of the three major blood vessels supply-ing the viscera—the celiac axis, the su-perior mesenteric artery, and the inferior mesenteric artery. Although angiography in the anteroposterior projection often fails to reveal the origins of these vessels, it sometimes shows the presence of a meandering mesenteric artery, a reliable sign of major occlusive disease of the ce-liac axis and superior mesenteric artery. A meandering mesenteric artery is the en-larged anastomotic channel between the middle colic and left colic arteries (i.e., between the superior mesenteric and in-ferior mesenteric arterial beds) (Fig. 9-1). This channel is also called the arc of Rio-lan, the artery of Gonzales, or the artery of Moskowitz. It is *not* the peripheral marginal artery of Drummond, which runs immediately adjacent to the colon and may also link the left and middle colic arterial systems. A lateral aortogram is needed to show the origins of the un-paired anterior aortic branches—the ce-

liac axis, the superior mesenteric artery, and the inferior mesenteric artery.

Atherosclerotic occlusion of stenosis of these vessels may be discovered during investigation of other arterial problems without any symptoms of mesenteric is-chemia being present.[10,11] That is, the ex-tensive collateral network of the gut is usually sufficient to provide adequate in-testinal blood supply (Fig. 9-2). In 1966, Morris et al.[12] were the first to suggest that occlusion or major stenosis of at least two of these three arteries was necessary to compromise the collateral supply and to produce symptoms of ischemia. This idea is currently accepted, and very few cases of symptomatic single-vessel le-sions have been reported in any series.[6,9] Single-vessel lesions become important when previous intraabdominal surgery has interrupted the collateral pathways.

The surgeon operating on patients with chronic visceral ischemia aims to relieve the disabling postprandial pain, thereby enabling resumption of normal diet with weight gain, and to prevent massive in-testinal infarction, which is usually fatal. A retrospective analysis by Perdue and Smith[13] found that approximately 50 per-cent of patients with intestinal infarction have premonitory abdominal pain. The onset of intestinal angina is a warning of imminent disaster, as most of these pa-tients progress to infarction within a few months.

PATHOLOGIC CONDITIONS CAUSING VISCERAL ISCHEMIA

Chronic Visceral Ischemia

The pathologic conditions causing chronic visceral ischemia include athero-sclerosis as well as fibromuscular hyper-

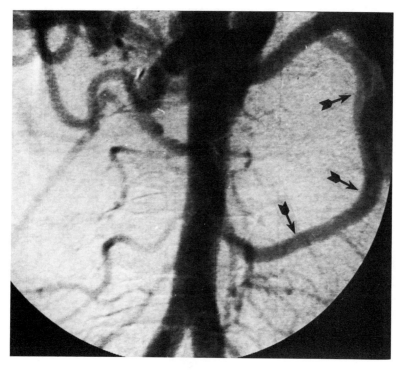

Fig. 9-1. Digital subtraction angiogram of the abdominal aorta showing a "meandering mesenteric artery" (arrows).

plasia, inflammatory arteriopathies, external compression, and atherosclerotic aneurysms.

Atherosclerosis

As mentioned earlier, most *symptomatic* mesenteric arterial disease is caused by atherosclerotic narrowing of the origins of the three major visceral vessels. Such disease usually originates as aortic atheroma that extends into the origins of the aortic branches. Atheroma rarely extends more than 1 to 2 cm into the visceral arteries and has a well-defined endpoint.[5,14] Although the distal thoracic aorta is often spared, atherosclerotic disease of the infrarenal vasculature is common. A lesion of superior mesenteric artery may be more extensive than a lesion of the celiac axis, and propagation of thrombus to the first major collateral pathway (the inferior

pancreaticoduodenal artery) often produces a relatively long segment of occlusion. Atherosclerosis of the superior mesenteric artery occasionally spares the origin of this vessel and causes stenosis several centimeters more distal, allowing clamping of the origin of the superior mesenteric artery without mobilization of the aorta.[1]

Because atheroma of distal segments of the aorta often involves the origin of the inferior mesenteric artery, this vessel is frequently ligated at the time of surgery for occlusive or aneurysmal disease of its origin. However, when severe celiac and superior mesenteric artery disease is present, the inferior mesenteric artery is often the principal collateral source for the mesenteric circulation. By revealing the existence of a meandering mesenteric artery, preoperative angiography in aneu-

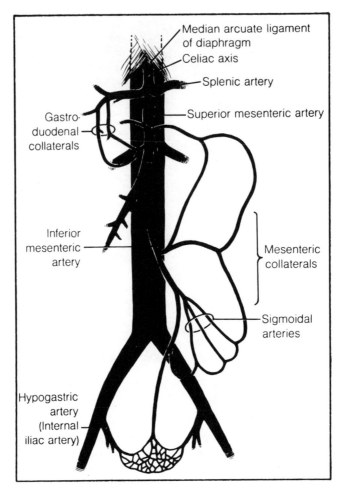

Fig. 9-2. Blood vessels and collateral pathways supplying the intestines. (From Stoney and Lusby,[14] with permission.)

rysmal and stenotic aortic disease usually reveals when preservation of the inferior mesenteric artery is necessary.

Fibromuscular Hyperplasia and Arteriopathies

Fibromuscular hyperplasia sometimes occurs in the celiac axis and superior mesenteric arteries and is rarely associated with symptomatic mesenteric insufficiency.[6,7,15] Of the various inflammatory arteriopathies, Takayasu's disease is the most likely to involve the mesenteric vascular supply.[16] This disease is a form of proliferative panarteritis occurring most frequently in children and young adults, predominantly female Orientals. It is characterized by stenosis, occlusion, or aneurysm formation, usually of the thoracic and abdominal aorta with its major branches. While the histologic picture of the diseased artery is not specific, the combination of histologic observations, geographic location, and pattern of involvement of vessels makes it readily distinguishable from other inflammatory arteriopathies such as polymyalgia rheumatica, giant cell arteritis, thromboangiitis obliterans, tuberculosis, and syphilis.

External Compression

A wide range of diseases can cause external compression of mesenteric vessels. In celiac artery compression syndrome (also called the median arcuate ligament syndrome), the celiac axis is compressed by the median arcuate ligament of the diaphragm.[14] Patients are usually women 20 to 40 years of age who present with intermittent epigastric pain. The onset of pain is not strongly associated with ingestion of food but may be related to posture. The duration and severity of pain vary; weight loss, nausea, vomiting, and altered bowel habit occur very inconsistently. The only objective sign is the presence of an epigastric bruit. Confirmation of diagnosis depends on radiologic evidence (by lateral aortography) of celiac axis compression, accentuated on inspiration; the aorta and its other major branches appear normal (Fig. 9-3). On rare occasion, the origin of the superior mesenteric artery may also be compressed.[8,14]

The pain in this syndrome may be caused by neurogenic pain produced by pressure of the median arcuate ligament on the celiac plexus. Other lesions causing external compression include neurofibromata and other fibrous bands extending over the origins of the artery.[6]

Splanchnic Aneurysms

Splanchnic aneurysms are uncommon and may affect any of the mesenteric vessels. This condition occurs predominantly in women, the average age being 52 years.[17] Although aneurysms of the celiac axis are the least common (3 percent) of visceral aneurysms, the risk of rupture and death is high.[16–19] Superior mesenteric aneurysms are rare but may undergo rupture or occlusion or may cause embolization of the gut (Figs. 9-4 and 9-5).

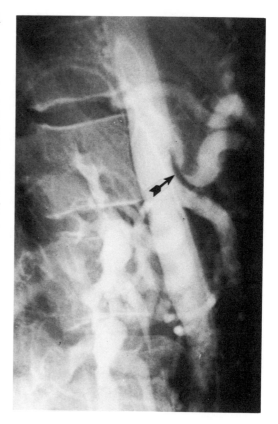

Fig. 9-3. Lateral aortogram showing celiac axis compression by the median arcuate ligament (arrow).

Acute Occlusion of Mesenteric Arteries

Acute mesenteric occlusion is either embolic or thrombotic in origin. Emboli usually have a cardiac source and may follow a recent myocardial infarction. Thrombi are usually caused by progressing atherosclerosis and sometimes aortic dissection or trauma. Sudden occlusion of the superior mesenteric artery when no collateral circulation exists can lead to bowel infarction within a few hours. Diagnosis is often difficult in the early phase of acute occlusion. The patient frequently complains of severe pain but has no specific signs until peritonitis occurs because of intestinal gangrene.

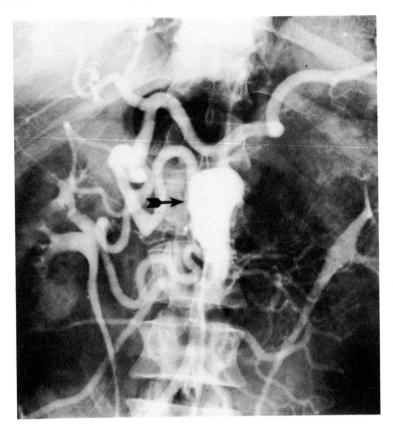

Fig. 9-4. Anteroposterior aortogram showing aneurysm (arrow) of the superior mesenteric artery.

Acute mesenteric occlusion should be strongly suspected in patients with prior cardiac disease who have sudden central abdominal pain, often severe, but few other abdominal signs for 4 to 6 hours. When this combination of conditions occurs, lateral aortography should be performed immediately. If an embolus can be removed and mesenteric blood supply restored before gangrene develops, the likelihood of death (more than 67 percent) would decrease.[17]

Acute mesenteric ischemia sometimes occurs in previously asymptomatic patients who undergo aortic reconstruction for occlusive or aneurysmal disease.[14,18] In the presence of occlusive disease of the celiac and superior mesenteric arteries, the major blood supply for the mesentery often consists of the inferior mesenteric artery via the marginal artery. Therefore, if the inferior mesenteric artery is not revascularized during corrective surgery (infrarenal aortic grafting), either intestinal or small bowel ischemia may occur. The incidences of significant intestinal or small bowel ischemia complicating aortic operations not including prophylactic mesenteric vascularization are relatively low—1 to 2 percent for colonic infarction and 0.15 percent for small bowel infarction.[17,18] However, the mortality rates associated with these complications are high (40 to 65 percent and 90 percent, respectively).[17,18]

Connolly and Kwaan[1] described a

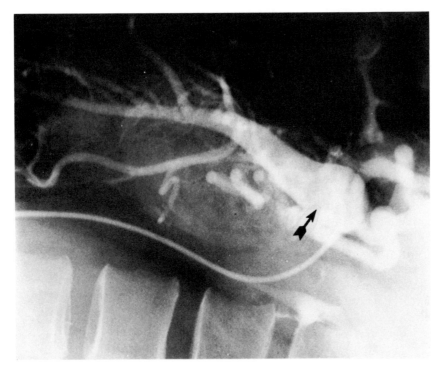

Fig. 9-5. Lateral aortogram showing aneurysm (arrow) of the superior mesenteric artery.

"mesenteric arterial steal phenomenon" in 13 patients who had intestinal ischemia after aortic reconstruction. These investigators suggested that the relatively higher blood flow to the distal circulation caused a "steal" in the presence of previously asymptomatic mesenteric stenotic disease. An additional cause of acute mesenteric ischemia in these patients may be inadvertent damage to the lumbar collateral pathways at the time of aortic mobilization.

Occult mesenteric stenosis may coexist with renovascular hypertension. Mesenteric perfusion may become inadequate after correction of renal artery stenosis and subsequent fall in systemic blood pressure. The importance of good preoperative arteriography and full assessment of all stenotic lesions prior to surgery cannot be overemphasized.

SURGERY

Criteria for Surgery and Factors Affecting Success

Indications for surgery differ greatly for chronic versus acute intestinal ischemia. The factors affecting the success of surgery also differ for these two conditions.

Chronic Visceral Ischemia

Long-term results of surgical management in chronic visceral ischemia depend on the extent of revascularization undertaken.[6] Because symptoms recur in 50 percent of patients undergoing single-vessel repair but in only 11 percent of patients undergoing full revascularization, the current practice in elective procedures is to perform as complete a revascularization as possible.[1,5,11,20,21]

Elective surgery for asymptomatic mesenteric occlusive disease is generally not justified, as the risk of surgery often outweighs the possible gain. The perioperative mortality rate ranges from 7.5 to 18 percent.[5,6,8,9,11] Cardiac disease, postoperative hemorrhage, and early graft occlusion with gut infarction are the major causes of perioperative death.

The exception to this general policy occurs when symptomatic infrarenal aortic disease is being repaired and asymptomatic but documented stenosis or occlusion of a major splanchnic vessel is also present. For example, Connolly and Kwaan[1,22] first reported the "aortoiliac steal syndrome" in 1965, and later documented late-onset symptomatic mesenteric ischemia after aortoiliac reconstruction. Their recommendation, supported by others,[8,9,21] is that revascularization of severely stenotic but asymptomatic mesenteric supply vessels should be performed if concomitant aortic or renal reconstruction is being undertaken. Under these circumstances, the expected incidence of visceral artery stenosis was approximately 3.5 percent after review of 200 angiograms for stenotic aortoiliac disease and approximately 2.5 percent after review of 200 angiograms for aneurysmal aortic disease.[1,22]

Acute Intestinal Ischemia

Acute gut ischemia is usually caused by sudden occlusion of the superior mesenteric artery.[11] If surgery is performed before gangrene of the bowel develops, revascularization will reduce the high mortality and morbidity associated with this progression of events. An embolus can usually be extracted from the superior mesenteric artery by balloon catheter with a direct approach to the proximal artery. Longitudinal arteriotomy requires vein patch angioplasty when closed.[11] Although fragmentation of the embolus with occlusion of the distal branches may

make full revascularization impossible, clearance of the major vessel will limit the extent of bowel infarction. Although administration of thrombolytic agents may prove useful for removing distal embolic fragments, this approach is still experimental.[23]

If surgery is delayed and some of the bowel has become infarcted, revascularization procedures may be able to salvage areas of marginal viability and thus reduce the amount of gut lost. However, when the whole small bowel has become infarcted, this approach is futile.

The procedures for revascularization in the acute situation are limited because of the potential for contamination. Synthetic graft materials should not be used, as the mortality rate associated with infection from such materials is high.[24] Therefore, embolectomy with vein patch angioplasty, endarterectomy, or autogenous vein bypass are the most used techniques; a "second-look" laparotomy is performed at 24 hours to check viability of the unresected bowel.[23] One experimental approach uses percutaneous angioplasty in such circumstances.[25] The use of vasodilating drugs such as papaverine at the time of revascularization appears to be beneficial in acute occlusion. Administration of vasodilating drugs may be the only form of treatment effective in nonocclusive mesenteric ischemia, such as occurs when cardiac output is low.[23]

Surgical Exposure

The surgical approach to the visceral arteries is determined by the vessels involved and the procedure to be used to restore adequate blood flow. The choice may depend on the surgeon's preference for either endarterectomy or bypass, or both.

Transabdominal Approach

In general, all of the visceral vessels can be exposed by a transabdominal approach; occasionally, a retroperitoneal procedure, with or without extension into the thoracic cavity, is necessary. Although a midline incision from the xiphoid process to the pubic symphysis is the most common procedure, transverse abdominal incisions and Pillsbury (curved thoracoabdominal retroperitoneal) incisions are also options. The celiac axis and superior mesenteric artery can be approached through the gastrohepatic ligament, a technique usually requiring mobilization of the left lobe of the liver, lateral retraction of the liver to the right, and lateral retraction of the stomach and esophagus to the left. Division of the median arcuate ligament, separation of the fibers of the left crus of the diaphragm, and excision of the fibers of the celiac plexus provide good exposure of the origins of these vessels and the lower thoracic aorta. Division of the fibrous origins of the median arcuate ligament helps to elevate the aorta at this site. Elevation and caudal displacement of the pancreas are needed to adequately control blood flow in the proximal superior mesenteric artery. Because of the risk of paraplegia from ischemic myelopathy, care should be taken not to damage intercostal and spinal canal arteries when mobilizing the lower thoracic aorta.

The superior mesenteric artery, renal arteries, infrarenal aorta, and inferior mesenteric artery are readily approached transabdominally and inferiorly to the transverse mesocolon through the posterior peritoneum. A long vertical midline incision or a long transverse supraumbilical incision provides this exposure. The small bowel is packed to the right, and the posterior peritoneum is opened to expose the aorta. Midline dissection superiorly exposes the left renal vein, which needs full mobilization and division of its tributaries, including the left suprarenal and gonadal veins, to allow safe retraction. Further dissection enables lifting of the transverse mesocolon and pancreas and exposure of the origin of the superior mesenteric artery and renal arteries. The base of the small bowel mesentery contains the superior mesenteric artery, which is easily exposed with this approach. The branches of the superior mesenteric artery should be treated with care, as the inferior pancreaticoduodenal artery is a major collateral channel when the superior mesenteric artery has undergone stenosis or occlusion. Care should also be taken to protect the inferior mesenteric artery and its branches to the left colon, as this vessel is frequently a major collateral source of mesenteric supply. If graft replacement of the infrarenal aorta is being performed, early decision to reimplant the inferior mesenteric artery allows preservation of the origin of this vessel during opening of the aorta (i.e., a disc of aortic wall containing the origin is excised and then, after endarterectomy, reattached to the aorta).

Thoracoabdominal Retroperitoneal Approach

A left thoracoabdominal incision and retroperitoneal dissection provide generous exposure of the thoracic and abdominal aorta and its major branches. Although this approach has been used with good results by Stoney et al.[5] and Wylie et al.[26] in relatively young, fit patients, most surgeons prefer the transabdominal route. The thoracoabdominal approach is needed for extensive occlusive or aneurysmal disease of the thoracic and abdominal aorta requiring graft replacement and for the lateral transaortic endarterectomy technique.[5,11]

In the thoracoabdominal approach, the incision is made over the eighth intercostal space and extended obliquely across the left abdomen toward the symphysis pubis. A retroperitoneal plane of dissection anterior to the left kidney exposes the abdominal aorta and diaphragm, which is divided circumferentially close to rib attachments to preserve innervation. Good exposure of the descending aorta to iliac artery bifurcations is obtained, and blood flow in all the major aortic branches can be controlled with this approach. However, dissection is more extensive than with a transabdominal approach, and entering of the left thoracic cavity incurs a higher risk of morbidity.

Endarterectomy

Transarterial Endarterectomy

In transarterial endarterectomy, one approaches the lesion through an arteriotomy at the site of the lesion. Single-vessel endarterectomy can be performed on either the celiac axis or superior mesenteric artery.

After exposure of these vessels, and with control of aortic blood flow above and below, the celiac axis is opened transversely at the distal extent of the palpable atheroma. A place of dissection is found, and retrograde endarterectomy of the aorta is performed. The arteriotomy is closed directly, and blood flow is restored. The difficulty of obtaining a clean endpoint in the distal aortic atheroma makes this technique less popular than other methods. However, in the acute situation in which synthetic grafting is not applicable, this procedure may be useful.

The superior mesenteric artery may be treated similarly by transarterial endarterectomy with either a transverse arteriotomy at the distal palpable limit of atheroma or a longitudinal arteriotomy through the atheroma. The transverse incision may be closed directly, but a longitudinal incision will need a patch closure, autogenous or synthetic, depending

on circumstances. Again, poor control of the aortic endpoint of the endarterectomy limits the application of this technique.

Although transarterial endarterectomy theoretically could be performed on the inferior mesenteric artery, the small size of this vessel makes this technique quite difficult. Exposure of the inferior mesenteric artery and adjacent aorta being relatively easy, this vessel is usually treated by transaortic endarterectomy and reimplantation.

Transaortic Endarterectomy

In transaortic endarterectomy, one approaches the lesion through the opened aorta. Owing to the difficulty of exposing the lower thoracic and upper abdominal aorta with a transperitoneal approach, in elective surgery, transaortic endarterectomy of the celiac axis and superior mesenteric artery is best performed with the thoracoretroperitoneal approach of Stoney et al.[5] and Wylie et al.[26] The procedure can be done through a midline abdominal, anterior aortic approach.[4] The lower thoracic aorta is clamped, and a "trapdoor" flap of anterior aorta is made. The trapdoor includes the orifices of both the celiac axis and the superior mesenteric artery. Eversion endarterectomy is then performed on the lesions in the orifices of either or both vessels. Using the anterior approach, the surgeon may need to convert the trapdoor into a free button of aortic wall to facilitate endarterectomy. Once completed, the button or trapdoor is sutured back into position, the clamp is released, and blood flow is reestablished.

This anterior transabdominal approach with transaortic trapdoor or button for endarterectomy of the inferior mesenteric artery is probably the easiest approach for revascularization of the inferior mesenteric artery. The inferior mesenteric artery button is resutured to the aorta or to the graft replacement of that section of diseased aorta, if necessary.

The thoracoretroperitoneal approach gives excellent exposure of the descending thoracic and abdominal aorta. All major branches of this section can be treated, and this approach is needed for complex thoracoabdominal aortic replacement for stenotic or aneurysmal disease. In these major grafting procedures, the visceral branches are excised from the parent aorta with a button of aortic wall. If needed, endarterectomy of these branch vessels is performed before their attachment to small openings cut in the graft at appropriate positions.[11]

When aortic replacement is not performed, endarterectomy of any or all of the major branches may be performed with this exposure. The celiac axis and superior mesenteric artery can be approached through a trapdoor by a left lateral aortic incision. This incision is extended across the anterior aorta above and below this pair of vessels, leaving the trapdoor attached on the right side. When lifted up, endarterectomy of this segment of aorta is performed, and with gentle dissection, the place of separation is extended into the celiac or superior mesenteric artery orifices, or both. Traction on the lifted intima and continued dissection of the plane of separation evert the branch vessels until separation at the endpoint of the atheroma occurs. The trapdoor is then sutured closed and blood flow is reestablished. When occluded, the superior mesenteric artery often has a column of thrombus between the endpoint of the atheroma and the first major branch, the inferior pancreaticoduodenal artery. To clear this thrombus, the surgeon may need to make a separate longitudinal incision in the proximal superior mesenteric artery after reestablishing aortic blood flow. After clearance, the superior mesenteric artery is closed with a patch.

Should stenoses of the orifices of the renal arteries also be present, the thoracoretroperitoneal approach enables distal extension of the left lateral aortotomy in an oblique course between the superior mesenteric artery and the left renal artery toward the anterior aortic surface. Endarterectomy of this section of aorta, including the origins of the celiac axis, superior mesenteric artery, and left and right renal arteries, is readily performed in one procedure. The aortic incision is then closed directly and blood flow is reestablished. Should infrarenal aortic procedures also be necessary (as occurs in as many as 47 percent of cases), the aorta is then clamped below the renal arteries and further endarterectomy or grafting procedures are performed as necessary.[4,8,9]

Bypass Grafts

Two major controversies still exist regarding bypass options in mesenteric vascular disease. The first controversy concerns site of the origin of the graft; and the second, the graft material.

Site of Graft Origin, Anastomosis, and Antegrade Blood Flow

The positioning and site of origin of the bypass graft and its anastomosis to the recipient vessel are important considerations. All synthetic grafts should be kept retroperitoneal and should have a live tissue buffer (e.g., omentum) separating them from any bowel sections (e.g., duodenum) to minimize the risk of enteric fistulae. The lie of the graft in an anatomic position allowing antegrade blood flow minimizes turbulence and lessens the potential for graft occlusion. Antegrade flow is best achieved with a supraceliac graft origin and end-to-end anastomosis to the recipient vessel(s).

Supraceliac Aorta as a Site of Graft Origin. Although the supraceliac aorta is usually relatively free of atheroma, and a graft from this site would provide antegrade flow at all times, exposure of this segment of the aorta is more difficult than exposure of the infrarenal aorta. Most surgeons have limited experience in this region and are naturally hesitant to use this area. Probably the greatest concern relates to the need for suprarenal clamping and the risk of ischemic renal damage. This complication may prove fatal to the elderly patient with arterial disease, and it is this added risk that prevents routine use of supraceliac grafting. Some surgeons report that suprarenal clamps usually are needed for less than 30 minutes and that supraceliac grafting is no more hazardous than infrarenal grafting.[4,5]

Infrarenal Aorta as a Site of Graft Origin. Infrarenal graft origins may be made from any healthy vessel. There is little point in taking a graft from a heavily diseased vessel, as progression of atheroma will compromise the mesenteric reconstruction.[27] Potential sites of origin are the healthy aorta, the aorta after endarterectomy, the graft replacement of aorta, and the common iliac or external iliac artery.

With infrarenal graft origins, a long curved course for the graft and end-to-end anastomosis allow direct antegrade flow into the superior mesenteric artery.[28] A direct line to the superior mesenteric artery and end-to-side anastomosis would probably produce maximum turbulence and the greatest chance of graft kinking.

Revascularizing the celiac axis with an infrarenal graft origin does not allow an easy, direct anastomosis to the recipient vessel. Instead, it is easier to anastomose the graft end-to-side to the splenic or common hepatic branches of the celiac axis.[11,28] The graft is tunnelled through the base of the transverse mesocolon either in front of or behind the pancreas.

Intraoperative graft assessment is possible with electromagnetic flowmeters or duplex scanning.[29,30]

Bypass Materials

The bypass conduit may be autogenous or synthetic. Autogenous materials consist of arteries (usually the internal or external iliac artery) or veins (the long saphenous or cephalic vein). Synthetic material is unsuitable in cases of potential contamination, as commonly occurs in acute mesenteric occlusion with ischemic or infarcted bowel. In fact, for graft replacement of the superior mesenteric artery in the acute situation, use of the external iliac artery would be preferable to use of a synthetic material.[14]

Autogenous Grafts. Arterial autografts are rarely used in visceral vascular surgery. For one thing, in acute mesenteric occlusion, the internal iliac artery may be an important collateral source and therefore not available as graft material. Also, one of the reasons for using an arterial autograft—the ability of the repaired vessel to grow as a young patient grows— is usually not an issue in patients with mesenteric vascular disease. In addition, if the arterial autograft requires extensive endarterectomy to be an adequate conduit, the large denuded luminal surface is significantly thrombogenic. Finally, autogenous material does not appear to retain its presumed superiority when graft patency rates are examined.

Autogenous vein has been a superior conduit to synthetic material in femoropopliteal or tibial bypass, and one would expect it to maintain this advantage in other situations. However, some series report disappointing results with autogenous vein for mesenteric bypass procedures.[5,11,31] On the other hand, some series claim satisfactory results.[1,6,8] In the Mayo Clinic series, Hollier et al.[6] found no statistical difference in long-term patency rates between autogenous and synthetic grafts.

Synthetic Grafts.   Dacron grafts are probably the most commonly used bypass conduits for mesenteric revascularization. In this situation, graft lengths are usually short and flow volumes large, a combination that gives graft patency rates equivalent to or better than those for autogenous vein.[5] Revascularization of both the celiac axis and the superior mesenteric artery can be accomplished by using a small bifurcation graft (12 by 6 mm) with a supraceliac or infrarenal origin.

From a supraceliac origin, the lie of the graft enables end-to-end anastomosis and antegrade flow to both mesenteric vessels. This combination is believed least likely to induce neointimal hyperplasia, and long-term patency rates are good.[5]

From an infrarenal origin, the limb to the celiac axis is best anastomosed to either the splenic or common hepatic artery in an end-to-side fashion. The limb to the superior mesenteric artery can be direct with end-to-side anastomosis or curved to allow end-to-end anastomosis and antegrade flow.[28]

The major problems with revascularization of the superior mesenteric artery from an infrarenal graft origin with end-to-side anastomosis in the base of the small bowel mesentery are the mobility of the mesentery and the tendency for such grafts to kink and encourage thrombus formation. These problems do not occur with supraceliac grafts with end-to-end anastomosis. To overcome the problem of kinking from the infrarenal position, externally supported polytetrafluoroethylene (Gortex) has been used successfully by Jaxheimer et al.[21] Another possible solution is to construct a very short H-style anastomosis from anterior aortic wall to proximal superior mesenteric artery in the manner of a portocaval shunt with a very short but wide (10-mm) tube.[28]

The inferior mesenteric artery can undergo bypass grafting in a manner similar to that used for the celiac axis and superior mesenteric artery. However, the inferior mesenteric artery is easily approached transabdominally and is quite suitable for orifice endarterectomy and reimplantation, these two options being the most commonly used. In chronic mesenteric occlusive disease of the celiac axis and superior mesenteric artery, it is important to remember that the inferior mesenteric artery may be the major source of blood supply to the entire bowel. Therefore, when infrarenal aortic grafting or endarterectomy is being performed, due consideration should always be given to preservation of the inferior mesenteric artery.

In elective revascularization for chronic mesenteric ischemia, a period of preoperative hyperalimenation by intravenous feeding should be considered to halt the catabolic process and to enhance immunologic function.[21,27]

SUMMARY

Major stenotic or occlusive disease of the celiac axis, superior mesenteric artery, and inferior mesenteric artery is quite common in our aging population. The usual cause is atherosclerosis, primarily of the aorta, with extension into the orifices of these three branch arteries. Symptomatic intestinal ischemia is uncommon because of extensive collateral development between the branches of the three major vessels of mesenteric supply. Unless other surgery has interrupted the collateral network, symptoms usually do not occur until at least two of the three vessels are diseased.

Patients with chronic ischemia present with postprandial abdominal pain, weight loss, and minimal abdominal signs apart from epigastric bruit. Surgery is required to relieve pain, allow weight gain, and avert the progression to massive intestinal infarction, which is usually fatal.

Acute mesenteric ischemia is often caused by emboli from the heart and presents with acute, severe abdominal pain but few, if any, other abdominal signs in the first 4 to 6 hours before development of gut infarction and peritonitis. Surgery is urgently required to revascularize the gut, to limit or prevent gut infarction, and to resect nonviable tissue.

Surgical results in acute mesenteric occlusion improve if all diseased mesenteric vessels are revascularized. A transabdominal approach is satisfactory for most procedures including supraceliac grafting. A left thoracoretroperitoneal approach is advantageous for transaortic endarterectomy of the celiac axis and superior mesenteric artery; however, because of the extensiveness of the incision, this approach might be reserved for younger, less debilitated patients.

Surgery is recommended only for patients who are symptomatic, and for a small group of asymptomatic patients with proven major occlusive disease of the mesenteric vessels who are undergoing intraabdominal procedures likely to interrupt collateral pathways. Such procedures include aortic reconstruction for occlusive or aneurysmal disease and resections of the colon, small bowel, or stomach.

Much controversy still exists as to the most effective surgical approach. Although endarterectomy is favored by some, most surgeons prefer grafting techniques; both produce satisfactory long-term results. The autogenous vein bypass does not appear to have a clear advantage in visceral vascular disease; for nonemergency surgery, many surgeons prefer synthetic conduits, which have less chance of kinking. In an acute situation having the potential for contamination of the abdominal cavity, endarterectomy and autogenous grafting are the only safe options.

Transluminal balloon angioplasty and administration of thrombolytic agents are potentially useful new options for patients who have visceral vascular disease. Awareness of mesenteric ischemia as a possible cause of abdominal pain needs to increase. Less invasive diagnostic tests with digital subtraction angiography and duplex scanning should encourage earlier evaluation of mesenteric vessels in these patients.

REFERENCES

1. Connolly JE, Kwaan JHM: Management of chronic visceral ischemia. Surg Clin North Am 62:345–356, 1982
2. Dunphy JE: Abdominal pain of vascular origin. Am J Med Sci 192:109–113, 1936
3. Mikkelsen WP: Intestinal angina. Its surgical significance. Am J Surg 94:262–269, 1957
4. Rapp JH, Reilly LM, Qvarfordt PG et al: Durability of endarterectomy and antegrade grafts in the treatment of chronic visceral ischemia. J Vasc Surg 3:799–806, 1986
5. Stoney RJ, Ehrenfeld WK, Wylie EJ: Revascularization methods in chronic visceral ischemia caused by atherosclerosis. Ann Surg 186:468–476, 1977
6. Hollier LH, Bernatz PE, Pairolero PC et al: Surgical management of chronic intestinal ischemia: a reappraisal. Surgery 90:940–946, 1981
7. Reul GJ, Jr., Wukasch DC, Sandiford FM et al: Surgical treatment of abdominal angina: review of 25 patients. Surgery 75:682–689, 1974
8. Stanton PE, Jr., Hollier PA, Seidel TW et al: Chronic intestinal ischemia: diagnosis and therapy. J Vasc Surg 4:338–344, 1986
9. Baur GM, Millay DJ, Taylor LM, Jr., Porter JM: Treatment of chronic visceral ischemia. Am J Surg 148:138–144, 1984

10. Reiner L, Jimenez FA, Rodriguez FL: Atherosclerosis in the mesenteric circulation: observations and correlations with aortic and coronary atherosclerosis. Am Heart J 66:200–209, 1963

11. Crawford ES, Morris GC, Jr., Myhre HO, Roehm JOF, Jr: Celiac axis, superior mesenteric artery, and inferior mesenteric artery occlusion: surgical considerations. Surgery 82:856–866, 1977

12. Morris GC, Jr., De Bakey ME, Bernhard V: Abdominal angina. Surg Clin North Am 46:919–930, 1966

13. Perdue GD, Jr., Smith RB, III: Intestinal ischemia due to mesenteric arterial disease. Am Surg 36:152–156, 1970

14. Stoney RJ, Lusby RJ: Surgery of celiac and mesenteric arteries. p. 813–825. In Haimovici H (ed): Vascular Surgery. Principles and Techniques. 2nd Ed. Appleton-Century-Crofts, Norwalk, CT, 1984

15. Golden DA, Ring EJ, McLean GK, Freiman DB: Percutaneous transluminal angioplasty in the treatment of abdominal angina. AJR 139:247–249, 1982

16. Scott D, Awang H, Sulieman B et al: Surgical repair of visceral artery occlusions in Takayasu's disease. J Vasc Surg 3:904–910, 1986

17. Rogers DM, Thompson JE, Garrett WV et al: Mesenteric vascular problems. A 26-year-old experience. Ann Surg 195:554–565, 1982

18. Bergqvist D, Bowald S, Eriksson I et al: Small bowel necrosis after aorto-iliac reconstruction. Br J Surg 73:28–30, 1986

19. Graham JM, McCollum CH, DeBakey ME: Aneurysms of the splanchnic arteries. Am J Surg 140:797–801, 1980

20. Zelenock GB, Graham LM, Whitehouse WM, Jr et al: Splanchnic arteriosclerotic disease and intestinal angina. Arch Surg 115:497–501, 1980

21. Jaxheimer EC, Jewell ER, Persson AV: Chronic intestinal ischemia. The Lahey Clinic approach to management. Surg Clin North Am 65:123–130, 1985

22. Connolly JE, Kwaan JHM: Prophylactic revascularization of the gut. Ann Surg 190:514–522, 1979

23. Boley SJ, Borden EB: Acute mesenteric vascular disease. p. 659–671. In Wilson SE, Veith FJ, Hobson RW, II, Williams RA (eds): Vascular Surgery. Principles and Practice. McGraw-Hill, New York, 1987

24. Coleman M, Burnett J, Barratt LJ, Dupont P: Glomerulonephritis associated with chronic infection of a Dacron arterial prosthesis. Clin Nephrol 20:315–320, 1983

25. Martin LG, Price RB, Casarella WJ et al: Percutaneous angioplasty in clinical management of renovascular hypertension: initial and long-term results. Radiology 155:629–633, 1985

26. Wylie EJ, Stoney RJ, Ehrenfeld WK: Visceral atherosclerosis. p. 207–232. In Manual of Vascular Surgery. Vol. 1. Springer-Verlag, New York, 1980

27. Connelly TL, Perdue GD, Smith RB, III et al: Elective mesenteric revascularization. Am Surg 47:19–25, 1981

28. Eidemiller LR, Nelson JC, Porter JM: Surgical treatment of chronic visceral ischemia. Am J Surg 138:264–268, 1979

29. Okuhn SP, Reilly LM, Bennett JB, III et al: Intraoperative assessment of renal and visceral artery reconstruction: the role of duplex scanning and spectral analysis. J Vasc Surg 5:137–147, 1987

30. Qamar MI, Read AE: Intestinal blood flow (editorial). Q J Med 56:417–419, 1985

31. Rob C: Surgical diseases of the celiac and mesenteric arteries. Arch Surg 93:21–32, 1966

10

Anesthesia Goals for Surgery to Relieve or Prevent Visceral Ischemia

Michael F. Roizen

The goals of anesthesia for surgery to relieve or prevent visceral ischemia are to maximize surgical benefit and to minimize patient morbidity. I believe that an understanding of the pathophysiologic consequences of surgical manipulations and of the causes of postoperative morbidity greatly facilitates meeting these goals. Perhaps in no other surgical endeavor can the anesthesiologist have as great an effect in reducing morbidity as in supraceliac abdominal aortic reconstruction. Also, in no other area has morbidity probably decreased as quickly: the mortality rate of more than 25 percent by 6 days after major aortic reconstructions in the mid-1960s has decreased to 1 to 4 percent today.

MORBIDITY AND MORTALITY OF VISCERAL VASCULAR SURGERY

Aneurysmal versus Occlusive Disease

Reconstruction of the supraceliac abdominal aorta is performed either to replace a segment having degenerative aneurysmal disease or to increase blood flow to and from a vessel having stenosing occlusive disease. Although the natural histories of the two types of disease differ, the segmental nature of the disease processes (i.e., the vessels above and below the lesion are relatively normal) provides the basis for reconstruction for both types of disease.

Aneurysmal Disease

Patients undergoing aortic surgery for aneurysmal disease are twice as likely to die or have perioperative morbidity as are patients undergoing aortic surgery for occlusive disease; also, median survival time (5.8 verus 10.7 years) is lower.[1,2] Given these figures, one might ask, Should patients be subjected to surgery for *asymptomatic* aneurysms? The answer is yes; because of an unpredictable tendency to rupture or embolize, aneurysms pose an ever-present threat to the life of the patient. Therefore, aggressive surgical management is warranted even when symptoms are not present.[3–5] Several facts support this practice. First, because of the likelihood of rupture, mortality is high if surgery is not undertaken. Unoperated patients with aneurysms of the abdominal aorta have an 80 percent mortality rate 5 years after diagnosis.[6-8] The risk of rupture is related to size of the aneurysm: the larger the diameter, the greater the risk. Specifically, the 5-year incidence of rupture is approximately 25 percent for lesions 4 to 7 cm in diameter, 45 percent for those 7 to 10 cm, and 60 percent for those exceeding 10 cm.[8] The larger the aneurysm, the greater the likelihood of sudden rupture: 71.8 percent of fatal ruptures of larger lesions occur in the first 2 years, whereas 39.1 percent of fatal ruptures of smaller lesions occur during that same time period.[9]

Second, mortality is high if the aneurysm ruptures and emergency surgery is undertaken. Since the 1960s, the mortality rate after surgery for ruptured aortic aneurysm has remained high—25 to 75 percent.[9-11]

The third factor justifying surgical intervention for all aortic aneurysms is that elective surgical repair incurs low mortality. Because of improvements in surgical and anesthetic management, perioperative mortality has decreased steadily, from approximately 17 percent before 1960 to 2 to 5 percent since 1980, despite an increase in the number of procedures performed in older and/or sicker patients.[12-14] Successful surgical repair of an abdominal aortic aneurysm also appears to prolong life.[4,5,7,12,15] In 1966, Szilagyi et al.[15] showed that surgical repair of aneurysms exceeding 6 cm in diameter approximately doubled life expectancy. Today, even patients with abdominal aortic aneurysms smaller than 6 cm in diameter are considered candidates for aortic reconstructive surgery.

To summarize, three factors account for the current lack of hesitancy in repairing all aortic aneurysms surgically: (1) the morbidity of elective repair is now much lower than in the 1960s; (2) mortality is much greater when aortic reconstruction is performed on an emergency basis (25 to 90 percent); and (3) the tendency of the aneurysm to enlarge and rupture is unpredictable[1,2,16,17] (in the series described by Szilagyi et al.,[15] 19 percent of aneurysms smaller than 6 cm in diameter ruptured and caused death).

Occlusive Disease

Occlusive disease tends to be progressive, with compromise of the distal circulation leading to disabling claudication or limb-threatening ischemia. In contrast to aneurysmal disease, in which surgery is warranted whenever the disease is present, occlusive disease requires surgical intervention only for the relief of disabling symptoms.[3]

In setting out to correct symptomatic occlusive disease of the aortoiliac segment, the surgeon endeavors to return inflow to the limbs at the groin to near normal levels while maintaining flow to the internal iliac and visceral branches. The mean age of patients undergoing aortoiliac reconstruction is 54 years; these patients are, on average, more than 10 years younger than those with aneurysmal disease of the aorta.[18]

Symptomatic disease of the mesenteric artery is usually caused by atherosclerotic narrowing of the origins of the three major vessels supplying the viscera: the celiac, superior mesenteric, and inferior mesenteric arteries. Other, less common causes of viscereal ischemia include fibromuscular dysplasia, in association with superior mesenteric insufficiency[19]; Takayasu's arteritis[20]; or external compression of the celiac axis by the median arcuate ligament of the diaphragm.[21] All three of these conditions occur most commonly in women 20 to 40 years of age. In contrast, both chronic atherosclerotic ischemia and acute occlusive disease occur in the elderly, who are often hypertensive, and in heavy cigarette smokers. Acute mesenteric occlusion is caused by either embolism or thrombosis. Embolism commonly originates in the heart and may follow a recent myocardial infarction. Thrombosis is occasionally caused by aortic dissection or trauma but is usually related to progressing atherosclerosis.

Elective surgery for *asymptomatic* mesenteric occlusive disease is generally not justified, as the risks of surgery often outweigh the possible gains. Specifically, perioperative mortality rates range from 7.5 to 18 percent[19,22-24]: cardiac disease, renal insufficiency, postopertaive hemorrhage, and early graft occlusion with bowel infarction are the major causes of perioperative death.

Central Nervous System, Renal, and Myocardial Ischemia

Cardiac problems are the most frequent causes of morbidity and mortality after operations for visceral ischemia and thoracoabdominal aortic reconstruction for aneurysms or atherosclerosis (Table 10-1).[12,15,25,26] Also, in almost every series, cardiac complications were the conditions limiting both perioperative and long-term survival (Table 10-1).[12,13,15-17,25-37] Other causes of morbidity after vascular surgery include pulmonary infections, graft infections, renal insufficiency and failure, hepatic failure, and spinal cord ischemia. The incidence of these types of morbidity has declined substantially over the past 20 years, with death from renal failure decreasing from 25 percent to less than 1 percent at present.[1,2,15-17,26,30,38-42] Much of the improvement in reducing renal failure has resulted from better perioperative management of fluids.[43-47]

Investigators have used sensory evoked potentials and the electroencephalogram (EEG) to gauge spinal cord and cerebral protection during coarctation repairs or resection of abdominal or thoracoabdominal aneurysms.[48] I find no evidence in the literature that monitoring of the EEG is of benefit in these procedures, and no evidence that stroke is a predictable consequence of even supraceliac or descending thoracic aortic reconstruc-

Table 10-1. Percentages of Perioperative Mortality Related to Cardiac Events during Aortic Reconstruction

Series	Deaths/Total No. of Patients	Mortality Caused by Cardiac Dysfunction (%)
Szilagyi et al.[15] (1966)	59/401	48
Hicks et al.[28] (1975)	19/225	53
Thompson et al.[12] (1975)	6/108	83
Young et al.[27] (1977)	7/144	100
Mulcare et al.[29] (1978)	14/140	79
Whittemore et al.[30] (1980)	1/110	100
Crawford et al.[31] (1981)	41/860	54
Hertzer[32] (1983)	22/523	64
Yeager et al.[33] (1986)	4/97	100
Benefiel et al.[26] (1986)	3/96	67

(Adapted from Roizen et al.,[108] with permission.)

tion. However, spinal cord ischemia does occur in 1 to 11 percent of operations involving repair of the distal descending thoracic aorta.[49]

The range of pressures over which autoregulation of blood pressure is in effect is similar for the spinal arteries as for other components of central nervous system (CNS) blood flow.[50,51] Because blood flow in the spinal arteries depends on collaterization and is often bidirectional, blood supply to the spinal cord can be "stolen" and redistributed to the rest of the body when blood pressures in other areas of the body are lower. Such a situation may arise when a single occluding clamp is applied high on the aorta. Thus, surgical techniques designed to minimize spinal cord ischemia include bypass shunts to supply blood to the lower extremities, femorofemoral extracorporeal bypass, double-clamping techniques, drainage of cerebrospinal fluid, preservation of the native aorta with its intercostal artery, magnesium therapy, hypothermia, and encouragement of faster surgery.[52–58] Nevertheless, only rarely will a patient have complications from spinal cord ischemia, a rare cause of morbidity and mortality in both published reports and anecdotal information.

Probably the greatest concern of surgeons is the need to clamp the aorta at the suprarenal level and the subsequent risk of ischemic damage to the kidneys. This complication may prove fatal to the elderly patient with arterial disease. It is this added potential for morbidity that precludes the routine use of supraceliac grafting. Although ischemic damage to the kidneys is a valid concern when occluding the aorta above the renal vessels, the potential for cardiac morbidity may be even more important. This larger concern arises because the hemodynamic consequences of temporary aortic occlusion are greater the more proximal the level of occlusion, the less well developed the collateral circulation, or the greater the occlusion of collateral circulation.[59] In addition, most patients needing surgery for visceral ischemia have atherosclerosis of the coronary arteries. In fact, the pathologic condition giving rise to chronic visceral ischemia is usually atherosclerotic occlusive disease, with its high incidence of coronary artery disease, and only rarely fibromuscular dysplasia, inflammatory arteriopathy, external compression, or aneurysmal atherosclerotic disease.

Therefore, because of the predominance of myocardial dysfunction as a source of morbidity and mortality, this chapter emphasizes the need to prevent myocardial damage in patients undergoing aortic surgery. This priority should be kept in mind when managing concurrent diseases such as hypertension, chronic obstructive lung disease, renal insufficiency, and diabetes. Indeed, the most important aspects of planning perioperative management of concurrent diseases may be understanding and searching for the end organ effects of these diseases and understanding the appropriate drug therapy.[60]

Having clearly established priorities helps the anesthetist when dealing with concurrent diseases under less-than-desirable conditions. For example, although it would be unusual to give anesthesia to patients with uncontrolled hypertension or metabolic disease, untreated pulmonary infections, or recent (within 3 to 6 months) myocardial infarction if other portions of the myocardium are still at risk,[60–63] an expanding aneurysm or threatened limb loss can make emergency surgery necessary. Attempts at rapid control of blood pressure or electrolytes may be more hazardous than leaving the condition untreated and trying to control the abnormality slowly. For instance, rapid reduction of blood pressure in a patient with renal or visceral insufficiency may precipitate renal failure or the death of bowel and should be postponed to the postoperative period (assuming that surgery cannot be delayed to permit gradual preoperative control of blood pressure). Similarly, discontinuing a drug may be more hazardous than continuing drug therapy and being aware of its effects.

Specific attempts have been made to identify, prior to surgery, patients at risk of myocardial injury.[60-64] However, until these procedures gain widespread acceptance, and until extensive trials demonstrate reduced overall mortality with a particular technique, the general goal of optimizing care—with the specific focus on minimizing myocardial morbidity— seems logical. This goal is based on the fact that patients with aortic disorders are likely to have preexisting coronary artery disease, and on the fact that cardiac dysfunction is the most frequent cause of morbidity and mortality after thoracoabdominal aortic and visceral reconstructive surgery.

ANESTHESIA GOALS FOR SURGERY FOR THORACOABDOMINAL AORTIC AND VISCERAL ARTERY RECONSTRUCTION

The surgical goal in operations for visceral ischemia is to permanently restore normal circulation to the viscera while at the same time minimizing the length of time of ischemia to the viscera and, more important, to the renal circulation. Attaining these goals is difficult, for each of the possible surgical approaches hampers some aspect of the overall plan while optimizing other aspects (see Ch. 9).

For minimal morbidity and mortality, my anesthesia goals are to provide a pain free environment conducive to surgical manipulations and preserve (1) myocardial, (2) renal, (3) pulmonary, (4) CNS, and (5) visceral organ function. To meet these goals, one needs to ensure an oxygen supply adequate to the needs of the myocardium; to reduce, if possible, the myocardial requirement for oxygen; and to maintain adequate perfusion to all other organs. The last objective usually requires preservation of adequate intravascular volume so that cardiac output can be maintained.

Effects of Occluding the Aorta at Various Levels

For a better understanding of the monitors used to meet these goals, it is helpful to be aware of the pathophysiologic events occurring on application and removal of aortic cross-clamps.

Occluding the aorta causes hypertension in the proximal segment and hypotension in the distal segment. During resection of a congenitally coarcted aorta, acute occlusion of the thoracic aorta has very little effect on cardiovascular variables because of the normal development, over years, of extensive collateral vessels around the coarctation. However, in patients who have an aortic aneurysm or atherosclerosis and no extensive collateral circulation, occlusion of the aorta increases afterload and peripheral vascular resistance. These increases occur in proportion to the level of the occlusion. Our group found that myocardial stress also varies with the level of occlusion.[59]

Myocardial performance and circulatory variables remain within an acceptable range after the aorta is occluded at infrarenal levels.[59] This conclusion agrees with earlier reports. For example, in 1968, Perry[65] demonstrated that the increase in afterload after temporary occlusion of the aorta at the infrarenal level had little effect on circulatory variables. The use of newer, more sophisticated techniques has shown that increasing the depth of anesthesia or administering vasodilating drugs at the time of infrarenal aortic occlusion keeps indices of myocardial performance within an acceptable range,[35-37,66] even in sick patients (in our series, 25 percent had severe left ventricular dysfunction before aortic surgery[59]). Abnormal wall motion and thickening, as well changes in ejection fraction, appear to be early signs of myocardial ischemia.[67] However, we did not detect abnormal wall motion in any of the patients undergoing infrarenal occlusion.[59]

Thus far, only one study has contradicted the view that myocardial well-being is preserved after infrarenal aortic occlusion. Attia et al.[16] reported a 30 percent incidence (3 of 10 patients) of myocardial ischemia after infrarenal occlusion. However, investigators from the same institution (Massachusetts General Hospital) later described a technique that allows infrarenal aortic occlusion without eliciting evidence of myocardial ischemia.[17] The technique consists of actively preventing an increase in myocardial oxygen demand by using sodium nitroprusside to avoid large increases in pulmonary capillary wedge pressure. Therefore, on the basis of these data, I consider it safe to assume that occlusion of the aorta at the infrarenal level increases afterload only slightly and that current techniques prevent much of the cardiac stress associated with such occlusion.

Few published reports describe the myocardial and cardiovascular effects of occluding the aorta at the supraceliac or infraceliac-suprarenal level in humans. After occluding the descending thoracic aorta in eight patients, Kouchoukos et al.[2] noted increases of 35, 56, 43, and 90 percent in mean arterial, central venous, mean pulmonary arterial, and pulmonary capillary wedge pressures, respectively, and a decrease of 29 percent in cardiac index. These hemodynamic effects are greater that those we found for supraceliac aortic occlusion and may be attributable to the more proximal level of thoracic aortic occlusion.[59] Occlusion at the supraceliac level caused substantially more myocardial stress, as evidenced by abnormal motion of the walls, than did occlusion at the infraceliac-suprarenal or infrarenal level (Table 10-2). Although systemic and pulmonary capillary wedge pressures were kept normal at all times in 10 of 12 patients who underwent occlusion at the supraceliac level, 11 of these patients had abnormal motion of the left ventricular wall, suggesting ischemia. Some of the factors contributing to this increase in resistance to myocardial ejection may have been the more than 100 percent increase in peripheral vascular resistance, the change in aortic impedance characteristics, the release of vasoactive substances with intestinal ischemia, or the activation of hormonal systems (see Ch. 11), all of which lead to ventricular dilation.

Despite low ejection fractions, these patients were able to maintain cardiac output and stroke volume via stretch (expansion) of the left ventricle muscle fibers. Pulmonary capillary wedge pressure frequently did not reflect this increased left ventricular end-diastolic volume accurately; however, two-dimensional transesophageal echocardiography (2D TEE) made possible the identification and treatment of myocardial dysfunction that was not detected by conventional monitoring techniques[59,66,68] (see Ch. 28). The most important information I have obtained using 2D TEE during vascular surgery is that dilating the heart through administration of fluids (as is often requested by surgeons for stimulation of urinary output) is a likely precursor of myocardial ischemia.

These pathophysiologic changes in hemodynamic variables could result from the effect that clamping has on normal

Table 10-2. Effect of Level of Aortic Occlusion on Percent Change in
Cardiovascular Variables during Vascular Surgery

Variable	% Change in Variable if Aorta Occluded at the:		
	Supraceliac Level	Infraceliac-Suprarenal Level	Infrarenal Level
Mean arterial blood pressure	54	5[a]	2[a]
Pulmonary capillary wedge pressure	38	10[a]	0[a]
End-diastolic area	28	2[a]	9[a]
End-systolic area	69	10[a]	11[a]
Ejection fraction	−38	−10[a]	−3[a]
Abnormal wall motion (% of patients)	92	33	0
New myocardial infarctions	8	0	0

[a] Statistically different ($P < 0.05$) from group undergoing aortic occlusion at the supraceliac level.
(Adapted from Roizen et al.,[108] with permission.)

patterns of flow to the arteries. For example, 22 percent of cardiac output usually goes to renal vessels, and 27 percent goes to the superior mesenteric vessels and celiac trunk.[69] Thus, the expected decrease in flow and the increase in afterload and peripheral vascular resistance after supraceliac aortic occlusion could cause left ventricular dilation. Other factors possibly contributing to myocardial dysfunction during operative supraceliac occlusion include release of vasoactive substances from ischemic areas and the presence of unmetabolized citrate from transfused blood.[70]

Results of studies on animals support the view that myocardial function is altered after occlusion of the descending thoracic aorta. Longo et al.[71] studied coronary and systemic hemodynamic changes in dogs during clamping and unclamping of the aorta at suprarenal and infrarenal levels. On application of the cross-clamp to the suprarenal aorta, peripheral resistance increased twofold to threefold, with immediate hypertension in the proximal segment, marked increases in coronary blood flow and pulse pressure, decreases in aortic blood flow and cardiac output, and little change in

pulse rate. These results were similar to ours.[59] In the study by Longo et al.,[71] the left ventricles of the dogs dilated on application of the cross-clamp. Mandelbaum and Webb[72] showed that occluding the descending thoracic aorta in dogs decreased left ventricular function. However, occluding the infrarenal aorta was much less stressful, the cardiovascular consequences being only slight (as they are in human patients with diseased hearts).[59,72]

In normal dogs, the renal artery can be occluded for an hour before the kidneys are injured even slightly.[47] Data from a study we performed on human subjects support this observationn.[45] Preoperative and postoperative renal function did not differ between patients who underwent less than 40 minutes of suprarenal cross-clamping and those who underwent infrarenal aortic occlusion.[45]

Hemodynamic Changes on Restoration of Aortic Blood Flow

Despite the negligible cardiovascular effects of temporarily occluding the aorta at an infrarenal level, hypotension (declamping shock) still occurs on restoration of aortic blood flow. This hemodynamic alteration occurs even when blood flow is restored to only one leg. Although severe hypotension occurs only rarely,[2,17,42] moderate hypotension (a decrease in systolic blood pressure of 40 mmHg) is not uncommon.

Two hypotheses offer explanations for such hypotension. The first suggests that myocardial depression is caused by the washout of acid, acid metabolites, and vasoactive substances from ischemic extremities on restoration of blood flow. This idea has been largely discredited in recent years.[2,36,46] However, many would say such factors play a role in the hypotension, especially during surgery where temporary occlusion has taken more than 30 minutes. The second hypothesis suggests a relative depletion of volume. Our own work with 2D TEE supports this theory.[59] Reactive hyperemia in the freshly revascularized area decreases total vascular resistance, venous return, and blood pressure. Thus, hypotension can be ameliorated by expansion of volume without a decrease in cardiac output; in fact, the expansion may increase cardiac output. However, if hypotension persists for more than 4 minutes after removal of the clamp, and if blood deficits have been replaced, I believe that other causes should be sought. A 2D TEE of the left ventricle often reveals that venous return is still inadequate (sometimes as a result of hidden persistent bleeding or misjudged replacement of blood deficits), or that a rare allergic reaction to graft material has occurred.[73]

Monitoring Devices and Techniques

Because of these complications, my monitoring practices stress preservation of myocardial, pulmonary, and renal function as well as intravascular volume. A catheter is almost always inserted into the radial artery of the nondominant hand (see Ch. 5 for a more complete discussion of this topic). In addition, urinary output and some form of ventricular filling pressure are monitored, the latter usually via pulmonary artery catheter. This catheter allows evaluation of systemic vascular resistance, cardiac output, and pulmonary capillary wedge pressure. I prefer the external jugular route for insertion, although many anesthetists use the internal jugular or subclavian route. I use a modified chest lead V_5 to monitor the electrocardiogram (ECG) during surgery, except when myocardial ischemia has been demonstrated in areas other than the anterior myocardial wall. Body temperature is almost always monitored and is maintained meticulously. This is accomplished by warming all fluids (starting preoperatively) and by placing the patient on a heating mattress on the operating room table. If necessary, anesthetic gases are humidified. For me, 2D TEE has been invaluable for monitoring the myocardial consequences of clamping and unclamping of the aorta, and I now use it routinely for procedures entailing temporary occlusion at the supraceliac level (see Ch. 28). A short-axis cross-sectional view of the left ventricle provides an excellent qualitative assessment of left ventricular filling volumes, global ventricular contractility, and regional ventricular function.[73,74] When a discrepancy has existed between pulmonary capillary filling pressures and filling pressures obtained by 2D TEE, I have found the latter to be more reliable and useful.[59,74,75]

To reduce the incidence of organ ischemia and pulmonary dysfunction, fluids are managed with the aim of preventing intraoperative hypotension and minimizing cardiac dilation. Although no data support this theory at present, I strongly believe that prehydration of patients undergoing vascular reconstructive surgery ensures adequate perfusion of vital organs and thus minimizes the hemodynamic fluctuations occurring on induction of anesthesia. During the early period of dissection, intravascular volume is kept at normal levels by noting cardiac filling on the 2D TEE or by sustaining a normal pulmonary capillary wedge pressure. To accomplish this, blood losses of less than 10 ml/kg and insensible losses (assumed to be 5 to 7 $ml \cdot kg^{-1} \cdot h^{-1}$ during dissection) are replaced with lactated Ringer's solution or saline.

Various indicators help assess perfusion of vital organs before cross-clamping of the aorta. Perfusion of the heart affects (1) myocardial contractility, as judged by global and regional motion of the wall on the 2D TEE[59,67,68]; (2) changes in ST segments on the modified chest lead V_5 of the ECG; and (3) cardiac output. Urinary output indicates perfusion of the kidneys. Although I believe that 2 ml/0.5 h per 70 kg of body weight is adequate, surgeons seem to be more confidant of the adequacy of perfusion if urinary output is 20 to 30 ml/0.5 h per 70 kg. Urinary flow almost always decreases during dissection around the renal vessels (see below, "Protecting the Kidneys"[45]). Eye signs are the most commonly used indicators of CNS perfusion. Although the EEG or sensory evoked potentials can be used, I have had little experience with these monitoring techniques for these operations. Finally, I use gas exchange to judge perfusion of the lungs.

Protecting the Myocardium

The difference in my management of aortic occlusion at different levels (e.g., supraceliac versus infrarenal) is that I am absolutely meticulous in planning my management and in executing that procedure for all occlusions occurring at or above the level of the renal vessels. I am only slightly less meticulous when temporary occlusion will occur at the infrarenal level.

Before Clamping of the Aorta

For the half hour immediately before cross-clamping and aortic occlusion, the patient is kept in a slightly hypovolemic state, accomplished by using 2D TEE to estimate ventricular volume or by keeping pulmonary or arterial pressure at 5 to 12 mmHg. At the time of occlusion, I am prepared to give a vasodilating drug through an intravenous line available specifically for that purpose. This precaution of using a specific intravenous line is taken to avoid hypotension caused by accidental bolus administration of vasodilator. The infusion site is often the third lumen of the pulmonary artery catheter.

During the early part of aortic dissection, I protect the heart by trying to keep hemodynamic variables within the preoperative range.[60] Without evidence to the contrary, a little hypertension must be assumed to be just as harmful as a little hypotension. For example, in extreme cases, systolic blood pressure might be allowed to decrease to as low as 90 mmHg or to rise to as high as 190 mmHg if the preoperative range was 110 to 170 mmHg. A contingency plan goes into effect should values approach or exceed these limits. If blood pressure reaches 150 mmHg, the amount of anesthetic is increased; at approximately 160 mmHg, nitroprusside is infused; at 165 or 175 mmHg, the table is tilted. If systolic blood pressure drops to 110 mmHg, the anesthetic is decreased and the possible causes of hypotension are reviewed. At 105 mmHg, the amount of anesthetic is decreased even more, and the patient is placed in a head-down position. At 100 mmHg, more fluid is infused, and the patient is titled in a steeper head-down position. The possible causes of hypotension are reviewed again, and, if possible, the cause is corrected. At 90 mmHg, a dilute drip infusion of phenylephrine is added: 10 mg of phenylephrine in 500 ml of saline is infused at a rate that increases systolic blood pressure to approximately 100 mmHg.

For heart rate, a range of acceptable values is again established based on preoperative determinations. Using a preoperative range of 60 to 90 beats/min as an example, I would initiate the following treatment if these limits were exceeded. Here, tachycardia is assumed to be of greater concern than bradycardia and would be prevented more aggressively. At 95 beats/min, I might increase the anesthetic, give more narcotic, or add an intravenous drip infusion of a β-adrenergic receptor-blocking drug. At 100 beats/min, a bolus might be given (or an intravenous drip infusion begun) of a β-adrenergic receptor-blocking drug, assuming intravascular fluid volume was acceptable. At 45 beats/min, the anesthetic might be decreased or a dilute solution of dopamine (200 mg in 500 ml of saline or 5 percent dextrose in water) administered. Again, bradycardia is tolerated to a greater extent than tachycardia during these operations, because, in my view, minimizing myocardial oxygen demand should be of primary importance. Use of 2D TEE gives some latitude in the range of acceptable values before intervention.

Pulmonary artery pressures are not allowed to remain abnormal (that is, below 5 or above 15 mmHg) during this procedure, assuming that these values are confirmed by echocardiographic values. Increases in pulmonary artery pressure are treated aggressively by administration of nitroglycerin or nitroprusside, depending on whether the suspected cause is an increase in preload or an increase in afterload.[76,77] For low pressures, more fluid is infused, except in the 1- or 2-minute interval immediately before application of the aortic cross-clamp.

During Temporary Occlusion of the Aorta

Application of a cross-clamp to the aorta at the supraceliac level probably produces the greatest hemodynamic stress normally experienced by surgical patients. In fact, 92 percent of the patients our group has studied had ischemia, as evidenced by abnormal motion and thickening of the wall[59] (Table 10-2). Temporary occlusion at more distal levels is less hemodynamically stressful. Stabilizing pulmonary artery pressure and systemic blood pressure by administering vasodilating drugs before and during suprarenal cross-clamping may not be sufficient. In one of our studies, myocardial ischemia (as indicated by abnormal global or regional motion of the wall) required additional administration of vasodilating drugs, to the point of bringing systolic blood pressure toward the low end of the normal preoperative range.[59] If this occurs and blood pressure is as low as possible (i.e., administration of nitroprusside has reduced afterload), I often attempt to decrease preload with nitroglycerin and, if necessary, to decrease heart rate with intravenous administration of esmolol; propranolol can also be given. If these maneuvers fail to prevent myocardial dysfunction on placement of the cross-clamp, the surgeon can be asked to unclamp the aorta partially until myocardial function is more stable. This is done before incision of the aorta or its branches. In our study, despite myocardial dysfunction in 11 of the 12 patients undergoing supraceliac cross-clamping, only 1 of the 11 had perioperative myocardial infarction.[59] Therefore, myocardial contractility seems to be affected most by ventricular size and by keeping vital signs within the normal preoperative range.

I try to avoid administering vasoconstrictors if at all possible. Although coronary and cerebral vessels are not as densely innervated as other areas of the body, α_1- and α_2-adrenergic agents can still induce coronary and cerebral vasoconstriction. In addition, α-adrenergic vasoconstriction appears to be important in maintaining an appropriate distribution of flow between the outer and inner myocardium.[77] Perhaps because of this, or perhaps for other reasons, myocardial ischemia occurs more than twice as frequently in patients who are deeply anesthetized and whose systemic pressure is maintained with infusion of phenylephrine than in those whose blood pressure is maintained simply by light anesthesia and endogenous vasoconstrictors.[79] Such ischemia appears to be related to the myocardial dilation induced by these agents (the problem of a stretched, dilated myocardium[79]).

In preparation for unclamping of the aorta, a different set of maneuvers is performed to reach the same goals. To ensure adequate volume when the cross-clamp is removed, I replace blood losses during occlusion by administering warmed blood, milliliter for milliliter. I normally have only four units of packed cells available during this procedure. The packed cells usually are diluted with normal saline or, less commonly, with lactated Ringer's solution (making sure to add enough lactated Ringer's solution to avoid clumping of the cells because of the calcium in that solution). Although my preference is to administer whole blood, it is not routinely available at our institution.[80]

When greater blood loss is anticipated (e.g., for patients previously operated on for the same condition), I often have autotransfusion available and a second person to operate the equipment. After the sixth unit of blood has been given and if more blood loss is anticipated, or after 8 units of blood have been administered, 10 units of platelets are requested for the patient (and occasionally 2 units of fresh frozen plasma). After giving 8 to 10 units of packed cells, I routinely administer a unit of fresh frozen plasma for each unit of packed cells (see Chs. 30 and 31 for a different point of view). When no more blood is at hand, and if it is absolutely necessary (that is, when colloid or crystalloid cannot be used), the best available type-specific, washed packed cells are administered. For example, if B-negative blood is needed but not available, B-positive blood is given. Blood filters are changed after every two units when transfusion blood is more than 10 days old, and after every four units when it is less than 10 days old.

Because a large part of the vascular tree is excluded from circulation during temporary occlusion of the aorta, blood loss can be considerable during cross-clamping at the supraceliac level, without onset of hypotension or tachycardia. Since maintenance of volume status is so important, I monitor more than pulmonary artery pressures or occlusion pressures. Observation of the surgical field is of key importance. When any blood vessel is dissected, the anesthetist and surgeon must communicate closely; blood loss can occur with astonishing rapidity, and the attention of the anesthetist may not be focused on the operative field. Watching the volume in the suction bottles or listening to the sound that suction of variable amounts of fluid makes supplements the data, as does observation of left ventricular cavity size on 2D TEE.

Blood loss into the pleural or retroperitoneal cavity may not be detected in the amounts that are measured every 5 to 10 minutes. In addition, evisceration of bowel, often necessary for optimal exposure of the thoracoabdominal aorta, further depletes intravascular volume. Thus, the anesthetist has to be guided closely by pulmonary artery pressures or echocardiographic estimates of left ventricular filling volumes, or both. Just before removal of the cross-clamp to reopen the aorta, blood pressure, pulmonary capillary wedge pressure, and filling volumes are allowed to rise as high as possible without the occurrence of myocardial ischemia. The surgeon then opens the aorta gradually to ensure that neither hypotension nor bleeding from the suture line is excessive.

During Removal of the Cross-Clamp

Pathophysiologic events on removal of the aortic cross-clamp may cause inadequate return of volume to the heart (that is, inadequate preload). Thus, immediately before and during removal of the cross-clamp, infusion of nitroprusside is discontinued and infusion of crystalloid or blood is begun; usually, 2 units of whole blood or 2 liters of crystalloid are pressured into venous access sites. Note, however, that the total volume of blood and crystalloid administered rarely exceeds the content of the suction bottles by more than 3 liters. Also, the usual aim is to have hematocrit from 28 to 32 percent at the end of surgery. Guided by filling pressures or echocardiographic estimates of volume, or both, I am careful not to dilate the left ventricle to an abnormal size. Another technique for maintaining normal volumes during cross-clamping is controlled volume depletion. That is, for a short time, a specific amount of blood is removed (see Ch. 30) from the patient just before or during application of the cross-clamp. Just before removal of the clamp, this amount is replaced. Although I have used this technique, I do not advocate its routine use.

A third technique for maintaining normal hemodynamic values employs halothane, enflurane, or isoflurane (rather than nitroglycerin or nitroprusside) as the vasodilating agent. This interesting technique is usually effective[81] but requires very close observation of pulmonary artery pressures, the echocardiogram, or both, or assurance that myocardial dilation and dysfunction do not occur. I do not recommend this technique for routine use.

As mentioned earlier, moderate hypotension may occur on removal of the aor-

tic cross-clamp. If hypotension persists for more than 4 minutes after removal of the clamp, and if blood pressure does not return to normal levels after blood deficits have been replaced, other causes should be sought. These include myocardial dysfunction caused by inadequate metabolism of the citrate present in replacement blood, if such blood has not yet gone to the liver, where citrate is metabolized. This problem can be treated by administering calcium, which antagonizes the effect of citrate.[70] Other causes include hidden, persistent bleeding or misjudged replacement of blood deficits: on the echocardiogram, the ventricular cavity would be devoid of volume; and on the oscilloscope, filling pressures reflecting pulmonary artery pressures would be low. If necessary, the surgeon can reclamp or occlude the aorta, preferably below the renal arteries. Thus, replacement and maintenance of volume are mainstays of therapy before, during, and immediately after removal of the supraceliac cross-clamp. When blood flow is opened up to the first extremity, replacement of volume should also be considered. Removal of the clamp from the second leg usually causes few hemodynamic effects, presumably because of the existence of collateral blood vessels across the pelvis.

Protecting the Central Nervous System

Other investigators have used sensory evoked potentials and the EEG to gauge protection of the brain and spinal cord.[48,82] Our group has found no benefit in examining the EEG and no evidence that stroke is a predictable consequence of aortic reconstruction, even at the supraceliac level. However, in rare instances, spinal cord ischemia is a predictable consequence of this procedure.

Although spinal cord sensory evoked potentials (see Ch. 26) may prove useful, I do not have much experience in using this technique. Animal experiments indicate that the period of time during which blood supply to the spinal cord can be temporarily disrupted before the occurrence of permanent neurologic injury may be longer with isoflurane than with other anesthetic agents. In this animal model, other halogenated anesthetics and intravenous anesthetics incur a shorter ischemic interval before permanent neurologic damage.[83]

Protecting the Kidneys

In one of our studies, intraoperative urinary output was not predictive of postoperative renal function.[45] We measured the hourly urinary output and calculated the lowest and mean urinary outputs for each of 137 patients undergoing aortic reconstruction (38 at the supraceliac level). Pulmonary capillary wedge pressure was kept within normal limits for each patient. When urinary output was less than 0.125 $ml·kg^{-1}·h^{-1}$, patients were given crystalloid (so that the pulmonary capillary wedge pressure increased to a high-normal level), or furosemide, mannitol, or nothing. For each patient, serum creatinine and blood urea nitrogen levels were assayed on postoperative days 1, 3, and 7. No significant correlation existed between mean intraoperative urinary output (or lowest hourly urinary output) and changes from preoperative to postoperative levels of creatinine or blood urea nitrogen (Fig. 10-1). Thus, urinary output, which is believed to be an index of perfusion and is therefore monitored routinely during surgery, had no predictive value regarding postoperative renal function in normovolemic patients undergoing aortic reconstruction.

Furthermore, no difference existed in

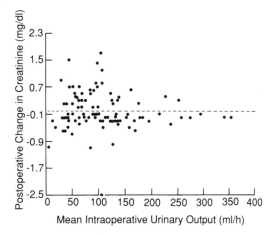

Fig. 10-1. Lowest hourly intraoperative urinary output did not correlate with maximum adverse change in renal function after surgery (i.e., change in creatinine levels from before aortic abdominal surgery to 7 days after surgery) in 137 patients. (From Alpert et al.,[45] with permission.)

postoperative renal function when aortic occlusion at the suprarenal level was compared with occlusion at the infrarenal level.[45]

Our results do not agree with those of other studies. Some investigations have found that pretreatment with mannitol lessened increases in creatinine levels after renal ischemia in patients and animals.[84–87] Direct infusion of mannitol into the renal artery sustained renal cortical perfusion (as assayed by the xenon washout technique) in mongrel dogs after infrarenal aortic occlusion.[84] In rabbits, pretreatment with mannitol prevented an increase in serum creatinine after 60 minutes of renal artery occlusion.[87] In dogs subjected to aortic clamping and unclamping, adequate replacement of blood with saline prevented a decrease in renal blood flow, an occurrence that is consistent with our findings (i.e., Alpert et al.[45]). Thus, furosemide and ethacrynic acid significantly increase both the total and the cortical components of renal blood flow, as demonstrated by studies of xenon 133 washout.[84] The use of mannitol, furosemide, or ethacrynic acid, however, has not been clearly shown to prevent renal failure. The difference between the results of Alpert et al.[45] and those of other investigators[84–87] may be due to variations among species, the maintenance of normal intravascular volume by Alpert and associates,[45] the insensitivity of urinary output as a measure of the adequacy of renal perfusion, or a combination of these factors. In my opinion, preoperative renal function, surgical speed and technique, and the maintenance of appropriate intravascular volume and normal myocardial function are the most important determinants of postoperative renal function.

It is important to monitor renal function because acute renal failure after aortic reconstruction incurs high morbidity and a mortality rate of more than 30 percent.[88] This complication occurs most frequently in patients with ruptured aneurysms who have signficant hypotension, and in those requiring clamping of the aorta at the suprarenal level. Despite our reported results, infusion of mannitol before clamping of the renal arteries is believed by some to be beneficial and is commonly used[89] (see Ch. 9). Furosemide, vasodilating drugs, and angiotensin-converting enzyme inhibitors may also be given before clamping of the renal artery. If prolonged renal ischemia is anticipated, selective profound hypothermia of the kidneys may decrease the incidence of postoperative renal impairment. It recently was suggested that infusion of verapamil into the renal arteries just before reperfusion might also be beneficial,[89] although the question has been raised whether any maneuver is more beneficial than good surgical technique.[45] However, my management is biased by results of my own studies. Thus, when intraoperative urinary output is less than 0.125

$ml \cdot kg^{-1} \cdot h^{-1}$, my procedure is to ensure that no mechanical problems exist in urine collection and that left-sided cardiac filling volumes or pressures are adequate. I then continue to monitor urinary output but do not treat low levels. Urinary output usually returns to acceptance levels within 2 hours. If it does not, or if I am uneasy about low urinary output, 2 to 5 mg of furosemide is administered intravenously for stimulation of urine production.[45]

Thus, virtually all investigators have concluded that maintenance of adequate intravascular volume and myocardial function largely prevents insufficiency of the kidneys or other organs from becoming major clinical problems and that this practice is the key to intraoperative perfusion of critical organs.

CHOICE OF ANESTHETIC AND ADJUVANT AGENTS

Almost all anesthetic techniques and drugs have been used for aortic reconstructive surgery. For this operative procedure, as for other types of vascular surgery, the skill of the anesthetist in maintaining hemodynamic equilibrium and in attending to detail appears to be more crucial to outcome than choice of drugs.[90] Although choice of agent and technique does indeed appear to affect outcome,[26,91,92] quality of care and the attentiveness of the anesthesiologist are, in my opinion, much more important.

Inhalation Anesthetics

Halothane, enflurane, and isoflurane are halogenated hydrocarbons having negative inotropic properties when administered to volunteers not undergoing surgery. However, during surgery, these agents act as vasodilators,[81,93,94] isoflurane being the most potent. Vasodilation is both advantageous and disadvantageous: it provides an additional way of controlling afterload and preload but can increase intravascular volume. This increased volume can be detrimental at the end of the procedure. As the amount of the anesthetic decreases, intravascular volume could return to the central compartment and cause relative hypervolemia and even pulmonary edema. To prevent this problem in patients given a volatile anesthetic or an epidural anesthetic, I simulate the situation of increased central blood volume that occurs with awakening. That is, I tilt the patient (head lower than feet) for the approximately 30 minutes of closure, and then slowly return the patient to the level position while either gradually reducing the concentration of the volatile anesthetic or letting the epidural anesthetic wear off. Tilting the patient allows me to predict the postanesthetic volume status and to make appropriate adjustments.

Volatile agents have several other advantages. They permit careful, deliberate induction, manipulation and monitoring of hemodynamic variables, and adjustment of dose. In addition, by providing a moderate degree of muscle relaxation, they decrease the need for muscle relaxants and increase the ease of reversing paralysis.

With the use of volatile hydrocarbon anesthetics, tracheal extubation usually can be accomplished by the end of surgery, at which time the patient is allowed to breathe spontaneously. Thus, the stressful stimuli and hypertension associated with continued intubation are avoided, and early assessment of neurologic function is facilitated. This process also allows evaluation of motor function and sensation of the limbs should I wish to place an epidural catheter for postoperative analgesia. Also, because extuba-

tion occurs at the end of surgery, the patient is able to report angina, for which nitroglycerin can then be given.

Since the introduction of isoflurane, I have tended to avoid using halothane. Occlusion of the aorta at the supraceliac level tends to make the liver hypoxic for a time; under this condition, halothane theoretically could create a hepatitis-like condition.[95] However, in one of our group's studies, 20 of the first 40 patients we anesthetized for supraceliac aortic revascularization were given halothane without any adverse effect attributable to that agent.[81]

Narcotic Anesthetics

All commonly used narcotics produce similar cardiovascular effects unless they are administered rapidly in large doses.[90] Induction of anesthesia with narcotic agents can be accomplished quickly and decreases cardiac index (cardiac output per square meter of surface area) by a small but statistically significant amount. In sufficient doses, narcotics produce analgesia and hypnosis, with only slight decreases in cardiac contractility and blood pressure.[90] By continuing to infuse narcotics or to administer other agents, one can maintain anesthesia throughout surgery. Surgical stimulation after such induction significantly increases heart rate, arterial blood pressure, and systemic vascular resistance. Nitroglycerin, nitroprusside, or a volatile anesthetic agent can be added to the narcotic for manipulation of circulation during clamping and unclamping of the aorta.

Nitrous oxide can be used with narcotics, as with the inhalational agents. It increases afterload and myocardial work, depresses myocardial inotropic performance and output, and decreases renal and splanchnic blood flow.[93,96] In addition, nitrous oxide may produce long-lasting toxicity by causing nutritional, neurologic, and immunologic deficits.[97] It can also distend the bowel.

A disadvantage of using narcotics is that they tend to linger in the patient into the postoperative period. This characteristic increases the likelihood that controlled ventilation will be needed after surgery. However, in more than 50 percent of the narcotic/nitrous oxide anesthetic techniques used for suprarenal aortic reconstruction, Benefiel et al.[26] were able to extubate the trachea in the operating room. An advantage of using high doses of narcotics as the anesthetic is that this method provides continued, excellent postoperative analgesia.

In a prospective controlled study at our institution, patients were randomly assigned to receive either a volatile agent (isoflurane) or a narcotic (sufentanil)-based anesthetic for aortic reconstruction.[26] During and after surgery, systemic and pulmonary capillary blood pressures and heart rates were kept within 20 percent of mean (baseline) preoperative ward values. Major morbidity was less with sufentanil anesthesia than with isoflurane anesthesia (Table 10-3). Because published rates of complications in patients undergoing aortic reconstruction[12,15,26,27] have been as high as or higher than those for the isoflurane group of Benefiel et al.,[26] my belief is that sufentanil has a protective effect. Further study is needed to determine whether all narcotics are protective, or whether the combination of sufentanil and isoflurane produces an outcome as good as, or better than, that with sufentanil alone.

Epidural Anesthetics

Epidural anesthesia has been used successfully for resection of infrarenal aortic aneurysms and aortic reconstruction.[98] It can also be combined with general anes-

thesia for supraceliac aortic reconstruction. A significant risk with epidural anesthetics is that administration of heparin might create an epidural hematoma and subsequent neurologic deficit.[99] Such a deficit could be confused with that caused by spinal cord ischemia, thereby delaying correct diagnosis, evacuation of the hematoma, and return of neurologic function. Thus, I am reluctant to use epidural anesthesia for supraceliac aortic reconstruction. In addition, the absence of sensation and movement of the leg after surgery might cause undue worry for the patient. This disadvantage can be ameliorated by administering (at the end of surgery) epidural anesthetic agents in concentrations that affect sensory but not motor fibers. A number of studies, including a large series of Rao and El-Etr[99] (see Ch. 24) and a study on use of epidural anesthesia even after full heparinization in cardiac surgery,[100] indicate that this potential problem is more theoretical than actual. Use of heparin does not appear to contraindicate the use of epidural anesthesia or even continuous epidural anesthesia.

Rao and El-Etr[99] believe that proper patient selection and atraumatic technique are important in ensuring a low rate of complications with regional anesthesia. Their protocol included postponement of elective vascular surgery for 24 hours if blood was aspirated from the epidural needle. This protocol was intended to allow clot formation in the epidural space before institution of intraoperative anticoagulation.[99] Other groups use a single-shot epidural or intrathecal technique with a 25- or 26-gauge needle to reduce the risk of postponement of surgery and to provide for postoperative pain relief by addition of a narcotic.[101] To reduce the incidence of pruritus and respiratory depression from such epidural or intrathoracic analgesia, some anesthesiologists routinely infuse

Table 10-3. Morbidity and Mortality Associated with Two Anesthetic Agents for Aortic Reconstruction

Morbidity and Mortality	No. of Instances of Morbidity after Aortic Surgery with:	
	Isoflurane-Based Anesthetic (n = 50)[a]	Sufentanil-Based Anesthetic (n = 46)[a]
Renal insufficiency	16	4[b]
Congestive heart failure	13	4[b]
Mechanical ventilation necessary for more than 24 hours	9	4
Pneumonia	2	1
Renal failure	3	1
Stroke	2	0
Myocardial infarction	0	1
Death	2	1
Important or severe complications	20	9[b]
Important or severe complications and failure	17	7[b]

[a] n = of patients
[b] $P < 0.05$, as determined by Fisher's exact test.
(Modified from Benefiel et al.,[26] with permission.)

naloxone (2 mg in 250 ml of saline, which equals 8 μg/ml, given at a rate of 0.5 to 1.5 $\mu g \cdot kg^{-1} \cdot h^{-1}$ or about 7 ml/h).[101,102] Because most patients who undergo aortic reconstruction have urinary catheters in place for at least 36 hours after surgery, retention of urine (another side effect of spinal or epidural narcotics) is not a major issue. Another potential disadvantage of epidural anesthesia is the possibility of a relative overload of fluid toward the end of the procedure. As with inhalational agents, the patient is tilted (head lower than feet) near the end of the procedure so that fluid status is normal as the anesthetic wears off.

One advantage of using epidural anesthesia is the possible decrease in myocardial ischemia.[100] However, most findings suggesting this advantage include a comparison group given a fixed dose of isoflurane rather than an individualized dose based on the patient's hemodynamic status.[100] Epidural anesthesia may also make myocardial ischemia worse.[78] Other advantages include excellent muscle relaxation, a smaller bowel (because of sympathectomy) that tends not to obstruct the operative field, and hemodynamic stability once the block is fully achieved.

The initiation of epidural anesthesia often decreases blood pressure, cardiac output, and possibly perfusion to the gut and kidney, which, in the stenotic state, may be pressure dependent. During clamping and unclamping of the aorta in a patient under epidural anesthesia, the circulation can be controlled by administration of volatile anesthetics or intravenous agents that reduce afterload.

In addition, Yeager and colleagues[92] compared epidural with general anesthesia regarding outcome after surgical procedures in 48 patients, some of whom had vascular operations. The incidence of cardiovascular and infectious disease complications, plus medical care costs, were lower with the combination of epidural anesthesia and general anesthesia than with general anesthesia alone. Similar results were obtained for patients given epidural analgesia after surgery.[101] Thus, epidural anesthesia appears not to be a risky technique and, in fact, may be advantageous for aortic reconstruction.

In view of certain characteristics of the Yeager et al.[92] study (the small number of patients studied, particularly vascular patients, and the little detail provided about the general anesthesia technique), another study verifying the findings of this group seems to be in order. The same need applies to our study showing a benefit for sufentanil compared with inhalational anesthetics.[26] The technique I use is inevitably influenced by my own studies.

Muscle Relaxants

The choice of muscle relaxants for aortic reconstruction consists of continuous infusion of succinylcholine or bolus injections of *d*-tubocurarine, metocurine, pancuronium, vecuronium, or atracurium. The newer neuromuscular relaxants vecuronium and atracurium have shorter half-lives and provide more hemodynamic stability than do the other agents. *d*-Tubocurarine is preferable to metocurine or pancuronium when the degree of hypertension is insignificant, the vagolytic effect of pancuronium is not desired, or renal insufficiency is great enough to prolong excretion of metocurine or pancuronium. I routinely titrate the muscle relaxant to the chronotropic cardiovascular effect I wish to achieve.

ONE APPROACH TO PROVIDING ANESTHESIA FOR SUPRARENAL AORTIC AND VISCERAL VASCULAR SURGERY

The following section describes my procedure for providing anesthesia for suprarenal aortic reconstruction. As soon as all oral intake has been restricted, prehydration is begun at maintenance rates. Although specific data are not available to support this view, my opinion is that maintenance of a normal hydration status reduces variations in blood pressure upon induction of anesthesia.

After the patient's preoperative condition has been optimized, the preoperative range of values for hemodynamic variables is determined for this particular patient. Then anesthesia management is planned so that intraoperative values are kept within 20 percent of this range, provided pulmonary capillary wedge pressure does not exceed 15 mmHg, heart rate does not exceed 100 beats/min, and no signs of organ ischemia are present. Premedication is requested and consists of a benzodiazepine and a narcotic—usually diazepam, 0.015 mg/kg, given 1.5 to 2 hours before incision; and morphine sulfate, 0.01 mg/kg, administered intramuscularly 1 hour before incision. These dosages are reduced for old age, debility, pulmonary disease, and other conditions.

All of the patient's usual medications are also requested. In my view, any drug therapy required chronically for wellbeing will most probably also be required during surgery. Omitting chronic drug therapy can worsen the condition of the disease after surgery. For example, tachycardia, angina, or both may occur if propranolol is omitted; aspiration of saliva or food, if levodopa is omitted; or accelerated hypertension, if clonidine is omitted. Thus, I believe that the patient should be given antihypertensive medication, including diuretics, before being brought to the operating room.[60] Many diabetic patients who require insulin are given an infusion of insulin throughout surgery, or half the usual dose on the morning of surgery. Preoperative considerations and drug therapy for diabetic patients are described elsewhere.[60] However, because no particular premedication seems indicated or contraindicated for most patients, the patient's anesthetist should determine what is appropriate. I avoid the use of anticholinergic drugs because they produce dry mouth and tachycardia, the former making the patient uncomfortable and the latter increasing myocardial oxygen consumption.

In the preoperative holding area and/or the operating room, I place the monitoring devices and lines I believe necessary for induction of anesthesia: usually, an 18-gauge radial artery catheter in the nondominant hand, a manual blood pressure cuff, a pulse oximeter, an electrocardiograph (leads II and modified chest lead V_5), an ST-segment trend monitor, a precordial stethoscope, a 16-gauge intravenous catheter, and a pulmonary artery line (or central venous pressure catheter if the patient shows no evidence of myocardial, pulmonary, or renal disease). Insertion of this last device can usually await until induction has been completed. Then, after 3 mg of *d*-tubocurarine has been given, infusion of 750 μg of sufentanil in 100 ml of saline is begun at a rate of approximately 15 to 50 μg/min per 70 kg of body weight. Also, the patient is coached regarding breathing of 100 percent oxygen from a face mask (ventilation will continue for the next 6 hours). After approximately 3 minutes, thiopental (75 mg/70 kg) is administered intravenously and a 3- to 5-minute intravenous infusion of pancuronium (0.1 mg/kg) or metocurine (0.5 mg/kg) is begun, depending on whether I want heart rate to increase or

stay the same. Other agents are chosen if the patient has renal insufficiency and a creatinine level above 2 mg/dl.

When depth of anesthesia is judged adequate (by lack of response to insertion of a Foley catheter or placement of another intravenous catheter, or by the existence of pinpoint pupils) and when muscle relaxation is adequate, the trachea is intubated and mechanical ventilation is begun with 0 to 60 percent nitrous oxide in oxygen. The rest of the period before cross-clamping is devoted to meticulous attention to maintaining various conditions. Temperature is maintained by use of a heating mattress, warming of all fluids, and if necessary, warming of ventilatory gases. Volume homeostasis is assessed by heart rate, blood pressure, pulmonary capillary or central venous pressure, and left ventricular end-diastolic volume (using 2D TEE). I ensure the absence of organ ischemia and monitor, but usually do not treat, urinary output. Also, systemic and pulmonary blood pressures and heart rate are kept within the patient's normal preoperative range. Every increase in blood pressure or heart rate is either anticipated or treated as soon as it occurs with 25 to 50 μg of sufentanil per 70 kg of body weight. Further increases are treated with repeated doses of sufentanil or with addition of nitroglycerin or nitroprusside, enflurane or isoflurane, or esmolol or propranolol, depending on the event and on my best estimate of cause. The rest of the patient's course is managed by the physiologic principles discussed above.

An earlier section ("Protecting the Myocardium") provided details about minimizing the risk of myocardial ischemia. This paragraph summarizes those ideas. Starting 0.5 hour before clamping of the aorta, the patient is kept in a slightly hypovolemic state. At the time of occlusion, I am prepared to give a vasodilating drug through an intravenous line placed specifically for that purpose, to avoid hypotension secondary to an accidental bolus administration of vasodilator. When stabilizing pulmonary artery and systemic blood pressures with administration of more sufentanil and vasodilating drugs before and during aortic clamping is not sufficient (i.e., when wall motion abnormalities or changes in ST segment indicate myocardial ischemia), additional vasodilating drugs are given until systolic blood pressure is at the low end of the normal preoperative range. Once afterload has been reduced as much as possible with nitroprusside, I often attempt to decrease preload with nitroglycerin and, if necessary, to decrease heart rate with esmolol or propranolol. If these maneuvers fail to prevent myocardial dysfunction on placement of the clamp, the surgeon is usually asked to unclamp the aorta partially until myocardial function becomes more stable. Close communication between surgeon and anesthetist and a mutual appreciation of the actions of the other are key, I believe, to facilitating the patient's course. Administration of vasoconstrictors is avoided at all times.[79]

Two practices ensure adequate volume at the time of removal of the clamp: replacing all blood lost during occlusion with warmed blood, and keeping hematocrit slightly above 30 percent (hematocrit will decrease to 30 percent after occlusion). My personal belief, substantiated by some data, is that 30 percent is the minimum acceptable hematocrit value for patients in this risk group.[103–106] Much of the transfused blood is either predeposited or autotransfused blood salvaged from the operative field. Immediately before and during removal of the cross-clamp, infusion of vasodilator is discontinued and infusion of crystalloid or blood is begun; usually, two units of whole blood are pressured into venous access sites. Guided by filling

pressures or echocardiographic estimates of volume, I am careful not to dilate the left ventricle to an abnormal size.

As discussed earlier, moderate hypotension sometimes occurs on removal of the aortic cross-clamp, regardless of whether the clamp is replaced below the renal vessels or such that blood flow to only one leg is obstructed. If hypotension persists for more than 4 minutes after removal of the clamp and does not return to normal levels after replacement of blood deficits, other causes are sought, for example, myocardial dysfunction or hidden blood loss. If necessary, the surgeon can reclamp or occlude the aorta, preferably below the renal arteries. Thus, volume replacement and maintenance are mainstays of therapy before, during, and immediately after removal of the aortic cross-clamp. When blood flow to the first extremity is restored, volume replacement should also be considered.

During closure, I again ensure adequate organ perfusion, as well as hemodynamic and temperature homeostasis, and reverse the effect of muscle relaxants. I often have infusions of nitroglycerin and/or esmolol available at this time and do not allow hemodynamic variations outside the patient's normal range. If spontaneous ventilation is adequate (and it usually is by 6 hours after the initial dose of sufentanil), the trachea is extubated. Otherwise, controlled ventilation continues until spontaneous ventilation is judged adequate. If an inhalational anesthesia is used, an epidural catheter is normally placed at the end of the operation, while the patient is still in the operating room, but only after the patient has demonstrated bilateral foot movement (with light anesthesia during closure). Epidural narcotics are administered to these patients; other pain therapy is rarely needed for 24 hours when the sufentanil-based technique described here is used. In my view, continuing care into the postoperative period is very important for patient outcome.

CONCLUSION

Outcome after suprarenal aortic reconstructive surgery has improved. As the mortality rate has decreased, the use of venous pressure (fluid)-monitoring devices has increased: from 13 percent for 1961 to 1969 to 100 percent after 1971. After 1975, the use of pulmonary artery thermodilution catheters also increased.[107] Thus, overall, mortality and morbidity for aortic reconstructive surgery have decreased greatly over the last three decades. Crawford et al.[31] attributed most of the reduction in morbidity in patients who had infrarenal resections before 1971 to improvement in operative techniques; and after 1981, to improvements in anesthesia, monitoring, and supportive care. However, perioperative mortality from supraceliac aortic reconstruction still exceeds 4 percent.

One of our studies showed that an 8 percent incidence of myocardial infarction, with no mortality, is possible in patients who have severe myocardial dysfunction monitored with 2D TEE.[59] However, the 4 percent mortality of Crawford et al.[31] and the even lower rate of Benefiel et al.[26] seem to me to be as good as one can expect to achieve using current techniques. Morbidity and mortality should be only negligible for patients who have isolated celiac artery disease and little dysfunction in other organs.

Perhaps in no other subspecialty can anesthesiologists have as great an influence on patient outcome as in anesthesia for suprarenal aortic reconstructive surgery. Patients undergoing vascular reconstruction are generally elderly. Because vascular disease is a generalized process, such patients are likely to have atherosclerotic disease elsewhere in their vascular system. Most have coronary artery disease. Many have a history of smoking, chronic obstructive pulmonary disease, renal insufficiency, or lipid abnormalities. Despite these concerns, it is the stress of clamping and unclamping of the suprarenal aorta on an already compromised heart that is responsible for most of the morbidity associated with vascular surgery. Therefore, my bias is to make the heart the major focus of attention. I believe the available data on aortic reconstruction suggest that ensuring intact myocardial function is probably the best way of making certain that spinal cord, visceral, and renal perfusion will be adequate.

Attempts have been made to identify (e.g., by dipyridamole-thallium imaging or coronary angiography) patients who have significant coronary artery disease and are therefore at high risk of myocardial events. The purpose is to have such patients undergo coronary artery bypass surgery before their vascular surgery. However, such approaches have not been demonstrated to reduce morbidity. Critics claim that identification of high-risk patients is useful but that coronary angiography and prophylactic coronary artery surgery are simply "survival tests" for vascular surgery. The future of such methods will be determined by results of studies on outcome. Until then, maintenance of normal hemodynamic variables and vigilance about myocardial well-being will remain my highest priorities. I also believe that consistent meticulous attention to details such as prehydration and use of warming mattresses are, in the long run, far more important to outcome than is the occasional brilliant therapeutic maneuver.

Although my biases regarding both monitoring and anesthetic techniques are evident, it should also be clear that many other approaches can be used for avoiding myocardial dysfunction. Perhaps it is most important to remember that the best patient results are probably achieved when the great vigilance shown during surgery is also applied before and especially after surgery.

REFERENCES

1. Plecha FR, Avellone JC, Beven EG et al: A computerized vascular registry: experience of The Cleveland Vascular Society. Surgery 86:826–835, 1979
2. Kouchoukos NT, Lell WA, Karp RB, Samuelson PN: Hemodynamic effects of aortic clamping and decompression with a temporary shunt for resection of the descending thoracic aorta. Surgery 85:25–30, 1979
3. DeBakey ME: Changing concepts in vascular surgery. J Cardiovasc Surg 27:367–409, 1986
4. May AG, DeWeese JA, Frank I et al: Surgical treatment of abdominal aortic aneurysms. Surgery 63:711–721, 1968
5. Hollier LH, Reigel MM, Kazmier FJ et al: Conventional repair of abdominal aortic aneurysm in the high-risk patient: a plea for abandonment of nonresective treatment. J Vasc Surg 3:712–717, 1986
6. Estes EJ, Jr: Abdominal aortic aneurysm. A study of one hundred and two cases. Circulation 2:258–264, 1950
7. Foster JH, Bolasny BL, Gobbel WG, Jr., Scott HW, Jr: Comparative study of elective resection and expectant treatment of abdominal aortic aneurysm. Surg Gynecol Obstet 129:1–9, 1969
8. Darling RC, Messina CR, Brewster DC, Ottinger LW: Autopsy study of unoperated abdominal aortic aneurysms. The case for early resection. Circulation, 56: (suppl. 2), II-161 to II-164, 1977
9. Szilagyi DE, Elliott JP, Smith RF: Clinical fate of the patient with asymptomatic abdominal aortic aneurysm and unfit for surgical treatment. Arch Surg 104:600–606, 1972
10. Khaw, H, Sottiurai VS, Craighead CC, Batson RC: Ruptured abdominal aortic aneurysm presenting as symptomatic inguinal mass: report of six cases. J Vasc Surg 4:384–389, 1986
11. Lambert ME, Baguley P, Charlesworth D: Ruptured abdominal aortic aneurysms. J Cardiovasc Surg 27:256–261, 1986
12. Thompson JE, Hollier LH, Patman RD, Persson AV: Surgical management of abdominal aortic aneurysms: factors influencing mortality and morbidity—a 20-year experience. Ann Surg 181:654–661, 1975
13. Thurmond AS, Semler HJ: Abdominal aortic aneurysm: incidence in a population of risk. J Cardiovasc Surg 27:457–460, 1986
14. Reigel MM, Hollier LH, Kazmier FJ et al: Late survival in abdominal aortic aneurysm patients: the role of selective myocardial revascularization on the basis of clinical symptoms. J Vasc Surg 5:222–227, 1987
15. Szilagyi DE, Smith RF, DeRusso FJ et al: Contribution of abdominal aortic aneurysmectomy to prolongation of life. Ann Surg 164:678–699, 1966
16. Attia R, Murphy JD, Snider M et al: Myocardial ischemia due to infrarenal aortic cross-clamping during aortic surgery in patients with severe coronary artery disease. Circulation 53:961–965, 1976
17. Silverstein PR, Caldera DL, Cullen DJ et al: Avoiding the hemodynamic consequences of aortic cross-clamping and unclamping. Anesthesiology 50:462–466, 1979
18. Brewster DC, Darling RC: Optimal methods of aortoiliac reconstruction. Surgery 84:739–748, 1978
19. Hollier LH, Bernatz PE, Pairolero PC et al: Surgical management of chronic intestinal ischemia: a reappraisal. Surgery 90:940–946, 1981
20. Rogers DM, Thompson JE, Garrett WV et al: Mesenteric vascular problems. A 26-year experience. Ann Surg 195:554–565, 1982
21. Stoney RJ, Lusby RJ: Surgery of celiac and mesenteric arteries. p. 813–825. In

Haimovici H. (ed): Vascular Surgery. Principles and Techniques. 2nd Ed. Appleton-Century-Crofts, Norwalk, CT, 1984

22. Stoney RJ, Ehrenfeld WK, Wylie EJ: Revascularization methods in chronic visceral ischemia caused by atherosclerosis. Ann Surg 186:468–476, 1977

23. Baur GM, Millay DJ, Taylor LM, Jr., Porter JM: Treatment of chronic visceral ischemia. Am J Surg 148:138–144, 1984

24. Crawford ES, Morris GC, Jr., Myhre HO, Roehm JOF, Jr: Celiac axis, superior mesenteric artery, and inferior mesenteric artery occlusion: surgical considerations. Surgery 82:856–866, 1977

25. Roizen MF, Ellis JE, Smith JS et al: Anesthesia for major vascular surgery. p. 183–196. In Estafanous FG (ed): Anesthesia and the Heart. Butterworth, Stoneham, MA, 1988

26. Benefiel DJ, Roizen MF, Lampe GH et al: Morbidity after aortic surgery with sufentanil vs isoflurane anesthesia (abstract). Anesthesiology 65:A516, 1986

27. Young AE, Sandberg GW, Couch NP: The reduction of mortality of abdominal aortic aneurysm resection. Am J Surg 134:585–590, 1977

28. Hicks GL, Eastland MW, DeWeese JA et al: Survival improvement following aortic aneurysm resection. Ann Surg 181:863–869, 1975

29. Mulcare RJ, Royster TS, Lynn RA, Conners RB: Long-term results of operative therapy for aortoiliac disease. Arch Surg 113:601–604, 1978

30. Whittemore AD, Clowes AW, Hechtman HB, Mannick JA: Aortic aneurysm repair. Reduced operative mortality associated with maintenance of optimal cardiac performance. Ann Surg 192:414–421, 1980

31. Crawford ES, Saleh SA, Babb JW, III et al: Infrarenal abdominal aortic aneurysm. Factors influencing survival after operation performed over a 25-year period. Ann Surg 193:699–709, 1981

32. Hertzer NR: Myocardial ischemia. Surgery 93:97–101, 1983

33. Yeager RA, Weigel RM, Murphy ES et al: Application of clinically valid cardiac risk factors to aortic aneurysm surgery. Arch Surg 121:278–281, 1986

34. Roizen MF: Anesthesia for vascular surgery. p. 93–104. In Benumof JL (ed): Clinical Frontiers in Anesthesiology. Grune & Stratton, Orlando, FL, 1983

35. Carroll RM, Laravuso RB, Schauble JF: Left ventricular function during aortic surgery. Arch Surg 111:740–743, 1976

36. Lunn JK, Dannemiller FJ, Stanley TH: Cardiovascular responses to clamping of the aorta during epidural and general anesthesia. Anesth Analg 58:372–376, 1979

37. Meloche R, Pottecher T, Audet J et al: Haemodynamic changes due to clamping of the abdominal aorta. Can Anaesth Soc J 24:20–34, 1977

38. DeBakey ME, Creech O, Jr., Morris GC, Jr: Aneurysm of thoracoabdominal aorta involving the celiac, superior mesenteric, and renal arteries. Report of four cases treated by resection and homograft replacement. Ann Surg 144:549–573, 1956

39. Burnham SJ, Johnson G, Jr., Gurri JA: Mortality risks for survivors of vascular reconstructive procedures. Surgery 92:1072–1076, 1983

40. Denlin A, Ohlsén H, Swedenborg J: Growth rate of abdominal aortic aneurysms as measured by computed tomography. Br J Surg 72:530–532, 1985

41. Darling RC: Ruptured arteriosclerotic abdominal aortic aneurysms. A pathologic and clinical study. Am J Surg 119:397–401, 1970

42. Sabawala PB, Strong MJ, Keats AS: Surgery of the aorta and its branches. Anesthesiology 33:229–259, 1970

43. Barry KG, Mazze RI, Schwartz FD: Prevention of surgical oliguria and renal-hemodynamic suppression by sustained hydration. N Engl J Med 270:1371–1377, 1964

44. Wheeler CG, Thompson JE, Kartchner MM et al: Massive fluid requirement in surgery of the abdominal aorta. N Engl J Med 275:320–322, 1968

45. Alpert RA, Roizen MF, Hamilton WK et al: Intraoperative urinary output does not predict postoperative renal function

in patients undergoing abdominal aortic revascularization. Surgery 95:707–711, 1984

46. Bush HL, Jr., LoGerfo FW, Weisel RD et al: Assessment of myocardial performance and optimal volume loading during elective abdominal aortic aneurysm resection. Arch Surg 112:1301–1306, 1977

47. Moyer JH, Heider C, Morris GC, Jr., Handley C: Renal failure. I. The effect of complete renal artery occlusion for variable periods of time as compared to exposure to sub-filtration arterial pressures below 30 mm Hg for similar periods. Ann Surg 145:41–58, 1957

48. Laschinger JC, Cunningham JN, Jr., Catinella FP et al: Detection and prevention of intraoperative spinal cord ischemia after cross-clamping of the thoracic aorta: use of somatosensory evoked potentials. Surgery 92:1109–1117, 1982

49. Crawford ES, Walker HSJ, III, Saleh SA, Normann NA: Graft replacement of aneurysm in descending thoracic aorta: results without bypass or shunting. Surgery 89:73–85, 1981

50. Marcus ML, Heistad DD, Ehrhardt JC, Abboud FM: Regulation of total and regional spinal cord blood flow. Circ Res 41:128–134, 1977

51. Kobrine AI, Doyle TF, Rizzoli HV: Spinal cord blood flow as affected by changes in systemic arterial blood pressure. J Neurosurg 44:12–15, 1976

52. Connolly JE: Prevention of paraplegia secondary to operations on the aorta. J Cardiovasc Surg 27:410–417, 1986

53. Wadouh F, Arndt C-F, Oppermann E et al: The mechanism of spinal cord injury after simple and double aortic cross-clamping. J Thorac Cardiovasc Surg 92:121–127, 1986

54. Vacanti FX, Ames A, III: Mild hypothermia and Mg^{++} protect against irreversible damage during CNS ischemia. Stroke 15:695–698, 1984

55. Coles JG, Wilson GJ, Sima AF et al: Intraoperative management of thoracic aortic aneurysm. Experimental evaluation of perfusion cooling of the spinal cord. J Thorac Cadiovasc Surg 85:292–299, 1983

56. Katz NM, Blackstone EH, Kirlin JW, Karp RB: Incremental risk factors for spinal cord injury following operation for acute traumatic aortic transection. J Thorac Cardiovasc Surg 81:669–674, 1981

57. Svensson LG, Loop FD: Prevention of spinal cord ischemia in aortic surgery. p. 273–285. In Bergan JJ, Yao JST (eds): Arterial Surgery. New Diagnostic and Operative Techniques. Grune & Stratton, Orlando, FL, 1988

58. Svensson LG, Rickards E, Coull A et al: Relationship of spinal cord blood flow to vascular anatomy during thoracic aortic cross-clamping and shunting. J Thorac Cardiovasc Surg 91:71–78, 1986

59. Roizen MF, Beaupre PN, Alpert RA et al: Monitoring with two-dimensional transesophageal echocardiography. Comparison of myocardial function in patients undergoing supraceliac, suprarenal-infraceliac, or infrarenal aortic occlusion. J Vasc Surg 1:300–305, 1984

60. Roizen MF: Anesthetic implications of concurrent diseases. p. 255–357. In Miller RD (ed): Anesthesia. 2nd ed. Vol. 1. Churchill Livingstone, New York, 1986

61. Boucher CA, Brewster DC, Darling RC et al: Determination of cardiac risk by dipyridamole-thallium imaging before peripheral vascular surgery. N Engl J Med 312:389–394, 1985

62. Leppo J, Plaja J, Gionet M et al: Noninvasive evaluation of cardiac risk before elective vascular surgery. J Am Coll Cardiol 9:269–276, 1987

63. Eagle KA, Singer DE, Brewster DC et al: Dipyridamole-thallium scanning in patients undergoing vascular surgery. Optimizing preoperative evaluation of cardiac risk. JAMA 257:2185–2189, 1987

64. Hertzer NR, Beven EG, Young JR et al: Coronary artery disease in peripheral vascular patients. A classification of 1000 coronary angiograms and results of surgical management. Ann Surg 199:223–233, 1984

65. Perry MO: The hemodynamics of tem-

porary abdominal aortic occlusion. Ann Surg 168:193–200, 1968

66. Kalman PG, Wellwood MR, Weisel RD et al: Cardiac dysfunction during abdominal aortic operation: the limitations of pulmonary wedge pressures. J Vasc Surg 3:773–781, 1986

67. Pandian NG, Kerber RE: Two-dimensional echocardiography in experimental coronary stenosis. I. Sensitivity and specificity in detecting transient myocardial dyskinesis: comparison with sonomicrometers. Circulation 66:597–602, 1982

68. Smith JS, Cahalan MK, Benefiel DJ et al: Intraoperative detection of myocardial ischemia in high-risk patients: electrocardiography versus two-dimensional transesophageal echocardiography. Circulation 72:1015–1021, 1985

69. Guyton AC: Textbook of Medical Physiology. 6th Ed. p. 230–243. WB Saunders, Philadelphia, 1981

70. Olinger GN, Hottenrott C, Mulder DG et al: Acute clinical hypocalcemic myocardial depression during rapid blood transfusion and postoperative hemodialysis. A preventable complication. J Thorac Cardiovasc Surg 72:503–511, 1976

71. Longo T, Marchetti G, Vercellio G: Coronary hemodynamic changes induced by aortic cross-clamping. J Cardiovasc Surg 10:36–42, 1969

72. Mandelbaum I, Webb MK: Left ventricular function during cross-clamping of the descending thoracic aorta. JAMA 186:229–231, 1963

73. Roizen MF, Rodgers GM, Valone FH et al: Anaphylactoid reaction to vascular graft material. Anesthesiology (in press).

74. Schlüter M, Langenstein BA, Polster J et al: Transoesophageal cross-sectional echocardiography with a phased array transducer system. Technique and initial clinical results. Br Heart J 48:67–72, 1982

75. Beaupre PN, Cahalan MK, Kremer PF et al: Does pulmonary artery occlusion pressure adequately reflect left ventricular filling during anesthesia and surgery (abstract)? Anesthesiology 59:A3, 1983

76. Flaherty JT, Magee PA, Gardner TL et al: Comparison of intravenous nitroglycerin and sodium nitroprusside for treatment of acute hypertension developing after coronary artery bypass surgery. Circulation 65:1072–1077, 1982

77. Gerson JI, Allen FB, Seltzer JL et al: Arterial and venous dilation by nitroprusside and nitroglycerin—is there a difference? Anesth Analg 61:256–260, 1982

78. Feigl EO: The paradox of adrenergic coronary vasoconstriction. Circulation 76:737–745, 1987

79. Smith JS, Roizen MF, Cahalan MK et al: Does anesthetic technique make a difference? Augmentation of systolic blood pressure during carotid endarterectomy: effects of phenylephrine *versus* light anesthesia and of isoflurane *versus* halothane on the incidence of myocardial ischemia. Anesthesiology 69:846–853, 1988

80. Office of Medical Applications, National Institutes of Health: Perioperative red blood cell transfusion. Consensus Development Conference, June 27–29, 1988. JAMA 260:2700–2703, 1988

81. Roizen MF, Hamilton WK, Sohn YJ: Treatment of stress-induced increases in pulmonary capillary wedge pressure using volatile anesthetics. Anesthesiology 55:446–450, 1981

82. Rampil IJ, Correll JW, Rosenbaum SH et al: Computerized electroencephalogram monitoring and carotid artery shunting. Neurosurgery 13:276–279, 1983

83. Koike M, Roizen MF, Zivin J et al: Naloxone ameliorates adverse effects of some anesthetics on CNS injury (abstract). Anesthesiology 59:A333, 1983

84. Abbott WM, Austen WG: The reversal of renal cortical ischemia during aortic occlusion by mannitol. J Surg Res 16:482–489, 1974

85. Barry KG, Cohen A, Knochel JP et al: Mannitol infusion. II. The prevention of acute functional renal failure during resection of an aneurysm of the abdominal aorta. N Engl J Med 264:967–971, 1961

86. Flores J, DiBona DR, Beck CH, Leaf A: The role of cell swelling in ischemic

renal damage and the protective effect of hypertonic solute. J Clin Invest 51:118–126, 1972

87. Hanley MJ, Davidson K: Prior mannitol and furosemide infusion in a model of ischemic acute renal failure. Am J Physiol 241:F556–F564, 1981

88. Ostri P, Mouritsen L, Jørgensen B, Frimodt-Møller C: Renal function following aneurysmectomy of the abdominal aorta. J Cardiovasc Surg 27:714–718, 1986

89. Miller DC, Myers BD: Pathophysiology and prevention of acute renal failure associated with thoracoabdominal or abdominal aortic surgery. J Vasc Surg 5:518–523, 1987

90. Roizen MF: Does choice of anesthetic (narcotic vs. inhalational) significantly affect cardiovascular surgery? p. 180–189. In Estafanous FG (ed): Opioids in Anesthesia. Butterworth, Stoneham, MA, 1984

91. Reiz S, Bålfors E, Sørensen MB et al: Isoflurane—a powerful coronary vasodilator in patients with coronary artery disease. Anesthesiology 59:91–97, 1983

92. Yeager MP, Glass DD, Neff RK, Brinck-Johnsen T: Epidural anesthesia and analgesia in high-risk surgical patients. Anesthesiology 66:729–736, 1987

93. Smith NT, Eger EI, II, Stoelting RK et al: The cardiovascular and sympathomimetic responses to the addition of nitrous oxide to halothane in man. Anesthesiology 32:410–421, 1970

94. Smith JS, Cahalan MK, Benefiel DJ et al: Fentanyl versus fentanyl and isoflurane in patients with impaired left ventricular function (abstract). Anesthesiology 63:A18, 1985

95. Shingu K, Eger EI, II, Johnson BH et al: Effect of oxygen concentration, hyperthermia, and choice of vendor in anesthetic-induced hepatic injury in rats. Anesth Analg 62:146–150, 1983

96. Eisele JH, Smith NT: Cardiovascular effects of 40 percent nitrous oxide in man. Anesth Analg 51:956–963, 1972

97. Koblin DD, Watson JE, Deady JE et al: Inactivation of methionine synthetase by nitrous oxide in mice. Anesthesiology 54:318–324, 1981

98. Cunningham FO, Egan JM, Inahara T: Continuous epidural anesthesia in abdominal vascular surgery. A review of 100 consecutive cases. Am J Surg 139:624–627, 1980

99. Rao TLK, El-Etr AA: Anticoagulation following placement of epidural and subarachnoid catheters: an evaluation of neurologic sequelae. Anesthesiology 55:618–620, 1981

100. Reiz S, Bålfors E, Sørensen MB et al: Coronary hemodynamic effects of general anesthesia and surgery: modification by epidural analgesia in patients with ischemic heart disease. Reg Anesth 7:S8–S20, 1982

101. Isaacson IJ, Berry AJ, Venner DS et al: Beneficial effects of intrathecal morphine on patients for abdominal aortic surgery. Anesthesiology (in press)

102. Jones RDM, Jones JG: Intrathecal morphine: naloxone reverses respiratory depression but not analgesia. Br Med J 281:645–646, 1980

103. Lundsgaard-Hansen P: Hemodilution—new clothes for an anemic emperor. Vox Sang 36:321–336, 1979

104. Most AS, Ruocco NA, Jr., Gewirtz H: Effect of a reduction in blood viscosity on maximal myocardial oxygen delivery distal to a moderate coronary stenosis. Circulation 74:1085–1092, 1986

105. Weisel RD, Charlesworth DC, Mickleborough LL et al: Limitations of blood conservation. J Thorac Cardiovasc Surg 88:26–38, 1984

106. Crystal GJ, Salem MR: Myocardial oxygen consumption and segmental shortening during selective coronary hemodilution in dogs. Anesth Analg 67:500–508, 1988

107. Scobie TK, Masters RG: Changing factors influencing abdominal aortic aneurysm repair. J Cardiovasc Surg 23:309–313, 1982

108. Roizen MF, Sohn YJ, Stoney RJ: Intraoperative management of the patient requiring supraceliac aortic occlusion. p. 312–321. In Wilson SE, Veith FJ, Hobson RW, II, Williams RA (eds): Vascular Surgery. Principles and Practice. McGraw-Hill, New York, 1987

11

Anesthesia for Visceral Arterial Reconstruction: One Approach at the Mayo Clinic

Jeffrey J. Lunn
Michael Nugent

Chronic visceral ischemia has evolved as a recognizable clinical syndrome over the last 100 years. In 1869, Chiene[1] first described the pathologic conditions of mesenteric artery occlusive disease. However, the relationship of these conditions to the signs and symptoms of visceral ischemia that are now generally recognized continue to be somewhat controversial. In the 1930s, Conner[2] and Dunphy[3] suggested that a history of chronic abdominal pain on ingestion of food (called abdominal or intestinal angina[4]) arose from mesenteric arterial occlusive disease and bowel infarction. Although extensive progress has been made since that time in recognizing and treating chronic intestinal ischemia, diagnosis and surgical intervention remain to be standardized.

Chronic visceral ischemia almost always occurs after atherosclerotic lesions produce high-grade stenosis or occlusion of arterial blood flow.[5] Although splanchnic vessel disease is quite common[6,7] and is often asymptomatic, the clinical syndrome of "intestinal angina" is distinctly uncommon. Indeed, many patients are asymptomatic despite occlusion of all three major vessels supplying the gut.[8,9] On rare occasions, occlusion results from arteritis,[10] fibromuscular dysplasia,[11] or amyloidosis.[12] Another less common cause of chronic visceral ischemia is extrinsic vascular compression by either the median arcuate ligament or other structures.[13–15]

Because the vast majority of patients with chronic visceral ischemia have atherosclerosis as the cause, our discussion will focus on this challenging group.

COEXISTING CONDITIONS

Undoubtedly the most common condition associated with chronic visceral ischemia is atherosclerosis. As many as 50 percent of patients underoing surgery for visceral ischemia have had or will have other vascular surgical reconstruction. Rapp et al.[16] reported that of 67 patients with chronic visceral ischemia, 49 had other peripheral vascular disease, 23 had symptomatic coronary disease, and 35 had prior vascular reconstructions. Cerebrovascular disease is also common: Zelenock et al.[17] reported that 5 of 23 patients with chronic visceral ischemia also had symptomatic cerebrovascular disease.

Coronary Artery Disease

Coronary artery disease, either symptomatic or asymptomatic, is of most concern because it is a common cause of morbidity and mortality.[16,18] In three studies of patients undergoing surgery for chronic visceral ischemia, symptomatic coronary artery disease was recognized preoperatively in 26 to 39 percent of the patients.[16–18] More bothersome are the data of Reiner et al.[7] With the exception of four cases of intestinal infarction, the 88 adult patients in this autopsy study were entirely unselected and largely consecutive. Of these patients, more than two-thirds of those with severe mesenteric artery disease had severe coronary disease (i.e., at least 76 percent reduction in vessel lumen by atherosclerotic plaques). The chance of severe mesenteric vascular disease being associated with either severe coronary artery stenosis or occlusion was two to two and one-half times greater than the converse. Lapiccirella and Weber[19] noted a similar correlation between mesenteric and coronary artery disease. The implication of these data seems clear. Just as with patients who have aortic aneurysms,[20,21] the absence of signs or symptoms of cardiac disease in patients who have chronic ischemia of the mesenteric artery is no indication that cardiac morbidity or mortality will not occur.

How, then, do we determine the presence and severity of coronary artery disease preoperatively? We consider the history, physical findings, 12-lead electrocardiogram (ECG), and chest radiograph essential. Several other diagnostic techniques may add useful information. Positive results on treadmill exercise testing correlate with the occurrence of adverse cardiac events after peripheral vascular surgery.[22,23] However, such testing does not identify all patients at risk.[24,25] Nuclear scanning (with thallium 201) at rest and during exercise may add useful information and complement treadmill testing.[26] Dipyridamole-thallium imaging, a recently developed noninvasive method, detects nonviable areas of myocardium and, far more important, viable areas at risk of ischemia.[27] A major advantage is that it does not require exercise and is therefore useful for patients with peripheral vascular insufficiency who cannot exercise. Clinical assessment is less accurate than dipyridamole-thallium imaging, which also evaluates the functional aspects of coronary artery disease without incurring the risk of angiography. Patients who are identified as having areas of myocardium at risk may then be assessed for coronary angiography and surgery. Echocardiography and radionuclide angiocardiography remain very useful in the noninvasive assessment of left ventricular function.[28–30] Cardiac catheterization remains the ultimate diagnostic method of detecting and quantifying coronary artery disease and ventricular function. Some physicians advocate catheterizing the heart almost routinely prior to peripheral vascular surgery, a practice they believe justified by the frequent presence of surgically correctable coronary stenosis in this population.[20,31]

To what extent preoperative cardiac investigation is indicated remains controversial. In view of the incidence and extent of cardiac disease in patients with mesenteric artery ischemia, however, noninvasive evaluation of coronary perfusion and left ventricular function seems an appropriate minimum to us. This approach allows one to optimize cardiac status preoperatively and to assess cardiac status for management of hemodynamic responses to surgery.

Respiratory Disease

Use of tobacco is one of the most consistent risk factors in chronic visceral ischemia.[32] In one study of 23 patients undergoing surgery for symptomatic splanchnic arteriosclerotic occlusive disease, all but one (96 percent) were "heavy" smokers averaging 44 pack-years.[17] In another study, 16 of 23 patients with chronic visceral ischemia were cigarette smokers. Smokers and others at risk of postoperative pulmonary dysfunction (the obese, the elderly, and those with concurrent pulmonary disease) should be identified and evaluated by history and physical examination; pulmonary function should be quantitated, in many instances, by spirometry. Reversible conditions (e.g., infection, bronchospasm) should be corrected preoperatively. Also, preoperative pulmonary preparation (antibiotics, postural drainage, bronchodilators, and incentive spirometry) decreases morbidity in patients at risk.[33,34]

Renal Disease

Renal dysfunction and renal artery stenosis are also concerns in chronic visceral ischemia. Baur et al.[18] reported a 35 percent incidence of stenosis or occlusion of one or both renal arteries; Rapp et al.[16] reported an almost identical incidence for 67 patients. Additionally, 25 percent of the patients reported by Rapp and colleagues[16] had abnormally high preoperative levels of creatinine. Acute perioperative renal failure, which occurs most frequently in patients with preexisting renal dysfunction,[35,36] is a complication with high mortality. During the angiographic investigation of chronic visceral ischemia, the renal arteries are visualized routinely. About one-third of our patients require renal arterial procedures in addition to visceral revascularization.

Other Conditions

Diabetes mellitus, hypertension, electrolyte abnormalities, malnutrition, and preexisting drug regimens are additional problems and considerations common among patients with chronic visceral ischemia. These additional factors also deserve special attention in the preoperative evaluation and preparation period.

THE SURGICAL APPROACH

Numerous surgical solutions have been devised to correct visceral ischemia. At this institution, the type of procedure used depends on the location and extent of atherosclerotic disease, the coexisting diseases, and surgical preference. Only symptomatic patients undergo surgery, unless aortic reconstruction is planned and the patient is believed to be at risk of intestinal ischemia as a result. In this circumstance, visceral revascularization is done prophylactically at the time of aortic replacement. Undoubtedly, the most important surgical events for the anesthetist to manage are periods of either supraceliac or lower aortic occlusion. Associated with temporary aortic occlusion are the problems of organ ischemia and the hemodynamic responses to increasing impedance to left ventricular ejection. Communication about the proposed surgical procedure and any intraoperative changes in the surgical plan facilitate the safe conduct of anesthesia in these patients.

Our surgeons agree that complete revascularization is ideal in multiple-vessel disease. This approach produces the best long-term results.[37] There are three basic methods for visceral revascularization. The first, reimplantation, is often difficult because of an inability to reimplant the normal vessel into a disease-free segment of aorta. Subsequently, reimplantation is performed only rarely. The second method, bypass grafting, is the most commonly used. To allow for antegrade flow, our surgeons prefer antegrade (as opposed to retrograde) placement of grafts; this is done through a midline abdominal incision with exposure of the supraceliac aorta. The graft is usually placed with a clamp partially occluding the aorta. In rare instances of gross circumferential aortic disease, complete occlusion of the aorta by a clamp would be required. Both autogenous vein and Dacron prostheses can be used for these grafts. Vein is often used in vessels of smaller caliber ($\leq$5 mm), or when the potential for sepsis at the site is evident.

The third method of visceral revascularization, endarterectomy (both transarterial and transaortic), is performed frequently. Transaortic endarterectomy is particularly useful in patients with occlusion of the superior mesenteric artery and coexisting renal artery disease but no significant cardiac or pulmonary disease. Although surgeons at our institution are most experienced with abdominal incisions, the thoracoabdominal approach advocated by Stoney et al.[38] is becoming more popular. These procedures require more surgical exposure and dissection as well as a period of complete aortic occlusion (usually not longer than 30 minutes). Although Stoney and Olcott[39] report no neurologic complications suggestive of cord ischemia, the potential for this complication must be realized.

THE MESENTERIC CIRCULATION

Because the gut and mesenteric vasculature are the objects of surgical intervention, this discussion describes factors affecting intestinal blood flow.

Physiology

The small intestine receives most of its blood flow from the superior mesenteric artery (which delivers approximately 12 percent of the cardiac output),[40] with minor collateral support normally coming from the celiac and inferior mesenteric arteries. The mucosa, being metabolically the most active, receives over 50 percent of the total mesenteric blood flow.[41] Although the mucosa is sensitive to ischemia, 3 hours of severe reduction in blood flow may occur before pathologic mucosal changes develop.[42,43] We believe it is important to remember that although the mucosa is sensitive to injury, this membrane is able to repair itself to a great extent. Although the muscle layers are far less sensitive to ischemia, stricture and transient disturbances in motility may result from ischemia of these tissues. Ischemia progressing to infarction is a life-threatening event that is unlikely to occur within the time of surgery.

Mesenteric flow is regulated intrinsically by vasodilatory metabolites, intrinsic neurotransmitters (e.g., substance P, vasoactive intestinal peptide, enkephalins), paracrine substances, intrinsic hormones (e.g., secretin, gastrin, glucagon), and myogenic control.[43,44] Extrinsic regulation is provided by circulating substances such as glucagon and cholecystokinin, as well as both sympathetic and parasympathetic innervation.[43] Vagal parasympathetics have little or no direct effect on flow but do affect secretion and motility. Resting sympathetic nervous system influences on the mesenteric circulation are not prominent, but sympathetic stimulation promptly increases vascular tone and resistance, thereby decreasing flow.[43] Sustained sympathetic stimulation (neural, angiotensin II, or catecholamines) results in autoregulatory "escape"[40]; the initial sharp decrease in flow is transient, and blood flow returns toward normal despite continuous constrictor input.

Intraoperative Influences

Several intraoperative events decrease mesenteric blood flow, the greatest reduction occurring with intraabdominal surgical manipulation.[45] Positive-pressure ventilation,[46] positive end-expiratory pressure (PEEP),[47] hypocapnia,[48] metabolic acidosis,[49] and drugs such as α-adrenergic receptor agonists, β-adrenergic blocking agents, and digoxin[44,47,50,51] also decrease mesenteric blood flow. Increases in mesenteric flow can be obtained with agents such as isoproterenol, calcium antagonists, nitroglycerin, and dopamine (in low doses to 5 μg/kg/min).[40,52,53] Although vasodilators have been used successfully for nonocclusive bowel ischemia,[54,55] no evidence suggests that either local or systemic intraoperative administration of vasodilating drugs improves outcome in chronic atherosclerotic visceral ischemia. Persistent mesenteric vasoconstriction has been shown to occur after temporary occlusion of arterial inflow, however, and local arterial administration of vasodilators reverses this process experimentally.[54,55]

In general, anesthetic agents decrease splanchnic blood flow,[47] although to a much lesser degree than does surgical manipulation.[45] All inhaled agents in present use decrease arteriovenous oxygen content difference.[56] Isoflurane increases mesenteric vascular resistance and concomitantly reduces flow, possibly because of a release of catecholamines.[56-58] Halothane has been shown angiographically to cause splanchnic vasoconstriction,[59] but in high concentrations (greater than or equal to 2 MAC [MAC is the minimum alveolar concentration of an anesthetic necessary to produce a lack of response to a noxious stimulus in 50 percent of subjects]) it may produce mesenteric vasodilation.[56] Although enflurane decreases the metabolic rate, it does not change mesenteric vascular resistance or blood flow in isolated intestinal loops.[56] This characteristic may make enflurane the volatile agent of choice if only blood flow to the intestine is being considered.

Using the above principles to optimize patient care, one would ensure normal acid-base status, avoid hypothermia, and either avoid or minimize the use of PEEP. *When possible*, we avoid giving digitalis, particularly when calcium channel-blocking agents are suitable substitutes. However, we do not hesitate to use digitalis when specifically indicated. Glucagon may decrease the splanchnic vasoconstriction caused by administration of digoxin.[50] β-adrenergic receptor-blocking drugs also significantly decrease splanchnic blood flow and increase splanchnic vascular resistance. Decreases in splanchnic oxygen consumption accompany these effects.[51] Because we believe that supply-demand ratios are thus maintained, we continue to administer β-adrenergic receptor-blocking agents intraoperatively when appropriate. If pressor or inotropic support is needed dopamine (dose range, 0.5 to 5 μg/kg/min) is often initially chosen because it may increase mesenteric blood flow. When we administer an agent to increase α-adrenergic activity, we concomitantly begin administering dopamine in doses of 0.5 to 5 μg/kg/min to maintain renal and mesenteric blood flow through dopaminergic-induced splanchnic vasodilation. Because no evidence exists to encourage the intraoperative administration of vasodilating drugs to maintain visceral blood flow, we do not use such therapy unless indicated by analysis of cardiac function and hemodynamic variables.

In our opinion, the overriding objective of intraoperative care is the preservation of nonregenerative organs—the myocardium, the central nervous system, and the kidney. For these organs, infarction or even short periods of ischemia can cause significant morbidity and mortality.

MYOCARDIAL PROTECTION

Prevention and treatment of myocardial ischemia depends on how closely oxygen delivery meets the metabolic demand of the myocardium. We believe that controlling the factors influencing the supply and demand of oxygen is key in preventing or limiting myocardial injury or death. Several of these factors are amenable to therapy.

Increases in heart rate produce progressive elevations in myocardial oxygen consumption and contractility[60] (Bowditch's phenomena). Coronary blood flow (and therefore oxygen supply) is not constant. Blood flow to most cardiac muscle occurs predominantly during diastole, because the high intramyocardial pressures during systole effectively limit intramyocardial coronary blood flow. When the heart beats rapidly, diastole (perfusion time) decreases significantly, an effect that subsequently decreases oxygen delivery. In one study of patients with fixed coronary obstruction, increases in heart rate produced a greater degree of myocardial ischemia than did raising sys-

temic pressure, although both stresses produced similar increases in oxygen consumption.[61] Therefore, avoiding or correcting significant elevations in heart rate is an important goal in preventing or treating myocardial ischemia.

Perfusion pressure is another determinant of myocardial oxygen supply. In significant coronary artery stenosis, blood flow across the lesion becomes pressure dependent; reductions in pressure (particularly diastolic pressure) will decrease flow and may produce ischemia. For this reason, we believe preservation of adequate coronary artery perfusion pressure (distal coronary diastolic pressure minus left ventricular end-diastolic pressure [LVEDP]) is of considerable importance.

Left ventricular filling pressure (i.e., LVEDP) affects both coronary arterial inflow (supply) and myocardial oxygen consumption. In areas where flow is pressure dependent, increases in LVEDP will decrease the gradient between diastolic coronary pressure and the impeding intramyocardial pressure and will thus decrease flow. Increases in LVEDP may also increase heart size and, subsequently, wall tension and oxygen consumption.

Increases in myocardial contractility also increase myocardial oxygen demands. Undesirable increases in contractility (e.g., those during the combination of surgical stress and inadequate depth of anesthesia) must be avoided or controlled.

Afterload of the myocardium (that is, ventricular wall tension during systole) is often discussed but rarely monitored because no direct method of measuring afterload exists. Afterload is determined by wall thickness, left ventricular shape and size at end-diastole, and aortic blood pressure. Any change in these components that increases afterload also increases myocardial oxygen consumption. Therefore, controlling these components is part of the process of preventing and treating myocardial ischemia.

RENAL PROTECTION

Certain preoperative conditions (renal dysfunction or renal vascular disease) and intraoperative events (such as temporary occlusion of renal or aortic blood flow, hypotension, or embolization of plaque) may result in transient dysfunction or frank renal failure after surgery.

The cornerstone of renal protection is the provision of a stable hemodynamic state, represented by normal values for cardiac index, ventricular filling pressures, and systemic vascular resistance. We try to obtain this state with the appropriate administration of fluids, inotropic drugs, and/or vasodilating drugs. In one study of patients who had aortic reconstructive surgery, maintenance of optimal left ventricular filling pressure and ventricular performance was associated with better postoperative renal function than when intravascular volume was estimated by central venous pressure alone.[62] In another study, patients undergoing aortic reconstructive surgery were given either no treatment or administration of mannitol or furosemide, and/or fluids during periods of low urinary output.[63] If pulmonary capillary wedge pressure and systemic pressures were kept within "normal limits" during surgery, no difference in postoperative renal function occurred between patients given one of the treatments and those given no treatment. It is recognized that subnormal atrial filling pressures are strong stimuli for renal vasoconstriction[64,65]: raising subnormal pressures to a normal level can increase renal blood flow 50 to 100 percent at any given systemic blood pressure.[64,66] Raising left atrial pressure to above normal levels produces only

very weak renal vasodilation.[66] Atrial natriuretic peptide also is secreted in response to increased atrial pressures and results in diuresis, natriuresis, and decreased vascular resistance.[67–69] Whether these increases in urinary output result in a sustained benefit has been questioned by Alpert et al.[63] These investigators found that as long as filling volumes and systemic hemodynamics were in the normal range, urinary output during aortic reconstruction was not an accurate predictor of postoperative renal function.

Dopamine has effects that may be useful in renal protection. In low doses of 0.5 to 5 μg/kg/min, dopamine dilates renal blood vessels and increases renal blood flow, diuresis, and natriuresis.[53] Although the salt and water losses have been presumed to result from increases in blood flow,[53,70] these losses may be independent of the improvement in hemodynamics and flow.[71,72] Administration of dopamine after the ischemia of renal transplantation has been shown to increase renal blood flow, urine volume, and glomerular filtration rate significantly.[73] Dopamine also improves renal function in oliguric patients after cardiopulmonary bypass[74] and in patients undergoing orthotopic liver transplantation.[75]

Administration of diuretic drugs became a popular method of providing renal protection in the 1960s.[76] Mannitol improves glomerular filtration rate and renal blood flow in models of ischemia, possibly by attenuating endothelial swelling and maintaining patency of the tubules after ischemia.[77] Administration of mannitol also decreases blood viscosity, decreases renin release, and increases circulating volume and renal vasodilation initially.[78–80] Any or all of these events may account for the improvement in renal function. Clinically, evidence of mannitol-induced protection is controversial; however, mannitol is frequently used prophylactically before renal ischemia. Loop diuretics (i.e., those acting primarily in the loop of Henle) such as furosemide have been shown to have renal protective effects in some animal models. Little evidence, however, supports the use of loop diuretics for "protection" during surgery.[81]

For patients not undergoing a period of renal ischemia, and for those undergoing infrarenal aortic occlusion, the only therapy we normally use to protect renal function is optimization of hemodynamic status with drugs. For an occasional patient undergoing infrarenal aortic occlusion and for almost all patients requiring hemodynamic support with considerable α-adrenergic activity, we give low doses (2 μg/kg/min) of dopamine. For patients undergoing isolated renal artery occlusion or suprarenal aortic cross-clamping, we establish a solute diuresis with 0.25 to 0.5 g/kg of 20 percent mannitol, followed by 0.25 to 0.5 g/kg/h, prior to occlusion, until removal of the cross-clamp. If, after removal of the cross-clamp, the patient remains or becomes oliguric during a "normal" hemodynamic state, we continue the infusion of mannitol and start to administer dopamine (2 μg/kg/min). Although we rarely use furosemide, we may give it (beginning with small doses) if oliguria continues despite the above-described therapy. We double the administered amount of furosemide every 15 minutes until diuresis is established or excessive doses are approached.

PROTECTION OF THE CENTRAL NERVOUS SYSTEM

Although cerebrovascular occlusive disease is common in patients with chronic visceral ischemia, acute perioperative stroke is not. There is cumulative risk of a new stroke in patients who have asymptomatic carotid bruit, although the locations of the infarcts and bruits may not correlate.[82] A prospective study by Barnes and Marszalek[83] demonstrated no evidence that perioperative stroke occurs in patients who have no symptoms of cerebrovascular insufficiency. Despite these data, it seems sensible to maintain optimal cerebral perfusion. We make no attempt to monitor central nervous system (CNS) function specifically during visceral artery reconstruction. We maintain cerebral perfusion pressure by ensuring that mean arterial blood pressure is within the patient's normal range. We avoid hypercarbia, which may decrease blood flow to ischemic areas of the brain by intracerebral "steal."[84,85] Hypocarbia may also have adverse effects; cerebral lactate is higher and adenosine triphosphate levels lower (suggesting insufficient substrate delivery) in animals made hypocarbic.[86] Therefore, we adjust ventilation to maintain normal carbon dioxide levels.

MANAGEMENT OF DIABETES MELLITUS

The intraoperative management of insulin-dependent diabetes remains very controversial regarding acceptable levels of blood glucose during surgery. Although wound healing and wound infection rates may be improved with tight control of blood glucose levels during surgery,[87–89] there is no evidence that tight control improves morbidity or mortality.[90,91] Evidence is also accumulating that hyperglycemia may worsen neurologic outcome in patients or animals who have temporary CNS ischemia, although contradictory evidence has been presented from animal models of spinal cord, and focal CNS ischemia (see Ch. 5). Significant hypoglycemia, on the other hand, can be difficult to detect in the anesthetized patient and has devastating potential. Subsequently, we do not tightly control blood glucose levels during surgery and avoid hyperosmolar states, ketoacidosis, and hypoglycemia. We restrict patients from all oral intake after midnight and begin an intravenous infusion of glucose (5 percent dextrose in water or lactated Ringer's solution) about 6 A.M. We then give patients one-half of their usual dose of long-acting insulin. When the patient arrives at the operating room, we give 5 percent dextrose in lactated Ringer's solution at a rate of 125 ml/h/70 kg of body weight. The rest of the patient's fluid requirements are met with nondextrose-containing fluids. We measure blood glucose levels intermittently during surgery and generally treat glucose levels higher than 300 mg/dl with intravenous infusion of additional regular insulin.

MONITORING

The monitoring equipment we use routinely for patients undergoing surgery for aortic reconstruction consists of a five-lead electrocardiographic system, an automatic blood pressure cuff, a temperature probe, a precordial or esophageal stethoscope, a pulse oximeter, and a mass spectrometer for analysis of inspired and expired gases. We select electrocardiographic leads based on the location of the coronary stenosis, if known.[92] Otherwise, we use lead V_5, which most consistently detects ischemic changes (in one study, 89 percent of ischemic changes detected by a standard 12-lead ECG were observed in V_5[93]). We will soon be using a system that allows simultaneous observation of leads II and V_5.

In addition, we place arterial lines in all patients undergoing aortic reconstruction. We believe that beat-to-beat monitoring of arterial pressure is essential for patients who have cardiac or cerebrovascular disease and for those undergoing surgery requiring aortic occlusion. In addition, access for analysis of coagulation abnormalities and blood levels of gases, glucose, and electrolytes is frequently necessary. We generally choose the radial artery as the site for access because it is convenient and has a very low incidence of functionally significant complications.[94]

We believe that use of pulmonary artery catheters enhances management of patients undergoing aortic reconstruction. Such monitoring provides direct and derived data that are often the earliest indicators of myocardial ischemia. These data are vitally important in optimizing hemodynamic status for the prevention or treatment of myocardial ischemia. Whether the use of pulmonary artery catheters improves outcome in aortic reconstruction is unknown. However, they do improve outcome for patients at high risk of perioperative myocardial infarction[95] and for those undergoing aortic aneurysm resection.[96,97] Use of pulmonary artery catheters also improves renal function by optimizing extracellular volume and left ventricular performance.[62] It is our opinion that the information obtained from these monitors in general, and from pulmonary artery catheters in particular, greatly facilitates selection of the most appropriate intraoperative and postoperative therapies. Such information also allows one to judge the effectiveness of those therapies.

INDUCTION OF ANESTHESIA

On arrival of the patient at the operating suite, we place the standard monitors described earlier. We often insert epidural catheters (under local anesthesia) for postoperative analgesia, particularly in patients scheduled for thoracoabdominal incision. In peripheral vascular procedures, placement of an epidural catheter is a safe procedure as long as it precedes heparinization.[98] We then place any invasive monitoring devices and induce general anesthesia.

We believe maintenance of circulatory stability during induction is critical. We pay particular attention to avoid hypotension, or tachycardia and hypertension, in response to induction and endotracheal intubation. In patients with no history or evidence of coronary disease, administration of thiopental supplemented with 100 to 200 µg of fentanyl accomplishes our goals. When left ventricular function is impaired or the myocardium is obviously at risk of ischemia, we supplement a narcotic-based induction (produced by 500 to 1,000 µg of fentanyl or equivalent doses of sufentanil) with small doses of an amnestic drug such as midazolam, etomidate, diazepam, thiopental, or a potent inhalation agent.

To facilitate endotracheal intubation, we choose muscle relaxants based on their cardiovascular effects. Administration of vecuronium, atracurium, or the combination of metocurine with pancuronium[99] allows us to avoid producing tachycardia and provides stable systemic hemodynamics. Succinylcholine remains the standard if no contraindications are present. On very rare occasions, heart rate and mean arterial blood pressure increase slightly as a result of ganglionic stimulation.[100]

Lidocaine may be given intravenously, or by tracheal spray, to blunt the hemodynamic response to tracheal intubation.[101] A short-acting β-adrenergic receptor-blocking drug (such as esmolol) effectively controls increases in heart rate and blood pressure during intubation and other stressful stimuli.[102–104]

MAINTENANCE OF ANESTHESIA

For maintenance of anesthesia, we generally supplement moderate doses of narcotics (total doses of 10 to 20 µg/kg of fentanyl or equivalent) with a volatile agent. We prefer enflurane because it appears not to change mesenteric vascular resistance (see above)[56] and allows for controlled circulatory depression without evidence of coronary steal. Isoflurane has been associated with coronary steal in several studies of coronary artery disease.[105–110] The relevance of this coronary steal to humans with coronary artery atherosclerosis is controversial, however. In addition, because isoflurane increases mesenteric vascular resistance, it is probably less than ideal in this patient population. We often avoid nitrous oxide, which may be detrimental to patients with coronary stenosis.[111] Also, the potential increase in bowel gas volume that accompanies the use of nitrous oxide may make exposure more difficult. In this instance, we add air to decrease the fractional concentration of inspired oxygen.

Mechanical ventilation is instituted to keep carbon dioxide tension at 35 to 40 mmHg. Hypercapnia is avoided because it alters regional blood flow, perhaps by its sympathomimetic effects. We also avoid hypocapnia, which can decrease mesenteric blood flow,[48] increase myocardial oxygen extraction,[112] shift the oxyhemoglobin dissociation curve to the left,[113] decrease cerebral blood flow,[114] and decrease cardiac output.[115] Hemodynamic alterations are treated aggressively to keep heart rate, mean arterial blood pressure, cardiac index, preload, and systemic vascular resistance within "normal" limits. These goals frequently entail the use of β-adrenergic receptor-blocking drugs, nitroglycerin or sodium nitroprusside, and occasionally inotropic or vasoconstricting drugs.

We treat evidence of myocardial ischemia (changes in pulmonary capillary wedge pressure, waveforms, or ST segments) vigorously by correcting abnormal changes in hemodynamic status. Additionally, intravenous administration of nitroglycerin (0.5 to 1 μg/kg/min initially) is titrated to increase coronary blood flow by vasodilation,[116] to increase collateral flow,[117] and to correct elevations in left ventricular preload, thus decreasing myocardial fiber stretch.

The use of vasodilators needs to be individualized. Generally, we begin with nitroglycerin at doses of 0.5 to 1 μg/kg/min and titrate its administration to effect. When systemic resistance cannot be controlled with nitroglycerin alone, we infuse sodium nitroprusside. Because heart rate may increase significantly with these vasodilating drugs, we control such increases with β-adrenergic receptor-blocking drugs if no contraindications exist. Volume loading with lactated Ringer's solution, saline, or blood keeps left ventricular filling pressures at an optimum level.

TEMPORARY OCCLUSION OF THE AORTA

Temporary occlusion of the aorta (aortic cross-clamping) is a severe physiologic stress requiring detailed attention on the part of the anesthetist. Patients may have hypertension, myocardial ischemia, or congestive heart failure[118,119] in response to the increase in impedance to left ventricular ejection. Cardiac index may decrease and left ventricular filling pressures increase abruptly. In this situation, sodium nitroprusside may be used to decrease systemic vascular resistance and to control preload. However, this drug may be responsible for a coronary steal from potential ischemic zones.[120] The relevance of the steal by sodium nitroprusside (like that by isoflurane) in humans is not clear, and its potential benefit may outweigh its potential harm. During temporary aortic occlusion, nitroglycerin often improves cardiac index if left ventricular filling pressures are stable. Nitroglycerin may be advantageous in patients with ischemic heart disease, as it increases collateral coronary flow,[117] alleviates coronary artery spasm,[121] and redistributes a greater portion of coronary blood flow to the subendocardium.[122]

REMOVAL OF THE AORTIC CROSS-CLAMP

Systemic blood pressure and systemic vascular resistance often decrease significantly when aortic blood flow is restored after temporary occlusion of the aorta (aortic declamping). Several mechanisms have been proposed.[123,124] These decreases can be ameliorated by prior volume loading to optimize intravascular volume and cardiac function.[125,126]

We almost always give vasodilators prior to removal of the cross-clamp and increase left ventricular preload while continuing administration of vasodilators. Just before restoration of blood flow, the infusion is discontinued and the concentration of volatile anesthetic agent is reduced; we also adjust ventilation to normalize arterial blood gases. If blood pressure decreases greatly on unclamping of the aorta, the cross-clamp is partially or totally reapplied. If the drop in pressure is moderate and myocardial function has been normal prior to unclamping, we may give small doses (50 to 150 μg) of phenylephrine instead of partially reapplying the clamp. Most often, a severe drop in pressure is attributable to an underloaded left ventricle and indicates a need for greater volume administration. If additional therapy such as administration of inotropic drugs or vasoconstrictors is required, we select the drug based on measured and derived hemodynamic data. We do not routinely give bicarbonate "prophylactically" prior to unclamping, in anticipation of an acid load from ischemic tissue. The change in pH is usually not great[125]; also, if hemodynamics are adequate after unclamping, the change is self-limited by the metabolism of the lactic acid. Additionally, there is no correlation between the degree of acidosis on release of the clamp and the level of hypotension,[127] again indicating, we believe, the lack of rational basis for prophylactic administration of bicarbonate.

EARLY POSTOPERATIVE CARE

Certainly, not all patients undergoing suprarenal aortic reconstruction require prolonged respiratory support. Patients who are considered ready for tracheal extubation should be hemodynamically stable, not significantly hypothermic, free of surgical problems, and able to meet the usual criteria for postsurgical extubation.

We believe that all patients undergoing major vascular reconstruction should be admitted to an intensive care ward or other unit having equivalent nursing available postoperatively. We believe continued hemodynamic monitoring and therapy are imperative.

We also believe that adequate postoperative pain relief is extremely important to patient outcome. We have found that lumbar epidural administration of narcotics by continuous infusion (a 0.08 to 0.1 mg/kg bolus of morphine followed by an infusion at the rate of 0.008 to 0.01 mg/kg/h) is particularly effective, especially for patients with thoracoabdominal incisions. After extubation, we use respiratory maneuvers that assist in maintaining functional residual capacity and in decreasing alveolar hypoventilation.

SUMMARY

Patients undergoing mesenteric artery revascularization must be cared for with an appreciation for their coexisting conditions, particularly widespread atherosclerosis. We believe proper and thorough preoperative investigation and optimization of medical illness are beneficial to outcome. We construct anesthetic management around precepts that apply to any patient with cardiac disease undergoing noncardiac surgery. Cardioactive medications such as β-adrenergic receptor-blocking drugs or calcium channel-blocking agents are not discontinued prior to surgery. Invasive hemodynamic monitoring guides therapeutic decision-making. Induction and maintenance agents are tailored to cardiovascular status, and attempts are made to minimize undesirable changes in myocardial oxygen supply and demand. The patient is kept warm by use of blood warmers, heated, humidified gases, and manipulation of ambient temperature. We keep hemodynamic variables within a predetermined "normal" range for each patient. Administration of mannitol and/or dopamine should be considered (but not given routinely) to increase urinary output, particularly for patients undergoing temporary occlusion of the suprarenal aorta or renal arteries. On temporary occlusion of the aorta, appropriate unloading of the left ventricle is accomplished with sodium nitroprusside or nitroglycerin, or both. Left ventricular preload is kept normal during temporary occlusion. Just prior to restoring aortic blood flow, we institute volume loading to lessen the hemodynamic consequences of removing the cross-clamp. In our opinion, if the patient's condition allows, early extubation is desirable. High priority is given to adequate postoperative pain relief, with continued detailed hemodynamic monitoring and therapy to keep hemodynamic variables in a normal range individualized to the patient. This therapy mandates intensive postoperative care. If prolonged ventilation is necessary, we begin early enteral or parenteral nutrition, as most of these patients are somewhat malnourished preoperatively.

We do not wish to minimize the significance of chronic mesenteric ischemia or therapy directed toward improving blood flow to the gut during the intraoperative period. It is our belief, however, that attention to other diseased vascular beds (coronary, cerebral, and renal) is more important to outcome and supersedes that given to the mesenteric system. In fact, we believe that the assurance of adequate blood flow and pressure to the brain, heart, and kidneys by aggressive monitoring and pharmacologic and volume management does as much for mesenteric blood flow as does any other specific maneuver in the context of general anesthesia and intra-abdominal surgical manipulation.

REFERENCES

1. Chiene J: Complete obliteration of celiac and mesenteric arteries: viscera receiving their blood supply through extraperitoneal system of vessels. J Anat Physiol 3:63–72, 1869
2. Conner LA: A discussion of the role of arterial thrombosis in the visceral diseases of middle life, based upon analogies drawn from coronary thrombosis. Am J Med Sci 185:13–21, 1933
3. Dunphy JE: Abdominal pain of vascular origin. Am J Med Sci 192:109–113, 1936
4. Mikkelsen WP: Intestinal angina. Its surgical significance. Am J Surg 94:262–269, 1957
5. Crawford ES, Morris GC, Jr., Myhre HO, Roehm JOF, Jr: Celiac axis, superior mesenteric artery, and inferior mesenteric artery occlusion: surgical considerations. Surgery 82:856–866, 1977
6. Marston A: Patterns of intestinal ischaemia. Ann R Coll Surg Engl 35:151–181, 1964
7. Reiner L, Jiminez FA, Rodriguez FL: Atherosclerosis in the mesenteric circulation. Observations and correlations with aortic and coronary atherosclerosis. Am Heart J 66:200–209, 1965
8. Croft RJ, Menon GP, Marston A: Does "intestinal angina" exist? A critical study of obstructed visceral arteries. Br J Surg 68:316–318, 1981
9. Rob CG, Snyder M: Chronic intestinal ischemia: a complication of surgery of the abdominal aorta. Surgery 60:1141–1145, 1966
10. Hermanutz KD, Wahlen A, Sobbe A: Die klinische Bedeutung der Angiographie bei der Diagnose der Periarteriitis nodosa. (English abstract: The clinical importance of angiography in the diagnosis of periarteritis nodosa). Roentgenblaetter 28:339–349, 1975
11. Stanley JC, Gewertz BL, Bove EL et al: Arterial fibrodysplasia. Histopathologic character and current etiologic concepts. Arch Surg 110:561–566, 1975
12. Jennette JC, Sheps DS, McNeill DD: Exclusively vascular systemic amyloidosis with visceral ischemia. Arch Pathol Lab Med 106:323–327, 1982
13. Lawson JD, Ochsner JL: Median arcuate ligament syndrome with severe two-vessel involvement. Arch Surg 119:226–227, 1984
14. Potashov LV, Sedov VM, Ignashov AM et al: Surgical treatment of chronic ischemia of the digestive organs caused by compressive stenosis of the celiac trunk. Int Angiogr 4:189–192, 1985
15. Stanley JC, Fry WJ: Median arcuate ligament syndrome. Arch Surg 103:252–258, 1971

16. Rapp JH, Reilly LM, Qvarfordt PG et al: Durability of endarterectomy and antegrade grafts in the treatment of chronic visceral ischemia. J Vasc Surg 3:799–806, 1986

17. Zelenock GB, Graham LM, Whitehouse WM, Jr. et al: Splanchnic arteriosclerotic disease and intestinal angina. Arch Surg 115:497–501, 1980

18. Baur GM, Millay DJ, Taylor LM, Jr., Porter JM: Treatment of chronic visceral ischemia. Am J Surg 148:138–144, 1984

19. Lapiccirella V, Weber G: La claudicazione mesenterica sindrome di allarme della malattia coronarica; con ricerche sistematiche anatomoistologiche correlative tra localizzazione coronarica e localizzazione gastromesenterica del processo arteriosclerotico. (Mesenteric claudication and alarm syndrome due to coronary disease; anatomohistologic systematic studies on coronary and gastromesenteric localization of arteriosclerotic process). Arch De Vecchi Anat Patol Med Clin 19:1123–1142, 1953

20. Hertzer NR, Bevan EG, Young JR et al: Coronary artery disease in peripheral vascular patients. A classification of 1000 coronary angiograms and results of clinical management. Ann Surg 199:223–233, 1984

21. Tomatis LA, Fierens EE, Verbrugge GP: Evaluation of surgical risk in peripheral vascular disease by coronary arteriography: a series of 100 cases. Surgery 71:429–435, 1972

22. Cutler BS, Wheeler HB, Paraskos JA, Cardullo PA: Applicability and interpretation of electrocardiographic stress testing in patients with peripheral vascular disease. Am J Surg 141:501–506, 1981

23. von Knorring J, Lepäntalo M: Prediction of perioperative cardiac complications by electrocardiographic monitoring during treadmill exercise testing before peripheral vascular surgery. Surgery 99:610–613, 1986

24. Goldschlager N, Selzer A, Cohn K: Treadmill stress tests as indicators of presence and severity of coronary artery disease. Ann Intern Med 85:277–286, 1976

25. Gage AA, Bhayana JN, Balu V, Hook N: Assessment of cardiac risk in surgical patients. Arch Surg 112:1488–1492, 1977

26. Ritchie JL, Zaret BL, Strauss HW et al: Myocardial imaging with thallium-201: a multicenter study in patients with angina pectoris or acute myocardial infarction. Am J Cardiol 42:345–350, 1978

27. Boucher CA, Brewster DC, Darling RC et al: Determination of cardiac risk by dipyridamole-thallium imaging before peripheral vascular surgery. N Engl J Med 312:389–394, 1985

28. Limacher MC, Quinones MA, Poliner LR et al: Detection of coronary artery disease with exercise two-dimensional echocardiography. Description of a clinically applicable method and comparison with radionuclide ventriculography. Circulation 67:1211–1218, 1983

29. Federman J, Brown ML, Tancredi RG et al: Multiple-gated acquisition cardiac blood-pool isotope imaging. Evaluation of left ventricular function correlated with contrast angiography. Mayo Clin Proc 53:625–633, 1978

30. Feigenbaum H: Echocardiography. p. 88. In Braunwald E (ed): Heart Disease: A Textbook of Cardiovascular Medicine. 2nd ed. WB Saunders, Philadelphia, 1984

31. Hertzer NR: Myocardial ischemia. Surgery 93:97–101, 1983

32. Connolly JE, Kwaan JHM: Management of chronic visceral ischemia. Surg Clin North Am 62:345–356, 1982

33. Gracey DR, Divertie MB, Didier EP: Preoperative pulmonary preparation of patients with chronic obstructive pulmonary disease. A prospective study. Chest 76:123–129, 1979

34. Stein M, Cassara EL: Preoperative pulmonary evaluation and therapy for surgery patients. JAMA 211:787–790, 1970

35. Hermreck AS: The pathophysiology of acute renal failure. Am J Surg 144:605–610, 1982

36. Luft FC, Hamburger RJ, Dyer JK et al: Acute renal failure following operation for aortic aneurysm. Surg Gynecol Obstet 141:374–378, 1975

37. Hollier LH, Bernatz PE, Pairolero PC et

al: Surgical management of chronic intestinal ischemia: a reappraisal. Surgery 90:940–946, 1981

38. Stoney RJ, Ehrenfeld WK, Wylie EJ: Revascularization methods in chronic visceral ischemia caused by atherosclerosis. Ann Surg 186:468–476, 1977

39. Stoney RJ, Olcott C, IV: Visceral artery syndromes and reconstructions. Surg Clin North Am 59:637–647, 1979

40. Jacobson ED: Physiology of the mesenteric circulation. Physiologist 25:439–443, 1982

41. Granger DN, Richardson PDI, Kvietys PR, Mortillaro NA: Intestinal blood flow. Gastroenterology 78:837–863, 1980

42. Robinson JWL, Mirkovitch V, Winistörfer L, Saegesser F: Response of the intestinal mucosa to ischaemia. Gut 22:512–527, 1981

43. Parks DA, Bulkley GB, Granger DN et al: Ischemic injury in the cat small intestine: role of superoxide radicals. Gastroenterology 82:9–15, 1982

44. Banks RO, Gallavan RH, Jr., Zinner MJ et al: Vasoactive agents in control of the mesenteric circulation. Fed Proc 44:2743–2749, 1985

45. Gelman SI: Disturbances in hepatic blood flow during anesthesia and surgery. Arch Surg 111:881–883, 1976

46. Cooperman LH, Warden JC, Price HL: Splanchnic circulation during nitrous oxide anesthesia and hypocarbia in normal man. Anesthesiology 29:254–258, 1968

47. Andreen M: Inhalation versus intravenous anaesthesia. Effects on the hepatic and splanchnic circulation. Acta Anaesthesiol Scand, suppl., 75:25–31, 1982

48. Hughes RL, Mathie RT, Fitch W, Campbell D: Liver blood flow and oxygen consumption during hypocapnia and IPPV in the greyhound. J Appl Physiol 47:290–295, 1979

49. Juhl B, Einer-Jensen N, Madsen T: Effect of non-carbonic acidosis on total splanchnic perfusion and cardiac output during anaesthesia with O_2-N_2O-barbiturate-relaxant. Acta Anaesthesiol Scand 23:149–155, 1979

50. Levinsky RA, Lewis RM, Bynum TE, Hanley HG: Digoxin induced intestinal vasoconstriction. The effects of proximal arterial stenosis and glucagon administration. Circulation 52:130–136, 1975

51. Price HL, Cooperman LH, Warden JC: Control of the splanchnic circulation in man. Role of beta-adrenergic receptors. Circ Res 21:333–340, 1967

52. Walus KM, Fondacaro JD, Jacobson ED: Effects of calcium and its antagonists on the canine mesenteric circulation. Circ Res 48:692–706, 1981

53. Goldberg LI: Cardiovascular and renal actions of dopamine: potential clinical applications. Pharmacol Rev 24:1–29, 1972

54. Athanasoulis CA, Wittenberg J, Bernstein R, Williams LF: Vasodilatory drugs in the management of nonocclusive bowel ischemia. Gastroenterology 68:146–150, 1975

55. Britt LG, Cheek RC: Nonocclusive mesenteric vascular disease: clinical and experimental observations. Ann Surg 169:704–711, 1969

56. Tverskoy M, Gelman S, Fowler KC, Bradley EL: Intestinal circulation during inhalation anesthesia. Anesthesiology 62:462–469, 1985

57. Gelman S, Fowler KC, Smith LR: Regional blood flow during isoflurane and halothane anesthesia. Anesth Analg 63:557–565, 1984

58. Gelman S, Fowler KC, Smith LR: Liver circulation and function during isoflurane and halothane anesthesia. Anesthesiology 61:726–730, 1984

59. Benumof JL, Bookstein JJ, Saidman LJ, Harris R: Diminished hepatic arterial flow during halothane administration. Anesthesiology 45:545–551, 1976

60. Braunwald E: Control of myocardial oxygen consumption. Physiologic and clinical considerations. Am J Cardiol 27:416–432, 1971

61. Loeb HS, Saudye A, Croke RP et al: Effects of pharmacologically-induced hypertension on myocardial ischemia and coronary hemodynamics in patients with fixed coronary obstruction. Circulation 57:41–46, 1978

62. Bush HL, Jr., Huse JB, Johnson WC et

al: Prevention of renal insufficiency after abdominal aortic aneurysm resection by optimal volume loading. Arch Surg 116:1517–1524, 1981

63. Alpert RA, Roizen MF, Hamilton WK et al: Intraoperative urinary output does not predict postoperative renal function in patients undergoing abdominal aortic revascularization. Surgery 95:707–711, 1984

64. Kahl FR, Flint JF, Szidon JP: Influence of atrial distention on renal vasomotor tone. Am J Physiol 226:240–246, 1974

65. Brosnihan KB, Bravo EL: Graded reductions of atrial pressure and renin release. Am J Physiol 235:H175–H181, 1978

66. Mason JM, Ledsome JR: Effects of obstruction of the mitral orifice or distention of the pulmonary vein-atrial junctions on renal and hindlimb vascular resistance in the dog. Circ Res 35:24–32, 1974

67. Sagnella GA, MacGregor GA: Cardiac peptides and the control of sodium excretion. Nature 309:666–667, 1984

68. Needleman P, Currie MG, Geller DM et al: Atriopeptins: potential mediators of an endocrine relationship between heart and kidney. Trends Pharmacol Sci 5:506–509, 1984

69. Tikkanen I, Fyhrquist F, Metsärinne K, Leidenius R: Plasma atrial natriuretic peptide in cardiac disease and during infusion in healthy volunteers. Lancet 2:66–69, 1985

70. Beregovich J, Bianchi C, Rubler S et al: Dose-related hemodynamic and renal effects of dopamine in congestive heart failure. Am Heart J 87:550–557, 1974

71. Bello-Reuss E, Higashi Y, Kaneda Y: Dopamine decreases fluid reabsorption in straight portions of rabbit proximal tubule. Am J Physiol 242:F634–F640, 1982

72. Hilberman M, Maseda J, Stinson EB et al: The diuretic properties of dopamine in patients after open-heart operation. Anesthesiology 61:489–494, 1984

73. Grodin W, Scantlebury V, Warmington N: Dopaminergic stimulation of renal blood flow and renal function after transplantation (abstract). Anesthesiology 61:A129, 1984

74. Davis RF, Lappas DG, Kirklin JK et al: Acute oliguria after cardiopulmonary bypass: renal functional improvement with low-dose dopamine infusion. Crit Care Med 10:852–856, 1982

75. Polson RJ, Park GR, Lindop MJ et al: The prevention of renal impairment in patients undergoing orthotopic liver grafting by infusion of low dose dopamine. Anaesthesia 42:15–19, 1987

76. Barry KG, Cohen A, Knochel JP et al: Mannitol infusion. II. The prevention of acute functional renal failure during resection of an aneurysm of the abdominal aorta. N Engl J Med 264:967–971, 1961

77. Flores J, DiBona DR, Beck CH, Leaf A: The role of cell swelling in ischemic renal damage and the protective effect of hypertonic solute. J Clin Invest 51:118–126, 1972

78. Blantz RC: Effect of mannitol on glomerular ultrafiltration in the hydropenic rat. J Clin Invest 54:1135–1143, 1974

79. Golberg AH, Lilienfield LS: Effects of hypertonic mannitol on renal vascular resistance. Proc Soc Exp Biol Med 119:635–642, 1965

80. Bastron RD: Diuretics. p. 325. In Kaplan JA (ed): Cardiovascular Pharmacology. Vol. 2 of Cardiac Anesthesia series. Grune & Stratton, Orlando, FL, 1983

81. Levinsky NG, Bernard DB, Johnston TA: Mannitol and loop diuretics in acute renal failure. p. 712. In Brenner BM, Lazarus JM (ed): Acute Renal Failure. WB Saunders, Philadelphia, 1983

82. Heyman A, Wilkinson WE, Heyden S et al: Risk of stroke in asymptomatic persons with cervical arterial bruits. A population study in Evans County, Georgia. N Engl J Med 302:838–841, 1980

83. Barnes RW, Marszalek PB: Asymptomatic carotid disease in the cardiovascular surgical patient: is prophylactic endarterectomy necessary? Stroke 12:497–500, 1981

84. Brawley BW: The pathophysiology of intracerebral steal following carbon dioxide inhalation, an experimental study. Scand J Lab Clin Invest, suppl., 102:XIII:B, 1968

85. Boysen G, Ladegaard-Pedersen HJ,

Henriksen H et al: The effects of $PaCO_2$ on regional cerebral blood flow and internal carotid arterial pressure during carotid clamping. Anesthesiology 35:286–300, 1971

86. Michenfelder JD, Sundt TM, Jr: The effect of $PaCO_2$ on the metabolism of ischemic brain in squirrel monkeys. Anesthesiology 38:445–453, 1973

87. Rosenthal S, Lerner B, DiBiase BS, Enquist IF: Relation of strength to composition in diabetic wounds. Surg Gynecol Obstet 115:437–442, 1962

88. Rossini AA: Why control blood glucose levels? Arch Surg 111:229–233, 1976

89. Bagdade JD: Phagocytic and microbicidal functions in diabetes mellitus. Acta Endocrinol, 83:suppl. 205, 27–33, 1976

90. Galloway JA, Shuman CR: Diabetes and surgery. A study of 667 cases. Am J Med 34:177–191, 1963

91. Walsh DB, Eckhauser FE, Ramsburgh SR, Burney RB: Risk associated with diabetes mellitus in patients undergoing gallbladder surgery. Surgery 91:254–257, 1982

92. Robertson D, Kostuk WJ, Ahuja SP: The localization of coronary stenosis by 12 lead ECG response to graded exercise test: support for intercoronary steal. Am Heart J 91:437–444, 1976

93. Blackburn H, Taylor HL, Okamoto N et al: Standardization of the exercise electrocardiogram. A systematic comparison of chest lead configurations employed for monitoring during exercise. p. 101–133. In Karvonen MJ, Barry AJ (ed): Physical Activity and the Heart. Proceedings of a symposium, Helsinki, Finland. Charles C Thomas, Springfield, IL, 1967

94. Slogoff S, Keats AS, Arlund C: On the safety of radial artery cannulation. Anesthesiology 59:42–47, 1983

95. Rao TLK, Jacobs KH, El-Etr AA: Reinfarction following anesthesia in patients with myocardial infarction. Anesthesiology 59:499–505, 1983

96. Cohen JL, Wender R, Maginot A et al: Hemodynamic monitoring of patients undergoing abdominal aortic surgery. Am J Surg 146:174–177, 1983

97. Whittemore AD, Clowes AW, Hechtman HB, Mannick JA: Aortic aneurysm repair. Reduced operative mortality associated with maintenance of optimal cardiac performance. Ann Surg 192:414–421, 1980

98. Rao TLK, El-Etr AA: Anticoagulation following placement of epidural and subarachnoid catheters: an evaluation of neurologic sequelae. Anesthesiology 55:618–620, 1981

99. Lebowitz PW, Ramsey FM, Savarese JJ et al: Combination of pancuronium and metocurine: neuromuscular and hemodynamic advantages over pancuronium alone. Anesth Analg 60:12–17, 1981

100. Goat VA, Feldman SA: The dual action of suxamethonium on the isolated rabbit heart. Anaesthesia 27:149–153, 1972

101. Stoelting RK: Blood pressure and heart rate changes during short-duration laryngoscopy for tracheal intubation: influence of viscous or intravenous lidocaine. Anesth Analg 57:197–199, 1978

102. Menkhaus PG, Reves JG, Kissin I et al: Cardiovascular effects of esmolol in anesthetized humans. Anesth Analg 64:327–334, 1985

103. Ebert J, Gelman S, Coverman S et al: Effect of esmolol on the heart rate and blood pressure response during endotracheal intubation (abstract). Anesthesiology 63:A63, 1985

104. Newsome LR, Roth JV, Hugh CC, Jr., Nagle DM: Esmolol attenuates hemodynamic responses to intubation and surgical stimulation during open heart surgery (abstract). Anesthesiology 63:A62, 1985

105. Moffitt EA, Barker RA, Glenn JJ et al: Myocardial metabolism and hemodynamic responses with isoflurane anesthesia for coronary arterial surgery. Anesth Analg 65:53–61, 1986

106. Reiz S, Bålfors E, Sørenson MB et al: Isoflurane—a powerful coronary vasodilator in patients with coronary artery disease. Anesthesiology 59:91–97, 1983

107. Buffington CW, Romson JL, Duttlinger NC: Does isoflurance cause coronary steal (abstract)? Anesthesiology 63:A9, 1985

108. Reiz S, Östman M: Regional coronary hemodynamics during isoflurane-nitrous oxide anesthesia in patients with ischemic heart disease. Anesth Analg 64:570–576, 1985

109. Khambatta HJ, Sonntag H, Larsen R et al: Coronary artery disease: global and regional myocardial blood flow and metabolism during equipotent halothane and isoflurane anesthesia (abstract). Anesthesiology 65:A503, 1986

110. Goetz AE, Hobbhahn J, Conzen PFM et al: The myocardial microcirculation during anesthesia with isoflurane and enflurane: evidence of shunt perfusion at the capillary level (abstract). Anesthesiology 65:A262, 1986

111. Eisele JH, Reitan JA, Massumi RA et al: Myocardial performance and N_2O analgesia in coronary-artery disease. Anesthesiology 44:16–20, 1976

112. Vance JP, Brown DM, Smith G: The effect of hypocapnia on myocardial blood flow and metabolism. Br J Anaesth 45:455–463, 1973

113. Neill WA, Hattenhauer M: Impairment of myocardial O_2 supply due to hyperventilation. Circulation 52:854–858, 1975

114. Sørensen SC: Theoretical considerations on the potential hazards of hyperventilation during anaesthesia. Acta Anaesthesiol Scand, suppl., 67:106–110, 1978

115. Theye RA, Milde JH, Michenfelder JD: Effect of hypocapnia on cardiac output during anesthesia. Anesthesiology 27:778–782, 1966

116. Feldman RL, Pepine CJ, Conti CR: Magnitude of dilation of large and small coronary arteries by nitroglycerin. Circulation 64:324–333, 1981

117. Cohen MV, Downey JM, Sonnenblick EH, Kirk ES: The effect of nitroglycerin on coronary collaterals and myocardial contractility. J Clin Invest 52:2836–2847, 1973

118. Attia RR, Murphy JD, Snider M et al: Myocardial ischemia due to infrarenal aortic cross-clamping during aortic surgery in patients with severe coronary artery disease. Circulation 53:961–965, 1976

119. Carroll RM, Laravuso RB, Schauble JF: Left ventricular function during aortic surgery. Arch Surg 111:740–743, 1976

120. Goldstein RE: Coronary vascular responses to vasodilator drugs. Prog Cardiovasc Dis 24:419–436, 1982

121. Hillis LD, Braunwald E: Coronary-artery spasm. N Engl J Med 299:695–702, 1978

122. Macho P, Vatner SF: Effects of nitroglycerin and nitroprusside on large and small coronary vessels in conscious dogs. Circulation 64:1101–1107, 1981

123. Damask MC, Weissman C, Rodriguez J et al: Abdominal aortic cross-clamping. Metabolic and hemodynamic consequences. Arch Surg 119:1332–1337, 1984

124. Brant B, Armstrong RP, Vetto RM: Vasodepressor factor in declamp shock production. Surgery 67:650–653, 1970

125. Reiz S, Peter T, Rais O: Hemodynamic and cardiometabolic effects of infrarenal and common celiac artery declamping in man—an approach to optimal volume loading. Acta Anaesthesiol Scand 23:579–586, 1979

126. Silverstein PR, Caldera DL, Cullen DJ et al: Avoiding the hemodynamic consequences of aortic cross-clamping and unclamping. Anesthesiology 50:462–466, 1979

127. Baue AE, McClerkin WW: A study of shock: acidosis and the declamping phenomenon. Ann Surg 161:41–45, 1965

12

Anesthesia for Abdominal Aortic Reconstruction: One Approach at Massachusetts General Hospital

Michael T. Bailin
J. Kenneth Davison

SURGERY FOR ABDOMINAL AORTIC RECONSTRUCTION

Anesthesia, like surgery, has made great strides in recent years; very high risk patients now undergo surgical procedures previously deemed inadvisable. The combination of new anesthetic drugs and techniques, advanced monitoring, the treatments directed by such monitoring, and increased experience managing these patients perioperatively has produced satisfying results in very high risk patients. Elderly patients are also approached from a new perspective: ample studies reveal that values for both life expectancy and successful outcome after surgery in elderly patients are similar to values for other carefully selected patients.[1,2] As in all anesthetic practice, however, careful preoperative evaluation and assessment are vital to success.

Preoperative Assessment

Cardiovascular System

Despite improved outcome attained in aortic surgery, certain factors continue to cause morbidity and mortality in patients undergoing this type of surgery. The most common complications occurring soon after surgery involve the cardiovascular system, the incidence of myocardial infarction being 26 percent.[3] Vigorous assessment of the cardiovascular system before surgery is the basis of appropriate action to support the myocardium through the perioperative period.

Patients undergo vascular surgery because some aspect of vascular disease has become clinically apparent. Nevertheless, the diffuseness of atherosclerosis in these patients, who are usually elderly, suggests associated coronary involvement. A careful cardiac evaluation begins with the history, physical examination, electrocardiogram, and chest radiograph.

215

Assessment of the patient's tolerance to exercise is also valuable. The presence of hypertension, angina, congestive heart failure, and cardiomegaly and a history of myocardial infarction are all important factors in these patients. The importance of these determinants is discussed in other chapters.

Even a careful bedside examination (history and physical examination) may not reveal the existence of extensive coronary artery disease. At the Cleveland Clinic, routine coronary angiography for patients scheduled for aortic surgery showed that 35 to 40 percent had severe but correctable coronary artery lesions.[4] This study also showed that morbidity and mortality after vascular surgery was lower in patients who had undergone coronary revascularization before the vascular procedure than in those who had not. These figures did not include mortality associated with the coronary artery bypass grafting procedure.

At Massachusetts General Hospital, we include dipyridamole-thallium imaging as part of the initial evaluation. This technique has demonstrated a high incidence of severe coronary disease in patients whose initial history appeared relatively benign.[5] The presence of thallium redistribution on the delayed image suggests coronary artery disease. Patients with positive scans then undergo coronary angiography and subsequent angioplasty or bypass surgery, if feasible. Others are started on a medical regimen appropriate for severe coronary artery disease, including β-adrenergic receptor-blocking drugs, calcium channel-blocking drugs, and nitrates. This therapy is maintained throughout the perioperative period. Such risk stratification helps to determine the degree of invasive monitoring needed, plus postoperative requirements.

In our experience, the following conditions pose significant risk in major vascular surgery: (1) acute or recent myocardial infarction; (2) unstable angina (at rest, crescendo); and (3) uncontrolled or poorly controlled congestive heart failure.[6]

Recent Myocardial Infarction.   The timing of previous myocardial infarction does not appear to correlate as highly with risk at the time of vascular surgery as was once believed.[7] We have used the dipyridamole-thallium scan as an indicator of myocardium still at risk after an infarction. Whether the acquisition and application of this data can be used to decrease the frequency of perioperative cardiac events must still be determined.[8]

Unstable Angina.   At our institution, unstable angina is considered one of the most significant risk factors; therefore, every effort is made to revascularize (coronary revascularization) these patients before surgery. We direct optimal medical therapy at minimizing detrimental conditions that increase myocardial oxygen consumption, especially tachycardia.

Congestive Heart Failure.   Congestive heart failure always increases risk significantly, and certainly the patient with uncontrolled congestive heart failure is at very high risk. Although some studies correlate ejection fraction with outcome, these types of data should not dictate clinical practice.[9,10] Patients with extremely low ejection fractions (less than 20 percent) may undergo aortic operations with relative ease and do very well as a group. However, a positive dipyridamole-thallium scan for such patients would indicate significantly higher risk.

Renal System

Just as cardiac stability must be maintained for successful outcome, so must kidney function. Chronic renal insufficiency occurs frequently in these patients. Although acute renal failure should be a very infrequent occurrence during elective aortic surgery (especially infrarenal procedures), its occurrence perioperatively is associated with a dramatic increase in overall morbidity and mortality.

The risk factors associated with vascular disease also take their toll on the kidney. Hypertension, diabetes mellitus, and atherosclerotic renovascular disease alter renal function in this elderly patient population. Preoperatively, hypovolemia secondary to radiographic studies with dye, inadequate hydration, and use of bowel preparations and diuretics all compound the problem. Intraoperative hemodynamic changes and temporary aortic occlusion (either infrarenal and suprarenal) alter perfusion and jeopardize function. Thus, baseline renal function tests and electrolyte levels must be checked, and volume status and electrolyte balance must be preserved.

Pulmonary System

Partially because many of these patients have a long history of cigarette smoking, pulmonary involvement is common. We strongly discourage cigarette smoking for at least 2 weeks before surgery. Although a history and physical examination usually reveal the degree of respiratory compromise, leg claudication may prevent physical activity and mask symptoms of respiratory compromise. A productive cough, bronchospasm, and/or an elevated carbon dioxide partial pressure (PCO_2) (blood sample drawn while the patient is breathing room air) strongly suggests increased postoperative complications, and this possibility should be addressed.[11] If sputum is infected, we begin appropriate antibiotic treatment in conjunction with patient education about coughing techniques and breathing exercises. An elevated PCO_2 will dictate more intense postoperative respiratory care and may suggest the plan for a longer period of endotracheal intubation. Use of a retroper-

itoneal surgical incision instead of a transperitoneal incision may improve postoperative respiratory mechanics.

Endocrine Function

Many of these patients are diabetic, and management includes adjusting their daily insulin dosage (usually one-third to one-half their normal dose), administering adequate amounts of glucose, and checking blood sugar levels regularly. These patients may have a history of silent myocardial infarction (from autonomic neuropathy) or diabetic nephropathy and may be less resistant to infection.

Central Nervous System

Although patients undergoing aortic surgery often also have carotid artery disease, no evidence exists that correcting an asymptomatic carotid lesion improves outcome.[12] We believe it important to ascertain that the patient is asymptomatic when a bruit is found. Noninvasive studies can detect the degree of narrowing, and, in appropriate patients, the carotid lesion might be corrected prior to major abdominal vascular surgery.

Preoperative Visit

A comprehensive visit with the patient at least one day before surgery permits the anesthetist to assess the medical problems (discussed earlier) and to describe what the patient can expect perioperatively. Specifically, patient anxiety, type of premedication, use of invasive monitoring and epidural catheters, postsurgical care, possible adverse outcomes, and questions from the patient are the usual topics.

We perform a physical examination with special attention to checking blood pressure in each arm, pulse (for the efficacy of β-adrenergic receptor blockade), and the nasal airway (for nasal intubation, if ventilatory support is expected to exceed 24 hours). We also carefully check the mouth and neck (for ease of securing the airway), lungs and heart (for evidence of occult obstructive and restrictive lung disease and/or cardiovascular disease), and the back (for the apparentness of landmarks used for spinal-epidural catheter placement).

Premedication usually consists of diazepam (0.1 mg/kg orally) and morphine (0.1 mg/kg intramuscularly), a combination that allays anxiety and provides some analgesia during placement of catheters. Additional intravenous narcotic or benzodiazepine is titrated, as needed, in the induction area. Other drugs such as insulin, digoxin, heparin, and antianginal and bronchodilating drugs may be specifically ordered or omitted by the anesthetist.

Monitoring and Catheterization

At our institution, the patient is brought to an area adjacent to the operating room before surgery. There the anesthetist makes a final preoperative evaluation of the patient's chart, reviewing the last time and doses of medications, new laboratory data, recent progress notes, and vital signs. Any new concerns or symptoms are discussed with the patient. We place a 14- or 16-gauge intravenous catheter and a lumbar epidural catheter.

We believe continuous observation of systemic blood pressure, heart rate, electrocardiogram (ECG), and cardiac filling pressures is vitally important for patient management perioperatively. We also routinely monitor an esophageal stethoscope, oxygen saturation, temperature, and urinary output.

Continuous ECG (usually leads II and V_5), arterial blood pressure, and central venous pressure (CVP) or pulmonary artery pressure are displayed and recorded on paper. A printout of the electrocardiographic waveform allows comparison with the preoperative "control" ECG and better identification of subtle changes in rhythm and ST-T waves. We also record a seven-lead ECG (limb leads plus V_5) prior to induction. If we see new changes that relate to abnormal vital signs (increased blood pressure or tachycardia) prior to surgery, we institute antihypertensive, anti-ischemic drug therapy. If the patient remains ischemic or refractory to therapy, we admit the patient to the intensive care unit (ICU) for continued medical care before attempted aortic resection.

We insert a catheter (usually 18 gauge) percutaneously into the radial artery of the arm having the higher blood pressure, if a difference exists. If the radial artery is inaccessible, we cannulate the ipsilateral axillary artery with an 18-gauge, 6-inch catheter. For patients who have good ventricular function and exercise tolerance, we believe a central venous catheter is usually sufficient to measure right-sided filling pressure and to estimate volume status. Central venous access is also useful for drug infusion.

We use pulmonary artery catheterization for most patients and for all patients who have had recent myocardial infarction. We also catheterize the pulmonary artery in all patients who have had congestive heart failure or unstable or poorly controlled angina any time in their past. In our opinion, when preoperative evaluation is incomplete or nonspecific, knowledge of stroke volume, wedge pressure, and pulmonary artery pressure is sufficient to allow us to provide optimal care. In patients with significant renal, pulmonary, or hepatic disease, the ability to maximize cardiac output and to assess volume status more accurately is beneficial.

Induction of Anesthesia

In our practice, no set technique has been established for induction and maintenance of anesthesia for aortic surgery. Induction is strongly influenced by the patient's hemodynamic status (determined in the induction area) and by the anticipated hemodynamic effects of the anesthetic. In a teaching program, various techniques may be employed. Patients who pose challenges before or during induction (labile blood pressure, abnormal filling pressures, ischemia) continue to challenge the anesthetist throughout the perioperative course. We believe that vigilant hemodynamic assessment and therapy are critically important during induction and attempt to continue both through the ICU period until stability is attained.

After the initial data are collected in the induction area, patients are given either general anesthesia or epidural anesthesia combined with general anesthesia. General anesthesia is induced with a variety of drugs, each titrated to minimize undesirable cardiovascular responses. We typically administer morphine (0.1 to 0.2 mg/kg), in divided doses, or alfentanil (10 to 50 µg/kg) during induction. We also administer thiopental (1 to 3 mg/kg), establish an airway, and place a face mask. An intubating dose of a nondepolarizing relaxant is administered, as is 70 percent nitrous oxide in oxygen during controlled ventilation.

Relaxants are given slowly, and combinations are frequently used to minimize tachycardia or hypotension. We insert a urinary catheter and observe the response. If hemodynamic responses occur with oral airway insertion, gentle direction laryngoscopy, or tracheal spray, further anesthetic is given before intubation. Induction itself is therefore titrated against several stimuli and may proceed through surgical preparation and incision.

We sometimes use high-dose narcotic techniques (fentanyl or sufentanil) for patients with severe or inoperable coronary artery disease. The vagotonic effect of these narcotics can cause profound bradycardia on induction, especially when combined with preoperative β-adrenergic receptor blockade. Pancuronium may be used to support the heart rate. For these patients, we frequently use lumbar epidural catheters for postoperative pain control and as an aid in discontinuing mechanical ventilation.

Combining epidural and general anesthesia offers advantages, including inhibition of the stress response, profound abdominal muscle relaxation, rapid emergence from anesthesia, postoperative analgesia, and improved postoperative respiratory mechanics.[13] We give most of our patients this combined technique. We believe that systemic anticoagulation after epidural catheter placement is a safe technique. The epidural catheter is injected with approximately 10 to 12 ml of 0.75 percent bupivacaine before induction of general anesthesia. After ascertaining a satisfactory sensory level (usually T4 to T6), general anesthesia proceeds as above, although less narcotic is required. Epidural morphine is prepared and injected (typically 4 to 6 mg), usually within an hour of skin incision. We do not give additional bupivacaine, as the duration of action of the initial dose is usually adequate and does not therefore preclude postoperative extubation if deemed appropriate.

We infuse phenylephrine to keep blood pressure within 10 to 20 percent of baseline. When general anesthesia is used by itself, phenylephrine may or may not be required before skin incision, at which time absence of stimulation may lead to hypotension. In the combined technique, however, phenylephrine infusion becomes an integral part of our patient management.

Intraoperative Management

Good anesthetic management of patients undergoing aortic resection implies knowledge of the surgical maneuvers and anticipation of acute changes in blood volume and pressure. Effective treatment of ischemia, oliguria, dysrhythmias, and derangements caused by clamping and unclamping of the aorta depends on rapid and correct interpretation of available data.

Because tachycardia is poorly tolerated in these patients, who have a high incidence of coronary artery disease, we keep the heart rate within narrow limits intraoperatively. When tachycardia occurs, we search for its cause, considering hypovolemia, light anesthesia, severe anemia, withdrawal from β-adrenergic receptor-blocking drugs, and drug effect (e.g., pancuronium). We then treat tachycardia based on our best estimate of cause.

We infuse warmed crystalloid as appropriate, 750 to 1,000 ml/h being the average rate during surgery. Hypotension caused by moving of the intestines or by visceral traction is common and may be attributable to a combination of released vasodilators and vagal influence. Infusion of phenylephrine is efficacious during this transient phenomenon. Certain momentary deviations in blood pressure are unavoidable, and hypovolemia will accentuate the degree of these alterations in blood pressure. We continually assess volume status by monitoring blood pressure, cardiac filling pressures, urinary output, and blood loss.

Temporary Occlusion of the Aorta

Cross-clamping of the aorta causes hypertension proximal to the clamp. The increased work load from the increase in (apparent) systemic vascular resistance on the healthy left ventricle is well tolerated. Arterial blood pressure increases, but venous return and therefore CVP will decrease. Pulmonary artery pressures do not rise, and stroke volume will decrease. The wedge pressure and the ECG do not change. A low concentration of anesthetic vapor is sufficient to normalize systemic pressure. We do not believe that nitroglycerin or nitroprusside is required routinely to reduce blood pressure. Therefore, if ventricular function is normal, we do not give either drug prophylactically before or during cross-clamping of the aorta.

If ventricular function is abnormal because of coronary, valvular, or other disease, the pulmonary artery occlusion pressure and the pulmonary artery pressure usually rise after application of the cross-clamp. Central venous pressure will increase if the right ventricle cannot perform well with increased afterload. We examine the ECG for ischemia. New or larger V waves may be evident in the pulmonary capillary wedge pressure (PCWP) waveform. We often institute vasodilator therapy (usually intravenous nitroglycerin) at the first sign of ischemia or ventricular dysfunction with elevated filling pressures. We carefully titrate vasodilators to reduce arterial blood pressure and to lower PCWP. We use negative inotropic agents (anesthetic vapors, β-adrenergic receptor-blocking agents) with great caution in these patients.

Managing Decreased Urinary Output

Temporary occlusion of the infrarenal aorta decreases renal cortical blood flow. Because there is no routine intraoperative method of determining renal blood flow, we do not hesitate to establish brisk urinary output with drugs. After ensuring adequate intravascular volume and cardiac output, we administer mannitol (12.5 to 25 g intravenously) approximately 30 minutes before cross-clamping if urinary output is less than 1 ml/kg/h. If there is no response, we then give furosemide (5 to 20 mg intravenously). Loop diuretics are frequently necessary to establish urinary output for patients on chronic diuretic therapy.

For patients who remain oliguric during aortic occlusion, we may begin a low-dose infusion of dopamine after the graft is opened. We often use infusion of furosemide and mannitol for patients who have preexisting renal insufficiency or for those who are at high risk of perioperative renal dysfunction (diabetes, recent injection of radiocontrast agents, perirenal aortic surgery). Patients given combined epidural and general anesthesia may require infusion of phenylephrine for blood pressure support and are equally likely to have inadequate (as judged by arbitrary standards) urinary output. Attempts at establishing diuresis in this setting are the same as outlined earlier, provided intravascular volume is normal.

Blood Loss

In elective infrarenal aortic surgery, we usually monitor blood loss closely. We replace shed blood with crystalloid and autotransfusion until the hematocrit decreases to some critical level. Although we make this determination based on many factors, our general approach is to keep hematocrit in the "high 20s" in class 3 or 4 patients. In massive hemorrhage, we use 5 percent albumin or type specific red blood cells. Use of clotting factors, platelets, and fresh frozen plasma is not required in the routine care of these patients; however, these items are kept readily available for major blood loss.

Unclamping of the Aorta

Essential ingredients to successful unclamping of the aorta include anticipation of the surgeon's timing, discontinuation of vasodilating drugs and cardiac inotropic depressants well in advance, and aggressive volume loading in the 10 to 15 minutes before release of the cross-clamp. Picking an arbitrary value for PCWP or CVP has not been helpful in our practice. Rather, we try to achieve a gradual but definite increase in cardiac filling pressure (by means of volume loading) before the aorta is unclamped.

Reperfusion of the lower limbs causes a washout of lactate. Because the patient's normal buffering system is adequate, this event does not usually require administration of bicarbonate. It should be noted, however, that this buffering system decreases with hemodilution (see Ch. 30). As the aortic clamp is released, blood pressure invariably falls unless outflow is obstructed mechanically. For patients given general anesthesia alone, these decreases are minimal, and blood pressure rapidly returns to normal. Patients having a sympathetic block from epidural blockade often require phenylephrine support during this time. Occasional depression of myocardial contractility may occur and is caused by acidosis, diminished coronary perfusion, or other factors (not yet elucidated) circulating in the blood. We begin an infusion of nitroglycerin if PCWP remains elevated.

Hypothermia

We direct significant attention toward supporting the patient's temperature intraoperatively. Hypothermia caused by large incisions, prolonged surgery, and exposed viscera is virtually unavoidable. Hypothermia is associated with vasoconstriction that can accentuate hypertension at the end of surgery. Severe hypothermia may lead to depression of cardiac contractility, dysrhythmias, and coagulation disorders. Preservation of near-normal body temperature throughout surgery minimizes these problems and can be achieved with the use of fluid warmers, a heated humidifier, head covering, and warm irrigation.

Emergence from Anesthesia

In the past, most patients undergoing aortic surgery at our institution remain on mechanical ventilation. Now patients who have had uneventful surgery, and who have not been given narcotic doses that would preclude early tracheal extubation, are frequently extubated in the operating room or soon after arrival at the ICU. The use of epidural narcotics has been of benefit in this regard. Furthermore, some patients have had a retroperitoneal incision, which entails less respiratory compromise and fluid shifts; both advantages enable earlier tracheal extubation. Higher-risk patients (usually, those having severe cardiac or pulmonary disease) typically continue to receive mechanical ventilation after surgery. Anesthesia personnel and the ICU staff then decide the appropriate timing for extubation.

As consciousness returns, additional narcotic, relaxants, or antihypertensive drugs may be required. These prevent hypertension, tachycardia, or ischemia caused by pain, cold, and anxiety. Continuous monitoring of the ECG and arterial blood pressure is routine during our transfer of these high-risk patients from the operating room to the ICU.

SURGERY FOR THORACOABDOMINAL AORTIC ANEURYSMS

Repair of lesions involving both the thoracic and abdominal segments of the aorta presents difficult technical challenges for the vascular surgeon and additional problems for the anesthetist. Surgeons at our institution do not employ vascular shunts from the proximal aorta, as they believe no clear evidence has demonstrated a benefit from shunting in these cases.[14] The operating room team must be in close communication. We believe that optimal outcome depends on the anesthetist's understanding and anticipation of surgical maneuvers. Anticipation and treatment of myocardial dysfunction, massive hemorrhage, coagulopathy, profound acidosis secondary to visceral ischemia, renal and spinal cord ischemia, and extreme fluctuations in blood pressure are mandatory for successful management of these patients.

Monitoring

Monitoring devices include a radial or axillary artery catheter (optimally, right-sided), and a pulmonary artery line. Venous access must be sufficient to permit volume resuscitation if massive hemorrhage occurs. Volume lines consist of three large-bore intravenous cannulae or 8.5-Fr introducers, and volume is warmed prior to infusion. In addition to other routine monitors (pulse oximetry, urinary output, core temperature, esophageal stethoscope), the cerebrospinal fluid (CSF) pressure is generally monitored. A cathether is inserted into the lumbar subarachnoid space (same technique as for continuous spinal anesthesia) and is connected to a standard pressure transducer. No anesthetics are injected through this catheter, nor should a continuous flush system be attached. The usefulness of measuring CSF pressure is discussed below.

Anesthetic Considerations

We usually use a high-dose narcotic technique (normally, fentanyl, 50 to 75 μg/kg) for induction of anesthesia. Insertion of a double-lumen endotracheal tube allows deflation of the left lung and, thus, better surgical exposure during the proximal anastomosis. We give nondepolarizing muscle relaxants, expecting that in the absence of a spinal cord lesion, the patient will be able to demonstrate lower extremity motor function postoperatively. Because prolonged neuromuscular blockade may result from renal dysfunction secondary to suprarenal cross-clamping, we avoid using relaxants that depend on the kidneys for excretion. An infusion of atracurium is easily titrated to provide adequate muscle relaxation during surgical closure and is readily reversible, thereby permitting early neurologic assessment. After surgery is completed, we substitute a low-pressure, cuffed nasal or oral endotracheal tube for the double-lumen tube.

Temporary Occlusion of the Aorta

As the cross-clamp is applied, left ventricular decompensation may occur because of increased afterload, with or without severe arterial hypertension. The ECG and the PCWP waveform may indicate myocardial ischemia. Therefore, to lower systemic arterial pressure and PCWP before afterload increases acutely, we begin infusions of sodium nitroprusside and nitroglycerin prior to application of the thoracic aortic cross-clamp. Low concentrations of anesthetic vapor may be carefully added to vasodilator therapy to control severe hypertension after cross-clamping in patients with previously normal ventricular function.

Renal, hepatic, and bowel ischemia occur during cross-clamping of the supraceliac aorta. Sodium bicarbonate infusion and modest hyperventilation are instituted during the phase of visceral ischemia to offset the profound acidosis we find occurs with unclamping. We frequently assess pH. With hepatic and bowel revascularization, lactic acid and vasoactive and myocardial depressant substances are released, and dramatic hypotension may occur. Administration of sufficient volume, further bicarbonate, calcium chloride, and occasionally vasopressors in conjunction with slow release of the cross-clamp usually prevent prolonged hypotension.

Other Considerations

Massive intraoperative and postoperative bleeding is possible in these patients. Blood loss is replaced as it occurs with packed cells, 5 percent albumin, and autotransfusion. Crystalloid infusion is kept to a minimum. We believe that ready availability of fresh frozen plasma and platelets is mandatory. Transfusion of clotting factors should begin when large blood losses are associated with a clinically apparent lack of hemostasis. Clotting studies are requested to determine the magnitude of hemostatic derangement. Our surgeons do not administer heparin to patients because of the increased risk of bleeding inherent in this setting.

Renal failure or transient renal dysfunction occurs in a small percentage of cases. Prior to aortic cross-clamping, we administer mannitol and furosemide to institute diuresis; this combination is repeated after reperfusion. Our surgeons increase renal preservation with infusion of iced Ringer's solution through the renal arteries during the ischemic interval.

The incidence of paraplegia after these operations is 1 to 15 percent. Application of specific surgical and hemodynamic prinicples improves oxygen delivery to the spinal cord. The length of temporary occlusion of the aorta clearly influences the length of ischemia. Preservation of lumbar and intercostal arteries should decrease potential ischemia.

Spinal cord ischemia owing to hypoperfusion may be minimized by allowing proximal aortic pressure to remain high during clamping, thus promoting flow through collateral channels. As the cross-clamp is applied, intracranial pressure may increase secondary to systemic hypertension and profound vasodilation from intravenous administration of vasodilating drugs. This increase in pressure can be transmitted to the CSF and is measured by the CSF catheter. Spinal artery blood flow decreases because of two conditions—hypotension distal to the cross-clamp, and an increase in the CSF pressure surrounding the spinal cord. Therefore, to improve blood flow through the spinal arteries, we decrease CSF pressure by withdrawing CSF; this action affects the pressure gradient across the spinal arterial circulation. In our experience, withdrawal of 5 to 40 ml of CSF lowers spinal fluid pressure to preclamp levels.

Monitoring of spinal cord evoked potentials is another method of assessing the functional integrity of the spinal cord but is not in widespread use. The incidence of paraplegia increases greatly after emergency operations and with acute dissection.

SUMMARY

Successful outcome in aortic surgery requires a technically competent operation and careful attention to physiologic detail. Preoperative evaluation is geared toward improving patients' medical status (e.g., by means of coronary revascularization or rehydration after use of contrast agents) and recognizing their physiologic constraints. The use of invasive monitoring and vasoactive drugs enables intraoperative management to conform to the natural functioning of the body. Anticipation and rapid identification of cardiovascular changes allow treatment of one problem before sequelae or new problems supervene. Capable management of these patients is challenging but predicated on vigilance and communication in the operating room.

REFERENCES

1. O'Donnell TJ, Jr., Darling RC, Linton RR: Is 80 years too old for aneurysmectomy? Arch Surg: 111:1250–1257, 1976
2. Djokovic JL, Hedley-Whyte J: Prediction of outcome of surgery and anesthesia in patients over 80. JAMA 232:2301–2306, 1979
3. Cutler BS, Leppo JA: Dipyridamole thallium 201 scintigraphy to detect coronary artery disease before abdominal aortic surgery. J Vasc Surg 5:91–100, 1987
4. Hertzer NR: Clinical experience with preoperative coronary angiography. J Vasc Surg 2:510–514, 1985
5. Boucher CA, Brewster DC, Darling RC et al: Determination of cardiac risk by dipyridamole-thallium imaging before peripheral vascular surgery. N Engl J Med 312:389–394, 1985
6. Davison JK: Anesthesia for major vascular procedures in the elderly. Clin Anaesthesiol 4:931–957, 1986
7. Rao TLK, Jacobs KH, El-Etr AA: Reinfarction following anesthesia in patients with myocardial infarction. Anesthesiology 59:499–505, 1983
8. Eagle KA, Singer DE, Brewster DC et al: Dipyridamole-thallium scanning in patients undergoing vascular surgery. Optimizing preoperative evaluation of cardiac risk. JAMA 257:2185–2189, 1987
9. Fiser WP, Thompson BW, Thompson AR et al: Nuclear cardiac ejection fraction and cardiac index in abdominal aortic surgery. Surgery 94:736–739, 1983
10. Pasternak PF, Imparato AM, Bear G et al: The value of radionuclide angiography as a predictor of perioperative myocardial

infarction in patients undergoing abdominal aortic aneurysm resection. J Vasc Surg 1:320–325, 1984

11. Tisi GM: Preoperative identification and evaluation of the patient with lung disease. Med Clin North Am 71:399–412, 1987

12. Hertzer NR, Beven EG, Young JR et al: Incidental asymptomatic carotid bruits in patients scheduled for peripheral vascular reconstruction: results of cerebral and coronary angiography. Surgery 96:535–544, 1984

13. Yeager MP, Glass DD, Neff RK, Brinck-Johnsen T: Epidural anesthesia and analgesia in high-risk surgical patients. Anesthesiology 66:729–736, 1987

14. Crawford ES, Walker HSJ, III, Saleh SA, Normann NA: Graft replacement of aneurysm in descending thoracic aorta: results without bypass or shunting. Surgery 89:73–85, 1981

13

Anesthesia for Emergency Surgery for Visceral Ischemia

Michael F. Roizen

ACUTE VISCERAL ISCHEMIA

Without previous development of collateral vessels, sudden occlusion of the superior mesenteric artery can lead to bowel infarction within a few hours. Diagnosis is often difficult in the early phase. Frequently the patient has severe pain but no specific signs until peritonitis develops because of intestinal gangrene. Bowel infarction should be strongly suspected when a patient with prior cardiac disease suddenly has central abdominal pain, often severe, but few physical signs for 4 to 6 hours (see Ch. 9). If surgical intervention occurs before gangrene of the bowel develops, revascularization will reduce the otherwise high mortality and morbidity associated with bowel infarction.

Embolic and Thrombotic Sources of Acute Visceral Ischemia

Acute mesenteric occlusion is either embolic or thrombotic in origin. These emboli usually originate in the heart and may follow a recent myocardial infarction. Thrombosis occasionally results from aortic dissection or trauma but normally relates to progressing atherosclerosis in more than one vessel (see Ch. 9). Thrombosis rarely occurs in the other pathogenic conditions giving rise to chronic visceral ischemia: fibromuscular dysplasia, inflammatory arteriopathies, or external compressive disease.

An embolus can usually be extracted by Fogarty catheter from the superior mesenteric artery using a direct approach to the proximal artery. Surgeons worry that attempts to remove the embolus by Foley catheter may cause fragmentation of the embolus and subsequent occlusion of the distal branches, thus making full revascularization impossible. However, proponents of Fogarty embolectomy believe that clearance of major vessels limits the extent of bowel infarction. Although thrombolytic agents may prove useful in reducing ischemia from acute occlusion, use of these drugs has not yet been established.[1] For both acute and chronic visceral ischemia, the more common tendency is to perform surgery of a more invasive nature and to revascularize more than one vessel unless frank bowel infarction has already occurred (see Chs. 9 and 10).

227

Surgical Approaches

Two surgical approaches can be used for surgery for acute visceral ischemia: a left thoracotomy with a retroperitoneal approach, or a direct transabdominal dissection. In the first method, an incision is made over the eighth intercostal space and is extended obliquely across the left side of the abdomen toward the symphysis pubis. A retroperitoneal plane of dissection anterior to the left kidney exposes the abdominal aorta and the diaphragm, which is divided circumferentially close to the rib attachments so that innervation is preserved. This approach provides good exposure of the descending aorta to the bifurcations of the iliac arteries, plus control of all major branches of the aorta. However, a retroperitoneal dissection is more extensive than a transabdominal dissection, and the left thoracic cavity is entered. This combination of disadvantages may increase morbidity. In addition, and most important when discussing emergency operations in which dead bowel is possible, evaluation of the bowel is less optimal with a retroperitoneal approach than with a direct transabdominal approach, and often necessitates extension of the incision. For these reasons, and because most surgeons are more familiar with the transabdominal approach, that technique is the most popular for emergency visceral vascular surgery.

Probably the greatest concern in this procedure is the need for clamping of the aorta above the renal vessels. Occluding the aorta at this level places great hemodynamic stress on the heart. It also exposes the kidneys to the risk of ischemia. Either of these complications may prove fatal to the elderly patient who has arterial disease. Thus, although desirable from the standpoint of maintaining antegrade blood flow, the added potential for morbidity from hemodynamic stress prevents the routine use of grafting at the supraceliac level.

The Relative Urgency of Surgery for Ruptured Abdominal Aortic Aneurysm versus Acute Visceral Ischemia

Unlike a ruptured abdominal aortic aneurysm, in which the "trauma anesthetist" has time to do only a few things correctly and must hope for a bit of luck, emergency surgery for acute visceral ischemia does allow the anesthetist a little more time. Nevertheless, the urgent nature of acute visceral ischemia has definite implications for anesthesia management. For one thing, the time and delays inherent in providing ideal anesthesia care during elective suprarenal aortic reconstruction are just not possible. Also, concerns must be prioritized so that the little preparatory time that is available is used wisely. For example, some of the other causes of morbidity after emergency visceral vascular surgery besides cardiac problems include pulmonary infections, graft infections (this is particularly worrisome if synthetic grafts are used and bowel spillage or bowel resection is necessary), renal insufficiency and failure, hepatic failure, and spinal cord ischemia resulting in paraplegia. However, little time is available to worry about the relatively rare complication of spinal cord ischemia when death of the patient may be imminent. Thus, the use of somatosensory evoked potentials (SSEPs) or the electroencephalogram (EEG), often used by some investigators to gauge spinal cord and cerebral protection during resection of abdominal or thoracoabdominal aneurysms or coarctation repairs,[2,3] seems to me to become moot. Besides, I find no evidence in the literature that monitoring of the EEG is beneficial in these procedures, and no evidence that stroke is a predictable consequence of even supraceliac or descending thoracic aortic reconstruction.

On the other hand, blood flow in the spinal arteries depends on collateralization and is often bidirectional. Therefore, blood supply to the spinal cord can be "stolen" and given to the rest of the body when pressures in other areas of the body are lower. Such a situation may arise when a single occluding clamp is applied high on the aorta. As spinal cord ischemia does occur in 1 to 11 percent of procedures involving repair of the distal descending thoracic aorta,[4] some surgical techniques have been designed to minimize spinal cord ischemia—bypass shunts to supply blood to the lower extremities, femorofemoral extracorporeal bypass techniques, double-clamping techniques, drainage of cerebrospinal fluid, and preservation of the native aorta with its intercostal artery.[5,6] Because the surgeon's attention is usually riveted on restoring flow to an ischemic gut as rapidly and permanently as possible, only rarely will a patient with acute mesenteric occlusion develop complications from spinal cord ischemia.

In summary, despite the severe illness of patients presenting with acute mesenteric ischemia, this condition is less urgent than a rupturing aneurysm. In the latter situation, seconds count, whereas in acute mesenteric occlusion, the anesthetist may quite possibly have 15 to 30 minutes to optimize the situation. Thus, in acute mesenteric ischemia, my approach to preoperative hydration and optimal acid-base and hemodynamic equilibrium is usually more thorough.

ONE APPROACH TO PROVIDING ANESTHESIA FOR EMERGENCY VISCERAL VASCULAR SURGERY

Anesthesia Goals and Preoperative Preparation

As in all forms of elective vascular surgery, the most important sources of morbidity and mortality after acute visceral ischemia relate to the myocardium. Although the urgency of the surgical and anesthesia team to "get in there" and improve blood flow to the bowel is certainly appropriate, acute visceral ischemia allows a little more time than would rupture of an aneurysm. Most of this "extra" time is spent optimizing preload to the left ventricle. I believe that managing fluids with the aim of preventing intraoperative hypotension and minimizing cardiac dilation also reduces the incidence of ischemia to other organs and helps prevent pulmonary dysfunction. Although no supporting data currently exist, I strongly believe that by ensuring adequate perfusion of vital organs, prehydration of patients undergoing vascular reconstructive surgery minimizes the hemodynamic fluctuations occurring on induction of anesthesia.

Before induction, an extra 15 to 30 minutes are taken in the operating room to normalize filling pressures. I take into account the fact that patients with dead bowel or sepsis from visceral ischemia or abdominal perforation may be grossly dehydrated but that they may also have acute myocardial dysfunction. This careful balancing act is even more precarious and important in patients with mesenteric embolism from a recent myocardial infarction. Because of these concerns, my monitoring practices stress preservation of myocardial, pulmonary, and renal function as well as intravascular volume.

In contrast to surgery for rupture of an aortic aneurysm, in which almost all monitoring of filling pressures takes place after blood flow in the aorta has been controlled (see Ch. 18), in emergency visceral vascular surgery, most monitors are usually inserted before induction. I almost always insert a catheter into the radial artery of the nondominant hand. Urinary output and some form of ventricular filling pressure are usually monitored, the latter most frequently via pulmonary artery catheter. This catheter allows monitoring of systemic vascular resistance, cardiac output, and pulmonary capillary wedge pressure. For insertion, I prefer the external jugular route, although many anesthetists use the internal jugular or subclavian route. I use a modified chest lead V_5 to monitor the electrocardiogram (ECG) during surgery, except in those patients who have demonstrated myocardial ischemia in areas other than the anterior myocardial wall. In addition, body temperature is almost always monitored and is maintained meticulously by warming all fluids (starting preoperatively) and by placing the patient on a heating mattress on the operating room table.

After insertion of the pulmonary artery catheter, I carefully titrate fluid volume to a pulmonary capillary wedge pressure in the upper normal range (usually 12 to 15 mmHg). Titration can proceed at the rate of 100 to 200 ml of lactated Ringer's solution within 5 to 15 minutes. In my experience, these patients know they are sick and often have a high heart rate from both anxiety and depletion of intravascular volume. Nevertheless, I believe that if blood pressure and heart rate are stable when the patient arrives at the operating room, sterile preparation of the abdomen can begin. After that, intravascular volume status may be assessed by observing the patient for a decrease in systemic blood pressure and/or an increase in heart rate when the head is raised 10 to 15 degrees. Intravenous administration of a 50-mg bolus of thiopental may also aid in assessing volume. I ensure venous access and seek positive indications of acceptable volume loading by tilt test, administration of small doses of thiopental, or measurements from the pulmonary artery catheter. Thus, in this situation, a little extra time is spent inserting and attaching monitors, and ensuring normal or relatively normal volume status prior to induction.

Induction of Anesthesia

Preoxygenation is followed by either tracheal intubation in the conscious patient given topical anesthesia or, more often, by rapid-sequence induction of anesthesia. The latter consists of administration of small-to-moderate doses of fentanyl or sufentanil, small-to-moderate doses of thiopental (0.5 to 5 mg/kg, depending on the response to the test dose of thiopental), and a rapid-acting muscle relaxant; application of cricoid pressure; and endotracheal intubation. To blunt the hemodynamic effects of laryngeal visualization and endotracheal intubation during either awake intubation or rapid-sequence induction of anesthesia, one may administer an intravenous bolus of lidocaine, sodium nitroprusside, nitroglycerin, esmolol, or additional fentanyl, sufentanil, or thiopental.

If hypotension occurs after induction, I give 100 percent oxygen, elevate the patient's legs, and rapidly administer blood and fluids. If these measures fail to produce adequate blood pressure and perfusion, phenylephrine or dopamine is infused until the aorta can be occluded. This situation often means that the diagnosis of visceral ischemia was not complete and that aortic dissection, tear, or rupture may have occurred.

After induction of anesthesia, and

when blood pressure is stable, the surgeon will enter the abdomen rapidly, assess the extent and nature of disease, and try to dissect to the point where access to the diseased vessels can be obtained. Anesthetic management of this part of the procedure resembles that for elective visceral artery reconstruction (see Ch. 10) rather than that for emergency repair of ruptured aneurysms (see Ch. 18). Although repetitive of Chapter 10, a summary of the most salient points follows, so that the reader will not have to refer to Chapter 10.

Anesthetic Considerations during Surgery

Maintenance of anesthesia for emergency surgery for acute visceral ischemia is the same as for elective procedures (see Ch. 10). The following section describes my procedures for protecting the heart during this period.

During the early period of dissection, I keep intravascular volume at normal levels by noting cardiac filling on the two-dimensional transesophageal echocardiogram (see Chs. 10 and 28) or by sustaining a normal pulmonary capillary wedge pressure. To accomplish this, I replace blood losses of less than 10 ml/kg and insensible losses (assumed to be 5 to 7 ml/kg/h during this dissection phase) with lactated Ringer's solution or saline solution.

Various indicators are used for assessing perfusion of vital organs before cross-clamping of the aorta. Perfusion of the heart is indicated by myocardial contractility, as judged by global and regional motion of the wall on a two-dimensional transesophageal echocardiogram[7-10]; by changes in the ST segment on modified chest lead V_5 of the ECG; and by cardiac output. Perfusion of the kidneys is judged by urinary output. Although I believe that

output of 2 to 5 ml of urine per 0.5 hour per 70 kg is adequate in elective surgery, in emergency surgery, both the surgeons and I feel more confident if a brisk diuresis is produced. Diuresis probably does not actually help the patient, but because it is obtained with low-dose dopamine, with furosemide, or with mannitol given far enough in advance so that the drug does not increase preload while increasing afterload, diuresis probably does not harm the patient, either (see Ch. 10). To evaluate perfusion of the central nervous system, I observe eye signs. Even though the EEG and/or SSEPs can be used,[2,3] I have had little experience with these methods in this operative setting. In addition, there is little time to implement these techniques in such an urgent situation. Finally, perfusion of the lungs is assessed by noting gas exchange.

Protecting the Heart before Aortic Occlusion

During the early part of aortic dissection, I protect the heart by producing an adequate depth of anesthesia (i.e., one appropriate to the patient's potential or actual instability, but one ensuring a pain-free state) and by trying to keep hemodynamic variables within the preoperative range.[11] The difference between the emergency situation and an elective procedure is the frequent lack of "baseline-unstressed" preoperative values for the emergency patient. However, if preoperative values are available, I try to keep intraoperative hemodynamic values within or near the patient's normal preoperative range.

For example, if the patients heart rate ranged from 60 to 90 beats/min before surgery but exceeded these limits during surgery, treatment would be initiated. Here, tachycardia is assumed to be of greater concern than bradycardia and is avoided more aggressively. At 95 beats/min, I might increase the anesthetic, give more narcotic, or add a drip infusion of a β-adrenergic receptor-blocking drug. At 100 beats/min, I would give a bolus or begin a drip infusion of a β-adrenergic receptor-blocking drug, assuming values for intravascular fluid volume were acceptable. At 45 beats/min, I might decrease the anesthetic or administer a dilute solution of dopamine (200 mg in 500 ml of 5 percent dextrose in water) to keep heart rate within the acceptable range.

It is important to reemphasize that bradycardia is tolerated to a greater extent than tachycardia during vascular procedures, because, in my view, minimizing myocardial oxygen demand should be of primary importance. Use of two-dimensional transesophageal echocardiography (2D TEE) gives some latitude in the range of acceptable values before intervention. However, I do not allow pulmonary artery pressures to remain abnormal (that is, below 5 or above 15 mmHg) during this procedure, assuming that these values are confirmed by echocardiographic images. Increases in pulmonary artery pressure are treated aggressively by administration of nitroglycerin or nitroprusside, depending on whether the suspected cause is an increase in preload or an increase in afterload.[12,13] For low pressures, more fluid is infused, except in the 1- or 2-minute interval immediately before application of the aortic cross-clamp.

If at all possible, administration of exogenous vasoconstrictors is avoided. Although coronary and cerebral vessels are not as densely innervated as some other areas of the body, administration of α- and β2-adrenergic agents can still induce coronary and cerebral vasoconstriction. In addition, α-adrenergic vasoconstriction may affect the myocardium adversely in other ways. This characteristic appears to stem from the important role that α-adrenergic vasoconstriction plays in maintaining an appropriate distribution of blood flow between the outer and inner myocardium.[14] Because of this reason or others, the incidence of myocardial ischemia is twice as high in patients who are deeply anesthetized and whose systemic pressure is maintained with infusion of phenylephrine than in patients whose blood pressure is maintained with only light anesthesia and endogenous vasoconstrictors.[7] Such ischemia appears to be related to the myocardial dilation induced by these agents (the problem of the stretched, dilated myocardium).[7] In addition, because the gut is heavily innervated, α-adrenergic agents can cause mesenteric ischemia by themselves. In fact, one of the early treatments for visceral ischemia was administration of α-adrenergic receptor-blocking drugs.

Temporary Occlusion of the Aorta

Occlusion of the aorta causes hypertension in the proximal segment and hypotension in the distal segment. During resection of a congenitally coarcted aorta, acute occlusion of the thoracic segment of the aorta has very little effect on cardiovascular variables because of the normal development, over years, of extensive collateral vessels around the coarctation. However, when patients have aortic aneurysm or atherosclerosis but no extensive collateral circulation, occlusion of the aorta increases afterload and peripheral vascular resistance in proportion to the level of the occlusion. In one study, our group found that myocardial stress also varied with the level of occlusion.[8] Frequently, pulmonary capillary wedge pressure did not accurately reflect this increase in left ventricular end-diastolic volume. However, 2D TEE made possible the identification and treatment of myocardial dysfunction that was not detected by conventional monitoring techniques.[8,9] I have found 2D TEE to be an invaluable tool for monitoring the myocardial consequences of clamping and unclamping of the aorta and now use it routinely for all procedures entailing occlusion at the supraceliac level. Because the probe can be inserted and positioned rapidly (within 20 seconds to 5 minutes, the usual time being approximately 1.5 minutes), 2D TEE provides quick assessment capabilities in the anesthetized patient whose trachea is intubated. A short-axis, cross-sectional view of the left ventricle provides excellent qualitative assessment of left ventricular filling volumes, global ventricular contractility, and regional ventricular function.[10] In our studies, when a discrepancy has existed between pulmonary capillary filling pressures and filling pressures obtained by 2D TEE, we have found the latter to be more reliable and useful.[8,15]

The most important information I have obtained from using 2D TEE during vascular surgery is that dilating the heart with administration of fluid (as is often requested by surgeons for stimulation of urine output) is a likely precursor of myocardial ischemia.

These pathophysiologic changes in hemodynamic variables could result from the effect that clamping has on normal patterns of blood flow to the arteries. For example, 22 percent of cardiac output usually goes to renal vessels, and 27 percent goes to the superior mesenteric vessels and celiac trunk.[16] Thus, the likely decrease in flow and the almost certain increase in afterload and peripheral vascular resistance after aortic occlusion at the supraceliac level could dilate the left ventricle. Even when occlusion occurs in only one visceral vessel, the application of an aortic occluding clamp at the supraceliac level, or even of a side-biting clamp that occludes the aorta only partially, appears to increase impedance to blood flow, myocardial afterload, and myocardial work. Other factors that may contribute to myocardial dysfunction during op-erative occlusion at the supraceliac level include release of vasoactive substances from ischemic areas and the presence of unmetabolized citrate from transfused blood.[17]

Removal of the Aortic Clamp

During unclamping of the aorta, a different set of maneuvers is performed to reach the same goals. To ensure adequate volume when the cross-clamp is removed, I replace blood losses during occlusion, milliliter for milliliter, by administering warmed blood. I normally have only four units of packed cells available during this procedure. The packed cells usually are diluted with normal saline or occasionally with lactated Ringer's solution (being careful to provide enough lactated Ringer's solution to avoid clumping of the cells because of the calcium in that solution). Although I prefer administering whole blood (as that is what is lost), it is not routinely available at our institution.

Reactive hyperemia in the newly revascularized area decreases vascular resistance, venous return, and systemic blood pressure. If hypotension persists for more than 4 minutes after removal of the clamp and blood pressure does not return toward normal levels after blood deficits have been replaced, other causes should be sought. One possible source is myocardial dysfunction caused by inadequate metabolism of the citrate present in replacement blood. Such blood has not yet gone to the liver, where citrate is metabolized. This problem can be treated by administration of calcium, which antagonizes the effect of citrate.[17] Other possible causes of hypotension are hidden, persistent bleeding or misjudged replacement of blood deficits. On the echocardiogram, the ventricular cavity would be devoid of volume; on the oscilloscope, filling pressures reflecting pulmonary artery pressures would be low. If necessary, the surgeon can reclamp or occlude the aorta, preferably below the renal arteries. In this setting, an allergic reaction to graft material is another rare cause of inadequate myocardial preload.[18] Thus, replacement and maintenance of volume are mainstays of therapy before, during, and immediately after removal of the supraceliac cross-clamp.

Because of the possibility of bacterial contamination, I do not routinely use autotransfused blood in patients with acute visceral ischemia. After restoration of aortic and visceral flow, I determine whether prolonged (i.e., more than operative time plus, perhaps, 2 hours) postoperative ventilatory support will be necessary. This decision takes into account the pathologic conditions encountered (such as the presence or absence of dead bowel and the possibility of sepsis), the extent of surgical dissection, and the hemodynamic stability of the patient. Also, because of the possibility of sepsis and bacterial contamination, it is rare for me to institute epidural narcotic administration in this group of patients. Once a course for postoperative ventilatory care has been chosen, I administer sedatives and narcotics appropriate to that choice.

rapid surgical intervention to preserve gut, it does not require the instantaneous response or frame of mind of the "trauma anesthetist" during surgery for rupture of an aortic aneurysm. That is, even visceral vascular surgery performed on an emergency basis allows enough time to place monitoring lines and devices. I believe that organ dysfunction involving the heart can be minimized by keeping intraoperative hemodynamic values within the normal preoperative range, by ensuring that cardiac dilation does not occur at any point, and by minimizing episodes of tachycardia. Patients undergoing emergency surgery for acute visceral ischemia can be extremely sick from sepsis, acid-base and electrolyte disorders, and the consequences of bowel ischemia and infarction. They can also be only slightly less stable than the patient undergoing elective surgery. Once reconstruction has been completed, a plan for postoperative care should be established. Throughout the entire procedure, I try to provide enough anesthesia (and sedation-analgesia, sometimes with epidural narcotics, if bowel infarction has not occurred) to keep the patient from experiencing the end-organ effects of stress.

CONCLUSION

The primary goals of reconstruction for visceral ischemia are permanent restoration of normal visceral perfusion and gut salvage. Complications that occur during occlusion of the aorta can usually be linked to the heart, central nervous system, or kidneys. In the emergency setting of acute visceral ischemia, one has only a few minutes to obtain preoperative baseline values and to optimize preoperative hemodynamic, acid-base, and intravascular volume status. Although such a situation is an emergency necessitating

REFERENCES

1. Boley SJ, Borden EB: Acute mesenteric vascular disease. p. 659–671. In Wilson SE, Veith FJ, Hobson RW, II, Williams RA (ed): Vascular Surgery. Principles and Practice. McGraw-Hill, New York, 1987
2. Laschinger JC, Cunningham JN, Jr., Catinella FP et al: Detection and prevention of intraoperative spinal cord ischemia after cross-clamping of the thoracic aorta: use of somatosensory evoked potentials. Surgery 92:1109–1117, 1982
3. Kaplan BJ, Friedman WA, Alexander JA, Hampson SR: Somatosensory evoked potential monitoring of spinal cord ischemia

during aortic operations. Neurosurgery 19:82–90, 1986

4. Crawford ES, Walker HSJ, III, Saleh SA, Normann NA: Graft replacement of aneurysm in descending thoracic aorta: results without bypass or shunting. Surgery 89: 73–85, 1981

5. Connolly JE: Prevention of paraplegia secondary to operations on the aorta. J Cardiovasc Surg 27:410–417, 1986

6. Wadouh F, Arndt C-F, Oppermann E et al: The mechanism of spinal cord injury after simple and double aortic cross-clamping. J Thorac Cardiovasc Surg 92: 121–127, 1986

7. Smith JS, Roizen MF, Cahalan MK et al: Does anesthetic technique make a difference? Augmentation of systolic blood pressure during carotid endarterectomy: effects of phenylephrine *versus* light anesthesia and of insoflurane *versus* halothane on the incidence of myocardial ischemia. Anesthesiology 69:846–853, 1988

8. Roizen MF, Beaupre PN, Alpert RA et al: Monitoring with two-dimensional transesophageal echocardiography. Comparison of myocardial function in patients undergoing supraceliac, suprarenal-infraceliac, or infrarenal aortic occlusion. J Vasc Surg 1:300–305, 1984

9. Smith JS, Cahalan MK, Benefiel DJ et al: Intraoperative detection of myocardial ischemia in high-risk patients: electrocardiography versus two-dimensional transesophageal echocardiography. Circulation 872:1015–1021, 1985

10. Schlüter M, Langenstein BA, Polster J et al: Transesophageal cross-sectional echocardiography with a phased array transduced system. Technique and initial clinical results. Br Heart J 48:67–72, 1982

11. Roizen MF: Anesthetic implications of concurrent diseases. p. 255–357. In Miller RD (ed): Anesthesia. Vol. 1. 2nd Ed. Churchill Livingstone, New York, 1986

12. Flaherty JT, Magee PA, Gardner TL et al: Comparison of intravenous nitroglycerin and sodium nitroprusside for treatment of acute hypertension developing after coronary artery bypass surgery. Circulation 65:1072–1077, 1982

13. Gerson JI, Allen FB, Seltzer JL et al: Arterial and venous dilation by nitroprusside and nitroglycerin—is there a difference? Anesth Analg 61:256–260, 1982

14. Feigl ED: The paradox of adrenergic coronary vasoconstriction. Circulation 76:737–745, 1987

15. Beaupre PN, Cahalan MK, Kremer PF et al: Does pulmonary artery occlusion pressure adequately reflect left ventricular filling during anesthesia and surgery (abstract)? Anesthesiology 59:A3, 1983

16. Guyton AC: Textbook of Medical Physiology. 6th Ed. pp. 230–243. WB Saunders, Philadelphia, 1981

17. Olinger GN, Hottenrott C, Mulder DG et al: Acute clinical hypocalcemic myocardial depression during rapid blood transfusion and postoperative hemodialysis. A prevention complication. J Thorac Cardiovasc Surg 72:503–511, 1976

18. Roizen MF, Rodgers GM, Valone FH et al: Anaphylactoid reaction to vascular graft material presenting with vasodilation and subsequent disseminated intravascular coagulation. Anesthesiology (in press)

SURGERY FOR ABDOMINAL AORTIC RECONSTRUCTION

14

Abdominal Aortic Reconstruction: Surgical Goals and Methods

Robert J. Lusby

Surgeons use abdominal aortic reconstruction to treat either degenerative aneurysmal or stenosing occlusive disease. The natural histories of these two processes differ in an essential way. Because of their unpredictable tendency to rupture or embolize, aneurysms pose an ever-present threat to the life of the patient. Therefore, aggressive surgical management is warranted, even if symptoms do not exist.[1-3]

Occlusive disease tends to be progressive, with compromise of the distal circulation leading to disabling claudication or limb-threatening ischemia. Surgical intervention is indicated for the relief of these disabling symptoms.[1] In both instances, the disease process tends to be segmental; the fact that the vessels above and below the lesion are relatively normal provides the basis for operability.

Modern reconstructive surgery for arterial disease dates from dos Santos's use of thromboendarterectomy in 1947.[4] Wylie[5] extended this technique to the aortoiliac vessels in 1952. In 1950, Oudot and Beaconfield[6] described their use of a homograft to bypass stenotic aortoiliac disease. In 1951, Dubost et al.[7] performed the first successful resection of an abdominal aortic aneurysm with homograft implantation to restore arterial continuity. At about the same time, Blakemore and Voorhees[8] were experimenting with synthetic grafts of Vinyon "N" cloth; good results in dogs and early use in humans were reported in 1954. Further development of synthetic grafts, with wide use in various arterial reconstructions, saw Dacron become the preferred arterial conduit.[1,9]

Since that time, experience has clarified the role of various treatment options, including thromboendarterectomy, excision with graft interposition, bypass grafting, and transluminal angioplasty. Bypass grafting has become the most popular and effective method of treating aortoiliac disease.[10] The prime objective of any aortic procedure is the long-term restoration of normal circulation to the viscera and distal vasculature.

CAUSES OF ANEURYSM OR OCCLUSION OF THE ABDOMINAL AORTA

Atherosclerosis

Atherosclerosis is the major pathologic cause of both occlusive and aneurysmal disease.[1] The mechanism by which atherosclerosis causes not only plaque that protrudes into the arterial lumen but also aneurysmal dilatation of arterial segments is not clear.[11] However, some investigators believe that atherosclerotic plaque formation in the intima produces protracted ischemia in the media of the avascular abdominal aortic wall and that such ischemia favors development of aneurysm.[12] That is, the media of the infrarenal segment of the aorta has approximately 28 elastic lamellar units and no vasa vasorum. Therefore, nutrition of the aortic wall occurs by diffusion from the lumen. Medial ischemia reduces the number of intact laminae, thereby increasing tension in the remaining lamellae. When tension exceeds a critical level, aneurysmal dilatation occurs.

Also, collagenase activity seems to increase in early aneurysmal disease. This event is probably not a primary metabolic defect but rather a response to altered hemodynamic conditions or mechanical injury as a result of the atherosclerotic process.[13] The altered balance of collagen breakdown and replacement may lead to weakening of the wall and subsequent rupture. This process is observed in aneurysms that enlarge after other abdominal procedures such as cholecystectomy.[14] In accordance with the law of Laplace (T = P × R, T being tension, P being pressure, and R being the radius of the vessel), as the radius of a vessel increases, so does wall tension. Therefore, the larger the radius, the greater the risk of rupture.

Nonspecific Aortoarteritis

Although uncommon, nonspecific aortoarteritis (Takayasu's arteritis) can also cause aortic aneurysms and occlusion, plus the tendency of the aneurysm to rupture.[15] This condition is characterized by panarteritis and heavy lymphocyte infiltration of the media by histiocytes, plasma cells, and foreign body giant cells. These signs also occur in other inflammatory arteriopathies, such as polymyalgia rheumatica, giant cell arteritis, thromboangiitis obliterans, tuberculosis, and syphilis. However, the combination of histologic data, distribution of lesions in the thoracic and abdominal aorta and their major branches, and the tendency of the disease to occur in young Asian women distinguishes Takayasu's arteritis from similar inflammatory arteriopathies.

Embolic or Thrombotic Processes

Sudden occlusion of the infrarenal aorta and iliac vessels may result from embolic or thombotic processes. Emboli usually come from the heart and relate to mural thrombus in areas of infarction or to atrial fibrillation.[16] Thrombotic occlusion and embolization occasionally occur after angiographic catheter studies. On rare occasion, infective endocarditis produces infective emboli. Occlusive symptoms occur early, but mycotic aneurysms may form later.[17,18]

Other Causes

On rare occasion, intimal damage caused by blunt trauma produces aortic occlusion.[16,19] Presentation is usually acute, with marked distal ischemia requiring urgent revascularization. Penetrating trauma usually causes acute arterial injury manifested by brisk hemorrhage. Occasionally, covert arterial injury produces late development of false aneurysm or arteriovenous fistula. Anastomotic stenoses and dehiscences with false aneurysm formation are sometimes seen as late complications of aortoiliac reconstruction. These false aneurysms may be infective or sterile and may pose special problems in safe reconstruction of arterial circulation.[9]

ABDOMINAL AORTIC ANEURYSM

Mortality Rates

Predominantly because of rupture of the aneurysm, 80 percent of unoperated patients who have aneurysms of the abdominal aorta die within 5 years of diagnosis.[20-22] The larger the diameter of the aneurysm, the greater the risk of rupture: the incidence of rupture within 5 years of diagnosis is approximately 25 percent for lesions 4 to 7 cm in diameter, 45 percent for lesions 7 to 10 cm in diameter, and 60 percent for lesions larger than 10 cm in diameter.[22] Also, the larger the aneurysm, the greater the chance of early rupture: 71.8 percent of fatal ruptures of larger lesions occurred within 2 years of diagnosis, whereas only 39.1 percent of fatal ruptures of smaller lesions occurred within that time[23] (Fig. 14-1).

Successful surgical repair of an abdominal aortic aneurysm appears to increase life expectancy.[2,3,11,21,24] Improvements in surgical and anesthetic management are the chief reasons why perioperative mortality after elective surgery has declined steadily (from approximately 17 percent before 1960 to 2 to 5 percent since 1980), despite the fact that the indications for surgery have become more numerous.[11,25,26] During the same time, however, the mortality rate after surgery for ruptured aneurysms has remained high, from 25 to 75 percent.[2,27-29]

Many studies show the extreme seriousness of aortic rupture. In one particularly illustrative study, a series of 180 patients presented to a hospital with a diagnosis of ruptured abdominal aortic aneurysm and had immediate surgery.[29] Eighteen percent of the patients died before surgery; 10.5 percent died during surgery before completion of anastomosis; and 1.9 percent died during surgery after completion of grafting. Eight percent of aneurysms were inoperable. The overall in-hospital mortality was 75 percent; many patients who survived died later of multisystem failure. This study includes many patients who are often excluded from other reports. Also, because the mortality rate does not include those who died before reaching the hospital, it understates the mortality associated with rupture of an aortic aneurysm.

Risk Factors

Careful assessment of cardiac, renal, and pulmonary status is essential in the preoperative evaluation of patients undergoing aortic surgery.

Myocardial Ischemia

Coronary artery disease remains the most frequent cause of perioperative and late death in elective surgery for abdominal aortic aneurysm. Despite appreciation of this problem, controversy still exists as to the best management strategy for patients who have both abdominal aortic and coronary artery disease. The controversy centers around the routine or selective use of coronary angiography and the performance of coronary artery bypass in such patients.

Routine coronary angiography shows significant coronary disease in a large

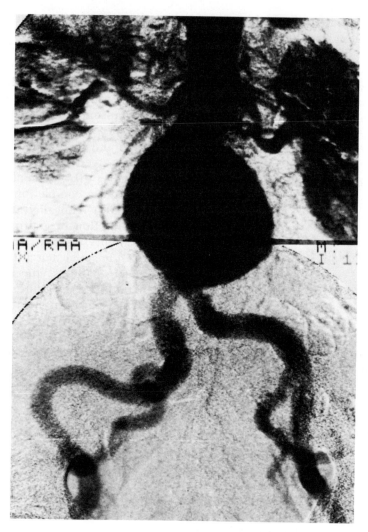

Fig. 14-1. Digital subtraction angiogram showing large infrarenal abdominal aortic aneurysm with uninvolved iliac arteries. Renal artery origins are clearly seen well above the aneurysm.

number of patients who have aortic disease.[30] However, delay in aortic reconstruction, especially aneurysm repair, and the relative hypotension during coronary artery bypass result in significant mortality (7.7 percent) from other vascular lesions.[30] Coronary angiography also carries significant morbidity, as does coronary bypass surgery; such morbidity may be higher in patients with aortic dis-

ease than in those not having peripheral vascular disease.

Studies indicate that perioperative mortality may be lower if coronary angiography is done selectively rather than routinely. A 1981 series used selective coronary angiography for patients with severe or unstable cardiac ischemia.[31] Although extensive invasive monitoring and cardiac support equipment were used, the in-hospital mortality from myocardial ischemia was only 2.9 percent. A 1986 study with the same criteria showed that high-risk cardiac patients undergoing elective surgery for abdominal aortic aneurysm had an acceptably low in-hospital mortality of 5.7 percent.[3]

Elective surgery for abdominal aortic aneurysm appears to be relatively safe for patients with no history of coronary artery disease. Among those who have known cardiac disease, selective coronary angiography and coronary artery bypass grafting are probably advantageous in a small percentage.[31] Our current practice in preoperative coronary evaluation of patients for abdominal aortic surgery is to perform coronary angiography only in those with marked myocardial ischemia on history or stress electrocardiogram. We believe that patients with both diseases would profit by first undergoing abdominal aortic aneurysm repair with suitable support measures and then, if warranted by cardiac symptoms alone, coronary artery revascularization. Although we believe that long-term survival rates after coronary artery bypass grafting will be higher in these high-risk cardiac patients, this belief has been difficult to document without a controlled prospective trial.[23]

Hypertension

Hypertension clearly accelerates the development of atherosclerosis. Uncontrolled hypertension increases the risk of rupture of the aneurysm and perioperative mortality.[23,24,32] Control of hypertension may be important in decreasing morbidity from cardiovascular and cerebrovascular disease.

Congestive Heart Failure

Congestive heart failure (manifested by pulmonary edema either clinically or radiologically) within 30 days of aneurysm resection is associated with increased perioperative mortality.[3,33] Left ventricular ejection fraction is a good indicator of the heart's ability to tolerate aortic surgery. In one series, a left ventricular ejection fraction of less than 35 percent was associated with an 80 percent incidence of perioperative myocardial infarction and 20 percent mortality.[34]

Renal Failure

Postoperative renal failure is associated with high morbidity and mortality.[35] A number of factors probably contribute to this event, including hypotension, microembolic "trashing" of the kidneys, and prolonged occlusion times. Preoperative renal failure, however, does not necessarily prohibit successful aortic surgery, provided adequate steps are taken to preserve renal function. Patients with preoperative renal failure on established dialysis do not appear to have increased morbidity with abdominal aortic aneurysm repair.[36] In contrast, compensated renal failure (serum creatinine levels higher than 4 mg/dl) managed without preoperative dialysis commonly requires postoperative dialysis and incurs high morbidity and mortality. This subgroup should be considered for dialysis—instituted before elective aortic surgery—to reduce postoperative problems.

Pulmonary Disease

Chronic pulmonary disease is closely associated with postoperative morbidity.[3] Pain, distension, and limitations induced by the abdominal wound all add to postoperative respiratory problems. None of the effort-independent pulmonary function tests used for predicting the need for postoperative ventilatory support is reliable. The least unreliable is the mean forced expiratory flow over the middle half of the forced vital capacity ("FEF25–

75%").[37] At our center, a value of less than 50 percent of the predicted value indicates a high probability of serious postoperative pulmonary complications. Preoperative preparation with bronchodilators, incentive spirometry, chest physiotherapy, and cessation of smoking may help to lessen postoperative problems; the lack of controlled studies lessens the certainty with which this statement can be made.[3,37] Transverse and oblique abdominal incisions, which tend to produce less postoperative pain and facilitate postoperative respiratory effort, should be considered in high-risk patients.

Age

Although age is believed to be significant risk factor in aortic surgery, the age at which individuals are accepted for surgery seems to be increasing.[3,23,33,34,37,38] In 1972, Szilagyi et al.[23] reported using 75 years as the age limit for surgical intervention, whereas in 1986 Hollier et al.[3] used 85 years. Wylie and Stoney (personal communication) have virtually no age limit, 105 years being the age of their oldest surgical patient. Nonetheless, advanced age is usually associated with a higher incidence of major disease and hence a higher operative risk. On the other hand, elective surgery always incurs less risk than emergent surgery. One study of patients over 80 years of age who had surgery for abdominal aortic aneurysm reported mortality rates of 37 percent for ruptured aneurysm, 27 percent for urgent aneurysm resections, and 3 percent for elective resections.[39] These figures are quite acceptable in view of the expected survival of 7.5 years for an 80-year-old person. Thus, age alone should not preclude a patient from undergoing repair of an abdominal aortic aneurysm.[22,26,31,32]

Preoperative Investigation

Although the clinical diagnosis is usually reliable, radiologic tests may be necessary to diagnose abdominal aortic aneurysm. The initial diagnosis is frequently made radiologically during unrelated investigations. The need for routine radiologic assessment of aneurysms of the abdominal aorta remains controversial. Most physicians now agree that assessment of the size of the aneurysm is important in estimating the risk of rupture. Because palpation usually overestimates the size by 20 percent or more in obese patients, accurate size estimation requires other methods.

Currently, both ultrasonography and computed tomography (CT) provide very accurate estimations of the size of abdominal aortic aneurysms.[40,41] Ultrasonography is quicker, less costly, incurs no hazard from ionizing radiation, and is well suited to mass screening and regular follow-up programs[25] (Fig. 14-2). However, computed tomographic scanning provides superior detail and better estimation of the location of the renal artery, the presence of intraluminal thrombus, contained aortic rupture, venous anomalies, and other pathologic conditions in the abdomen[41,42] (Figs. 14-3 and 14-4). Because both methods have specific limitations, rational use of each gives optimum information.[41]

Although size of the aneurysm is still the most important risk factor for rupture, stenotic atherosclerotic arterial disease is often also present. In one study, as many as 25 percent of patients with abdominal aortic aneurysm had, in addition, significant occlusive disease of the iliac arteries[11] (Fig. 14-5). Significant stenotic disease is poorly demonstrated by CT scanning and ultrasonography. Arteriography remains the best method for this evaluation, and intravenous digital subtraction angiography enables luminal as-

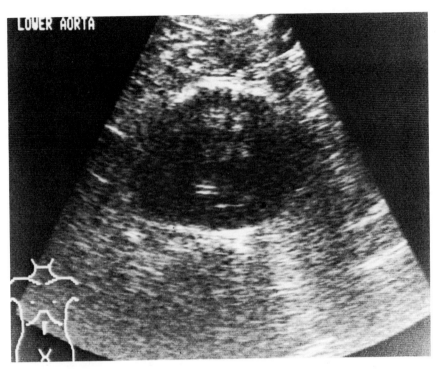

Fig. 14-2. Ultrasonographic image of an abdominal aortic aneurysm in the coronal plane.

sessment without arterial catheterization.[43,44] Use of digital subtraction angiography lessens the morbidity associated with emboli and thrombosis.

A prospective study by Bunt and Cropper[45] of routine angiography in preoperative evaluation of abdominal aortic aneurysms found that routine angiography provided decisive information in 18 percent of patients and potentially helpful information in an additional 14 percent. The additional information obtained from angiography includes the presence of the following: iliac aneurysmal or occlusive disease; juxtarenal or suprarenal extension of the aneurysm; aneurysmal or occlusive disease of the renal arteries; lesions of the visceral arteries, including the presence of a "meandering mesenteric artery"; horsehoe kidney; accessory renal arteries; arteriovenous fistula; and disease of other organs (Fig. 14-6).

Preliminary studies with magnetic resonance imaging have found good quality imaging of luminal detail and arterial wall pathology without the use of ionic contrast. The expectation is that quantifiable measurements of blood flow also will be possible with this noninvasive technique. With refinement in machinery and production of faster and cheaper scanners, magnetic resonance imaging may rapidly gain acceptance for preoperative aortic evaluation.[46]

Surgery for Abdominal Aortic Aneurysm

Surgical Exposure

The most popular surgical exposure for abdominal aortic aneurysm is through a vertical anterior midline abdominal incision with a transperitoneal approach to

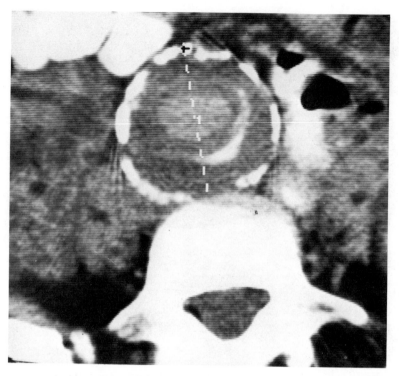

Fig. 14-3. Computed tomographic scan of abdominal aortic aneurysm. Contrast shows central channel of flowing blood distinct from thick laminated thrombus lining the aneurysm. Aneurysm is lying on the anterior longitudinal ligament.

the retroperitoneal structures. This approach allows a versatile surgical plan and provides access to all major arteries between diaphragm and pelvis. Also, other abdominal organs can be inspected easily. Most surgeons feel comfortable with this approach, and access can be rapid, if necessary, for control of ruptured aneurysms.

A transverse abdominal incision, immediately supraumbilical, gives good exposure for a transperitoneal approach to the abdominal aorta. It is a slower entry but postoperatively less painful than the vertical incision.

Among the disadvantages of the transperitoneal approach are the exposure of abdominal organs and their manipulation, which result in major heat and fluid losses and contribute to postoperative ileus.[47] Also, upper abdominal incisions

cause major postoperative discomfort and increase postoperative pulmonary morbidity.[37] With these problems in mind, various retroperitoneal approaches have been used to provide a smoother postoperative course.[47–51] The fact that the retroperitoneal approach is not used universally indicates the relative satisfaction most surgeons have with the transperitoneal procedure.

Although Dubost et al.[7] used the retroperitoneal approach in 1951 for the first abdominal aortic aneurysm repair, little attention was focused on this technique until Rob[50] evaluated a large series in 1963. He concluded that the incidences of respiratory and wound complications were less, that the degree of ileus was lower, and that patients were discharged earlier when a retroperiteoneal approach was used.

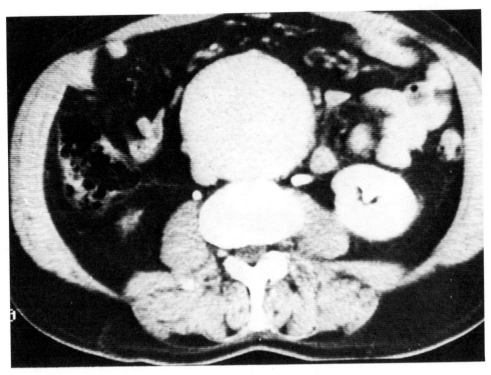

Fig. 14-4. Computed tomographic scan of abdominal aortic aneurysm in Fig. 14-1. Contrast shows entire lumen and no laminated thrombus.

The retroperitoneal approach anterior to the kidney was developed by Stoney and Wylie[52] for access to proximal aortic lesions. Williams et al.[47] used an extended left flank incision similar to that used for nephrectomy, with retroperitoneal dissection posterior to the kidney to enable higher exposure of the suprarenal aorta. This technique enables good exposure to the supraceliac aorta after division of the left crus of the diaphragm and is quite adequate for endarterectomy of renal and visceral arteries as well as aortic grafting.

Studies have compared variables during aortic procedures performed by transperitoneal and retroperitoneal approaches.[49,51] In general, retroperitoneal procedures incur less blood loss and lower intraoperative fluid requirements. Postoperatively, the degree of ileus seems to be less, and oral intake can be resumed earlier. Less pain is experienced (as judged by narcotic requirements) and fewer pulmonary complications appear to occur, with shorter hospital stays.

Graft Replacement

After surgical exposure of the aorta and iliac arteries, graft replacement of the aneurysmal segment of aorta is performed. If the graft is to be preclotted, the harvesting of blood for preclotting must be done before any administration of heparin.

Infrarenal aortic aneurysmal disease usually involves the aorta and common iliac arteries. An aortic bifurcation graft is used with end-to-end anastomoses to the proximal aortic neck and distal anastomoses to the common iliac arteries just short of their bifurcations[32] (Fig. 14-7).

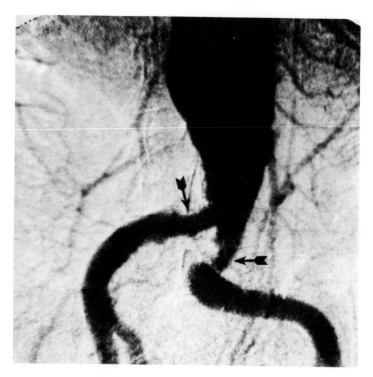

Fig. 14-5. Digital subtraction angiogram showing abdominal aortic aneurysm and mild stenotic disease of common iliac arteries (arrows).

When the iliac vessels are not aneurysmal or stenotic, use of a tube graft to replace the diseased aorta shortens the procedure and incurs less blood loss.[53]

Antibiotics. Prophylactic administration of systemic antibiotics is now an accepted practice for all implantation surgery.[54] The choice of antibiotic is determined by the likely contaminants. Prophylaxis against staphylococci, streptococci, and gram-negative organisms usually consists of administration of an appropriate broad-spectrum antibiotic, usually a cephalosporin. The antibiotic is commonly given at about the time of induction of anesthesia. Antibiotic seeding of vascular prostheses may offer an alternative in the near future.[54]

Heparinization. Systemic heparinization is a common practice that attempts to prevent distal thrombotic complications during and after temporary occlusion of

the aorta. However, distal ischemia complicating aortic surgery is now recognized as being related to the dislodgement of atheroemboli from the diseased aorta. The recognition of the embolic nature of distal ischemia prompted Starr et al.[55] to perform aneurysm resection without heparin administration. Instead, these investigators paid particular attention to minimal manipulation of the vessels before clamping, immediately after clamping of the artery proximally, and after release of the clamps after reconstruction. Copious flushing from proximal and distal vessels just before completion of anastomoses was also part of their procedure. Only one embolic event occurred among 434 procedures. In the absence of major distal occlusive disease, heparinization may be unnecessary in abdominal aortic aneurysm repair, careful technique probably

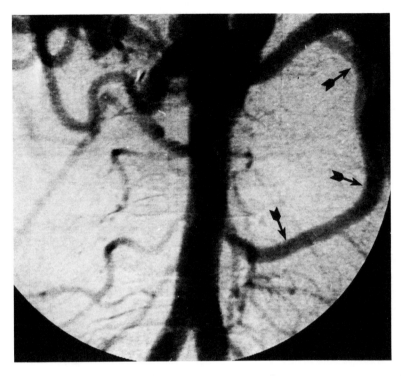

Fig. 14-6. Digital subtraction angiogram showing a "meandering mesenteric artery" (arrows).

being the more important factor in avoiding distal ischemia.[53,55]

Synthetic Grafts. A wide range of synthetic grafts are currently available. Most hospitals, however, carry only the limited variety representing their surgeons' preference. The standard material used since the late 1950s has been either knitted or woven Dacron.[1] More recently, polytetrafluoroethylene grafts, which are less porous, have become available.

Both knitted and woven Dacron grafts have advantages and disadvantages. The knitted grafts are quite porous and require preclotting before implantation. They develop more pseudointima and, as a result, may have more resistance to late infection than woven grafts.[47] These grafts are relatively pliable, easy to suture, and do not fray when cut. On the other hand, woven Dacron grafts are nonporous and do not require preclotting. This feature is quite an advantage in instances of ruptured aneurysm or bleeding diathesis. If cut by sharp instruments, woven Dacron tends to fray; however, this disadvantage can be overcome by using electrocautery to cut the graft. Woven grafts are more rigid and not as easy to manipulate as knitted grafts.

To make knitted grafts impervious, various sealing compounds such as albumin and gelatin have been developed. Grafts impregnated with these materials appear to have reduced blood loss at the time of implantation. Most recent work has been aimed at developing an antibiotic impregnation and endothelial cell seeding of grafts to lessen the risk of infection and thrombosis.[54,56,57]

Temporary Occlusion of the Aorta. Aortic cross-clamping adversely affects cardiac function and, by increasing afterload, increases wall stress on the left ventricle and pulmonary capillary wedge pressure.[58] Whether there is a direct as-

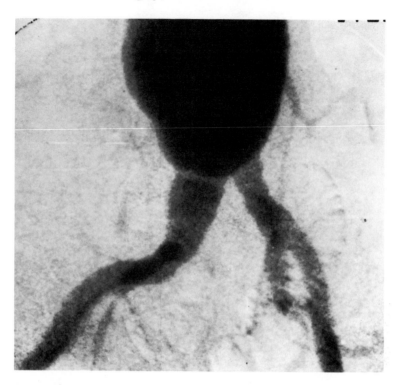

Fig. 14-7. Digital subtraction angiogram demonstrating abdominal aortic aneurysm extending to involve the right common iliac artery.

sociated decrease in cardiac function from some neurogenic or hormonal source secondary to aortic cross-clamping or its resulting gut or leg ischemia remains controversial.[58–60] The effects of temporary arterial occlusion on cardiac function are more marked with supraceliac occlusion than with infrarenal occlusion. Although the healthy heart normally tolerates infrarenal clamping for prolonged periods,[60] a diseased heart is vulnerable to these changes. Sophisticated monitoring with Swan-Ganz catheters, arterial pressure lines, and transesophageal echocardiography permits some control of adverse effects through appropriate volume loading and the use of vasodilating drugs.

Although most aortoiliac surgery can be performed with infrarenal clamping of the aorta, many situations require supra-

renal (usually supraceliac) occlusion of the aorta. Aneurysms of the abdominal aorta involve the pararenal aorta in as many as 20 percent of cases.[61] Because significant renal artery stenoses may coexist with an abdominal aortic aneurysm of infrarenal or pararenal site, correction of these renal artery lesions may well occur in conjunction with aneurysm repair.[61,62] Significant stenoses of the celiac trunk or superior mesenteric artery may similarly be addressed at the time of aortic reconstruction. Aortic surgery in the patient who has previously undergone aortic surgery frequently necessitates revision to a higher graft origin, and problems of infection in prosthetic materials may demand a clean site for a new graft origin. Ruptured aneurysms often require supraceliac clamping for initial control of blood flow. Thus, many conditions require aortic cross-clamping more cephalad than the usual infrarenal position. Renal function is most at risk in these situations; patients known to have preoperative renal insufficiency are at greatest risk of acute postoperative renal failure.

Postoperative renal failure in this patient group has a mortality rate of 67 percent, even with modern supportive care and the use of hemodialysis.[63] Various intraoperative maneuvers try to prevent this disastrous complication: avoidance of hypotension, infusion of mannitol, use of diuretics, and use of angiotensin-converting enzyme inhibitors.[64] Despite these practices and the use of intraoperative shunts or cold renal perfusion techniques, morbidity and mortality remain high for combined aortic reconstruction and renal revascularization.[62]

Inflammatory Aneurysms
Inflammatory aneurysms of the abdominal aorta occur in only 5 percent of aneurysms.[65–68] The thick, white inflammatory reaction in the retroperitoneum, seemingly centered on an abdominal aortic aneurysm, varies in extent. It may involve retroperitoneal structures and obstruct the ureter. Intraperitoneal organs may be adherent, particularly the duodenum and jejunum. The inflammatory reaction obliterates normal tissue planes, making dissection difficult and hazardous. Because the wall of the aneurysm is greatly thickened anteriorly and laterally but not posteriorly, these lesions may rupture posteriorly.[65,68] The reaction usually does not extend cephalad to the aneurysm. Management of these lesions entails dissection above and below the process for application of controlling clamps, with no attempt to dissect structures adherent to the reaction.[65,66] This procedure frequently requires supraceliac aortic cross-clamping. Once blood flow is controlled, the aneurysm is opened with electrocautery and the graft is inserted; suturing occurs from within the opened aorta. Of interest is the fact that once the aneurysm is repaired, the inflammatory reaction may subside with no signs of ureteral obstruction or retroperitoneal fibrosis.[65,68] The usefulness of preoperative steroid therapy has not yet been established. An early report by Hedges and Bentley[69] suggests that such treatment alleviates symptoms and reduces fibrosis but possibly increases the risk of rupture.[65]

Postoperative Problems

Aneurysm repair is a major stress to the body of elderly patients, who may have widespread atherosclerosis and decreased respiratory function. Major morbidity and mortality commonly result from associated coronary artery, cerebrovascular, and respiratory diseases. Special problems may arise from major arterial hemorrhage, coagulopathy, distal thromboembolic occlusions, visceral ischemia, spinal cord ischemia, renal failure, graft sepsis, graft occlusion, and aortoenteric fistula formation.

Hemorrhage
Acute arterial hemorrhage may occur soon after surgery. Arterial suture lines and porous grafts are liable to leak at this time; also, damaged lumbar vessels, mesenteric artery branches, and any other vessel encountered during surgery may bleed at this time. The cause of bleeding may be dislodgement of hemostatic plugs and elevated blood pressure, suture fracture, suture displacement, or reactionary bleeding. Whatever the cause, reoperation may be required to control hypotension through increased administration of stored blood. The significantly higher morbidity and mortality associated with hemorrhage after aneurysm repair em-

phasize the need for careful hemostasis at the time of the initial procedure.[11,33]

Coagulation Defects

Coagulation defects may occur in aortic reconstruction for a variety of reasons—often, the ingestion of aspirin, which should not be taken for at least 1 week before surgery (see Ch. 31). If necessary, one unit of platelets can be given preparatorily. This practice of administering a few platelets appears to be effective in normalizing clotting, as only a few platelets are required to begin the aggregation reaction that is inhibited by heparin (see Ch. 31). Preoperative coagulation disorders, if recognized, may be correctable, thereby enabling uncomplicated surgery. Excessive alcohol intake is associated with anemia, thrombocytopenia, abnormal liver function, and low production of vitamin K-dependent coagulation factors. Cogenital coagulation disorders are associated most frequently with deficiencies of factors VIII and IX.[70] Specific component therapy is available for most of these problems. Occasionally, consumption of clotting factors within the lumen of an abdominal aortic aneurysm may cause the preoperative syndrome of disseminated intravascular coagulation, although this syndrome is more commonly diagnosed during or after surgery.[71]

Notwithstanding these problems, the most common cause of coagulopathy in aortic surgery is that associated with large volume transfusion of stored blood; such transfusions occur in surgery for ruptured aneurysms or in prolonged, complex reconstructive procedures.[72–74] In elective surgery, autologous blood may be collected before surgery, thus overcoming a number of problems, such as transmission of disease (especially non-A, non-B hepatitis and acquired immune deficiency syndrome) and cross-matching errors. If possible, antiplatelet agents and anticoagulants should be discontinued before surgery to decrease perioperative blood loss. Rupture of aneurysms in patients taking oral anticoagulants presents a special problem, and administration of fresh frozen plasma or cryoprecipitate is usually required to correct the defect.

When the anticipated use of stored blood is greater than eight units, administration of platelets and/or fresh frozen plasma is advised (the ratio being one unit of platelets for each unit of blood, and one unit of fresh frozen plasma for each three or four units of blood). Specific platelet infusions are commonly used after cardiopulmonary bypass but also may be needed in large aortic aneurysms and after control of acute bleeding. Although very fresh whole blood is preferable to blood that has been stored for a time, the former is seldom available. A newer approach is the use of intraoperative autotransfusion of blood.[74,75] Although the necessary machinery is costly, significant advantages apparently exist in reducing homologous blood use and its attendant problems; however, no randomized, "blinded," controlled trial showing such a benefit yet exists.

Distal Ischemia

Distal ischemia after aortic reconstruction is a well-recognized embolic phenomenon.[55] When dissecting the aneurysmal aorta, loose friable atheroma or thrombus may be dislodged, thereby producing the multiple microemboli responsible for the "trash foot" syndrome (digital gangrene). Macroemboli lodging in large vessels may produce acute ischemia requiring further operative measures (balloon catheter embolectomy) for limb salvage. Certain techniques have proved effective in minimizing this problem, even without the use of heparin during and after aortic clamping: application of the clamp from distal vessel to proximal vessel, minimal handling of diseased vessels, and copious flushing with heparinized saline before completion of anastomoses.[55]

Renal Failure

Preoperative renal dysfunction indicates potential postoperative impairment. Despite intensive monitoring, careful fluid management, and use of hemodialysis, acute renal failure after aortic reconstruction still carries high morbidity and a mortality rate of more than 30 percent.[35] This complication occurs most frequently in ruptured aneurysm accompanied by significant hypotension and in suprarenal aortic clamping. Some investigators believe that performing renal revascularization at the time of aortic reconstruction may increase renal morbidity and should therefore be restricted to patients fulfilling very specific criteria.[61,62]

Miller and Myers[64] describe current methods of lessening the risk of acute renal failure after aortic reconstruction. Of major importance is the avoidance of repeated episodes of hypovolemia and hypotension. Normal intravenous volume status should be ensured before and after renal ischemia. Many believe that infusion of mannitol before clamping of the renal arteries is beneficial. Use of furosemide, vasodilating drugs, and angiotensin-converting enzyme inhibitors before renal artery clamping may also be beneficial. I believe that infusion of sodium nitroprusside for control of hypertension should be avoided. If prolonged renal ischemia is anticipated, selective profound hypothermia of the kidneys may crease the incidence of postoperative renal impairment. Although a recent report also suggests possible benefits from infusion of verapamil into the renal arteries just before reperfusion,[64] other data indicate that no practice lessens the risk of acute renal failure more than good surgical technique.[76]

Visceral Ischemia

Visceral ischemia, an uncommon complication of aortic reconstruction, usually affects the inferior mesenteric circulation and, on rare occasion, the superior mesenteric circulation. After aortic surgery, ischemic colitis occurs in 1 to 2 percent of patients and small bowel infarction occurs in 0.15 percent of patients; these figures may be higher after ruptured aortic aneurysm.[77] Mortality associated with these complications is as high as 90 percent.[77]

Preoperative aortography may show a "meandering artery" when the inferior mesenteric artery, via its collateral anastomoses, is the major source of blood supply to the superior mesenteric circulation (see Ch. 9). Under these circumstances, even without the existence of symptoms of visceral ischemia, elective aortic surgery carries a high risk of precipitating visceral ischemia. Therefore, the surgeon will plan to revascularize the inferior mesenteric artery during aortic repair[77–79] (see Ch. 9).

Spinal Cord Ischemia

Spinal cord ischemia is another rare complication of abdominal aortic surgery.[80] In the normal configuration, the major blood supply of the spinal cord occurs through the anterior spinal artery fed by medullary branches from the aorta, the largest of which arises between the T9 and T12 vertebral levels. The spinal arteries are frequently poorly collateralized. Therefore, the sacral supply to distal cord segments by branches of the internal iliac artery systems becomes important. To protect this important collateral pathway, the surgeon tries to preserve at least one internal iliac artery at the time of aortoiliac bifurcation grafting.[80] Occasionally, the major medullary supply to the anterior spinal artery is located in a pararenal position and is liable to injury if aortic procedures involve this area. Large lumbar vessels in this area should be preserved, if possible.[81]

Graft Infection

Late complications of aortic reconstruction are thankfully few. Graft infection is probably the most calamitous, carrying a mortality of up to 75 percent.[82] Fortunately, the incidence is low—approximately 2 percent in most series. Infection can be minimized by prophylactic administration of systemic antibiotics given perioperatively, avoidance of groin anastomoses, preservation of colonic perfusion, and careful attention to hemostasis. Emergency procedures and repeat operations carry higher rates of sepsis.[47]

Even though treatment of established graft infection is difficult, in general, the infected graft segment must be excised. Revascularization of the distal circulation may not be necessary if collateral blood supply is adequate. However, extra-anatomic bypass in which clean grafts are routed through noninfected tissues are usually needed. Despite such attempts, major amputation is necessary in approximately 30 percent of cases.[82] Specific antibiotic therapy is dictated from cultures of the infected graft; generally, at least 6 weeks of therapy are necessary. If the aortic suture line is infected (whether associated with aortoenteric fistula or not), a major cause of death is persistent sepsis in the area of the aortic stump after graft removal, with secondary hemorrhage a common terminal event. If infection is limited to one limb and distal anastomosis of an aortobifemoral graft, the infected limb of the graft may be removed and a prolonged specific antibiotic course given in the hope of eradicating sepsis without the need for total graft removal[82] (Fig. 14-8).

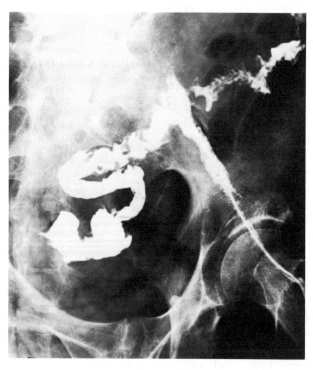

Fig. 14-8. Left groin sinogram demonstrating Dacron graft causing an enteric fistula.

Late graft infection may be caused by seeding of the prosthetic material from an infection in the distal circulation. The risk of bacteremic seeding of cardiac prosthetic valves has long been recognized; recent evidence suggests that similar problems exist with other prosthetic implants, including arterial grafts.[57] Occluded arterial conduits appear more susceptible to infection than do functioning grafts.[57] The need for prophylactic administration of antibiotics during surgical procedures known to cause bacteremia seems prudent, and most surgeons advise their patients accordingly. Such procedures include any involving manipulation of the oral, gastrointestinal, or genitourinary tracts.

Long-Term Results

Many large studies with long-term follow-up have documented an excellent survival rate for patients undergoing abdominal aortic aneurysm repair: the figure approximates the value found on the expected survival curve for a normal population of similar age.[1–3,11,21,23,24,32,33,39,83] This observation is in great contrast to the high mortality associated with nonresected aneurysms, the single most frequent cause of death being rupture of the aneurysm and the second being myocardial infarction.[24] In one study, the life expectancy of the patient with abdominal aortic aneurysm who had surgical repair was approximately twice that of the patient who had nonresective management, despite the higher mortality and morbidity associated with this surgical procedure in the 1960s.[24] Modern surgical and anesthetic techniques, plus the advent and improvement in intensive care facilities, produce an acceptably low perioperative mortality of 2 to 5 percent for aneurysm repair.[25,26,34,39,83] These improvements in surgery, anesthesia, and intensive care have advanced faster than medical management and have probably increased the longevity advantage of surgical repair well beyond the twofold range of the 1960s.

After abdominal aortic aneurysm repair, the major cause of late death is coronary artery disease (38 percent), followed by cerebral atherosclerosis (11 percent), graft failure (9 percent), cancer (7 percent), and renal failure (4 percent).[24]

AORTOILIAC OCCLUSIVE DISEASE

Whereas surgery for aneurysmal disease is frequently performed on asymptomatic patients because of the disastrous results that can follow rupture of an aneurysm, surgery for aortoiliac occlusive disease is performed only if patients become symptomatic. The indications for surgery are as follows: disabling claudication (which occurs in approximately two-thirds of patients), ischemic rest pain and/or pregangrenous conditions (approximately one-fifth), and ischemic gangrene (approximately one-eighth).[9] The mean age for aortoiliac reconstruction is 54 years, whereas the mean age for patients undergoing surgery for aortic aneurysmal disease is at least 10 years older. Patients having surgery for aortoiliac occlusive disease tend to have fewer preoperative risk factors than those with aneurysmal disease.[83] The operative courses for the two groups are very similar, except that blood transfusion requirements are higher in aneurysm repair. The postoperative courses of the two groups are also very similar, the major morbidity arising from cardiovascular complications.[83]

Concomitant Vascular Disease

Aortoiliac occlusive disease may occur in conjunction with intraabdominal aneurysmal disease and distal occlusive disease (Fig. 14-9).[11] In chronic aortoiliac occlusion, the likelihood of collateral flow development is high. As a result, stenotic lesions restricted to this segment hardly ever threaten limb viability. Patients with critical limb ischemia who have stenotic aortoiliac disease usually have concomitant occlusive lesions of the femoral, popliteal, or tibial vessels.[9,10] The incidence of distal femoropopliteal occlusive disease is much higher in patients undergoing occlusive aortoiliac procedures (45 percent or higher) than in those undergoing repair of abdominal aortic aneurysm (approximately 11 percent).[9,10,32,84] The patency of aortobifemoral bypass depends on the status of distal occlusive disease in the femoral segment.[9,85] The need for subsequent femoropopliteal bypass can be reduced greatly if the profunda femoris artery is opened by profundoplasty performed concomitantly with aortobifemoral bypass.[84,86]

Bypass surgery for occlusive disease employs femoral anastomoses more frequently than does surgery for aneurysm repair, which usually employs distal anastomoses to the common iliac arteries. The need to extend the bypass to the groin incurs a higher incidence of false aneurysms and graft sepsis.[47] Progression of distal disease may result in a significant number of further reconstructive procedures and the higher incidence of sepsis

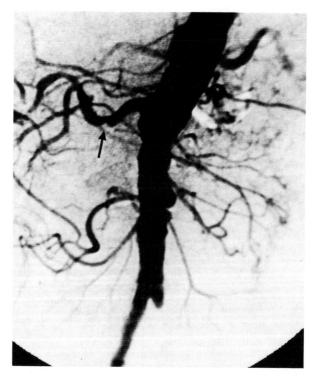

Fig. 14-9. Digital subtraction angiogram demonstrating aortoiliac occlusive disease with right renal artery stenosis (arrow) and absent left renal artery.

associated with repeat groin procedures.[47]

Hypoplastic Aortoiliac Syndrome

The hypoplastic aortoiliac syndrome is an unusual variant of stenotic arterial disease. This condition occurs predominantly in women (mean age, 43 years) who have a history of excessive smoking. Systemic hypertension and diabetes mellitus are usually not associated with this syndrome. Presentation normally consists of claudication, angiography demonstrating a narrow infrarenal aorta (average external diameter, 11.25 mm) often having an "hourglass" constriction just above its bifurcation. The aortic bifurcation is high; the small common iliac arteries (average external diameter, 5.25 mm) run a straight course without the usual lateral bowing around the pelvic brim. Collateral vessels are poorly formed, and symptoms tend to be more severe than expected from the extent of disease shown by arteriography.[87]

Surgery for Aortoiliac Occlusive Disease

In correcting occlusive disease of the aortoiliac segment, the surgeon tries to return the blood flow to the limbs at the groin to near normal while at the same time maintaining flow to the internal iliac and visceral branches.

Surgical exposure for aortoiliac procedures is similar to that for aortic aneurysm resection described above. Although transperitoneal approaches remain the most popular, advantages of retroperitoneal exposures are being increasingly documented.[47–51,88,89]

Because there is no need for exclusion of a segment of artery from the circulation, the proximal graft-to-aorta anastomosis is often an end-to-side configuration after excision of an ellipse of anterior aortic wall. Any suggestion of early aneurysmal dilatation, however, would necessitate exclusion of this segment. Similarly, advanced dengenerative changes in the infrarenal aorta may dictate the need for an end-to-end placement of the graft to avoid subsequent embolization of atheromatous debris. In either case, because of the expected progression of disease, the origin of any graft should be placed as close as possible to the renal arteries.[90] To minimize outflow resistance, the surgeon may perform bilateral lumbar sympathectomies in conjunction with aortoiliac surgery for occlusive disease.[90]

Endarterectomy

Aortoiliac endarterectomy is an alternative to bypass procedures in occlusive disease. Before suitable prosthetic grafts were widely available, endarterectomy was a popular method of repair, and long-segment aortoiliac procedures were performed. However, the incidence of early failure has been higher with endarterectomy of these vessels than with bypass grafting.[10] Early failure is probably attributable to inappropriate selection of patients who have occlusive atheroma extending into the external iliac arteries. Endarterectomy of these vessels is technically difficult, and an adequate endpoint is not readily achieved. Also, owing to the longer time required for this technique, the surgeon tends to limit endarterectomy to one iliac system.[10]

Because of the proven long-term patency of synthetic grafts, bypass grafting has largely replaced endarterectomy, although the latter is still used for stenosing atheroma restricted to the distal aorta and proximal common iliac arteries. Endarterectomy also provides an alternative for revascularization after removal of an infected aortic graft and in instances of potential contamination.[10,90]

Bypass Grafting

The development of synthetic materials suitable for arterial bypass grafting occurred in the early 1960s, with Dacron becoming the preferred fabric.[8-10] Because bypass grafting is quicker and incurs less blood loss than endarterectomy, it soon became the preferred surgical technique, especially for the aortoiliac system. The standard procedure for aortoiliac stenosis is arterial replacement with a Dacron aortobifemoral synthetic graft. Although the symmetrical nature of the disease process usually warrants a bilateral procedure (Fig. 14-10),[1] in unusual circumstances a unilateral aortofemoral bypass may be performed. Short- and long-term results

for surgery in this area are better with bypass grafting than with endarterectomy.[10] Synthetic arterial replacement is indicated for the following conditions: any suggestion of aneurysmal aortoiliac disease; aortic occlusion to the level of the renal arteries; the hypoplastic aortoiliac syndrome; and extensive stenotic disease with extension into or beyond the external iliac arteries.[10,87]

Special precautions are necessary in total occlusion (either chronic or acute) of the distal aorta. Thrombi develop and propagate proximally, frequently to the level of the renal arteries, even though the greatest occlusion occurs at the aortic bifurcation. In chronic occlusion, even if disabling claudication is not present, the risk of embolic disease to the kidneys is high, and surgery should be performed to reestablish distal aortic flow. In operative

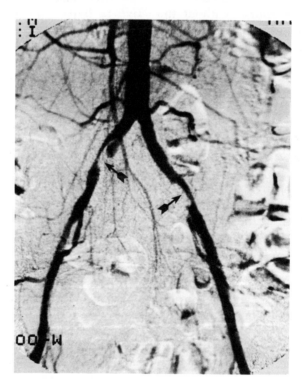

Fig. 14-10. Digital subtraction angiogram demonstrating bilateral localizing common iliac artery stenoses (arrows).

manipulation and clamping, great care must be taken not to dislodge material into the renal arteries. I find it advisable initially to clamp the aorta above the level of the renal vessels, open the infrarenal aorta, clear out the thrombus, and then move the aortic clamp to an infrarenal position before proceeding with bypass grafting from the infrarenal aorta.[90]

Percutaneous Transluminal Angioplasty

Another treatment modality available for stenotic disease but not aneurysmal disease is percutaneous transluminal angioplasty. Most reports find consistently good early and late results for short-segment iliac occlusive atheroma subjected to this procedure. For more peripheral arteries, early and late results are worse with transluminal angioplasty than with operative replacement or endarterectomy.[91–96] Combined iliac angioplasty with femoropopliteal bypass is possible with the intraoperative extrusion balloon catheter developed by Fogarty et al.[97]

Laser Angioplasty

The use of laser vaporization to clear occluded arterial segments has great potential. The combination of this technique with angioscopy and transluminal angioplasty is starting to be used clinically and may revolutionize the management of occlusive arterial disease.[98]

Extra-Anatomic Bypasses

Conventional reconstructive arterial surgery has developed with a principle of anatomic correctness. Generally, the surgeon takes a direct "anatomic" approach to diseased vessels by grafting and/or endarterectomizing vessel segments. Although an anatomic approach is usually the easiest and best method, some situations require a less conventional solution. Extra-anatomic grafts occur not, as the name implies, outside the body but

in unusual locations or at sites remote from the disease.[99] Conditions warranting extra-anatomic grafts include repeat surgery; surgery for graft infection; the presence of contraindications to transabdominal surgery (sepsis, adhesions, radiation, malignancy); and the need for less traumatic surgical options in frail, usually elderly, high-risk patients. In general, the price of using these alternative techniques is reduced long-term patency.

The most popular extra-anatomic bypass for aortoiliac reconstruction consists of axillofemoral bypass with synthetic material passed through a subcutaneous tunnel.[100,101] The major advantage is that perioperative morbidity and mortality are much less with this technique.[100,101] Surgery involves exposure of relatively superficial arteries in the axilla and groin and establishment of a long subcutaneous tract between the arteries. Either general anesthesia (without muscle relaxation) or local anesthesia is adequate. The need for extensive skin preparation and exposure limits access for the anesthetist and is thus a disadvantage. Axillofemoral bypass has other more important disadvantages. Long-term patency is significantly poorer for axillofemoral grafts than for aortofemoral grafts, although surgical revision may be performed with good results.[101] Graft thrombosis occurs in as many as 38 percent of patients within 21.5 months (mean value), the primary patency rate being only 54 percent at 3 years.[100,102]

The thoracic aorta is another option for graft origin. However, the use of a thoracic origin requires opening the thoracic cavity and thus increases morbidity. Although this choice seems inappropriate in an acute situation with a very ill patient, descending thoracic aorta-to-femoral artery bypass has been used successfully for conversion of axillofemoral grafts that recurrently fail.[103] Although the site of origin from the thoracic aorta varies and depends on numerous factors, the descending thoracic aorta is quite readily approached, and use of side-biting clamps eliminates the need for cardiopulmonary bypass.[103]

Femorofemoral bypass is another option for reconstruction of unilateral iliac occlusive disease; it can also be used in combination with axillounifemoral or aortounifemoral bypass.[101] Femorofemoral bypass is appropriate for the occasional patient who has asymmetrical rather than the usual symmetrical aortoiliac occlusive disease. Although some physicians believe that long-term patency may be compromised by the likely development of occlusive atheroma on the donor side, this opinion has not been confirmed in follow-up studies.[104,105] Most late graft failures appear to be caused by progression of distal occlusive disease.

The special problem of groin sepsis requiring reconstruction of arterial supply has prompted development of two other types of extra-anatomic grafts: the obturator foramen bypass to the profunda femoris artery or the distal superficial femoral artery, and extra-anatomic grafts to the popliteal artery.[106,107] Even though long bypasses with synthetic material are probably not ideal, they may well be the only practical alternative in acute sepsis.

SUMMARY

Surgical repair of abdominal aortic aneurysm and bypass procedures for symptomatic aortoiliac occlusive disease are well-established techniques. Operative mortality and morbidity are acceptably low, although high-risk patients require more extensive preoperative evaluation and intraoperative management. The major source of morbidity and mortality remains cardiovascular disease, a reflection of the generalized nature of atherosclerosis.

Although the most popular surgical approach for either abdominal aortic aneurysmal or occlusive disease remains a transperitoneal exposure, documented advantages exist for retroperitoneal procedures. Aortic replacement for aneurysmal disease necessarily requires implantation of exogenous material, synthetic Dacron conduits being the most popular. Occlusive disease may be managed by endarterectomy, synthetic bypass, or angioplasty. The first procedure is now reserved for isolated lesions of iliac origins or in unusual situations in which synthetic material is contraindicated, such as sepsis. In general, bypass procedures have proved to be long-lasting and very satisfactory for occlusive disease.

Long-term surgical resection (as opposed to nonsurgical management) of abdominal aortic aneurysms more than doubles life expectancy. Long-term patency and limb salvage rates are very good for bypass surgery for aortoiliac occlusive disease. Increasing severity of distal occlusive disease is associated with poorer patency rates. Sepsis, associated with groin incisions and repeat surgery, remains a major challenge for successful treatment. The current development of transluminal treatments for occlusive disease, including laser angioplasty and percutaneous transluminal angioplasty, has great potential. New grafts also promise improvements in the shorter term, with various agents that decrease porosity, the technique of antibiotic impregnation, and endothelial cell seeding all being developed.

REFERENCES

1. DeBakey ME: Changing concepts in vascular surgery. J Cardiovasc Surg 27:367–409, 1986

2. May AG, DeWeese JA, Frank I et al: Surgical treatment of abdominal aortic aneurysms. Surgery 63:711–721, 1968

3. Hollier LH, Reigel MM, Kazmier FJ et al: Conventional repair of abdominal aortic aneurysm in the high-risk patient: a plea for abandonment of nonresective treatment. J Vasc Surg 3:712–717, 1986

4. dos Santos JC: Sur la désobstruction des thromboses artérielles anciennes. Mem Acad Chir 73:409–411, 1947

5. Wylie EJ: Thromboendarterectomy for arteriosclerotic thrombosis of major arteries. Surgery 32:275–292, 1952

6. Oudot J, Beaconsfield P: Thrombosis of the aortic bifurcation treated by resection and homograft replacement. Report of five cases. Arch Surg 66:365–374, 1953

7. Dubost C, Allary M, Oeconomos N: Resection of an aneurysm of the abdominal aorta. Reestablishment of continuity by a preserved human arterial graft, with result after five months. Arch Surg 64:405–408, 1952

8. Blakemore AH, Voorhees AB, Jr: Aneurysm of the aorta: a review of 365 cases. Angiology 5:209–231, 1954

9. Szilagyi DE, Elliott JP, Jr., Smith RF et al: A thirty-year survey of the reconstructive surgical treatment of aortoiliac occlusive disease. J Vasc Surg 3:421–436, 1986

10. Brewster DC, Darling RC: Optimal methods of aortoiliac reconstruction. Surgery 84:739–748, 1978

11. Thompson JE, Hollier LH, Patman RD, Persson AV: Surgical management of abdominal aortic aneurysms: factors influencing mortality and morbidity—a 20-year experience. Ann Surg 181:654–661, 1975

12. Zatina MA, Zarins CK, Gewertz BL, Glagov S: Role of medial lamellar architecture in the pathogenesis of aortic aneurysms. J Vasc Surg 1:442–448, 1984

13. Zarins CK, Runyon-Hass A, Zatina MA et al: Increased collagenase activity in early aneurysmal dilatation. J Vasc Surg 3:238–248, 1986

14. Swanson RJ, Littooy FN, Hunt TK, Stoney RJ: Laparotomy as a precipitating factor in the rupture of intra-abdominal aneurysms. Arch Surg 115:299–304, 1980

15. Robbs JV, Human RR, Rajaruthnam P: Operative treatment of nonspecific aortoarteritis (Takayasu's arteritis). J Vasc Surg 3:605–616, 1986

16. Littooy FN, Baker WH: Acute aortic occlusion—a multifaceted catastrophe. J Vasc Surg 4:211–216, 1986

17. Swensson EE, Willman VL, Peterson GJ: Acute aortic occlusion from aspergillosis in a healthy patient with survival. J Vasc Surg 4:187–191, 1986

18. Vo NM, Russell JC, Becker DR: Mycotic emboli of the peripheral vessels: analysis of forty-four cases. Surgery 90:541–545, 1981

19. Perry MO: Arterial injuries caused by blunt trauma. p. 329–338. In Veith FJ (ed): Critical Problems in Vascular Surgery. Appleton-Century-Crofts, East Norwalk, CT, 1981

20. Estes JE, Jr: Abdominal aortic aneurysm: a study of one hundred and two cases. Circulation 2:258–264, 1950

21. Foster JH, Bolasny BL, Gobbel WG, Jr., Scott HW, Jr: Comparative study of elective resection and expectant treatment of abdominal aortic aneurysm. Surg Gynecol Obstet 129:1–9, 1969

22. Darling RC, Messina CR, Brewster DC, Ottinger LW: Autopsy study of unoperated abdominal aortic aneurysms: the case for early resection. Circulation, 56: (suppl. 2,) II-161 to II-164, 1977

23. Szilagyi DE, Elliott JP, Smith RF: Clinical fate of the patient with asymptomatic abdominal aortic aneurysm and unfit for surgical treatment. Arch Surg 104:600–606, 1972

24. Szilagyi DE, Smith RF, DeRusso FJ et al: Contribution of abdominal aortic aneurysmectomy to prolongation of life. Ann Surg 164:678–699, 1966

25. Thurmond AS, Semler HJ: Abdominal aortic aneurysm: incidence in a population at risk. J Cardiovasc Surg 27:457–460, 1986

26. Reigel MM, Hollier LH, Kazmier FJ et al: Late survival in abdominal aortic aneurysm patients: the role of selective

myocardial revascularization on the basis of clinical symptoms. J Vasc Surg 5:222–227, 1987

27. Darling RC: Ruptured arteriosclerotic abdominal aortic aneurysms. A pathologic and clinical study. Am J Surg 119:397–401, 1970

28. Khaw H, Sottiurai VS, Craighead CC, Batson RC: Ruptured abdominal aortic aneurysm presenting as symptomatic inguinal mass: report of six cases. J Vasc Surg 4:384–389, 1986

29. Lambert ME, Baguley P, Charlesworth D: Ruptured abdominal aortic aneurysms. J Cardiovasc Surg 27:256–261, 1986

30. Hertzer NR, Young JR, Kramer JR, et al: Routine coronary angiography prior to elective aortic reconstruction. Results of selective myocardial revascularization in patients with peripheral vascular disease. Arch Surg 114:1336–1344, 1979

31. Brown OW, Hollier LH, Pairolero PC et al: Abdominal aortic aneurysm and coronary artery disease. A reassessment. Arch Surg 116:1484–1488, 1981

32. De Bakey ME, Crawford ES, Cooley DA et al: Aneurysm of abdominal aorta. Analysis of results of graft replacement therapy one to eleven years after operation. Ann Surg 160:622–639, 1964

33. Bjerkelund CE, Smith-Erichsen N, Solheim K: Abdominal aortic reconstruction. Prognostic importance of coexistent diseases. Acta Chir Scand 152:111–115, 1986

34. Pasternack PF, Imparato AM, Bear G et al: The value of radionuclide angiography as a predictor of perioperative myocardial infarction in patients undergoing abdominal aortic aneurysm resection. J Vasc Surg 1:320–325, 1984

35. Ostri P, Mouritsen L, Jørgensen B, Frimoldt-Møller C: Renal function following aneurysmectomy of the abdominal aorta. J Cardiovasc Surg 27:714–718, 1986

36. Cohen JR, Mannick JA, Couch NP, Whittemore AD: Abdominal aortic aneurysm repair in patients with preoperative renal failure. J Vasc Surg 3:867–870, 1986

37. Gracey DR, Divertie MB, Didier EP: Preoperative pulmonary preparation of patients with chronic obstructive pulmonary disease. A prospective study. Chest 76:123–129, 1979

38. Purdy RT, Beyer FC, III, McCann WD, et al: Reduced aortic cross-clamp time in high-risk patients with abdominal aortic aneurysm. J Vasc Surg 3:820–823, 1986

39. Harris KA, Ameli FM, Lally M et al: Abdominal aortic aneurysm resection in patients more than 80 years old. Surg Gynecol Obstet 162:536–538, 1986

40. Hansen HJB: Elective surgery for abdominal aortic aneurysm. p 44–58. In Bergan JJ (ed): Arterial Surgery. Churchill Livingstone, Edinburgh, 1984

41. Bernstein EF, Harris ED, Leopold GR: Echography and computed tomography in the diagnosis and evaluation of abdominal aortic aneurysms p. 31–44. In Veith FJ (ed): Critical Problems in Vascular Surgery. Appleton-Century-Crofts, East Norwalk, CT, 1981

42. Papanicolaou N, Wittenberg J, Ferrucci JT, Jr et al: Preoperative evaluation of abdominal aortic aneurysms by computed tomography. AJR 146:711–715, 1986

43. Thomas ML, Bowles JN: The value of intravenous digital subtraction angiography (IV-DSA) in the pre-operative assessment of abdominal aortic aneurysms. J Cardiovasc Surg 27:461–465, 1986

44. Buonocore E, Meaney TF, Borkowski GP et al: Digital subtraction angiography of the abdominal aorta and renal arteries. Comparison with conventional aortography. Radiology 139:281–286, 1981

45. Bunt TJ, Cropper L: Routine angiography for abdominal aortic aneurysm: the case for informed operative selection. J Cardiovasc Surg 27:725–727, 1986

46. Flak B, Li DKB, Ho BYB et al: Magnetic resonance imaging of aneurysms of the abdominal aorta. AJR 144:991–996, 1985

47. Williams GM, Ricotta J, Zinner M, Burdick J: The extended retroperitoneal approach for treatment of extensive atherosclerosis of the aorta and renal vessels. Surgery 88:846–855, 1980

48. Shepard AD, Scott GR, Mackey WC et al: Retroperitoneal approach to high-risk abdominal aortic aneurysms. Arch Surg 121:444–449, 1986

49. Sicard GA, Freeman MB, VanderWoude JC, Anderson CB: Comparison between the transabdominal and retroperitoneal approach for reconstruction of the infrarenal abdominal aorta. J Vasc Surg 5:19–27, 1987

50. Rob C: Extraperitoneal approach to the abdominal aorta. Surgery 53:87–89, 1963

51. Peck JJ, McReynolds DG, Baker DH, Eastman AB: Extraperitoneal approach for aortoiliac reconstruction of the abdominal aorta. Am J Surg 151:620–623, 1986

52. Stoney RJ, Wylie EJ: Surgical management of arterial lesions of the thoracoabdominal aorta. Am J Surg 126:157–164, 1973

53 Burnett JR, Gray-Weale AC, Byrne K et al: The place of systemic heparin in elective aortic aneurysm repair (abstract). J Cardiovasc Surg, suppl., 28:7, 1987

54. Webb LX, Myers RT, Cordell AR et al: Inhibition of bacterial adhesion by antibacterial surface pretreatment of vascular prostheses. J Vasc Surg 4:16–21, 1986

55. Starr DS, Lawrie GM, Morris GC, Jr: Prevention of distal embolism during arterial reconstruction. Am J Surg 138:764–769, 1979

56. Herring M, Baughman S, Glover J et al: Endothelial seeding of Dacron and polytetrafluoroethylene grafts: the cellular events of healing. Surgery 96:745–755, 1984

57. Birinyi LK, Douville EC, Lewis SA et al: Increased resistance to bacteremic graft infection after endothelial cell seeding. J Vasc Surg 5:193–197, 1987

58. Falk JL, Rackow EC, Blumenberg R et al: Hemodynamic and metabolic effects of abdominal aortic crossclamping. Am J Surg 142:174–177, 1981

59. Dunn E, Prager RL, Fry W, Kirsh MM: The effect of abdominal aortic crossclamping on myocardial function. J Surg Res 22:463–468, 1977

60. Gooding JM, Archie JP, Jr., McDowell H: Hemodynamic response to infrarenal aortic cross-clamping in patients with and without coronary artery disease. Crit Care Med 8:382–385, 1980

61. Qvarfordt PG, Stoney RJ, Reilly LM et al: Management of pararenal aneurysms of the abdominal aorta. J Vasc Surg 3:84–93, 1986

62. Tarazi RY, Hertzer NR, Beven EG et al: Simultaneous aortic reconstruction and renal revascularization: risk factors and late results in eighty-nine patients. J Vasc Surg 5:707–714, 1987

63. Crawford ES, Crawford JL, Safi HJ et al: Thoracoabdominal aortic aneurysms: preoperative and intraoperative factors determining immediate and long-term results of operations in 605 patients. J Vasc Surg 3:389–404, 1986

64. Miller DC, Myers BD: Pathophysiology and prevention of acute renal failure associated with thoracoabdominal or abdominal aortic surgery. J Vasc Surg 5:518–523, 1987

65. Crawford JL, Stowe CL, Safi HJ et al: Inflammatory aneurysms of the aorta. J Vasc Surg 2:113–124, 1985

66. Goldstone J, Malone JM, Moore WS: Inflammatory aneurysms of the abdominal aorta. Surgery 83:425–430, 1978

67. Hall RG, Coupland GAE, Appleberg M: Inflammatory aneurysms of the abdominal aorta. Aust NZ J Surg 55:189–193, 1985

68. Pennell RC, Hollier LH, Lie JT et al: Inflammatory abdominal aortic aneurysms: a thirty-year review. J Vasc Surg 2:859–869, 1985

69. Hedges AR, Bentley PG: Resection of inflammatory aneurysm after steroid therapy. Br J Surg 73:374, 1986

70. Krieger JN, Hilgartner MW, Redo SF: Surgery in patients with congenital disorders of blood coagulation. Ann Surg 185:290–294, 1977

71. Thompson RW, Adams DH, Cohen JR et al: Disseminated intravascular coagulation caused by abdominal aortic aneurysm. J Vasc Surg 4:184–186, 1986

72. Collins JA: Problems associated with the massive transfusion of stored blood. Surgery 75:274–295, 1974

73. Worthington MM: Progress in transfusion therapy and treatment of bleeding problems in aortic aneurysm surgery. World J Surg 4:521–526, 1980

74. Brewster DC, Ambrosino JJ, Darling RC et al: Intraoperative autotransfusion in major vascular surgery. Am J Surg 137:507–513, 1979

75. Hallett JW, Jr., Popovsky M, Ilstrup D: Minimizing blood transfusions during abdominal aortic surgery: recent advances in rapid autotransfusion. J Vasc Surg 5:601–606, 1987

76. Alpert RA, Roizen MF, Hamilton WK et al: Intraoperative urinary output does not predict postoperative renal function in patients undergoing abdominal aortic revascularization. Surgery 95:707–711, 1984

77. Rogers DM, Thompson JE, Garrett WV et al: Mesenteric vascular problems. A 26-year experience. Ann Surg 195:554–565, 1982

78. Connolly JE, Kwaan JHM: Prophylactic revascularization of the gut. Ann Surg 190:514–522, 1979

79. Connelly TL, Perdue GD, Smith RB III et al: Elective mesenteric revascularization. Am Surg 47:19–25, 1981

80. Picone AL, Green RM, Ricotta JR et al: Spinal cord ischemia following operations on the abdominal aorta. J Vasc Surg 3:94–103, 1986

81. Connolly JE: Prevention of paraplegia secondary to operations on the aorta. J Cardiovasc Surg 27:410–417, 1986

82. O'Hara PJ, Hertzer NR, Beven EG, Krajewski LP: Surgical management of infected abdominal aortic grafts: review of a 25-year experience. J Vasc Surg 3:725–731, 1986

83. Sumio BE, Traquina DN, Gusberg RJ: Results of aortic grafting in occlusive vs aneurysmal disease. Arch Surg 120:817–819, 1985

84. Simma W, Bassiouny H, Haril P, Brücker P: Evaluation of profundoplasty in reconstructions of combined aorto-iliac and femoro-popliteal occlusive disease. J Cardiovasc Surg 27:141–145, 1986

85. Sladen JG, Gilmour JL, Wong RW: Cumulative patency and actual palliation in patients with claudication after aortofemoral bypass. Prospective long-term follow-up of 100 patients. Am J Surg 152:190–195, 1986

86. Poulias GE, Polemis L, Skoutas B et al: Bilateral aorto-femoral bypass in the presence of aorto-iliac occlusive disease and factors determining results. Experience and long term follow up with 500 consecutive cases. J Cardiovasc Surg 26:527–538, 1985

87. DeLaurentis DA, Friedmann P, Wolferth CC, Jr et al: Atherosclerosis and the hypoplastic aortoiliac system. Surgery 83:27–37, 1978

88. Johnson JN, McLoughlin GA, Wake PN, Helsby CR: Comparison of extraperitoneal and transperitoneal methods of aorto-iliac reconstruction. Twenty years experience. J Cardiovasc Surg 27:561–564, 1986

89. Helsby R, Moossa AR: Aorto-iliac reconstruction with special reference to the extraperitoneal approach. Br J Surg 62:596–600, 1975

90. Wylie EJ, Stoney RJ, Ehrenfeld WK: Aortoiliac atherosclerosis p. 107–157. In Manual of Vascular Surgery. Vol. 1. Springer-Verlag, New York, 1980

91. Knight RW, Kenney GJ, Lewis EE, Johnston GG: Percutaneous transluminal angioplasty. Results and surgical implications. Am J Surg 147:578–582, 1984

92. Katzen BT, Chang J, Knox WG: Percutaneous transluminal angioplasty with the Grüntzig balloon catheter. Arch Surg 114:1389–1399, 1979

93. Burnett JR, Walsh JA, Howard PR et al: Transluminal balloon angioplasty in diabetic peripheral vascular disease. Aust NZ J Surg 57:307–309, 1987

94. Cole SEA, Baird RN, Horrocks M et al: The role of balloon angioplasty in the management of lower limb ischaemia. Eur J Vasc Surg 1:61–65, 1987

95. Johansen K, Ricketts H, Wales LR, Morishima M: Combined arterial reconstruction and transluminal dilatation: therapeutic teamwork to combat vascular insufficiency. World J Surg 5:653–658, 1981

96. Blankensteijn JD, van Vroonhoven TJ,

Lampmann L: Role of percutaneous transluminal angioplasty in aorto-iliac reconstruction. J Cardiovasc Surg 27:466–468, 1986

97. Fogarty TJ, Chin A, Shoor PM et al: Adjunctive intraoperative arterial dilation. Simplified instrumentation technique. Arch Surg 116:1391–1398, 1981

98. Grundfest WS, Litvack F, Hickey A, et al: The current status of angioscopy and laser angioplasty. J Vasc Surg 5:667–673, 1987

99. Brief DK, Brener BJ: Extraanatomic bypasses. p. 414–424. In Wilson SE, Veith FJ, Hobson RW, II, Williams RA (ed): Vascular Surgery. Principles and Practices. McGraw-Hill, New York, 1987

100. Donaldson MC, Louras JC, Bucknam CA: Axillofemoral bypass: a tool with a limited role. J Vasc Surg 3:757–763, 1986

101. Moore WS: Thrombosis of aortofemoral, axillofemoral, or femorofemoral grafts. p. 445–461. In Veith FJ (ed): Critical Problems in Vascular Surgery. Appleton-Century-Crofts, East Norwalk, CT, 1981

102. Kalman PG, Hosang M, Cina C et al: Current indications for axillounifemoral and axillobifemoral bypass grafts. J Vasc Surg 5:828–832, 1987

103. McCarthy WJ, Rubin JR, Flinn WR, et al: Descending thoracic aorta-to-femoral artery bypass. Arch Surg 121:681–688, 1986

104. Brief DK, Brener BJ, Alpert J, Parsonnet V: Crossover femorofemoral grafts followed up five years or more. An analysis. Arch Surg 110:1294–1299, 1975

105. Mannick JA, Maini BS: Femorofemoral grafting: indications and late results. Am J Surg 136:190–192, 1978

106. Guida PM, Moore SW: Obturator bypass technique. Surg Gynecol Obstet 128:1307–1316, 1969

107. Veith FJ, Moss CM, Daly V et al: New approaches to limb salvage by extended extra-anatomic bypasses and prosthetic reconstructions to foot arteries. Surgery 84:764–774, 1978

15

Anesthetic Management for Abdominal Aortic Reconstruction

George H. Lampe
Dennis T. Mangano

Although abdominal aortic surgery can improve and prolong life, patients requiring vascular surgery have significant underlying diseases and undergo extreme intraoperative challenges. Minimizing perioperative morbidity and mortality is the goal of all personnel involved in the care of these patients.

Anesthetic management of vascular patients begins with preoperative evaluation of the specific patient and the suspected underlying disease states. This preoperative assessment is the basis for an anesthetic plan that includes the choice of intraoperative monitors and anesthetic agents. Because the surgical procedure itself produces predictable stresses, the anesthetist must be prepared to treat the effects of such stresses (e.g., the hemodynamic response to occlusion and unclamping of the aorta) and to manage frequently encountered intraoperative events such as oliguria and myocardial ischemia.

ASSESSING THE VASCULAR PATIENT

Atherosclerotic vascular changes progress throughout life to produce life-threatening occlusive or aneurysmal disease. For many patients, such disease begins in the fifth decade. The average age of patients undergoing aortic reconstructive surgery peaks in the sixth decade.[1–3] In the future, more elderly patients may require vascular surgery as the general population ages. The mortality associated with vascular surgery in patients over 80 years of age approaches 12 percent, a figure that is more than twice the value for younger patients requiring similar surgery.[4,5]

Because atherosclerosis is a generalized process affecting the entire arterial tree, coronary artery disease is common in patients requiring vascular surgery.[3,6–9] In one study, coronary angiography revealed that more than half of the 1,000 patients undergoing elective peripheral vascular surgery had significant coronary artery disease (coronary stenosis exceeding 50 percent) and that approximately one-third had severe disease (coronary stenosis exceeding 70 percent).[3] Furthermore, the incidence of occult ischemic heart disease was high. Angiography has also revealed that 15 percent of patients who have no history or electrocardiographic (ECG) evidence of ischemic heart disease have severe coronary artery disease and that 22 percent of these seemingly "normal" patients have impaired left ventricular function.[3,10] These figures are of concern because perioperative myocardial infarction and cardiac failure remain the most frequent cause of postoperative death in elective vascular surgery.[1,2,5,11]

Preoperative assessment of the degree and potential significance of coronary artery disease in the individual patient is difficult. Routine cardiac testing is often insensitive and costly. Because of the expense and morbidity associated with invasive measures such as coronary angiography, most physicians use other methods to define the cardiac high-risk subset of the vascular surgery population. Exercise testing[11] and radionuclide angiography[12] are modestly successful in identifying patients with severe ischemic heart disease. However, the use of these tests in patients with vascular disease is limited, because both methods require vigorous exercise to achieve maximum sensitivity and specificity,[13] and claudication restricts the vascular patient's ability to exercise.

Dipyridamole-thallium imaging has been used successfully to identify vascular patients at high risk of postoperative cardiac complications.[14–17] In high doses, dipyridamole (Persantine) is a potent coronary artery vasodilator. Administered intravenously, it dilates functional coronary arteries, an action that redistributes blood flow away from the myocardium subserved by a maximally dilated coronary artery distal to a stenosis, thus inducing coronary artery "steal."[14,18,19] Therefore, when thallium 201 is administered intravenously, the delay in its uptake in poorly perfused myocardium helps identify areas at risk of ischemia or infarction.

Boucher et al.[14] were the first to use this imaging technique in vascular patients. Eight of 16 patients identified as "high risk" in a study with dipyridamole-thallium imaging had postoperative ischemic events. None of 32 "low-risk" patients with either normal scans or persistent defects (signifying healed infarct) experienced postoperative ischemia. Other investigators have confirmed the ability of dipyridamole-thallium imaging to reliably identify patients at high risk of perioperative myocardial ischemia.[15–17]

Because this technique induces coronary artery vasodilation pharmacologically, exercise testing is unnecessary, making dipyridamole-thallium imaging particularly useful for patients with vascular insufficiency. Although angina may occur during testing (the incidence being approximately 30 percent), pain can be relieved immediately by intravenous administration of aminophylline.[14,16] No instances of myocardial infarction related to testing have been reported. Vascular patients identified as high risk by dipyridamole-thallium imaging may then be referred for further cardiac evaluation and possible coronary artery angioplasty or bypass grafting prior to vascular surgery.

Vascular patients frequently have not only coronary artery disease but also pulmonary and renal insufficiency. Approximately 70 percent of vascular patients have a history of smoking, and 18 to 50 percent have clinically apparent chronic obstructive pulmonary disease.[1,2,20] Although the subset of patients at risk of postoperative pulmonary failure has not been adequately defined, one assumes that patients with chronic pulmonary disease may require prolonged postoperative mechanical ventilation. Chronic renal insufficiency is present in 5 to 17 percent of vascular patients.[1,2,20-22] Additionally, intraoperative events such as hemorrhage, massive volume shifts, and ischemia secondary to aortic occlusion may further compromise renal function. Therefore, invasive intravascular monitoring is often used to estimate intraoperative and postoperative volume requirements. A systematic approach to the evaluation and treatment of oliguria is described below.

CHOICE OF INTRAOPERATIVE MONITORING

Technical advances of the past decade have provided anesthetists with new tools for more accurately and continuously measuring basic physiologic functions. However, clear definition of the particular patient populations who benefit from application of these monitors does not yet exist. Rao et al.[23] suggest that increasing the period of intensive monitoring to 3 days following an operation and monitoring each patient more invasively with arterial lines and pulmonary artery catheters may reduce the incidence of perioperative myocardial infarction in patients who have had a previous infarction. In fact, no studies have adequately evaluated the ability of any monitoring device to reduce perioperative morbidity and mortality.

Typically, patients who have significant underlying cardiac or pulmonary disease are monitored more intensively and more invasively than those who do not. The other criteria for aggressive monitoring are the degree of stress expected from the surgery and the length of the procedure. Because severity of underlying disease and invasiveness of the planned surgery are arbitrary criteria for selecting intensive monitoring, vascular surgery patients are frequently monitored with the following instruments.

The heart is monitored electrocardiographically, ideally with a five-lead system permitting simultaneous display of leads II and V_5. A three-lead ECG system can be adapted to maximize the sensitivity for detecting ischemia by placing the left arm electrode on the anterior chest in the position of V_5 and selecting lead I on the ECG monitor to reflect a modified CS_5 lead.[24,25] The most sensitive monitor of myocardial ischemia is two-dimensional transesophageal echocardiography, which has greater sensitivity than electrocardiography (see Ch. 28). We routinely use this technique to monitor vascular patients.[20,26-30] Blood pressure is measured by an indwelling radial artery line, which allows continuous monitoring and easy access for sampling arterial blood. Arterial oxygen saturation is monitored continuously by pulse oximeter, as this group of patients has a high incidence of pulmonary disease. The pulse oximeter may be particularly useful in instances requiring selective lung ventilation via double-lumen endotracheal tubes during resection of thoracoabdominal aneurysms. Heart tones, breath sounds, and body temperature are monitored by esophageal stethoscope.

Because of the large abdominal incision required, vascular patients are predisposed to progressive heat loss throughout surgery. Additionally, these operations may be lengthy, lasting from two to several hours; they usually require administration of large volumes of fluid. To prevent heat loss and subsequent shivering, coagulopathy, and dysrhythmias, we place a warming blanket heated to 39°C on the operating room table prior to surgery. All fluids administered intraoperatively also are warmed to 39°C. We routinely use a humidification trapping system at the end of the endotracheal tube. If heat loss becomes severe, active warming of inspired gases by a heated humidifier is recommended.

Because of the length of surgery and the likelihood of significant fluid administration, we place a Foley catheter to drain the bladder. Although urinary output has been used as a measure of intravascular volume, oliguria frequently occurs during vascular surgery, even when there is no evidence of hypovolemia. Also, high urinary output may occur in response to hyperglycemia or mannitol-induced diuresis, even in hypovolemic patients. The limitations of using urine production to estimate volume status and renal function are discussed more extensively in a later section.

Intravascular volume may be monitored more specifically by means of a central venous pressure (CVP) or pulmonary artery (PA) catheter. We select one of these two monitors based on the level at which temporary aortic occlusion will occur, plus the patient's underlying cardiac disease. Patients requiring suprarenal aortic occlusion are susceptible to postoperative oliguria.[31] To guarantee the best possible index of intravascular volume, these patients are monitored with a PA line.[32–34] A CVP catheter is used in patients who require infrarenal cross-clamping and with no evidence of cardiac disease. A PA catheter is used in those patients who have impaired left ventricular function or severe pulmonary disease, as the CVP line often will be an inadequate monitor of left-sided cardiac filling pressures in these patients.[34]

CHOICE OF ANESTHETIC AGENTS

We know very little about how our choice of anesthetic agents affects patient outcome.[35,36] In the absence of controlled randomized clinical trials, anesthetists usually rely on their training and experience to select anesthetic agents. Two recent studies have compared regional with general anesthesia and narcotic with inhaled anesthesia in an attempt to determine whether choice of anesthetic technique affects patient outcome.

Yeager et al.[37] studied 22 patients requiring major vascular surgery. This group was a subset of 53 high-risk surgical patients randomly assigned to receive either epidural anesthesia and postoperative analgesia, or general anesthesia with postoperative parenteral narcotics. Patients given epidural anesthesia and analgesia had a significantly lower incidence of cardiovascular failure and major infections. Also, hospital costs were lower.

Limitations in this study may prevent widespread acceptance of epidural anesthesia and analgesia as the preferred anesthetic technique for abdominal aortic surgery. First, the size of the study population was small, and some believe that the perceived benefit of epidural anesthesia and analgesia did not, in fact, exist (this would represent an alpha error).[38] Second, the incidence of morbidity and mortality in patients given general anesthesia was higher at their institution than at other institutions using a similar anesthetic regimen. For example, 40 percent of patients given general anesthesia at their institution had a "major infection," whereas only 3 to 10 percent of patients in other series had major infections.[2,20]

More specific concerns also apply to the use of continuous epidural anesthesia for vascular patients given anticoagulants intraoperatively. The reported incidence of paraplegia related to systemic heparinization after epidural or lumbar puncture ranges from 0 to 1.46 percent.[39–42] In a study of 4,015 vascular patients managed with continuous epidural or spinal anesthesia, no instances of peridural hematoma leading to spinal cord compression or permanent neurologic compromise occurred.[39] However, certain precautions had been taken. Whenever blood was aspirated through the needle during placement of the epidural catheter, the surgical procedures were cancelled and performed with general anesthesia the next day; this happened four times. Additionally, heparin was titrated in small boluses, and anticoagulation was monitored frequently by activated clotting time. Finally, patients with a history of leukemia, hemophilia, blood dyscrasias, thrombocytopenia, or preoperative anticoagulation therapy had been excluded from this study. Another study of 1,000 vascular patients, all given oral anticoagulants preoperatively and heparin intraoperatively, found no permanent neurologic sequelae related to epidural anesthesia.[40] Patients were excluded from this study if they had neurologic disease, infection at the puncture site, blood dyscrasias, thrombocytopenia, prior heparinization, aspirin therapy, or a thrombotest below 10 percent. A third study reported that intrathecal administration of morphine in 40 patients given heparin for cardiac surgery caused no neurologic complications.[41] Patients with prolonged prothrombin times on the morning of surgery were excluded from their study.

Despite the absence of paraparesis in these studies of patients undergoing elective surgery, some risk of peridural hematoma exists in this clinical setting.[43,44] For these studies, the maximum risk of epidural hematoma calculated with 95 percent confidence limits would be as high as 0.075, 0.30, and 7.5 percent, respectively.

Of greatest concern is the reported 1.46 percent incidence (5 of 342) of paraparesis related to systemic heparinization after diagnostic lumbar puncture in patients with ischemic stroke.[42] Factors increasing the risk of paraparesis included traumatic lumbar puncture, initiation of anticoagulation within 1 hour of lumbar puncture, and aspirin therapy at the time of lumbar puncture.

If the clinician chooses to use epidural anesthesia, important differences in intraoperative systemic hemodynamics and volume requirements should be anticipated. One study comparing continuous epidural with general anesthesia for abdominal aortic surgery illustrates these differences.[45] Epidural anesthesia was associated with a lower mean arterial pressure (78 versus 96 mmHg), a lower systemic vascular resistance (1,396 versus 1,927 dynes/sec/cm^5), and a higher volume requirement (2,500 versus 1,531 ml) when fluids were infused to keep pulmonary capillary wedge pressure (PCWP) at preoperative levels prior to aortic cross-clamping. When the cross-clamp was removed, patients with epidural anesthesia had a dramatic decrease in mean arterial pressure (to 50 versus 78 mmHg), and 50 percent (2 of 4) had ischemic ECG changes. These catastrophic decreases in blood pressure associated with epidural anesthesia and aortic unclamping did not occur if PCWP was kept 3 to 4 mmHg above preanesthetic values by volume infusion.

Preventing adverse outcomes after epidural anesthesia depends on effective communication between the anesthetist and the providers of postoperative care. The physiologic changes in regional neural blockade must be appreciated by the postoperative team to prevent sudden mobilization of fluid from the vasodilated peripheral circulation into the central circulation as the anesthetic block recedes. Hypervolemia may cause hypertension and congestive heart failure. These conditions may be prevented or treated by reducing intravenous fluid infusions during the terminal phase of regional neural blockade and by treating clinical signs of volume overload with vasodilators.

Only one study has compared the effect of two different general anesthetic techniques on patient outcome.[20] One hundred patients were randomly assigned to receive either sufentanil or isoflurane as their anesthetic for aortic surgery. Of these patients, 3 percent died and 1 percent had myocardial infarction. This was a low rate of complication, considering the high risk factors for the group: 72 percent had chronic lung disease; 48 percent had prior myocardial infarction; and 53 percent had aortic cross-clamping at the suprarenal level. Patients given sufentanil had significantly lower incidences of postoperative renal insufficiency and congestive heart failure, despite identical intraoperative hemodynamic states, fluid administration, and episodes of myocardial ischemia.

INTRAOPERATIVE MANAGEMENT

Occluding the aorta excludes significant portions of the vascular tree from the circulation, an action that increases after-load and forces compensatory dilation of the left ventricle and the vascular bed proximal to the cross-clamp. Aortic occlusion may precipitate hypertension and myocardial ischemia. Three major factors can be used to predict blood pressure responses to application of an aortic cross-clamp: (1) the level of the cross-clamp; (2) the severity of underlying cardiac disease; and (3) the presence of aneurysmal versus occlusive disease. By far, the most significant factor is the level of aortic cross-clamping (Table 15-1). Infrarenal cross-clamping limits only flow to the lower extremities and consequently produces minimal changes in blood pressure, systemic vascular resistance, and stroke volume index.[26,45–50] In contrast, suprarenal aortic occlusion requires an additional redistribution of approximately 20 percent of the cardiac output (renal blood flow) to proximal vascular beds and may precipitate hypertension and myocardial ischemia.[26] Supraceliac cross-clamping excludes the liver, gut, kidneys, and lower extremities from the circulation and therefore produces the highest incidence of significant hemodynamic changes and myocardial ischemia.[26]

Table 15-1. Percent Change in Cardiovascular Variables on Initiation of Aortic Occlusion

| | Percent Change after Aortic Occlusion at: | | |
Variable	Supraceliac Level	Infraceliac-Suprarenal Level	Infrarenal Level
Mean arterial blood pressure	54	5[b]	2[b]
Pulmonary capillary wedge pressure	38	10[b]	0[b]
LV[a] end-diastolic area	28	2[b]	9[b]
LV end-systolic area	69	10[b]	11[b]
Ejection fraction	−38	−10[b]	−3[b]
Patients having wall motion abnormalities	92	33	0
New myocardial infarctions	8	0	0

[a] LV = left ventricular.
[b] Significantly ($P < 0.05$) different from group undergoing supraceliac aortic occlusion.
(From Roizen et al.,[26] with permission.)

Underlying cardiac disease can alter the effect of the aortic cross-clamp by impairing the heart's normal adaptive response to aortic occlusion. For example, because of limited left ventricular compliance, severe coronary disease combined with left ventricular dysfunction may result in dangerously elevated systemic and pulmonary arterial pressures during infrarenal aortic cross-clamping.[48,50] These hemodynamic alterations may be minimized by skillful anesthetic management (see below).[26]

The underlying aortic disease process also may influence the hemodynamic response to aortic cross-clamping. Occlusive disease can result in minimal distal aortic flow and extensive collateral circulation to the lower extremities, minimizing systemic hemodynamic changes when the aorta is occluded.[51] Aneurysmal disease, however, is characterized by a large volume of flow directed through the aorta, which may exaggerate proximal hemodynamic responses to aortic occlusion.[51-53]

Therefore, information available from the patient's chart the day before surgery, including the location of the aortic lesion, the patient's cardiac status, and the presence of occlusive or aneurysmal disease, allows for reasonably accurate estimations of the patient's hemodynamic response to aortic occlusion.

TREATING THE HEMODYNAMIC RESPONSE TO TEMPORARY OCCLUSION OF THE AORTA

If application of the aortic cross-clamp causes hypertension, myocardial ischemia, or increases in PCWP, three general techniques may be used to reduce the strain on the heart: (1) administration of nitroglycerin, (2) administration of sodium nitroprusside, or (3) increasing the concentration of the inhaled anesthetic.

In human subjects and in animal models of myocardial ischemia, administration of nitroglycerin usually minimizes the effects and improves the outcome of myocardial ischemia.[54-59] In contrast, nitroprusside worsens ischemic conditions.[55-57] Consequently, our first choice in treating adverse hemodynamic or ischemic responses to aortic occlusion is administration of nitroglycerin. The major limitation of nitroglycerin is that it is not as predictable as other agents in reducing systemic blood pressure during aortic occlusion. In a study of patients having coronary artery bypass surgery, high doses of intravenously administered nitroglycerin failed to lower blood pressure in 18 percent of patients.[60] Although the study was performed in a clinical setting that differed from that of aortic surgery, the study results confirmed our clinical impression that approximately 20 percent of vascular patients do not respond adequately to high doses of infused nitroglycerin. Therefore, our standard practice is to identify patients who will respond to such therapy. We do this by initiating an infusion of nitroglycerin during the relatively stable period of aortic dissection early in the case. However, the hemodynamic response to nitroglycerin depends on intravascular volume, which may change dramatically by the time aortic dissection is completed and the surgeon is ready to occlude the aorta. Consequently, our nitroglycerin "trial" provides only a rough estimate of patient response.

Although nitroglycerin has few systemic toxic effects, some important precautions need consideration. Infusion of nitroglycerin can cause methemoglobinemia.[59,61-63] Nitrates promote the oxidation of ferrous (Fe^{2+}) hemoglobin to the ferric (Fe^{3+}) state. Because the oxidized Fe^{3+} hemoglobin does not participate in oxygen transport, oxygen saturation and content decrease, and cyanosis (as evidence by a desaturated "chocolate brown" arterial blood sample) occurs if significant methemoglobinemia is present. Because oxygen solubility is unaffected, arterial oxygen partial pressure may be normal or quite high. In one instance, methemoglobinemia occurred acutely following a "low-dose" infusion of 90 µg of nitroglycerin per minute.[63] Two other cases of methemoglobinemia have been reported following prolonged infusion of 60 to 2,000 µg of nitroglycerin per minute.[61,62] The diagnosis of methemoglobinemia can be confirmed by measuring methemoglobin levels (normally less than 1 percent) by cooximetry.

Second, nitroglycerin is absorbed by polyvinylchloride tubing and fluid bags. Absorption varies between 40 and 80 percent and is not a self-limiting process. Because the amount of drug administered is titrated to an easily and continuously measured physiologic response (i.e., blood pressure), the fact that nitroglycerin is absorbed into the delivery system is of no clinical significance. To quantify the dose delivered to the patient more carefully, glass bottles and nonabsorbent tubing (Tridil) can be used.

Sodium nitroprusside also causes vasodilation and decreases the left ventricular strain associated with aortic cross-clamping. Its primary advantage is speed and predictability in decreasing systemic blood pressure.[60,64] One major disadvantage of sodium nitroprusside is that it may promote coronary artery steal and thus worsen myocardial ischemia in patients with occlusive coronary disease. Coronary artery steal occurs when vasodilation of functional coronary arteries redirects blood flow away from a vascular bed that is ischemic, maximally dilated, and distal to a stenosis.[55,57,65] Nitroprusside also increases the pulmonary shunt fraction more than does nitroglycerin,[60] thereby decreasing intraoperative oxygenation. High doses (greater than 10 µg/kg/min) of nitroprusside can cause cyanide and thiocyanate poisoning.[66,67] Because so many adverse responses may be associated with use of nitroprusside, we reserve administration of this drug for instances in which high aortic cross-clamping has provoked an intolerable hypertensive response in a patient unresponsive to nitroglycerin.

Finally, the potent inhaled anesthetics halothane, enflurane, and isoflurane decrease systemic blood pressure in a dose-related fashion. Halothane and enflurane decrease myocardial contractility,[68–70] and high concentrations of enflurane or isoflurane produce arterial vasodilation.[70–72]

It may seem that treating the increases in systemic pressure and PCWP with negative inotropes (i.e., inhaled anesthetics) might further impair cardiac function and thereby precipitate cardiac failure and myocardial ischemia. However, a study by Roizen and colleagues[73] examined the effects of increasing doses of enflurane and halothane to treat increases in PCWP (with and without depression of the ST segment) in vascular patients. All patients responded with a prompt decrease in peripheral vascular resistance, systolic blood pressure, and PCWP. All changes in ST segment returned to baseline. The authors suggest that during inadequate or light anesthesia, the benefits of increasing the concentration of anesthetic may outweigh the potential disadvantage of anesthetic-induced myocardial depression.[73] Such benefits include suppression of catecholamines and other vasoactive substances, reduction in systemic blood pressure, and reduction in peripheral and coronary vascular resistance.

PREPARING THE PATIENT FOR REMOVAL OF THE AORTIC CROSS-CLAMP

After surgical repair of the aorta has been completed and the aortic cross-clamp has been removed, hypotension invariably follows.[74] Appropriate anesthetic management tries to minimize the degree and length of hypotension. Hypotension occurs because the lower extremities have been ischemic and are therefore vasodilated maximally, a condition that results in peripheral pooling of blood.[32,45–47,75,76] In addition, high levels of lactate and other acids associated with anaerobic metabolism are washed into the central circulation and cause vasodilation.[49,75] Adequate volume loading to maintain normal or slightly elevated cardiac filling pressures is a way to avoid catastrophic decreases in blood pressure.[32,45,47,49,75,77] However, even with optimal volume management, removal of a high aortic cross-clamp may occasionally cause persistent hypotension. In this case, the surgeon may choose to reestablish aortic occlusion, and the anesthetist may choose to initiate aggressive volume infusion. If successive attempts at gradual unclamping of the aorta result in unacceptable levels of hypotension, administration of vasopressors such as phenylephrine (Neo-Synephrine) and bicarbonate to correct acidosis may be useful.

EVALUATION AND TREATMENT OF OLIGURIA

Postoperative renal insufficiency continues to be a life-threatening complication of aortic reconstruction.[2,20,26,32,78]

Suprarenal, infrarenal, and distal aortic occlusion can all cause renal insufficiency.[78]

Occluding the aorta at the suprarenal level interrupts renal blood flow and may cause ischemic renal insufficiency. Renal failure is most common in patients subjected to prolonged (greater than 55 minutes) suprarenal aortic occlusion.[31] Renal failure in patients undergoing shorter periods of renal ischemia may be related to embolization of atheromatous plaque, unsuccessful surgical repair, or other undefined factors. When the renal arteries are occluded, urine production stops. In 36 patients undergoing renal artery occlusion of 20 to 45 minutes, urinary flow resumed within a mean time of 25 minutes.[31]

Occluding the aorta at the infrarenal level impairs renal blood flow and increases vascular resistance. In patients given a continuous infusion of mannitol, renal blood flow decreased 38 percent and renal vascular resistance increased 75 percent during infrarenal cross-clamping.[79] These changes persisted for 1 hour after removal of the cross-clamp. The effect of infrarenal cross-clamping on regional blood flow within the kidney is controversial. Renal blood flow may be redistributed toward the renal cortex[79] or to the juxtamedullary nephrons,[80–82] or may not change at all.[83]

Oliguria has been defined variously as urinary output of less than 0.125 to 0.5 ml/kg/h.[21,84] Regardless of the level of aortic occlusion, oliguria frequently occurs during aortic surgery. In one study, more than half of the 137 patients undergoing aortic surgery had low urinary output (less than 30 ml/h) during surgery.[21] However, the presence of intraoperative oliguria failed to predict postoperative renal dysfunction. In addition, several studies have shown that high urinary output does not guarantee the preservation of renal function.[21,32]

As a measure of renal function, the occurrence of oliguria is too sensitive (many patients with oliguria will not have renal insufficiency) and not sufficiently specific (on rare occasion, a patient will have high-output renal failure) to be reliable. However, because it is our only intraoperative measure of renal function, oliguria should not be ignored. The mortality rate for patients experiencing postoperative renal failure ranges from 50 to 90 percent if renal failure occurs during rupture of an abdominal aneurysm.[85,86] In contrast, the expected mortality for vascular patients whose renal function has been preserved is 0 to 12 percent.[1,2,87]

A systematic approach to the evaluation and treatment of oliguria begins with elimination of the mechanical problems associated with urine collection. That is, patency of the Foley catheter and absence of obstructions in the collection system are verified. Second, volume status should be assessed and intravascular volume optimized by additional volume infusion to raise left-sided cardiac filling pressures into the high normal range.[88-90] Third, when blood pressure is within 20 percent of the preoperative baseline level, we observe the effects of additional volume infusion on cardiac output.

Despite 20 years of controversy and research, the effectiveness of administering drugs to treat oliguria is still poorly defined. There is no good evidence that reestablishing high urinary outflow with the use of diuretics changes the progression or prognosis of acute renal failure.[91-94] However, there is no doubt that converting a patient from an oliguric to a nonoliguric state makes postoperative fluid and electrolyte management much easier.

Mannitol is an osmotic diuretic that is freely filtered by the renal glomerulus but is not reabsorbed by the renal tubules. It indirectly increases intravascular volume and reduces blood viscosity, thereby increasing renal blood flow.[92,93,95] Mannitol has been administered prior to an expected episode of ischemia in an attempt to preserve renal cortical blood flow, to prevent acute postischemic tubular necrosis,[31,74,93,95] and to treat intraoperative and postoperative oliguria. At one institution, administration of mannitol resulted in a low incidence (4 percent) of postischemic renal failure after suprarenal aortic occlusion of 15 to 150 minutes.[31]

Potent "loop diuretics" such as furosemide inhibit tubular sodium absorption and force diuresis in patients with preserved glomerular filtration.[92] In patients experiencing oliguria either during or after aortic reconstructive surgery, small doses of furosemide (5 to 10 mg) are frequently effective in initiating diuresis.

The use of low doses of dopamine appears to be a reasonable intervention when other measures to treat oliguria (optimizing hemodynamic state and filling pressures) have failed.[92,93,96] Dopamine is an endogenous catecholamine that has, at low doses (1 to 5 μg/kg/min), predominantly β-adrenergic and dopaminergic actions. β-adrenergic stimulation increases contractility and decreases peripheral vascular resistance, thereby increasing cardiac output. Dopaminergic stimulation causes vasodilation of the renal and mesenteric arteries. The combination of these effects increases renal blood flow.[92,97] Whether dopamine reduces postischemic renal stress or speeds recovery is unknown.

MYOCARDIAL ISCHEMIA: MONITORING AND TREATMENT

Standard, multiple-lead, and Holter monitoring systems demonstrate a 20 to 79 percent incidence of intraoperative ischemia in patients with coronary disease who are undergoing surgery.[98–104] Because ischemic events appear to lead to postoperative complications,[102] we believe that monitoring of myocardial ischemia and intervention to terminate these episodes should be aggressive.

Methods for detecting intraoperative myocardial ischemia are evolving rapidly. Four principal methods are either in clinical use or under study: (1) single-lead, multiple-lead, and computerized ECG detection of changes in ST segment; (2) echocardiographic detection of wall motion abnormalities; (3) measurement of pulmonary wedge pressures for detection of changes in myocardial compliance; and (4) measurement of lactate levels for detection of changes in myocardial metabolism. Potentially, these techniques can provide sensitive measurements of the electrical, mechanical, and metabolic components of ischemic response.

The Electrocardiogram

Intraoperative ECG monitoring of myocardial ischemia has undergone a marked change over the last decade. Clinical practice has evolved from the use of single-lead to selective-, multiple-, and simultaneous-lead ECG monitoring systems. Recently, computerized signal processing has been used to detect variations in the ST segment.

For older patients at significant risk of intraoperative ischemia during major and prolonged surgery, five-lead ECG systems are in common use. For monitoring ischemia in awake humans undergoing exercise stress testing, lead V_5 best detects abnormalities in the ST segment.[24,105–107] Therefore, lead V_5 has been recommended for intraoperative use as well. To detect changes in ST segment, the diagnostic mode that filters frequencies below 0.14 Hz is more useful than the monitoring mode (see Ch. 3). However, all signals must be calibrated electrically. The criterion for ischemia evidenced by changes in the ST segment is a horizontal or downsloping depression of 1 mm or more occurring 80 msec beyond the J point. Other changes, such as isolated J-point depression with an upsloping ST segment, are usually rate related and may be a normal response. The depth of the depression in the ST segment has been related to subsequent coronary events. Certainly, a depression of 2 mm or more carries a more significant prognosis than lesser changes. In one study, the comparative height of the R wave, used as a normalizing factor, was reported to augment the validity of the standard measurement for change in the ST segment.[108] Although nonspecific changes in the ST segment and T wave (a deviation in the ST segment of less than 1 mm and flattening and inversion of the T wave) may also indicate ischemic events, these manifestations may be normal variants; they also may be associated with hyperventilation, strain patterns, or the effects of digitalis.[109]

The Echocardiogram

Significant advances in echocardiography have promoted its use in patients with ischemic heart disease. Both M-mode and two-dimensional echocardiography are noninvasive and may offer advantages over standard ECG techniques. With the development of wall motion abnormalities, systolic thinning may occur before abnormalities in the ST segment or increases in intracavitary left ventricular pressure occur.[28] Intraoperative use of two-dimensional transesophageal echocardiography is relatively straightforward and can provide an echo signal of higher quality than can the conventional precordial technique[110] (also see Ch. 28). The device consists of a single-element transducer (3.5 or 5 MHz) or a multielement phased-array transducer (3.5 MHz) attached to the tip of a commercially available gastroscope. The device can be easily advanced into the esophagus of the anesthetized patient. Images of the aortic and mitral valves, the four cardiac chambers, and the short axis and apex of the left ventricle can be displayed on a video monitor. Regional wall motion abnormalities, which are considered indicative of ischemia, can be detected and time sequenced during surgery by using the left ventricular short-axis view at the level of the papillary muscles (at approximately 45 cm from the teeth, as measured on the gastroscope).

Two-dimensional transesophageal echocardiography is superior to electrocardiography in providing information that is sensitive and specific to the diagnosis of intraoperative myocardial ischemia and infarction. Among 50 patients requiring cardiovascular surgery, echocardiography detected myocardial ischemia in 24 patients, and electrocardiography detected it in 6.[28] Intraoperative myocardial infarctions occurred in three patients, all of whom had persistent wall motion abnormalities detected by echocardiography; only one of these patients had an ECG change in the ST segment. In another study, 14 patients requiring coronary angioplasty of the left anterior descending coronary artery were studied during balloon inflation—a procedure that causes temporary ischemia to a large area of myocardium. All patients had immediate wall motion abnormalities visible on echocardiogram. A twelve-lead electrocardiogram indicated changes in ST segment in 86 percent of patients within 1 minute. A three-lead system (leads I, aVL, and V_5) indicated ischemic changes in only 57 percent at 1 minute.[29]

Transesophageal echocardiography has several possible disadvantages. First, diagnosing wall motion abnormalities requires ongoing attention to the video image. Therefore, attention may be focused away from the patient. Although *qualitative* assessment of segmental wall motion abnormalities (ischemia) is straightforward for the anesthetist or clinician, *quantitative* measurements are difficult to perform during surgery. Until computer software is developed to provide digitized information to the clinician as it actually occurs, the use of transesophageal echocardiography for quantitation of ejection fraction and intracardiac planar dimensions is limited to research applications. Finally, the initial cost ($50,000 to $200,000) and maintenance costs ($10,000 to $30,000 per year) of echocardiographic equipment are substantial. Therefore, the use of echocardiography in the clinical setting is not yet widespread. However, with resolution of cost and quantitation problems, this method of monitoring will become important to the intraoperative management of patients with cardiac disease who are undergoing major surgery.

The Pulmonary Capillary Wedge Pressure Measurement

Because increases in PCWP may precede ECG changes in the ST segment during intraoperative episodes of ischemia, measurement of PCWP may be another useful indicator of an ischemic event.[111] However, the sensitivity and specificity of the PCWP measurement relative to ECG changes in ST segment or to echocardiographic changes in wall motion has yet to be determined. The most significant problem with relying on PCWP to monitor ischemia is that acute increases in left ventricular end-diastolic pressure may occur but not be apparent on the PCWP reading.[112] PCWP would therefore be a relatively insensitive marker. Furthermore, the specific cause of sudden increases in PCWP in patients with coronary artery disease may be ambiguous, possibly reflecting either impaired diastolic relaxation or impaired systolic contraction, or volume overload. Nevertheless, sudden increases in PCWP suggest either ischemia or left ventricular dysfunction; we treat both conditions aggressively in patients with coronary artery disease. Reduction of PCWP can be accomplished by using nitrates or diuretics to reduce preload, dobutamine to improve contractility and promote pulmonary vascular dilation, and vasodilators to reduce both pulmonary and systemic vascular resistance.

Lactate Levels

The intraoperative determination of metabolic markers of ischemia is currently limited to the research setting. Methods consist of determinations of coronary sinus lactate and radiolabeled lactate, assays of free fatty acid and carbohydrates, and magnetic resonance spectroscopy. The coronary sinus has been catheterized in a number of studies addressing principally the comparative effects of anesthetic agents on the ischemic state.[113–118] For clinical purposes, routine catheterization is neither practical nor warranted. In the future, several of these techniques (particularly magnetic resonance spectroscopy) may find clinical application. However, the benefits of any of these methods must first be evaluated fully and related to those in current use, such as electrocardiography and echocardiography. As with all methods of detecting ischemia, we must determine whether the use of these new monitors truly affects morbidity before we consider widespread clinical use.

Treatment of Myocardial Ischemia

The relationship of intraoperative ischemia to postoperative outcome is suggested by a study that reports the risk of postoperative infarction to be two to three times higher in patients who have intraoperative ischemia during coronary artery bypass grafting surgery.[102] We therefore advocate aggressive treatment of myocardial ischemia when it is detected intraoperatively.

We first try to normalize blood pressure and left ventricular filling pressures and to slow heart rate. Once these hemodynamic variables return to preoperative baseline levels, we add nitroglycerin and β-adrenergic blocking agents, as tolerated, to optimize the balance between oxygen supply and demand. Several studies have shown that nitrates and β-adrenergic blocking agents limit the size of myocardial infarctions. Administration of calcium channel-blocking agents does not appear to improve outcome from myocardial infarction.[119]

Effective prevention of myocardial ischemia with drugs is a desirable yet unproven intervention. Ample documentation shows that abrupt withdrawal of β-adrenergic blocking agents causes rebound tachycardia and an acute worsening of myocardial ischemia.[120–124] One prospective, double-blinded, cross-over study reported that discontinuation of β-adrenergic blocking agents in 10 patients was associated with six serious or fatal consequences.[123] Two patients died: one had myocardial infarction, and one was a "sudden death." A third patient had ventricular tachycardia, and three others had accelerated unstable angina. Although continuation of all antihypertensive and antianginal drugs to the morning of surgery is widespread clinical practice, patients having abdominal vascular surgery will have all oral intake restricted for many hours and possibly days. Prophylactic administration of β-adrenergic blocking drugs has not been studied in this patient population but may lower the incidence of myocardial ischemia in these high-risk patients.

Several studies of prophylactic infusion of nitroglycerin show variable rates of success in preventing myocardial ischemia.[99,101,125]

CONCLUSION

Minimizing the morbidity and mortality of vascular surgery patients is one of the greatest challenges facing anesthetists. Preoperative testing with dipyridamole-thallium imaging may identify a particularly high-risk subgroup who may benefit from invasive cardiac diagnosis and therapy prior to aortic surgery. Two-dimensional transesophageal echocardiography is a more sensitive monitor of intraoperative myocardial ischemia and, when used with prompt intervention with nitroglycerin and β-adrenergic blocking agents, may help reduce perioperative myocardial complications.

From collective studies, we can predict that certain patients are more likely to have severe hypertension or myocardial ischemia following aortic occlusion: those subjected to high temporary aortic occlusion, those with poor left ventricular function, and those with aneurysmal disease. Hypertension and myocardial ischemia may be treated with administration of nitroglycerin or nitroprusside or by increasing the concentration of potent inhalational anesthetics. Adequate volume loading is the most important step in avoiding prolonged hypotension associated with unclamping of the aorta.

We have only begun to address the important question of whether choice of anesthetic technique affects patient outcome. Small studies suggest that either epidural anesthesia and analgesia or narcotic-based general anesthesia reduces patient morbidity. However, these results must be confirmed before such techniques could be recommended as being superior to other commonly used methods.

REFERENCES

1. Young AE, Sandberg GW, Couch NP: The reduction of mortality of abdominal aortic aneurysm resection. Am J Surg 134:585–590, 1977
2. Diehl JT, Cali RF, Hertzer NR, Beven EG: Complications of abdominal aortic reconstruction. An analysis of perioperative risk factors in 557 patients. Ann Surg 197:49–56, 1983
3. Hertzer NR, Beven EG, Young JR et al: Coronary artery disease in peripheral vascular patients. A classification of 1000 coronary angiograms and results of surgical management. Ann Surg 199:223–233, 1984
4. Crawford ES, Saleh SA, Babb JW III et al: Infrarenal abdominal aortic aneurysm. Factors influencing survival after operation performed over a 25-year period. Ann Surg 193:699–709, 1981
5. Plecha FR, Bertin VJ, Plecha EJ et al: The early results of vascular surgery in patients 75 years of age and older: an analysis of 3259 cases. J Vasc Surg 2:769–774, 1985
6. Kannel WB, McGee D, Gordon T: A general cardiovascular risk profile: the Framingham Study. Ann J Cardiol 38:46–51, 1976
7. Criqui MH: Epidemiology of atherosclerosis: an updated overview. Am J Cardiol 57:18C–23C, 1986
8. Tomatis LA, Fierens EE, Verbrugge GP: Evaluation of surgical risk in peripheral vascular disease by coronary arteriography: a series of 100 cases. Surgery 71:429–435, 1972
9. Gage AA, Bhayana JN, Balu V, Hook N:

Assessment of cardiac risk in surgical patients. Arch Surg 112:1488–1492, 1977

10. Hertzer NR, Young JR, Beven EG et al: Late results of coronary bypass in patients with peripheral vascular disease. I. Five-year survival according to age and clinical cardiac status. Cleveland Clin Q 53:133–143, 1986

11. Cutler BS: Prevention of cardiac complications in peripheral vascular surgery. Surg Clin North Am 66:281–303, 1986

12. Jain KM, Patil KD, Doctor US, Peck SL: Preoperative cardiac screening before peripheral vascular operations. Am Surgeon 51:77–79, 1985

13. Rozanski A, Diamond GA, Berman D et al: The declining specificity of exercise radionuclide ventriculography. N Engl J Med 309:518–522, 1983

14. Boucher CA, Brewster DC, Darling RC et al: Determination of cardiac risk by dipyridamole-thallium imaging before peripheral vascular surgery. N Engl J Med 312:389–394, 1985

15. Brewster DC, Okada RD, Strauss HW et al: Selection of patients for preoperative coronary angiography: use of dipyridamole-stress—thallium myocardial imaging. J Vasc Surg 2:504–510, 1985

16. Cutler BS, Leppo JA: Dipyridamole thallium 201 scintigraphy to detect coronary artery disease before abdominal aortic surgery. J Vasc Surg 5:91–100, 1987

17. Eagle KA, Singer DE, Brewster DC et al: Dipyridamole-thallium scanning in patients undergoing vascular surgery. Optimizing preoperative evaluation of cardiac risk. JAMA 257:2185–2189, 1987

18. Albro PC, Gould KL, Westcott RJ et al: Noninvasive assessment of coronary stenoses by myocardial imaging during pharmacologic coronary vasodilation. III. Clinical trial. Am J Cardiol 42:751–760, 1978

19. Leppo J, Boucher CA, Okada RD et al: Serial thallium-201 myocardial imaging after dipyridamole infusion: diagnostic utility in detecting coronary stenoses and relationship to regional wall motion. Circulation 66:649–657, 1982

20. Benefiel DJ, Roizen MF, Lampe GH et al: Morbidity after aortic surgery with sufentanil vs isoflurane anesthesia (abstract). Anesthesiology 65:A516, 1986

21. Alpert RA, Roizen MF, Hamilton WK et al: Intraoperative urinary output does not predict postoperative renal function in patients undergoing abdominal aortic revascularization. Surgery 95:707–711, 1984

22. Lausten GS, Engell HC: Postoperative complications in abdominal vascular surgery. Acta Chir Scand 150:457–461, 1984

23. Rao TLK, Jacobs KH, El-Etr AA: Reinfarction following anesthesia in patients with myocardial infarction. Anesthesiology 59:499–505, 1983

24. Kaplan JA, King SB, III: The precordial electrocardiographic lead (V_5) in patients who have coronary-artery disease. Anesthesiology 45:570–574, 1976

25. Kaplan JA, Wells PH: Electrocardiographic monitoring. p. 163–205. In Ream AK, Fogdall RP (eds): Acute Cardiovascular Management: Anesthesia and Intensive Care. JB Lippincott, Philadelphia, 1982

26. Roizen MF, Beaupre PN, Alpert RA et al: Monitoring with two-dimensional transesophageal echocardiography. Comparison of myocardial function in patients undergoing supraceliac, suprarenal-infraceliac, or infrarenal aortic occlusion. J Vasc Surg 1:300–305, 1984

27. Schlüter M, Hanrath P: The clinical application of transesophageal echocardiography. Echocardiography 1:427–442, 1984

28. Smith JS, Cahalan MK, Benefiel DJ et al: Intraoperative detection of myocardial ischemia in high-risk patients: electrocardiography versus two-dimensional transesophageal echocardiography. Circulation 72:1015–1021, 1985

29. Wohlgelernter D, Cleman M, Highman HA et al: Regional myocardial dysfunction during coronary angioplasty. Evaluation by two-dimensional echocardiography and 12 lead electrocardiography. J Am Coll Cardiol 7:1245–1254, 1986

30. Benefiel DJ, Roizen MF, Schiller NB: Monitoring with transesophageal echo-

cardiography. Appl Cardiol 14:9–13, 1986

31. Crawford ES, Snyder DM, Cho GC, Roehm JOF, Jr: Progress in treatment of thoracoabdominal and abdominal aortic aneurysms involving celiac, superior mesenteric, and renal arteries. Ann Surg 188:404–422, 1978

32. Bush HL, Jr., Huse JB, Johnson WC et al: Prevention of renal insufficiency after abdominal aortic aneurysm resection by optimal volume loading. Arch Surg 116:1517–1524, 1981

33. Rice CL, Hobelman CF, John DA et al: Central venous pressure or pulmonary capillary pressure as the determinant of fluid replacement in aortic surgery. Surgery 84:437–440, 1978

34. Mangano DT: Monitoring pulmonary arterial pressure in coronary-artery disease. Anesthesiology 53:364–370, 1980

35. Keats AS: The Rovenstine Lecture, 1983: Cardiovascular anesthesia: perceptions and perspectives. Anesthesiology 60:467–474, 1984

36. Roizen MF: But what does it do to outcome (editorial)? Anesth Analg 63:789–790, 1984

37. Yeager MP, Glass DD, Neff RK, Brinck-Johnsen T: Epidural anesthesia and analgesia in high-risk surgical patients. Anesthesiology 66:729–736, 1987

38. McPeek B: Inference, generalizability, and a major change in anesthetic practice (editorial). Anesthesiology 66:723–724, 1987

39. Rao TLK, El-Etr AA: Anticoagulation following placement of epidural and subarachnoid catheters: an evaluation of neurologic sequelae. Anesthesiology 55:618–620, 1981

40. Odoom JA, Sih IL: Epidural analgesia and anticoagulant therapy. Experience with one thousand cases of continuous epidurals. Anaesthesia 38:254–259, 1983

41. Mathews ET, Abrams LD: Intrathecal morphine in open heart surgery (letter). Lancet 1:543, 1980

42. Ruff RL, Dougherty JH, Jr: Complications of lumbar puncture followed by anticoagulation. Stroke 12:879–881, 1981

43. Owens EL, Kasten GW, Hessel EA, II: Spinal subarachnoid hematoma after lumbar puncture and heparinization: a case report, review of the literature, and discussion of anesthetic implications. Anesth Analg 65:1201–1207, 1986

44. Hanley JA, Lippman-Hand A: If nothing goes wrong, is everything all right? Interpreting zero numerators. JAMA 249:1743–1745, 1983

45. Lunn JK, Dannemiller FJ, Stanley TH: Cardiovascular responses to clamping of the aorta during epidural and general anesthesia. Anesth Analg 58:372–376, 1979

46. Carroll RM, Laravuso RB, Schauble JF: Left ventricular function during aortic surgery. Arch Surg 111:740–743, 1976

47. Silverstein PR, Caldera DL, Cullen DJ et al: Avoiding the hemodynamic consequences of aortic cross-clamping and unclamping. Anesthesiology 50:462–466, 1979

48. Gooding JM, Archie JP, Jr., McDowell H: Hemodynamic response to infrarenal aortic cross-clamping in patients with and without coronary artery disease. Crit Care Med 8:382–385, 1980

49. Falk JL, Rackow EC, Blumenberg R et al: Hemodynamic and metabolic effects of abdominal aortic crossclamping. Am J Surg 142:174–177, 1981

50. Attia RR, Murphy JD, Snider M et al: Myocardial ischemia due to infrarenal aortic cross-clamping during aortic surgery in patients with severe coronary artery disease. Circulation 53:961–965, 1976

51. Johnston WE, Balestrieri FJ, Plonk G et al: The influence of periaortic collateral vessels on the intraoperative hemodynamic effects of acute aortic occlusion in patients with aorto-occlusive disease or abdominal aortic aneurysm. Anesthesiology 66:386–389, 1987

52. Dunn E, Prager RL, Fry W, Kirsh MM: The effect of abdominal aortic cross-clamping on myocardial function. J Surg Res 22:463–468, 1977

53. Meloche R, Pottecher T, Audet J et al: Haemodynamic changes due to clamping of the abdominal aorta. Can Anaesth Soc J 24:20–34, 1977

54. Bussmann W-D, Passek D, Seidel W, Kaltenbach M: Reduction of CK and CK-MB indexes of infarct size by intravenous nitroglycerin. Circulation 63:615–622, 1981

55. Chiariello M, Gold HK, Leinbach RC et al: Comparison between the effects of nitroprusside and nitroglycerin on ischemic injury during acute myocardial infarction. Circulation 54:766–773, 1976

56. Endrich B, Franke N, Peter K, Messmer K: Induced hypotension: action of sodium nitroprusside and nitroglycerin on the microcirculation. A micropuncture investigation. Anesthesiology 66:605–613, 1987

57. Mann T, Cohn PF, Holman BL et al: Effect of nitroprusside on regional myocardial blood flow in coronary artery disease. Result in 25 patients and comparison with nitroprusside. Circulation 57:732–738, 1978

58. Borer JS, Redwood DR, Levitt B et al: Reduction in myocardial ischemia with nitroglycerin or nitroglycerin plus phenylephrine administered during acute myocardial infarction. N Engl J Med 293:1008–1012, 1975

59. Hill NS, Antman EM, Green LH, Alpert JS: Intravenous nitroglycerin. A review of pharmacology, indications, therapeutic effects and complications. Chest 79:69–76, 1981

60. Flaherty JT, Magee PA, Gardner TL et al: Comparison of intravenous nitroglycerin and sodium nitroprusside for treatment of acute hypertension developing after coronary artery bypass surgery. Circulation 65:1072–1077, 1982

61. Gibson GR, Hunter JB, Raabe DS, Jr et al: Methemoglobinemia produced by high-dose intravenous nitroglycerin. Ann Intern Med 96:615–616, 1982

62. Zurick AM, Wagner RH, Starr NJ et al: Intravenous nitroglycerin, methemoglobinemia, and respiratory distress in a postoperative cardiac surgical patient. Anesthesiology 61:464–466, 1984

63. Robicsek F: Acute methemoglobinemia during cardiopulmonary bypass caused by intravenous nitroglycerin infusion. J Thorac Cardiovasc Surg 90:931–934, 1985

64. Gerson Jl, Allen FB, Seltzer JL et al: Arterial and venous dilation by nitroprusside and nitroglycerin—is there a difference? Anesth Analg 61:256–260, 1982

65. Warltier DC, Gross GJ, Brooks HL: Coronary steal-induced increase in myocardial infarct size after pharmacologic coronary vasodilation. Am J Cardiol 46:83–90, 1980

66. Tinker JH, Michenfelder JD: Sodium nitroprusside: pharmacology, toxicology and therapeutics. Anesthesiology 45:340–354, 1976

67. Cohn JN, Burke LP: Nitroprusside. Ann Intern Med 91:752–757, 1979

68. Bahlman SH, Eger EI, II, Halsey MJ et al: The cardiovascular effects of halothane in man during spontaneous ventilation. Anesthesiology 36:494–502, 1972

69. Eger EI, II, Smith NT, Stoelting RK et al: Cardiovascular effects of halothane in man. Anesthesiology 32:396–409, 1970

70. Calverly RK, Smith NT, Prys-Roberts C et al: Cardiovascular effects of enflurane anesthesia during controlled ventilation in man. Anesth Analg 57:619–628, 1978

71. Stevens WC, Cromwell TH, Halsey MJ et al: The cardiovascular effects of a new inhalation anesthetic, Forane, in human volunteers at constant arterial carbon dioxide tension. Anesthesiology 35:8–16, 1971

72. Cromwell TH, Stevens WC, Eger EI II et al: The cardiovascular effects of compound 469 (Forane) during spontaneous ventilation and CO_2 challenge in man. Anesthesiology 35:17–25, 1971

73. Roizen MF, Hamilton WK, Sohn YJ: Treatment of stress-induced increases in pulmonary capillary wedge pressure using volatile anesthetics. Anesthesiology 55:446–450, 1981

74. Sabawala PB, Strong MJ, Keats AS: Surgery of the aorta and its branches. Anesthesiology 33:229–259, 1970

75. Reiz S, Peter T, Rais O: Hemodynamic and cardiometabolic effects of infrarenal aortic and common iliac artery declamping in man—an approach to optimal volume loading. Acta Anaesthesiol Scand 23:579–586, 1979

76. Eklöf B, Neglén P, Thomson D: Temporary incomplete ischemia of the legs induced by aortic clamping in man. Effects on central hemodynamics and skeletal muscle metabolism by adrenergic block. Ann Surg 193:89–98, 1981

77. Wheeler CG, Thompson JE, Kartchner MM et al: Massive fluid requirement in surgery of the abdominal aorta. N Engl J Med 275:320–322, 1966

78. McCombs PR, Roberts B: Acute renal failure following resection of abdominal aortic aneurysm. Surg Gynecol Obstet 148:175–178, 1979

79. Gamulin Z, Forster A, Morel D et al: Effects of infrarenal aortic cross-clamping on renal hemodynamics in humans. Anesthesiology 61:394–399, 1984

80. Abbott WM, Cooper JD, Austen WG: The effect of aortic clamping and declamping on renal blood flow distribution. J Surg Res 14:385–392, 1973

81. Abbott WM, Austen WG: The reversal of renal cortical ischemia during aortic occlusion by mannitol. J Surg Res 16:482–489, 1974

82. Gelman S, Navar LG: Infrarenal aortic cross-clamping and renal hemodynamics (letter). Anesthesiology 63:223–224, 1985

83. Cronenwett JL, Lindenauer SM: Distribution of intrarenal blood flow following aortic clamping and declamping. J Surg Res 22:469–482, 1977

84. Dritz RA: Surgery on the aorta and peripheral arteries. p. 728. In Ream AK, Fogdall RP (ed): Acute Cardiovascular Management: Anesthesia and Intensive Care. JB Lippincott, Philadelphia, 1982

85. Tilney NL, Bailey GL, Morgan AP: Sequential system failure after rupture of abdominal aortic aneurysms: an unsolved problem in postoperative care. Ann Surg 178:117–122, 1973

86. Abbott WM, Abel RM, Beck CH, Jr., Fischer JE: Renal failure after ruptured aneurysm. Arch Surg 110:1110–1112, 1975

87. Hertzer NR, Avellone JC, Farrell CJ et al: The risk of vascular surgery in a metropolitan community. With observations on surgeon experience and hospital size. J Vasc Surg 1:13–21, 1984

88. Kahl FR, Flint JF, Szidon JP: Influence of left atrial distention on renal vasomotor tone. Am J Physiol 226:240–246, 1974

89. Wilkes BM, Mailloux LU: Acute renal failure. Pathogenesis and prevention. Am J Med 80:1129–1136, 1986

90. Zager RA: Alterations of intravascular volume: influence on renal susceptibility to ischemic injury. J Lab Clin Med 108:60–69, 1986

91. Lucas CE, Zito JG, Carter KM et al: Questionable value of furosemide in preventing renal failure. Surgery 82:314–320, 1977

92. Tiller DJ, Mudge GH: Pharmacologic agents used in the management of acute renal failure. Kidney Int 18:700–711, 1980

93. Fink M: Are diuretics useful in the treatment or prevention of acute renal failure? South Med J 75:329–334, 1982

94. Brezis M, Rosen S, Silva P, Epstein FH: Renal ischemia: a new perspective (editorial). Kidney Int 26:375–383, 1984

95. Barry KG, Cohen A, Knochel JP et al: Mannitol infusion. II. The prevention of acute functional renal failure during resection of an aneurysm of the abdominal aorta. N Engl J Med 264:967–971, 1961

96. Davis RF, Lappas DG, Kirklin JK et al: Acute oliguria after cardiopulmonary bypass: renal functional improvement with low-dose dopamine infusion. Crit Care Med 10:852–856, 1982

97. Goldberg LI: Cardiovascular and renal actions of dopamine: potential clinical applications. Pharmacol Rev 24:1–29, 1972

98. Roy WL, Edelist G, Gilbert B: Myocardial ischemia during non-cardiac surgical procedures in patients with coronary-artery disease. Anesthesiology 51:393–397, 1979

99. Coriat P, Daloz M, Bousseau D et al: Prevention of intraoperative myocardial ischemia during noncardiac surgery with intravenous nitroglycerin. Anesthesiology 61:193–196, 1984

100. Coriat P, Harari A, Daloz M, Viars P: Clinical predictors of intraoperative myocardial ischemia in patients with

coronary artery disease undergoing non-cardiac surgery. Acta Anaesthesiol Scand 26:287–290, 1982

101. Thomson IR, Mutch WAC, Culligan JD: Failure of intravenous nitroglycerin to prevent intraoperative myocardial ischemia during fentanyl-pancuronium anesthesia. Anesthesiology 61:385–393, 1984

102. Slogoff S, Keats AS: Does perioperative myocardial ischemia lead to postoperative myocardial infarction? Anesthesiology 62:107–114, 1985

103. Kotrly KJ, Kotter GS, Mortara D, Kampine JP: Intraoperative detection of myocardial ischemia with an ST segment trend monitoring system. Anesth Analg 63:343–345, 1984

104. Kotter GS, Bernstein JS, Kotrly KJ: ECG changes detect coronary artery bypass graft occlusion without hemodynamic instability. Anesth Analg 63:1133–1135, 1984

105. Blackburn H, Taylor HL, Okamato N et al: Standardization of the exercise electrocardiogram. A systematic comparison of chest lead configurations employed for monitoring during exercise. p. 101. In Karvonen MJ, Barry AJ (ed): Physical Activity and the Heart. Proceedings of a Symposium, Helsinki, Finland. Charles C Thomas, Springfield, II, 1967

106. Fuchs RM, Achuff SC, Grunwald L et al: Electrocardiographic localization of coronary artery narrowings: studies during myocardial ischemia and infarction in patients with one-vessel disease. Circulation 66:1168–1176, 1982

107. Chaitman BR, Bourassa MG, Wagniart P et al: Improved efficiency of treadmill exercise testing using a multiple lead ECG system and basic hemodynamic exercise response. Circulation 57:71–79, 1978

108. Hollenberg M, Budge WR, Wisneski JA, Gertz EW: Treadmill score quantifies electrocardiographic response to exercise and improves test accuracy and reproducibility. Circulation 61:276–285, 1980

109. Marriott HJL: Coronary insufficiency and related matters. p. 415. Practical Electrocardiography. 7th ed. Williams & Wilkins, Baltimore, 1983

110. Schlüter M, Langenstein BA, Polster J et al: Transesophageal cross-sectional echocardiography with a phased array transducer system. Technique and initial clinical results. Br Heart J 48:67–72, 1982

111. Kaplan JA, Wells PH: Early diagnosis of myocardial ischemia using the pulmonary arterial catheter. Anesth Analg 60:789–793, 1981

112. Rahimtoola SH, Loeb HS, Ehsani A et al: Relationship of pulmonary artery to left ventricular diastolic pressures in acute myocardial infarction. Circulation 46:283–290, 1972

113. Reiz S, Bålfors E, Friedman A et al: Effects of thiopentone on cardiac performance, coronary hemodynamics and myocardial oxygen consumption in chronic ischemic heart disease. Acta Anaesthesiol Scand 25:103–110, 1981

114. Reiz S, Bålfors E, Gustavsson B et al: Effects of halothane on coronary haemodynamics and myocardial metabolism in patients with ischaemic heart disease and heart failure. Acta Anaesthesiol Scand 26:133–138, 1982

115. Reiz S, Häggmark S, Östman M: Invasive analysis of non-invasive indicators of myocardial work and ischaemia during anaesthesia soon after myocardial infarction. Acta Anaesthesiol Scand 25:303–311, 1981

116. Sonntag H, Larsen R, Hilfiker O et al: Myocardial blood flow and oxygen consumption during high-dose fentanyl anesthesia in patients with coronary artery disease. Anesthesiology 56:417–422, 1982

117. Sonntag H, Merin RG, Donath U et al: Myocardial metabolism and oxygenation in man awake and during halothane anesthesia. Anesthesiology 51:204–210, 1979

118. Moffitt EA, Sethna DH, Gary RJ et al: Nitrous oxide added to halothane reduces coronary flow and myocardial oxygen consumption in patients with coronary disease. Can Anaesth Soc J 30:5–9, 1983

119. Yusuf S: Interventions that potentially limit myocardial infarct size: overview of clinical trials. Am J Cardiol 60:11A–17A, 1987

120. Slome R: Withdrawal of propranolol and myocardial infarction (letter). Lancet 1:156, 1973

121. Diaz RG, Somberg J, Freeman E, Levitt B: Myocardial infarction after propranolol withdrawal. Am Heart J 88:257–258, 1974

122. Alderman EL, Coltart DJ, Wettach GE, Harrison DC: Coronary artery syndromes after sudden propranolol withdrawal. Ann Intern Med 81:625–627, 1974

123. Miller RR, Olson HG, Amsterdam EA, Mason DT: Propranolol-withdrawal rebound phenomenon. Exacerbation of coronary events after abrupt cessation of antianginal therapy. N Engl J Med 293:416–418, 1975

124. Houston MC, Hodge R: Beta-adrenergic blocker withdrawal syndromes in hypertension and other cardiovascular diseases. Am Heart J 116:515–523, 1988

125. Coriat P, Mundler O, Bousseau D et al: Response of left ventricular ejection fraction to recovery from general anesthesia: measurement by gated radionuclide angiography. Anesth Analg 65:593–600, 1986

16

Anesthesia for Abdominal Aortic Reconstruction: One Approach at Dartmouth Medical School

Mark P. Yeager
D. David Glass

Abdominal aortic reconstructive surgery prolongs life.[1-3] The relatively high in-hospital mortality rate from early operative series has decreased to its present level of 1 to 5 percent.[4-6] Morbidity has also declined.[5-8] A marked increase in effort is now required to improve operative results even slightly. Therefore, as long as certain established principles of management prevail, considerable variability exists for anesthetic and surgical practice. The principles and practices advocated routinely at one center may be anathema at another. We now describe the preferences at Dartmouth regarding management of these difficult patients. We limit our discussion to issues that are often controversial because of the variety of management options available. A more general discussion of anesthetic care of patients undergoing abdominal aortic reconstruction can be found elsewhere in this text.

Although all patients undergoing abdominal aortic surgery should be evaluated and managed with their uniqueness in mind, in many ways these patients are relatively homogeneous. For example, they are generally in the sixth to eighth decades of life (rarely younger or older), they usually have atherosclerosis at several sites, they frequently have lung disease, and they often take several potent medications. Operative procedures and perioperative events are also similar. The procedures tend to be long, to involve significant blood loss and other "fluid shifts," to stress global cardiovascular function greatly, and perhaps to reduce global or regional perfusion of several organs. For these reasons, it is possible, and even desirable, to use an anesthetic plan that varies little from one operation to the next.

PREOPERATIVE CONSIDERATIONS

Few patients need more careful preoperative planning and evaluation than those undergoing abdominal aortic surgery. The following paragraphs describe some of the more common issues arising before surgery and our management of these matters.

Evaluation of the Cardiovascular System

By the time surgery has been scheduled, a diagnosis of cardiovascular disease has already been made. Several questions naturally arise: (1) What is the extent of disease, and does it involve the coronary, renal, cerebral, mesenteric, or spinal arterial blood supply? (2) Has the function of any of these organs already been reduced? (3) Are these organs at risk of further reduction in function?

Evaluating the coronary arteries and the functional state of the heart is the single most common preoperative problem. From the standpoint of postoperative morbidity, it is also the most important.[5,9] What is the best way to proceed? Some believe that all patients having abdominal aortic surgery should also undergo intensive preoperative cardiac evaluation.[10] This approach is designed to be very sensitive in detecting those patients most likely to have perioperative cardiac morbidity. Unfortunately, specificity is low, because one does not necessarily identify the patients who will do well. Also, this method has not been shown to be cost-effective, although one could argue that even a single perioperative myocardial infarction can be very expensive. Finally, such an approach tends to impugn the value of good clinical judgment. The opposite tack would be for the anesthetist simply to assume that all patients undergoing abdominal aortic reconstruction also have myocardial or coronary disease and to manage them accordingly. This approach is, of course, neither sensitive nor specific.

We prefer to take an intermediate position by using a clinically directed preoperative evaluation of the cardiovascular system. To streamline this system and minimize delays in evaluation and scheduling, we have developed a simple algorithm that indicates who should receive more intensive evaluation by a cardiologist prior to surgery (Fig. 16-1). Once referral is made to the cardiology service, appropriate questions need to be asked: What is the diagnosis? What is the functional state of the myocardium? Is there significant valvular disease? What is the likely functional state of the coronary arteries? The methods by which the cardiologist answers these questions are based on personal preference. Certainly, many tests have been shown to correlate well with perioperative cardiac morbidity.[11-22] Although test results can be used for reassurance, their primary usefulness should be the physiologic information they supply.

Performance of Coronary Artery Surgery before Aortic Surgery

Patients undergoing major noncardiac vascular surgery often have, in addition, significant coronary artery disease (CAD).[10] Because coronary artery bypass grafting (CABG) is valuable in treating CAD, it is important to ask what effect this procedure may have on patients who must undergo further vascular procedures. Certainly, patients who have already undergone, and recovered from, CABG seem to tolerate subsequent procedures quite well.[23] The issue then becomes whether or not they tolerate subsequent procedures so well that one should consider CABG surgery before proceeding with other kinds of vascular surgery (for example, abdominal aortic reconstructive surgery). Some centers have

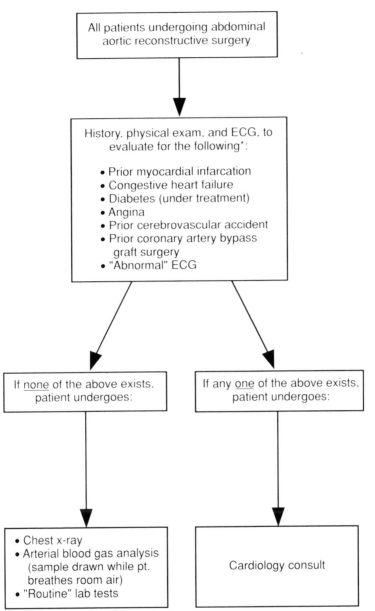

Fig. 16-1. Algorithm used to decide which patients undergoing abdominal aortic reconstructive surgery need more intensive cardiac evaluation. *At Dartmouth, the existence or discovery of any of the following conditions does not warrant full cardiac evaluation: hyperglycemia not requiring treatment, hypertension under treatment, chronic obstructive pulmonary disease, carotid bruits on examination, and previous carotid endarerectomy. Abnormal ECG = an electrocardiogram indicating cardiac rhythm other than sinus, more than five premature ventricular contractions a minute, or evidence of ischemia.

advocated that this sequence be strongly considered.[24-26]

This approach entails several problems. The first problem is the small but finite mortality and morbidity associated with CABG in even the best of hands. Does "prophylactic" CABG before abdominal aortic reconstructive surgery actually lower *overall* morbidity and mortality? This question is impossible to answer without conducting a proper randomized controlled clinical trial, and this has not been done. The second problem relates to the constant introduction of new management techniques for patients with CAD. For example, even if results from an earlier study have suggested benefit from CABG for some patients, what is the role of coronary angioplasty for these patients at this time? Finally, there is the issue of timing. What should be done, and when? Having cared for patients with known abdominal aortic aneurysms that have ruptured while the patient was recovering from CABG surgery, we believe that this question is not moot. We also believe that the answer to the question of whether CABG surgery should be performed before other procedures is best answered by applying good clinical judgment to each case. If the aneurysm is small and CAD is clinically unstable, we believe CAD should be corrected. Conversely, if the aneurysm is large and the patient has stable, well-controlled angina with good myocardial function, we first repair the aneurysm. For the many situations between these two extremes, our position is that the best management for each situation comes from using a clinical, and not a statistical, approach.

Pulmonary Artery Catheterization

Catherization of the pulmonary artery provides many benefits: the ability to obtain information regarding both right and left ventricular systolic and diastolic function and cardiac output; access for central venous infusions; and a way of monitoring real-time mixed venous oxygen saturation. Of these, a central venous catheter provides only information on right ventricular diastolic function plus a port for infusions. The relationship between central venous pressure and pulmonary artery pressure is poor.[27] The often sought-for correlation between central venous pressure and blood volume is also very poor. The clinical and economic risks of pulmonary artery catheterization are well known. The direction in which the balance between risks and benefits will lean varies with each institution and each patient.

Our practice is to place pulmonary artery catheters having the ability to measure mixed venous oxygen saturation in all patients undergoing abdominal aortic reconstructive surgery. We base this decision on clinical data demonstrating that preoperative,[12] intraoperative,[7,28-31] and postoperative[32] use of the pulmonary artery catheter provides information that lowers morbidity. We believe that the risks—both economic and clinical—are small when viewed in the context of an expensive surgical procedure for which one would want central venous access at the very least. Once the risk and expense of a central venous catheter are agreed upon, the added risk and expense of a pulmonary artery catheter become even less significant.

INTRAOPERATIVE MANAGEMENT

Blood Replacement

Some of these procedures entail high operative blood loss. In the past, this was a problem primarily of procurement and availability of adequate donor blood. However, the issue of blood transfusion has recently become considerably more complex. First, the concern over transmission of disease, notably acquired immune deficiency syndrome, is prominent. Not only are patients fearful of receiving transfusions, but some volunteers are even afraid to donate blood, thus decreasing the blood supply at blood banks. Perhaps even more important from a clinical point of view is the increasing awareness that transfusion of homologous blood products causes a measurable and clinically significant depression of immune function. This effect may translate into clinically significant depression of postoperative immunity.[33-37] Finally, blood transfusions cost money. In the current era of cost containment, this fact must be part of the decision-making process.

For these reasons, we use a blood-scavenging device for all patients undergoing abdominal aortic surgery. Economically, this practice is justifiable if one can prevent the transfusion of approximately two to four units of homologous red blood cells. However, the economic benefit also depends on how the costs of the two options (homologous transfusion or blood scavenging) are calculated.

Preinduction Preparations

Given that patients undergoing major vascular surgery belong to the same patient population as those undergoing CABG surgery and given that the magnitude of the surgery is roughly equivalent, it is appropriate to manage these patients comparably in the preoperative period. This means that they should be given a particularly careful explanation of what to anticipate before and after the operation. Such patients generally benefit from preoperative medication given either before or shortly after arrival at the induction room. Because placement of monitoring lines can be physically and psychologically discomforting, we administer a combination of analgesic and anxiolytic medications. Small increments of thiopental provide transient but reliable amnesia during difficult periods of preoperative preparation.

Before induction of general anesthesia, we insert an epidural catheter, usually in a high lumbar or low thoracic interspace. Although there is good evidence that this is a safe procedure to perform even in the presence of warfarin-type anticoagulation,[38] we prefer not to place an epidural catheter unless the prothrombin time, the partial thromboplastin time, and the platelet count are all close to normal. (Many would argue that only prothrombin time is necessary for patients given warfarin who do not have a history of bleeding.) The preoperative use of platelet-inhibiting drugs such as aspirin does not preclude the use of an epidural catheter, and we do not routinely check bleeding time.

Induction of Anesthesia

After arrival of the patient at the operating room, we measure baseline data from all hemodynamic monitors. A test dose of 3 ml of local anesthetic (usually 1.5 percent lidocaine because of its rapid onset of action) with 1:200,000 epinephrine is given through the epidural catheter as soon as the electrocardiogram and arterial blood pressure are monitored. The rest of preinduction preparation can then take place while the effects of the test dose are being evaluated. Subsequently, we give 6 to 10 ml of local anesthetic solution to establish a partial block prior to induction of general anesthesia. Partial block allows confirmation that the epidural catheter is functioning properly without creating the hemodynamic instability that can attend induction of general anesthesia during a full epidural block.

We then induce general anesthesia using incremental doses of narcotics (typically 100 to 200 μg of fentanyl), 60 to 70 percent nitrous oxide in oxygen, 50- to 100-mg increments of thiopental, and an "intubating dose" of a nondepolarizing muscle relaxant. Graded stimuli are then applied, and the patient's responses are evaluated. Such stimuli include initiation of positive-pressure ventilation, establishment of an oral airway, catheterization of the urinary bladder, laryngoscopy, and tracheal intubation. The goal is to maintain hemodynamic stability, especially stability and/or control of the determinants of myocardial oxygen consumption. We also frequently use a lidocaine tracheal spray prior to intubation, even if lidocaine is used for the epidural block, as the time course of systemic absorption from the two sites differs.

Maintenance of general anesthesia is then accomplished; we use controlled positive-pressure ventilation and monitoring of the end-tidal concentration of carbon dioxide to keep arterial CO_2 partial pressure at approximately 35 mmHg and thus avoid cardiovascular stimulation caused by acidemia. We allow the nondepolarizing muscle relaxant to wear off if possible and rely on the epidural local anesthetic to supply muscle relaxation for procedures below the renal arteries. This technique has the advantage of allowing patient movement if the light general anesthetic we are using becomes so light that awareness is a problem. One can also avoid the muscarinic effects of reversal agents; these effects may be profound during sympathetic block induced by a local anesthetic. We also try to avoid giving further doses of narcotics, especially if we plan to give epidural narcotics postoperatively for pain control. Avoidance of

narcotics usually requires that anesthesia be maintained with nitrous oxide and occasional small increments of thiopental during periods of maximal stimulation (such as bowel manipulation and packing) or with the addition of small concentrations of a potent inhalation agent.

After general anesthesia is induced and before surgical incision, we administer local anesthetic solution through the epidural catheter to a total volume of 15 to 22 ml, depending on factors such as patient age, body habitus, and site of catheter insertion. This dose produces a good, dense somatic afferent block as well as blockade of most of the visceral afferent nerve fibers, thus creating maximum inhibition of the endocrine stress response to surgery.[39,40] The block is continued with a continuous, or virtually continuous, infusion of 6 to 8 ml/h of 1.5 percent lidocaine solution. We prefer this infusion to bolus administration because infusion eliminates the need to respond to a decrease in the local anesthetic block. Although the patient is asleep and we are unable to check the level of blockade, we have not yet had a patient for whom the level of block was too high at the end of surgery.

A second reason for using continuous epidural infusion is that it eliminates the increase in cerebrospinal fluid pressure seen with bolus administration of medication in the epidural space.[41,42] For most patients, perfusion of the spinal cord represents a physiologic "waterfall" in which cerebrospinal fluid pressure, and not spinal venous pressure, is an important component of spinal cord perfusion pressure.[43] In patients with occlusive arterial disease who undergo temporary occlusion of the aorta, spinal arterial pressure may become dangerously low, so that spinal cord perfusion pressure is critically affected by cerebrospinal fluid pressure.[44–48]

While administering local anesthetic

through the epidural catheter, we usually begin an infusion of dopamine in "renal" doses. Infusion of dopamine has the dual effect of maintaining urinary output (the value of this practice is admittedly still unclear[49]) and of providing support of myocardial contractility. Use of an epidural catheter in this patient population may impair myocardial performance because of interruption of the cardiac sympathetic innervation and/or a systemic effect of the local anesthetic.[50-53] The use of small doses of dopamine seems to offset these effects.

Once anticoagulation is initiated, we frequently monitor activated clotting time as a measure of both the adequacy of anticoagulation and as a protection against excessive anticoagulation while an epidural catheter is in place. With this safeguard, the intraoperative use of an epidural catheter appears to be quite safe.[54]

Temporary Occlusion of the Aorta

Temporary occlusion of the abdominal aorta has an unpredictable effect on cardiovascular function. Although numerous reports have studied hemodynamic variables before and after cross-clamping, and even though some of these studies have demonstrated clear-cut trends depending on study design,[29,31,55,56] there is no way to predict with certainty what the physiologic effect of the clamp will be in an individual patient. This variability is one of the principle reasons behind our decision to use pulmonary artery catheters in all patients. However, the information derived from hemodynamic monitors may have implications that vary constantly. For example, a pulmonary artery occlusion pressure that is considered adequate before the aortic cross-clamp is applied may be wholly inadequate before it is removed.[31] In addition, it has become

clear with the use of intermittent or on-line monitors of ventricular volume that diastolic compliance and systolic performance may change during abdominal aortic surgery.[57] Finally, depending on where the cross-clamp is placed and whether or not diastolic function changes, systolic wall stress may vary significantly without measured changes in the total peripheral resistance.[58] All these potential effects must be kept in mind when evaluating cardiovascular function after application of the cross-clamp.

As mentioned, we frequently use dopamine to provide renal (and mesenteric) arteriolar vasodilation. The use of other agents such as mannitol or furosemide is beneficial in animals.[59] The value of these drugs in humans for anticipated renal ischemia has not been proved[60,61] but perhaps can be justified from a physiologic point of view. For example, furosemide has the interesting quality of decreasing oxygen consumption (by enzyme inhibition) in the metabolically active region of the renal tubule. Because this area of the nephron has the most tenuous oxygen supply, the use of furosemide may protect the kidneys by decreasing oxygen demand rather than by increasing urine volume.[62]

Removal of the aortic cross-clamp can be dangerous if adequate preparations are not made. By far, the most important preparation is establishing adequate volume status before removal of the cross-clamp. To us, this goal usually means keeping pulmonary artery occlusion pressure from 12 to 16 mmHg. We correct any significant base deficit that exists before removal of the clamp but do not routinely give sodium bicarbonate prior to clamp removal. We believe that the hemodynamic consequences of clamp removal can be managed adequately with volume loading (and, if necessary, transient inotropic support). Also, the metabolic acid released from ischemic regions should be rapidly buffered and/or metabolized with normal cardiac output and hepatic perfusion. Gradual removal of the clamp by the surgeon also helps keep the physiologic excitement of this maneuver under control.

Emergence from Anesthesia

After release of the cross-clamp and before the end of the operation, we make a series of observations and decisions. First, we reestablish overall hemodynamic function using either volume infusion or vasoactive drugs, or both. Even with continuous epidural block with local anesthetics, peripheral vascular resistance and/or myocardial contractility frequently increase on emergence from anesthesia. Either condition may require treatment. The usual treatment consists of administration of either analgesics or vasodepressor agents. We prefer the latter, because we try to avoid giving sedating medications at the time of emergence. Second, the postoperative use of epidural narcotics, if planned, should be initiated approximately 1 hour before emergence. We find that spinal or epidural administration of narcotics works far better if used in a prophylactic or prospective manner. Third, if the plan is to extubate the patient shortly after surgery, the kinetics of current and planned drug administration need to be evaluated so that this goal can be accomplished. Finally, a quick evaluation of metabolic variables likely to have been disrupted by the operation is in order. Have coagulation factors been depleted, and should they be restored? Has preoperative potassium depletion or intraoperative β-adrenergic activation[63] lowered serum potassium to a level requiring treatment? What is the core temperature, and is it low enough to affect emergence decisions?

Table 16-1. Physiologic Effects of Hypothermia

System	Effect
Cardiovascular	Decreased cardiac output
	Ventricular irritability
	Negative dromotropic effect
Respiratory	Depressed mentation
	Depressed cough reflex
	Increased affinity of hemoglobin for oxygen
Metabolism	Increased oxygen requirement (e.g., from shivering)
	Increased production of lactic acid
	Decreased tissue perfusion and acid buffering
	Decreased hepatic function

The last question is frequently linked to the decision regarding extubation, although the reasons for doing so are usually unclear. Review of the physiologic effects of hypothermia (Table 16-1) shows that none is improved by endotracheal intubation and positive-pressure ventilation, although therapeutic efforts directed at these effects may necessitate mechanical ventilation. The one concern we have relates to the additive cerebral depressant effect of hypothermia and sedative medications. Small amounts of sedation have an augmented effect in the hypothermic patient. Therefore, if extubation is planned early in the postoperative period, it is particularly important to avoid additional sedation as much as possible. The question of when to extubate patients after major vascular procedures is discussed in Chapter 29. Because we plan to use epidural analgesia to control postoperative pain, we routinely extubate patients either in the operating room or within the first hour or two in the intensive care unit.

POSTOPERATIVE MANAGEMENT

Early experience with aortic reconstructive surgery taught anesthetists and surgeons a great deal regarding optimal care of their patients. Operative problems and complications were common. Today it is unusual for a major intraoperative problem to determine the ultimate outcome of the procedure. Postoperative care, which had a less spectacular historic development, has emerged as the most important determinant of overall operative outcome: it is after surgery that most complications occur.[5] Therefore, even if not involved in the early postoperative care of vascular surgical patients, the anesthetist should still pay particular attention to the transfer of care and to the possible effects that intraoperative anesthetic management may have on postoperative events.

We transfer patients from the operating room with continuous monitoring of electrocardiogram and arterial blood pressure, plus administration of supplemental oxygen. Intraoperative events and administration of medication are discussed carefully with the intensive care staff, which is usually under the medical direction of an anesthesiologist. Particular attention is paid to plans regarding control of hemodynamic variables and techniques of postoperative analgesia.

We care for all patients in the intensive care unit for at least 24 to 48 hours. The exact length of time depends on many factors. With the epidural-light general anesthesia technique, many patients look so well clinically that there is a strong temptation to discharge them from the intensive care unit early. It is important to remember that many postoperative complications, especially cardiac complications, appear 2 or 3 days after surgery[5,9] and that the ability to decrease the frequency of complications may require several days of intensive care.[32]

We use epidural administration of narcotics to control postoperative pain. Decisions consist of what agent to use, how to administer the narcotic, and whether or not to use adjunctive medications. Almost all of our patients receive morphine as the narcotic of choice. We give morphine because it is currently the only federally approved narcotic for epidural administration, and because it has a long duration of action. More lipid-soluble narcotics such as fentanyl have a faster onset of action and a shorter duration of action. Lipophilicity may also increase the likelihood of a high serum concentration of the drug. A higher concentration would increase the risk of respiratory depression. Although, to date, we have used intermittent dosing schedules for epidural administration of narcotics, we are beginning to use infusion pumps for continuous administration. Continuous administration has the potential advantage of providing more consistent pain relief and a decrease in the risk of respiratory depression owing to high transient concentrations of narcotic in the cerebrospinal fluid. Finally, it seems that the concomitant administration of both a dilute solution of local anesthetic agent (e.g., 0.125 percent bupivacaine) and a narcotic may work synergistically to improve analgesia. Synergism would permit administration of both drugs at lower total dosages to decrease their side effects. It is important to allow return of sensorimotor function in the lower extremities early in the postoperative period so that assessment of spinal cord function is possible. Once the decision is made to discontinue epidural administration of a narcotics, we find that many patients become good candidates for patient-controlled analgesia for continued pain control. The question of how long to monitor for respiratory depression after administration of epidural narcotics is difficult to answer. We use basically the same variables that other institutions have used in making this decision,[64] and we generally monitor major vascular surgical patients for 12 to 18 hours after their last epidural dose of morphine.

SUMMARY

The provision of optimal anesthetic care for patients undergoing abdominal aortic surgery requires an appreciation of two factors. The first is that one can understand the physiologic disturbances engendered by the anesthetic and the operation. Second, this information can be applied uniquely to each patient. With this approach, patient care approaches the ideal.

REFERENCES

1. Foster JH, Bolasny BL, Gobbel WG, Jr., Scott HW, Jr: Comparative study of elective resection and expectant treatment of abdominal aortic aneurysm. Surg Gynecol Obstet 129:1–9, 1969
2. Estes JE, Jr: Abdominal aortic aneurysm: a study of one hundred and two cases. Circulation 2:258–264, 1950
3. Couch NP, Lane FC, Crane C: Management and mortality in resection of abdominal aortic aneurysms. A study of 114 cases. Am J Surg 119:408–416, 1970
4. Whittemore AD, Clowes AW, Hechtman HB, Mannick JA: Aortic aneurysm repair. Reduced operative mortality associated with maintenance of optimal cardiac performance. Ann Surg 192:414–421, 1980
5. Diehl JT, Cali RF, Hertzer NR, Beven EG: Complications of abdominal aortic reconstruction. An analysis of perioperative risk factors in 557 patients. Ann Surg 197:49–56, 1983
6. Inahara T, Geary GL, Mukherjee D, Egan JM: The contrary position to the nonresective treatment for abdominal aortic aneurysm. J Vasc Surg 2:42–48, 1985
7. Bush HL, Jr., Huse JB, Johnson WC et al: Prevention of renal insufficiency after abdominal aortic aneurysm resection by optimal volume loading. Arch Surg 116:1517–1524, 1981
8. Pasternack PF, Imparato AM, Baumann FG et al: The hemodynamics of β-blockade in patients undergoing abdominal aortic aneurysm repair. Circulation, 76: suppl. III, III-1 to III-7, 1987
9. Hertzer NR: Fatal myocardial infarction following abdominal aortic aneurysm resection. Three hundred forty-three patients followed 6–11 years postoperatively. Ann Surg 192:667–673, 1980
10. Hertzer NR, Beven EG, Young JR et al: Coronary artery disease in peripheral vascular patients. A classification of 1000 coronary angiograms and results of surgical management. Ann Surg 199:223–233, 1984
11. Cutler BS, Wheeler HB, Paraskos JA, Cardullo PA: Assessment of operative risk with electrocardiographic exercise testing in patients with peripheral vascular disease. Am J Surg 137:484–490, 1979
12. Del Guercio LRM, Cohn JD: Monitoring operative risk in the elderly. JAMA 243:1350–1355, 1980
13. Hakki A-H, DePace NL, Colby J, Iskandrian AS: Implications of normal exercise electrocardiographic results in patients with angiographically documented coronary artery disease. Correlation with left ventricular function and myocardial perfusion. Am J Med 75:439–444, 1983
14. Weiner DA, McCabe CH, Dagostino G et al: Cardiokymography during exercise testing: a new device for the detection of coronary artery disease and left ventricular wall motion abnormalities. Am J Cardiol 51:1307–1311, 1983
15. Pasternack PF, Imparato AM, Bear G et al: The value of radionuclide angiography as a predictor of perioperative myocardial infarction in patients undergoing aortic aneurysm resection. J Vasc Surg 1:320–325, 1984

16. Boucher CA, Brewster DC, Darling RC et al: Determination of cardiac risk by dipyridamole-thallium imaging before peripheral vascular surgery. N Engl J Med 312:389–394, 1985

17. Cutler BS, Leppo JA: Dipyridamole thallium 201 scintigraphy to detect coronary artery disease before abdominal aortic surgery. J Vasc Surg 5:91–100, 1987

18. Tillisch J, Brunken R, Marshall R et al: Reversibility of cardiac wall-motion abnormalities predicted by positron tomography. N Engl J Med 314:884–888, 1986

19. Morise AP, McDowell DE, Savrin RA et al: The prediction of cardiac risk in patients undergoing vascular surgery. Am J Med Sci 293:150–158, 1987

20. Labovitz AJ, Pearson AC: Evaluation of left ventricular diastolic function: clinical relevance and recent Doppler echocardiographic insights. Am Heart J 114:836–851, 1987

21. Fusejima K: Noninvasive measurement of coronary artery blood flow using combined two-dimensional and Doppler echocardiography. J Am Coll Cardiol 10:1024–1031, 1987

22. Jacobson HG (ed): Magnetic resonance imaging of the cardiovascular system: present state of the art and future potential. Council on Scientific Affairs. Report of the Magnetic Resonance Imaging Panel. JAMA 259:253–259, 1988

23. Cruchley PM, Kaplan JA, Hug CC, Jr et al: Non-cardiac surgery in patients with prior myocardial revascularization. Can Anaesth Soc J 30:629–634, 1983

24. Ruby ST, Whittemore AD, Couch NP et al: Coronary artery disease in patients requiring abdominal aortic aneurysm repair. Selective use of a combined operation. Ann Surg 201:758–764, 1985

25. David TE: Combined cardiac and abdominal aortic surgery. Circulation, 72: suppl. II, II-18 to II-21, 1985

26. Hertzer NR, Young JR, Beven EG et al: Late results of coronary bypass in patients with infrarenal aortic aneurysms. The Cleveland Clinic study. Ann Surg 205:360–367, 1987

27. Ansley DM, Ramsay JG, Whalley DG et al: The relationship between central venous pressure and pulmonary capillary wedge pressure during aortic surgery. Can J Anaesth 34:594–600, 1987

28. Bush HL, Jr., LoGerfo FW, Weisel RD et al: Assessment of myocardial performance and optimal volume loading during elective abdominal aortic aneurysm resection. Arch Surg 112:1301–1306, 1977

29. Silverstein PR, Caldera DL, Cullen DJ et al: Avoiding the hemodynamic consequences of aortic cross-clamping and unclamping. Anesthesiology 50:462–466, 1979

30. Reiz S, Peter T, Rais O: Hemodynamic and cardiometabolic effects of infrarenal aortic and common iliac artery declamping in man—an approach to optimal volume loading. Acta Anaesthesiol Scand 23:579–586, 1979

31. Lunn JK, Dannemiller FJ, Stanley TH: Cardiovascular responses to clamping of the aorta during epidural and general anesthesia. Anesth Analg 58:372–376, 1979

32. Rao TLK, Jacobs KH, El-Etr AA: Reinfarction following anesthesia in patients with myocardial infarction. Anesthesiology 59:499–505, 1983

33. Keane RM, Munster AM, Birmingham W et al: Suppression of lymphocyte function after aortic reconstruction. Use of nonimmunosuppressive anesthesia. Arch Surg 117:1133–1135, 1982

34. Foster RS, Jr., Costanza MC, Foster JC et al: Adverse relationship between blood transfusions and survival after colectomy for colon cancer. Cancer 55:1195–1201, 1985

35. Clarke PJ, Tarin D: Effect of pre-operative blood transfusion on tumour metastases. Br J Surg 74:520–522, 1987

36. Waymack JP, Gallon L, Barcelli U et al: Effect of blood transfusions on immune function. III. Alterations in macrophage arachidonic acid metabolism. Arch Surg 122:56–60, 1987

37. Blumberg N, Agarwal MM, Chuang C: Relation between recurrence of cancer of the colon and blood transfusion. Br Med J 290:1037–1039, 1985

38. Odoom JA, Sih IL: Epidural analgesia and anticoagulant therapy. Experience with

one thousand cases of continuous epidurals. Anaesthesia 38:254–259, 1983

39. Engquist A, Brandt MR, Fernandes A, Kehlet H: The blocking effect of epidural analgesia on adrenocortical and hyperglycemic responses to surgery. Acta Anaesthesiol Scand 21:330–335, 1977

40. Møller IW, Hjortsø E, Krantz T et al: The modifying effect of spinal anaesthesia on intra- and postoperative adrenocortical and hyperglycaemic response to surgery. Acta Anaesthesiol Scand 28:266–269, 1984

41. Usubiaga JE, Usubiaga LE, Brea LM, Goyena R: Effect of saline injections on epidural and subarachnoid space pressures and relation to postspinal anesthesia headache. Anesth Analg 46:293–296, 1967

42. Hilt H, Gramm H-J, Link J: Changes in intracranial pressure associated with extradural anaesthesia. Br J Anaesth 58:676–680, 1986

43. Griffiths IR, Pitts LH, Crawford RA, Trench JG: Spinal cord compression and blood flow. I. The effect of raised cerebrospinal fluid pressure on spinal cord blood flow. Neurology 28:1145–1151, 1978

44. Blaisdell FW, Cooley DA: The mechanism of paraplegia after temporary thoracic aortic occlusion and its relationship to spinal fluid pressure. Surgery 51:351–355, 1962

45. Grace RR, Mattox KL: Anterior spinal artery syndrome following abdominal aortic aneurysmectomy. Case report and review of the literature. Arch Surg 112:813–815, 1977

46. Wadouh F, Lindemann E-M, Arndt CF et al: The arteria radicularis magna anterior as a decisive factor influencing spinal cord damage during aortic occlusion. J Thorac Cardiovasc Surg 88:1–10, 1984

47. Wadough F, Arndt C-F, Oppermann E et al: The mechanism of spinal cord injury after simple and double aortic cross-clamping. J Thorac Cardiovasc Surg 92:121–127, 1986

48. Dasmahapatra HK, Coles JG, Taylor MJ et al: Identification of risk factors for spinal cord ischemia by the use of monitoring of somatosensory evoked potentials using coarctation repair. Circulation, 76: suppl. III, III-14 to III-18, 1987

49. Alpert RA, Roizen MF, Hamilton WK et al: Intraoperative urinary output does not predict postoperative renal function in patients undergoing abdominal aortic revascularization. Surgery 95:707–711, 1984

50. Wattwil M, Sundberg A, Arvill A, Lennquist C: Circulatory changes during high thoracic epidural anaesthesia—influence of sympathetic block and of systemic effect of the local anaesthetic. Acta Anaesthesiol Scand 29:849–855, 1985

51. Bunt TJ, Manczuk M, Varley K: Continuous epidural anesthesia for aortic surgery: thoughts on peer review and safety. Surgery 101:706–714, 1987

52. Sundberg A, Wattwil M, Wiklund L: Haemodynamic effects of intravenous bupivacaine during high thoracic epidural anaesthesia. Acta Anaesthesiol Scand 31:143–147, 1987

53. Lundberg J, Norgren L, Thomson D, Werner O: Hemodynamic effects of dopamine during thoracic epidural analgesia in man. Anesthesiology 66:641–646, 1987

54. Rao TLK, El-Etr AA: Angicoagulation following placement of epidural and subarachnoid catheters: an evaluation of neurologic sequelae. Anesthesiology 55:618–620, 1981

55. Dunn E, Prager RL, Fry W, Kirsh MM: The effect of abdominal aortic cross-clamping on myocardial function. J Surg Res 22:463–468, 1977

56. Johnston WE, Balestrieri FJ, Plonk G et al: The influence of periaortic collateral vessels on the intraoperative hemodynamic effects of acute aortic occlusion in patients with aorto-occlusive disease or abdominal aortic aneurysm. Anesthesiology 66:386–389, 1987

57. Kalman PG, Wellwood MR, Weisel RD et al: Cardiac dysfunction during abdominal aortic operation: the limitations of pulmonary wedge pressures. J Vasc Surg 3:773–781, 1986

58. Roizen MF, Beaupre PN, Alpert RA et al: Monitoring with two-dimensional transesophageal echocardiography. Comparison of myocardial function in patients

undergoing supraceliac, suprarenal-infraceliac, or infrarenal aortic occlusion. J Vasc Surg 1:300–305, 1984

59. Abbott WM, Austen WG: The reversal of renal cortical ischemia during aortic occlusion by mannitol. J Surg Res 16:482–489, 1974

60. Gamulin Z, Forster A, Morel D et al: Effects of infrarenal aortic cross-clamping on renal hemodynamics in humans. Anesthesiology 61:394–399, 1984

61. Brown CB, Ogg CS, Cameron JS: High dose frusemide in acute renal failure: a controlled trial. Clin Nephrol 15:90–96, 1981

62. Brezis M, Rosen S, Silva P, Epstein FH: Renal ischemia: a new perspective. Kidney Int 26:375–383, 1984

63. Brown MJ, Brown DC, Murphy MB: Hypokalemia from beta$_2$-receptor stimulation by circulating epinephrine. N Engl J Med 309:1414–1419, 1983

64. Ready LB, Oden R, Chadwick HS et al: Development of an anesthesiology-based postoperative pain management service. Anesthesiology 68:100–106, 1988

17

Anesthesia for Resection of Abdominal Aortic Aneurysm: One Approach at Baylor College of Medicine

Salwa A. Shenaq

Physicians often ask whether all abdominal aneurysms should be resected. Most vascular surgeons agree that surgery should be considered for every aneurysm.[1] Aortic aneurysm is a serious disease: the untreated aneurysm often ruptures and causes sudden death.[2] The classic study by Estes[3] in 1950 reported a 5-year survival rate of only 18.9 percent for 102 patients with abdominal aortic aneurysm who did not have surgery; 63.3 percent of the deaths resulted from rupture of the aneurysm.[3,4] Other studies on unoperated aneurysms reported survival rates of only 54.3 percent at 1 year and 17.2 percent at 5 years.[4,5] In a fourth study (68 patients), 39.7 percent lived less than 1 year after diagnosis, 29.4 percent were alive at the end of 2 years, 11.8 percent lived 4 years, and fewer than 5 percent lived 5 years.[6] Other reports confirm that aneurysm of the abdominal aorta is unpredictable and potentially fatal.[7]

Fortunately, operative mortality has decreased steadily since the first successful resection and graft replacement of an abdominal aortic aneurysm in 1951.[8]

Several factors are responsible: the increasing experience of surgeons; refinements in surgical techniques; and tremendous improvements in anesthesia, monitoring, and postoperative care.[2]

Operative mortality is now less than 1 percent; the 10-year survival rate has improved from 0 (with medical treatment) to 30 percent (with graft replacement), despite the advanced age of some patients.[2,9-11] Discussing the factors influencing survival, Crawford et al.[2] described 920 consecutive patients at Baylor who had graft replacement for infrarenal abdominal aortic aneurysm from 1955 to 1980. The survival rate for the 60 patients (6.5 percent) whose aneurysm had ruptured was 77 percent. The survival rate for the 860 patients (93.5 percent) whose aneurysm had not ruptured was 95 percent. Mortality within 30 days of surgery decreased from 18 percent in the 1950s to 1.43 percent in 1979 and 1980. Heart disease, hypertension, and advanced age were the chief risk factors associated with these early deaths. Over the 25 years of study, the mortality rate for patients having these risk factors decreased from 19.2 to 1.9 percent (Fig. 17-1).[2]

Therefore, the consensus among vascular surgeons seems to be that abdominal aortic aneurysm almost always warrants surgery, even when symptoms are absent. Two facts support this belief: (1) the life expectancy of patients undergoing such surgery has improved greatly; and (2) the operative mortality rate for patients who have asymptomatic aortic aneurysm has decreased.[1]

PATIENT PRESENTATION

For asymptomatic patients, aneurysm is often discovered accidentally as a pulsatile midabdominal mass during physical examination. If occlusive disease exists, a bruit may be heard. Other patients report abnormal pulsation. Routine abdominal roentgenography may show calcification in the wall of the aneurysm.

For some patients with angina, a pulsatile abdominal mass is discovered during evaluation and general examination. Sometimes aneurysm of the abdominal segment of the aorta is discovered during evaluation of a primary aneurysm elsewhere in the aorta. A small percentage of patients present for the first time with a ruptured or leaking aneurysm; of 1,110 patients with infrarenal abdominal aortic aneurysm, 6 percent were operated on for ruptured aneurysm.[12]

Yet another group of patients undergoes exploratory surgery that for some reason has to be terminated, with sub-

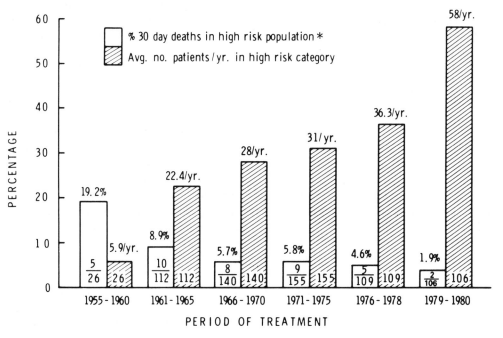

Fig. 17-1. Results from a study of 920 patients who had surgery for infrarenal abdominal aortic aneurysm at Baylor College of Medicine from 1955 to 1980. This graph provides data regarding early deaths among the 648 high-risk patients in the study, that is those who were elderly or had heart disease. Although the number of high-risk patients who were treated *increased* 10-fold over 25 years, the percentage of early deaths among such patients *decreased* 10-fold. *Significance at $P < 0.01$. (From Crawford et al.,[2] with permission.)

sequent transfer of the patient to our hospital for resection of the aneurysm. For example, the general condition of the patient may require extensive perioperative support not available at small, remote hospitals. Also, exploratory surgery may reveal that resection of the aneurysm is beyond the expertise of the surgeon performing the initial operation.

DIAGNOSIS OF ANEURYSM

Most patients with abdominal aortic aneurysm are referred by nonvascular surgeons and radiologists who diagnose the condition during study of the abdomen, that is, during procedures involving the gastrointestinal tract, back, kidney, bladder, ureter, and other areas.[12] For 75 percent of patients, abdominal aortic aneurysm can be diagnosed easily by palpating a pulsatile abdominal mass. However, for some patients (e.g., the obese or those having pain and tenderness), palpation of the aneurysm may be difficult. The presence of a calcified shadow in the abdomen around the aorta should alert the physician to the presence of an aneurysm.

Although ultrasonography performed for other abdominal complaints may reveal an aneurysm, the presence of gastrointestinal gas or radiopaque material may render results inaccurate. On the other hand, ultrasonography can be an excellent diagnostic tool for asymptomatic patients who have only minimal gastrointestinal air.[12] Despite significant improvements in ultrasonographic technique and equipment over the past 10 years, ultrasonography is still less accurate than computed tomography (CT) in diagnosing the size and extent of abdominal aortic aneurysms.[13]

The accuracy of aortography in diagnosing aneurysms depends on the expertise of the radiologist. Aortography is helpful in demonstrating the patency of aortic branches, the branches of greatest concern being the visceral vessels. Our goal in examining the aortogram is to exclude associated occlusion.[12] Also, the aortogram shows the proximity of the aneurysm to the renal arteries. Because it provides the surgeon with greater detail, digital subtraction angiography is becoming increasingly popular. In addition, this method uses less contrast medium and thus lessens the associated hazards.

Computed tomography is an extremely accurate method of diagnosing and evaluating the upper abdominal segment of the aorta.[12] Also, the use of thin-section (as opposed to conventional) CT improves detection of the origin of at least one renal artery to almost 100 percent.[13] For accurate diagnosis, our surgeons prefer CT scanning, aortography, or both.

EVALUATION OF ASSOCIATED CONDITIONS

To detect any associated conditions that increase surgical risk, we evaluate the patient thoroughly before surgery. Because myocardial infarction is the leading cause of death after major vascular surgery,[14] any patient with angina (of any degree) is also evaluated by a cardiologist. Of 860 patients who had surgery for nonruptured infrarenal abdominal aortic aneurysm, over half of the 41 deaths resulted from cardiac disease (2.4 percent)[2] However, we do not perform coronary angiography routinely for every aortic aneurysm (as recommended by Hertzer and colleagues[15]), but only when patients are symptomatic and have positive results on stress test. Noninvasive nuclear and echocardiographic studies performed before cardiac catherization help us determine the severity of coronary artery disease, the condition of the valves, and the nature of ventricular wall motion. Patients with severe coronary artery disease usually undergo myocardial revascularization before resection of the aneurysm.

Abdominal aortic aneurysm may be accompanied by decreased renal function. Although dissecting aneurysm involving the renal arteries is an uncommon event in abdominal aortic disease, the presence of this condition can impair renal function. Also, generalized atherosclerosis may involve the renal artery. If the aneurysmal process includes the renal artery, occlusion of the renal arteries is possible. An additional hazard is the nephrotoxic effect of contrast medium used for aortography. For these reasons, we evaluate renal function by measuring blood urea nitrogen (BUN) and creatinine levels in all patients with abdominal aortic aneurysm. Those who have elevated levels are evaluated by a nephrologist. Although we ensure proper hydration before surgery, we do not insert a pulmonary artery catheter preoperatively unless the patient has severe coronary artery disease. In addition, surgery and aortography are usually not performed on the same day. Infusion of sodium bicarbonate (50 mEq) with 25 g of mannitol in 1,000 ml of 5 percent dextrose in 0.2 percent saline during and after aortography decreases the possibility of nephrotoxic effects from contrast medium.[16]

In our view, proper control of hypertension is important in stabilizing hemodynamic status and avoiding major changes in blood pressure, especially during clamping and unclamping of the aorta. Therefore, most of our patients with aneurysms are now given calcium channel-blocking drugs and diuretics on the day of surgery. Before the widespread use of calcium channel-blocking drugs, most patients were given propranolol.

Pulmonary function is evaluated thoroughly. All pulmonary infections are treated aggressively to prevent postoperative pulmonary problems, to shorten the period of mechanical ventilation, and to minimize postoperative pulmonary infection. Patients with excessive pulmonary secretions undergo pulmonary toilet and physiotherapy. Patients are usually informed about the use of postoperative incentive spirometry and positive-pressure ventilation during the anesthetist's visit.

If the patient is diabetic, blood glucose levels are usually measured before and during surgery. If glucose exceeds 250 mg/dl, we administer 10 units of regular insulin and continue measuring glucose levels after surgery.

THE PREOPERATIVE VISIT

Our general practice is to acquaint ourselves with the patient and explain anesthesia and the preparation for surgery at least 36 hours before surgery. We also describe the use of an endotracheal tube, the postoperative intensive care unit (ICU) environment, and the purpose of mechanical ventilation and respiratory therapy. If, on occasion, the surgeon has not been able to discuss the procedure with the patient on the day before surgery, we are not able to visit the patient until the day of surgery.

The anesthetist usually reviews the record and laboratory tests to ensure that the patient is in the best possible condition before surgery. This practice minimizes the chance of cancellation of surgery or disagreement with the surgeon. Surgery is seldom canceled because of the general condition of the patient.

PREOPERATIVE SEDATION

After meeting with the patient, we select the premedication most appropriate for the general condition and age of the patient. Normally, light sedation is given while the patient is still in the room. As soon as the patient reaches the anesthesia holding area, an intravenous catheter is inserted for administration of extra sedation. The resulting heavy sedation decreases the apprehension that can cause angina, a tremendous increase in blood pressure, and even expansion of the aneurysm. During this period, the patient is monitored closely.

For the past few years, the most frequently used premedications at our institution have been diazepam (2.5 to 5 mg) and diphenhydramine (25 to 50 mg), given orally while the patient was still in the room or intravenously on arrival at the anesthesia holding area. Recently, however, we have been administering lorazepam (1 to 2 mg) orally about 1 to 2 hours prior to anticipated entry into the operating room, or intravenous midazolam, titrated slowly. Midazolam is usually diluted to 1 mg/ml, the average-size patient receiving 2.5 mg for sedation. Patients 75 years of age or older are given only diphenhydramine (25 mg) or no sedation. Diphenhydramine is an antihistamine and sedative having anticholinergic effects. Because histamine release is possible after administration of narcotics and some muscle relaxants, we believe that diphenhydramine has a place in the preoperative medication plan.

For a few patients, pressure exerted by the aneurysm causes pain, frequently in the back. Severe pain and tenderness are signs of leakage or impending rupture of the aneurysm. Patients given a small dose of narcotic (3 mg of morphine sulfate or 25 μg of fentanyl intravenously) to relieve pain are monitored closely in the holding area. Some patients may require administration of oxygen before surgery.

After inserting an intravenous catheter (usually 16 gauge), we administer sedation. When the patient is comfortable, a 20-gauge catheter is inserted into the radial artery of the arm having the better pulse.

A few patients may be admitted to the ICU the night before surgery because their condition is unstable or because they have advanced multisystem disease. These patients usually have venous catheters (peripheral and central) in place; most of them will also have a pulmonary artery catheter in place to guide management of hemodynamic variables. These patients usually remain in the ICU until surgery.

TRANSFER TO THE OPERATING ROOM

The anesthesiologist, anesthesia resident, and surgery resident normally accompany the patient to the operating room. If the patient was being given oxygen in the holding area, a portable oxygen tank is transferred with the patient. For critically ill patients, a portable monitor is used during transfer. On arrival at the operating room, oxygen is given while monitoring devices are applied. Baseline heart rate and blood pressure are recorded, and anesthesia is induced.

INDUCTION OF ANESTHESIA AND MONITORING

The patient is positioned supine with the arms placed alongside the trunk. Padding protects the elbows, and a folded towel usually supports the wrists. Aspiration confirms proper functioning of the arterial line. We induce anesthesia with 2.5 mg of midazolam, titrating a narcotic (fentanyl or sufentanil) until the lash reflex is abolished. (The average-size patient with good left ventricular function usually requires a total of 0.5 to 1 mg of fentanyl or 3 to 5 µg/kg of sufentanil.) To prevent chest rigidity, we generally administer 1 mg of pancuronium bromide before the narcotic. If these drugs do not produce sleep, 50 to 100 mg of thiopental is added before administration of muscle relaxant. As soon as the lash reflex is lost, we administer pancuronium bromide (0.1 mg/kg) intravenously to facilitate endotracheal intubation. We also give lidocaine (1 mg/kg) intravenously before intubation to obtund laryngeal reflexes. At this time, we ventilate the patient with 100 percent oxygen and insert a urinary catheter and temperature probe. After endotracheal intubation, the patient is placed in the Trendelenburg position.

Our usual practice is to insert a central venous catheter into the right or left subclavian vein for rapid administration of emergency drugs. Also, a pulmonary artery catheter is floated through the right internal jugular vein. We use both types of catheter because the latter is removed 24 or 48 hours after surgery, whereas the central venous catheter is left in place for 3 to 4 days. The peripheral venous catheter is usually removed on the second postoperative day.

A nasogastric tube is inserted and a baseline hemodynamic profile is recorded—heart rate; blood pressure; and central venous pressure, pulmonary artery pressure, and pulmonary capillary wedge pressure (PCWP). We also measure cardiac output and calculate peripheral vascular resistance. Electrocardiographic leads V_5 and II are monitored continuously. Although lead V_5 is believed to reveal myocardial ischemia, it is still an insensitive detector of early ischemia. Also, PCWP may be an inaccurate indicator of myocardial dysfunction in patients with stiff (noncompliant) left ventricles.[17] Although transesophageal echocardiography is a safe and sensitive indicator of myocardial dysfunction and ischemia, and although it has a rational basis for use during operative management of high-risk patients,[18] at this time it is not available to us for intraoperative use. We are in the process of investigating its use intraoperatively.

MAINTENANCE OF ANESTHESIA

Before starting the incision, extra doses of narcotics are administered together with a small amount (0.25 to 0.5 percent) of isoflurane or enflurane for maintenance of anesthesia. The patient is ventilated with 100 percent oxygen. In our opinion, these large doses of narcotics eliminate the need for nitrous oxide and thus the myocardial depressant effect of that agent.[19]

Four infusions are usually kept ready: nitroglycerin (100 µg/ml), dopamine (1,600 µg/ml), phenylephrine (100 µg/ml), and nitroprusside (100 µg/ml). These infusions are connected to the central venous line through small connection tubing (designed by us at this institution) having four entry sites.

Hemodynamic profiles are recorded at the following times: after incision, during exposure of the aneurysm, before and after clamping and unclamping of the aorta, and at the end of surgery. Recording of such profiles ensures that therapeutic decisions will be made and reviewed, at a minimum, at these key time periods.

INTRAOPERATIVE CONSIDERATIONS AND MANAGEMENT OF HEMODYNAMIC STATUS

To avoid hypothermia during surgery, we use blood warmers during administration of fluids and blood. The room is kept at a temperature tolerable to the surgical team and appropriate for the patient, and temperature is varied according to the individual needs of the patient. Use of a humidifier also prevents heat loss. We do not use warming blankets during surgery.

Clamping of the Aorta

Occluding the aorta not only increases blood pressure, systemic vascular resistance (SVR), afterload, pulmonary artery pressure, and PCWP but also decreases cardiac output. Administering a vasodilating drug such as sodium nitroprusside before or during aortic cross-clamping almost always reverses these deleterious effects. We always watch the surgeon in anticipation of aortic cross-clamping. The surgeon normally notifies us 30 seconds before clamping the aorta. As the aorta is being clamped slowly, we start the infusion of nitroprusside; blood pressure and pulmonary artery pressure change very little. During cross-clamping, we normally infuse a vasodilating drug even if blood pressure is not high. Although the dose is minimal, it allows us to give more volume without overload. We believe that such controlled volume loading helps prevent hypovolemia and hypotension upon removal of the aortic clamp.

After completion of the proximal anastomosis, the surgeon usually flushes the graft by temporarily removing the aortic clamp to ensure that there are no leaks at the suture line. The infusion of sodium nitroprusside is stopped momentarily and then resumed after the clamp is repositioned.

Because aortic cross-clamping is stressful, utmost attention to hemodynamic status is necessary to prevent left ventricular failure. This requirement is especially pertinent to patients with coronary artery disease (particularly compromised left ventricular function), as occlusion of the aorta may increase myocardial oxygen consumption and aggravate ischemia.[20,21]

As mentioned earlier, infusion of sodium nitroprusside prevents hypertension during aortic cross-clamping. For patients with coronary artery disease, we initially try to control blood pressure with infusion of nitroglycerin.[22] If this does not succeed, we add nitroprusside to minimize the intracoronary "steal" sometimes resulting from the use of sodium nitroprusside. After measuring cardiac output and calculating SVR, we may find that one of the situations shown in Table 17-1 exists; if so, we treat the condition as indicated in the table.

Unclamping of the Aorta

At the surgeon's 30-second notice of aortic unclamping, we stop infusing the vasodilating drug and increase volume infusion. Depending on the hemoglobin level (we try to keep it above 9 g/dl), the volume infused consists of Plasmalyte solution, autologous blood, or banked blood. We routinely transfuse autologous blood in all surgery for abdominal aneurysm. The device we use is the Baylor rapid autologous transfusion (BRAT) system, developed at Baylor for rapid blood salvage (Kardiothor, Inc., Houston, TX). BRAT has 1/4-inch-caliber tubing and a high-capacity roller pump that speeds processing of shed blood (Fig. 17-2).[23] The red blood cells are concentrated at a rate of 600 ml/min, washing is accomplished at a rate of 2 L/min, and the cells

Table 17-1. Treatment for Various Hemodynamic States during Occlusion of the Abdominal Aorta[a]

CO	BP	PCWP	SVR	Administer
↓	↓	↓	Ø	Volume
↓	↑	↑	↑	Vasodilating drug
↑	↓	↓	↓	Vasoconstricting drug
↓	↓	Ø or ↑	Ø	Cardiotonic drug

[a] CO = cardiac output; BP = blood pressure; PCWP = pulmonary capillary wedge pressure; and SVR = systemic vascular resistance. ↑ = increase; ↓ = decrease; and Ø = no change.

are reinfused to the bag at 1 L/min. With BRAT, the average time for salvaging a unit of shed blood decreases from 10 to 15 minutes to 2 to 3 minutes. The average number of units salvaged is two. Since the start of the use of BRAT, patients with uncomplicated infrarenal abdominal aortic aneurysm have not had to receive banked blood.

Despite volume infusion, hypotension usually occurs when the aorta is unclamped. Although the exact mechanism of declamping shock is not well understood, many causes have been suggested: sequestration and pooling of blood in the segment of the aorta below the clamp; release of vasodepressor substances; washout acidosis; and hypovolemia.[24] Another explanation is that hypertension during clamping of the aorta contributes to deterioration of myocardial function after the clamp is removed.[20,21]

Monitoring of urinary volume is important to ensure proper renal function during surgery. Our practice is not to use mannitol routinely for all patients with infrarenal aortic aneurysm but only for those with compromised renal function. In that instance, we infuse 25 g of mannitol 15 to 20 minutes before occlusion of the aorta.

Studies have produced conflicting results regarding other changes in renal hemodynamics during infrarenal aortic cross-clamping. Three studies reported no change in renal blood flow during infrarenal aortic cross-clamping.[25-27] A fourth study, however, reported a 75 percent increase in renal vascular resistance and a 38 percent decrease in renal blood flow.[28]

When an aneurysm is close to the renal arteries (juxtarenal aneurysm) and the aorta is clamped above the renal artery, renal ischemia occurs. Renal dysfunction may occur if the aorta is clamped for a long time. Mannitol may be beneficial for such patients and should be given, if you are going to give it, before aortic cross-clamping. For such patients, we commonly infuse small doses (2 to 3 μg/kg/min) of dopamine for its renal vasodilating effect.[29,30]

SURGICAL CONSIDERATIONS OF SPECIAL INTEREST TO THE ANESTHETIST

In routine infrarenal abdominal aortic aneurysm, aneurysmectomy is performed after cross-clamping of the aorta proximal and distal to the aneurysm. If possible, the proximal clamp is placed distal to the renal arteries. The distal clamps are usually placed to occlude the iliac arteries. The wall of the aneurysm is opened, and a tubular woven Dacron graft is sutured

In juxtarenal aneurysm, it is difficult to expose and clamp the aortic segment distal to the renal arteries. Therefore, the surgeon applies the aortic clamp proximal to the renal arteries at the hiatus of the diaphragm. Reconstruction is performed from inside the aneurysm and with minimal dissection around the aneurysm.[12] This technique also is used in two other circumstances: when the aneurysm has been explored recently and surgery has been aborted after dissection at the proximal end of the aneurysm; and when an aneurysm has ruptured and the aorta is clamped without dissection in order to control bleeding as quickly as possible.[12] In rare situations in which the patient has had multiple abdominal procedures in the past and in which extensive adhesions may be encountered, a retroperitoneal approach is used for exposure and resection of the aneurysm.

We generally do not administer heparin intravenously during resection of an abdominal aortic aneurysm and believe flushing of the graft is adequate to prevent clotting.

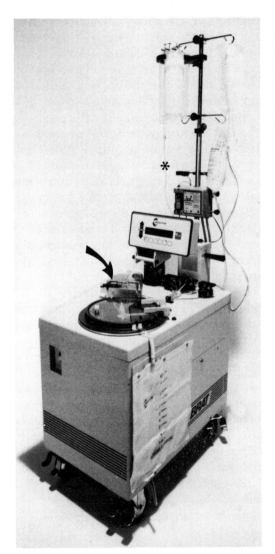

Fig. 17-2. Baylor rapid autologous transfusion (BRAT) system. The large-caliber tubing (*) and high-capacity roller pump (arrow) make possible rapid processing of shed autologous blood. (Courtesy of Kardiothor, Inc.)

in place. In 40 percent of patients, the aneurysm involves the aortic bifurcation and the iliac arteries.[12] This involvement may consist of either aneurysmal dilatation or atherosclerotic occlusive disease.[12] In this situation, a bifurcated graft is used.

TERMINATION OF THE OPERATION

After proper hemostasis at the suture line, the abdominal incision is closed. The muscle relaxant is not reversed, but the inhalation anesthetic is turned off. We do not extubate the trachea at the end of the procedure and usually continue mechanical ventilation for 4 to 6 hours postoperatively. If blood pressure is elevated, either sodium nitroprusside or nitroglycerin is infused during transport of the patient from the operating room to the ICU. Extra sedation may be required.

TRANSPORT OF THE PATIENT AND POSTOPERATIVE CARE

The period from the end of surgery to stabilization in the ICU can be hazardous if attention relaxes. Blood pressure may rise, or conversely, hypotension may occur because of lack of stimulation. These events can disturb the balance between left ventricular oxygen supply and demand and further compromise left ventricular function, especially in patients with coronary artery disease. This situation can be aggravated by hypothermia and shivering. Minimal movement of the patient and careful attention to cardiopulmonary status are important during this period. Before moving the patient from the operating table to the ICU bed, we check vital signs. If hemodynamic status is not stable, we postpone transfer to the ICU.

Attention to airway (endotracheal tube), monitoring devices, and intravenous tubing is important during transfer. We usually observe the electrocardiogram and blood pressure by portable monitor during transfer to the ICU. As soon as the monitoring lines are connected to the bedside monitor in the ICU, we again assess vital signs. The patient is ventilated mechanically with a volume-cycled ventilator (rate, 10 breaths/min; tidal volume, 10 ml/kg; and fractional concentration of inspired oxygen, 0.6).

Attention to urinary output is also important to us at this time. Normally, we measure urinary output every hour for the first 6 hours. Nurses generally draw our attention to renal function if urinary output is less than 30 ml/h for two consecutive hours.

To prevent gastric dilatation and ileus in patients undergoing surgery for aneurysm, we almost always insert a nasogastric tube during surgery and leave it in place until peristalsis starts. Irrigation of the tube with saline every few hours ensures patency. Auscultation of the abdomen for bowel sounds, usually present on the third or fourth postoperative day, is important in detecting ileus.

Because hypothermia usually occurs at the end of surgery, temperature monitoring continues postoperatively: the shivering that may accompany hypothermia can increase myocardial oxygen consumption tremendously.[31] We do not use warming blankets during surgery but do use them after surgery if necessary.

If excessive bleeding occurs, we perform a battery of coagulation tests (Coagulogram): determination of prothrombin time, partial thromboplastin time, fibrinogen level, platelet count, and Sonoclot (the Sonoclot instrument [Sienco, Inc., Morrison, Co] assesses platelet function by measuring clot impedance on a vibrating probe).[32]

In summary, successful surgery for aneurysm requires not only harmonious teamwork between surgeon and anesthetist but also careful attention to hemodynamic status, especially during clamping and unclamping of the aorta. Vigilance from the preoperative period into the postoperative period is, we believe, a key to successful outcome.

REFERENCES

1. Vollmar JF: What's new in surgical treatment of abdominal aortic lesions? J Cardiovasc Surg 23:202–204, 1982
2. Crawford ES, Saleh SA, Babb JW III et al: Infrarenal abdominal aortic aneurysm. Factors influencing survival after operation performed over a 25-year period. Ann Surg 193:699–709, 1981
3. Estes JE, Jr: Abdominal aortic aneurysm: a study of one hundred and two cases. Circulation 2:258–264, 1950

4. Lawrie GM, Crawford ES, Morris GC Jr, Howell JF: Progress in the treatment of ruptured abdominal aortic aneurysm. World J Surg 4:653–660, 1980

5. Ottinger LW: Ruptured arteriosclerotic aneurysms of the abdominal aorta. Reducing mortality. JAMA 233:147–150, 1975

6. Wright IS, Urdaneta E, Wright B: Reopening the case of the abdominal aortic aneurysm. Circulation 13:754–768, 1956

7. Szilagyi DE, Elliott JP, Smith RF: Clinical fate of the patient wth asymptomatic abdominal aortic aneurysm and unfit for surgical treatment. Arch Surg 104:600–606, 1972

8. Dubost C, Allary M, Oeconomos N: Resection of an aneurysm of the abdominal aorta. Reestablishment of the continuity by a preserved human arterial graft, with result after five months. Arch Surg 64:405–408, 1952

9. De Bakey ME, Crawford ES, Cooley DA et al: Aneurysm of abdominal aorta. Analysis of results of graft replacement therapy one to eleven years after operation. Ann Surg 160:622–639, 1964

10. Volpetti G, Barker CF, Berkowitz H, Roberts B: A twenty-two year review of elective resection of abdominal aortic aneurysms. Surg Gynecol Obstet 142:321–342, 1976

11. Whittemore AD, Clowes AW, Hechtman HB, Mannick JA: Aortic aneurysm repair. Reduced operative mortality associated with maintenance of optimal cardiac performance. Ann Surg 192:414–421, 1980

12. Crawford ES, Crawford JL: Degenerative infrarenal abdominal aortic aneurysm. p. 134–135. In: Diseases of the Aorta. Williams & Wilkins, Baltimore, 1984

13. Gomes MN, Choyke PL: Pre-operative evaluation of abdominal aortic aneurysms: ultrasound or computed tomography? J Cardiovasc Surg 28:159–166, 1987

14. Mauney FM, Jr., Ebert PA, Sabiston DC, Jr: Postoperative myocardial infarction: a study of predisposing factors, diagnosis and mortality in a high risk group of surgical patients. Ann Surg 172:497–503, 1970

15. Hertzer NR, Young JR, Kramer JR et al: Routine coronary angiography prior to elective aortic reconstruction. Results of selective myocardial revascularization in patients with peripheral vascular disease. Arch Surg 114:1336–1344, 1979

16. McEvoy J, McGeown MG, Kumar R: Renal failure after radiological contrast media. Br Med J 4:717–718, 1970

17. Hansen RM, Viquerat CE, Matthay MA et al: Poor correlation between pulmonary arterial wedge pressure and left ventricular end-diastolic volume after coronary artery bypass graft surgery. Anesthesiology 64:764–770, 1986

18. Gewertz BL, Kremser PC, Zarins CK et al: Transesophageal echocardiographic monitoring of myocardial ischemia during vascular surgery. J Vasc Surg 5:607–613, 1987

19. Eisele JH, Smith NT: Cardiovascular effects of 40 percent nitrous oxide in man. Anesth Analg 51:956–963, 1972

20. Dunn E, Prager RL, Fry W, Kirsh MM: The effect of abdominal aortic crossclamping on myocardial function. J Surg Res 22:463–468, 1977

21. Attia RR, Murphy JD, Snider M et al: Myocardial ischemia due to infrarenal aortic cross-clamping during aortic surgery in patients with severe coronary artery disease. Circulation 53:961–965, 1976

22. Zaidan JR, Guffin AV, Perdue G et al: Hemodynamics of intravenous nitroglycerin during aortic clamping. Arch Surg 117:1285–1288, 1982

23. Yawn DH, Crawford ES, Saleh S et al: An improved intraoperative red cell salvage system for rapid auto-transfusion (abstract). Transfusion 22:415(S43), 1982

24. Grindlinger GA, Vegas AM, Manny J et al: Volume loading and vasodilators in abdominal aortic aneurysmectomy. Am J Surg 139:480–486, 1980

25. Foster JH, Adkins RB, Chamberlain NO et al: The renal effects of lower abdominal aortic cross-clamping. Report of negative results in dogs and monkeys. JAMA 183:451–454, 1963

26. Abbott WM, Cooper JD, Austen WG: The effect of aortic clamping and declamping on renal blood flow distribution. J Surg Res 14:385–392, 1973

27. Cronenwett JL, Lindenauer SM: Distribution of intrarenal blood flow following aortic clamping and declamping. J Surg Res 22:469–482, 1977

28. Gamulin Z, Forster A, Morel D et al: Effects of infrarenal aortic cross-clamping on renal hemodynamics in humans. Anesthesiology 61:394–399, 1984

29. Goldberg LI: Cardiovascular and renal actions of dopamine: potential clinical applications. Pharmacol Rev 24:1–29, 1972

30. McNay JL, McDonald RH, Jr., Goldberg LI: Direct renal vasodilation produced by dopamine in the dog. Circ Res 16:510–517, 1965

31. Bernhard VM, Towne JB (eds): Complications in Vascular Surgery. Grune & Stratton, Orlando, FL, 1980

32. Saleem A, Blifeld C, Saleh SA: Viscoelastic measurement of clot formation: a new test of platelet function. Ann Clin Lab Sci 13:115–124, 1983

18

Anesthesia for Emergency Surgery for Abdominal Aortic Reconstruction

Michael F. Roizen

RUPTURE OF ABDOMINAL AORTIC ANEURYSMS

The most common reason for performing emergency reconstruction of the aorta is leakage or rupture of an aneurysm. (Emergency surgery for acute ischemia is discussed in Chapter 23.) Ruptured aneurysms can occur because of atherosclerosis, mycosis, syphilis, inflammatory disease, or Marfan's syndrome.[1-12] Although aortic aneurysms occur only four times more frequently in men than in women, aortic aneurysms rupture ten times more frequently in men.

Aortic aneurysms usually rupture into the retroperitoneum.[2-12] Even though this site permits tamponade of the hemorrhage, retroperitoneal hemorrhage and subsequent hematoma can displace the left renal vein, inferior vena cava, and gut. Such displacement makes damage to these structures possible during the surgical approach. Venous hemorrhage is often much more difficult to control than arterial hemorrhage.

Approximately 25 percent of aneurysms rupture into the peritoneal cavity, a site associated with a great degree of exsanguination. Other sites of rupture include adjacent structures after formation of fistulae with the inferior vena cava, iliac veins, or renal veins.[13-17]

Aortoenteric fistulae most commonly rupture into the fixed third portion of the duodenum.[18] These fistulae usually occur between the overlying bowel and a portion of the aorta that has previously undergone resection and grafting for an existing aneurysm. Mortality rates associated with such fistulae are high, often exceeding 50 percent. An abdominal aortic aneurysm may dissect proximally, resulting in hemopericardium.[19]

The overall mortality rates in published series vary from 15 to 90 percent,[3-12] the time from onset of symptoms to control of bleeding being the key to outcome. This fact gives credence to the inescapable sense of urgency that accompanies such events. Other factors adversely affecting outcome are a history of chronic hypertension, heart disease, renal insufficiency, a hematocrit below 32.5 percent at diagnosis, hypotension at diagnosis, surgery lasting more than 400 minutes, and blood loss greater than 11,000 ml.[6,7,12] Factors associated with poor outcome that may be influenced by anesthetic management are hypotension lasting longer than 110 minutes and systolic blood pressure below 100 mmHg at the end of surgery.

The interval from onset of symptoms to arrival at the hospital ranges from 0.3 to 22.5 hours, the mean interval being approximately 7 hours.[12] Describing 100 patients with ruptured abdominal aortic aneurysms, Ottinger[9] reported the following distribution of symptoms: pain, 92 patients; collapse, 17; faintness, 13; vomiting, 13; numbness in leg, 3; inability to void, 2; and weakness in leg, 1. For eight patients, an adequate history could not be obtained. Pain in the back and/or abdomen was almost always present. This pain resulted from "dissection of the aortic wall and retroperitoneal spaces by blood." Therefore, many surgeons believe that the combination of pain and the presence of a known abdominal aortic aneurysm or pulsatile abdominal mass indicates dissection or rupture and the need for immediate surgical exploration.

Shock also frequently accompanies rupture. May et al.[8] reported that 56 percent of patients with ruptured abdominal aortic aneurysms were in shock at the time of admission and had cold, clammy extremities or blood pressure of 100/60 mmHg or less. However, the absence of hypotension does not rule out the possibility of rupture, and shock may occur suddenly. Dissection of an aortic aneurysm may be accompanied by severe hypertension that must be controlled immediately if rupture is to be prevented.

ANESTHETIC MANAGEMENT DURING EMERGENCY SURGERY FOR RUPTURED ABDOMINAL AORTIC ANEURYSMS

In my view, rapid diagnosis and immediate laparotomy and control of the proximal portion of the aorta are of the highest priority. If systolic blood pressure is less than 90 mmHg, some clinicians advocate administration of oxygen by face mask, with endotracheal intubation occurring only after control of the proximal portion of the aorta has been achieved.[6] However, because experienced anesthesia personnel can usually intubate the trachea rapidly, and because the threat of aspiration pneumonitis is substantial, I usually do not follow these recommendations. Initially, I perform rapid-sequence endotracheal intubation. I believe this procedure causes little morbidity, creates only a slight delay, and prevents a potentially serious complication.

Marked Hypotension Unresponsive to Rapid Volume Infusion

If loss of consciousness and/or mental aberration occurs along with marked hypotension unresponsive to rapid volume infusion, the probability of rupture into the free peritoneal cavity is high. The trachea should be intubated immediately in a rapid-sequence fashion, usually with the aid of muscle relaxants and with only small doses of barbiturates or narcotics. Ventilation with 100 percent oxygen should also be started. Almost simultaneously, laparotomy begins so that the surgeon can clamp the aorta.

For this first type of patients, I try to replace volume to the point of normalizing systemic blood pressure. At this time during uncontained rupture, systemic blood pressure is often the only guide to volume replacement.

The patient is resuscitated quickly (before induction, if possible) with type-specific uncross-matched blood and crystalloid administered via large-bore venous catheters by roller pumps and/or pressurized bags. If type-specific blood is not available, O-negative washed red blood cells may be given.

Once the aorta is controlled with a cross-clamp and blood pressure and perfusion are restored, additional venous access is obtained if necessary. It is often helpful, indeed necessary, to have a second anesthetist secure these lines while the first is securing the airway, monitoring blood pressure, and administering volume into the intravenous sites that have been established. Peripheral arterial and pulmonary artery catheters are then inserted. At this point, volume administration is guided by means of filling pressures obtained from pulmonary artery catheter readings.

I do not administer diuretics routinely, although many clinicians do. If intraoperative oliguria (urinary output of 0.125 ml/kg/h or less) occurs, I first ensure that the urinary catheter and collection system are unobstructed and that left-sided cardiac filling pressures are adequate. When hypotension has occurred because of rupture, and perhaps low-output acute tubular necrosis is present, 12.5 to 25 mg of mannitol or 40 to 120 mg of furosemide is administered to increase urinary output.[20]

If these patients are hemodynamically stable, I do not hesitate to administer muscle relaxants for paralysis and large doses of narcotics, as such patients will usually require postoperative mechanical ventilation and sedation for minimizing cardiovascular stress.

Partially Controlled Hemorrhage

A second group of patients has pain and shock that diminish on volume administration. For such patients, it may be assumed that hemorrhage has been contained at least partially. However, because rapid exsanguination can occur at any time, patients are transported immediately to the operating room for emergency laparotomy, and the same sense of urgency is maintained.

If blood pressure and heart rate are stable when the patient arrives, sterile preparation of the abdomen is begun. Intravascular volume status may be assessed by looking for a decrease in systemic blood pressure and/or an increase in heart rate when the patient's head is raised 10 to 15 degrees. Intravenous administration of a 50-mg bolus of thiopental may also aid in assessing volume. Induction is delayed until the abdomen is prepared and draped and the surgeon is ready. Venous access is ensured, and positive indications of acceptable volume loading are demonstrated by tilt test, administration of small doses of thiopental, or measurements from a rapidly placed pulmonary artery catheter. Thus, in this situation, little time is spent inserting or attaching monitors.

Preoxygenation is followed by rapid-sequence induction: administration of small doses of fentanyl or sufentanil, small-to-moderate doses of thiopental (0.5 to 5 mg/kg, depending on the response to the test dose of thiopental), and a rapid-acting muscle relaxant; application of cricoid pressure; and endotracheal intubation. When I am concerned about the effects of narcotics on maintenance of blood pressure, I occasionally induce anesthesia with alfentanil. Although the short half-life of this agent is prolonged in these patients, it is still shorter than that of other drugs. This means that any untoward effect resulting from alfentanil would still be shorter than that with other narcotics. (Even though I have in the past used naloxone to reverse disastrous decrements in blood pressure associated with administration of narcotics, this practice has potential complications.) To blunt the hemodynamic effects of laryngeal visualization and endotracheal intubation, one may administer an intravenous bolus of lidocaine, sodium nitroprusside, nitroglycerin, esmolol, or additional fentanyl, sufentanil, or thiopental.

If hypotension occurs after induction, I administer 100 percent oxygen, elevate the patient's legs, and rapidly administer blood and fluids. If these measures fail to produce adequate blood pressure and perfusion, I infuse phenylephrine or dopamine until the aorta can be occluded.

During temporary aortic occlusion, I insert a pulmonary artery catheter (if it is not already in place) to guide volume administration. I believe that high-normal filling pressures are desirable for attenuation of hypotension following removal of the aortic clamp.

Because of the site of aortic occlusion, replacement blood may not pass through the liver in amounts adequate to allow for metabolism of citrate.[21] Therefore, if hypotension occurs because of coagulopathy or poor myocardial contractility, administration of calcium may be therapeutic.

Procedure after use of a MAST Suit

A third possibility is the patient who has been treated initially with application of a military antishock trouser (MAST) suit. This temporizing measure allows transport of the patient to the operating room with less hemorrhage and, some believe, with clot formation and temporary sealing of the aortic rent. If possible, pressure should be removed in stages (e.g., from the epigastrium, then from one leg, and then from the other leg) rather than all at once, and only after the surgeons are completely ready to begin. Reducing all pressure at once would allow increased blood flow (reactive hyperemia) to occur in all areas simultaneously, thereby causing a large and precipitous decrease in blood pressure and filling volumes of the heart.

Other Considerations

I routinely use autotransfusion in patients who have actual or suspected rupture of an aortic aneurysm. However, a separate team sets up and operates the autotransfusion devices, as the attention of the primary anesthetist should be directed to the patient's volume status, gas exchange, and depth of anesthesia. My mnemonic for treating such patients is the acronym "WOVCATH," which means "Wonder if the patient can tolerate an anesthetic; Oxygen; Vecuronium; Coagulation; Acid-base; Temperature; and Hemodynamics." This mnemonic lists, in reverse order, the important aspects of patient care that I try to remember when everything about these patients invites disorganization.

In elective resection, the most important determinant of outcome is maintenance of cardiac well-being, as cardiovascular complications account for more than 50 percent of all mortality in elective aortic reconstruction.[22–31] In contrast, if rupture has occurred, hypotension secondary to exsanguination is the primary cause of death.[1–12] Therefore, when rupture is suspected, rapid control of the proximal portion of the aorta is probably more important than optimizing the patient's various preoperative conditions.

CONCLUSION

In contrast to elective reconstruction of the aorta, in which preservation of myocardial function is the primary goal, in emergency resection, the crucial factors for patient survival are initial rapid control of blood loss and reversal of hypotension, and then preservation of myocardial function.

SUMMARY

Perhaps in no other surgical circumstance is the mettle of an anesthetist tested to a greater extent than when providing anesthesia for emergency vascular surgery. Under these circumstances, the shift in mental focus from responding to trauma to caring for the heart is a difficult challenge for the anesthetist. However, I believe this step should be undertaken as soon as hemodynamic stability occurs. I also believe that vigilance must continue into the postoperative period if the risks of morbidity or mortality are to be minimized.

REFERENCES

1. Scobie TK, Masters RG: Changing factors influencing abdominal aortic aneurysm repair. J Cardiovasc Surg 23:309–313, 1982
2. Butler MJ, Chant ADB, Webster JHH: Ruptured abdominal aortic aneurysms. Br J Surg 65:839–841, 1978
3. Darling RC, Messina CR, Brewster DC, Ottinger LW: Autopsy study of unoperated abdominal aortic aneurysms. The case for early resection. Circulation, 56: suppl. 2, II-161 to II-164, 1977
4. Friedman SA: The evaluation and treatment of patients with arterial aneurysms. Med Clin North Am 65:83–103, 1981
5. Gardner RJ, Gardner NL, Tarnay TJ et al: The surgical experience and a one to sixteen year follow-up of 277 abdominal aortic aneurysms. Am J Surg 135:226–230, 1978
6. Lawrie GM, Crawford ES, Morris GC, Jr., Howell JF: Progress in the treatment of ruptured abdominal aortic aneurysm. World J Surg 4:653–660, 1980
7. Lawrie GM, Morris GC, Jr., Crawford ES et al: Improved results of operation for ruptured abdominal aortic aneurysms. Surgery 85:483–488, 1979
8. May AG, DeWeese JA, Frank I et al: Surgical treatment of abdominal aortic aneurysms. Surgery 63:711–721, 1968
9. Ottinger LW: Ruptured arteriosclerotic aneurysms of the abdominal aorta. Reducing mortality. JAMA 233:147–150, 1975
10. Sabiston DC, Jr: Abdominal aortic aneurysms. p. 1672. In Sabiston DC, Jr. (ed): Davis-Christopher Textbook of Surgery. The Biological Basis of Modern Surgical Practice. Vol. 2. 10th Ed. WB Saunders, Philadelphia, 1972
11. Thompson JE, Garrett WV: Peripheral-arterial surgery. N Engl J Med 302:491–503, 1980
12. Wakefield TW, Whitehouse WM, Jr., Wu S-C et al: Abdominal aortic aneurysm rupture: statistical analysis of factors affecting outcome of surgical treatment. Surgery 91:586–596, 1982
13. Merrill WH, Ernst CB: Aorta-left renal vein fistula: hemodynamic monitoring and timing of operation. Surgery 89:678–682, 1981
14. Savrin RA, Gustafson R: Spontaneous aorto-vena caval fistula: hemodynamic monitoring. J Cardiovasc Surg 22:88–91, 1981
15. Schramek A, Hashmonai M, Better OS et al: Aortocaval fistula due to rupture of abdominal aortic aneurysm. Isr J Med Sci 16:733–734, 1980
16. Clowes AW, DePalma RG, Botti RE et al: Management of aortocaval fistula due to abdominal aortic aneurysm. Am J Surg 137:807–809, 1979
17. Cohen LJ, Sukov RJ, Boswell W, Ashor G: Spontaneous aorto-caval fistula. Report of 2 cases. Radiology 138:357–359, 1981
18. Connolly JE, Kwaan JHM, McCart PM et al: Aortoenteric fistula. Ann Surg 194:402–412, 1981
19. Snow N: Hemopericardium from retrograde dissection of an abdominal aortic aneurysm. Am Surg 46:589–592, 1980

20. Alpert RA, Roizen MF, Hamilton WK et al: Intraoperative urinary output does not predict postoperative renal function in patients undergoing abdominal aortic revascularization. Surgery 95:707–711, 1984

21. Olinger GN, Hottenrott C, Mulder DG et al: Acute clinical hypocalcemic myocardial depression during rapid blood transfusion and postoperative hemodialysis. A preventable complication. J Thorac Cardiovasc Surg 72:503–511, 1976

22. Young AE, Sandberg GW, Couch NP: The reduction of mortality of abdominal aortic aneurysm resection. Am J Surg 134:585–590, 1977

23. Hicks GL, Eastland MW, DeWeese JA et al: Survival improvement following aortic aneurysm resection. Ann Surg 181:863–869, 1975

24. Thompson JE, Hollier LH, Patman RD, Persson AV: Surgical management of abdominal aortic aneurysms: factors influencing mortality and morbidity—a 20-year experience. Ann Surg 181:654–661, 1975

25. Mulcare RJ, Royster TS, Lynn RA, Conners RB: Long-term results of operative therapy for aortoiliac disease. Arch Surg 113:601–604, 1978

26. Whittemore AD, Clowes AW, Hechtman HB, Mannick JA: Aortic aneurysm repair. Reduced operative mortality associated with maintenance of optimal cardiac performance. Ann Surg 192:414–421, 1980

27. Crawford ES, Saleh SA, Babb JW III et al: Infrarenal abdominal aortic aneurysm. Factors influencing survival after operation performed over a 25-year period. Ann Surg 193:699–709, 1981

28. Hertzer NR: Myocardial ischemia. Surgery 93:97–101, 1983

29. Yeager RA, Weigel RM, Murphy ES et al: Application of clinically valid cardiac risk factors to aortic aneurysm surgery. Arch Surg 121:278–281, 1986

30. Szilagyi DE, Smith RF, DeRusso FJ et al: Contribution of abdominal aortic aneurysmectomy to prolongation of life. Ann Surg 164:678–699, 1966

31. Benefiel DJ, Roizen MF, Lampe GH et al: Morbidity after aortic surgery with sufentanil vs isoflurane anesthesia (abstract). Anesthesiology 65:A516, 1986

Section V

SURGERY FOR PERIPHERAL VASCULAR INSUFFICIENCY OF THE LOWER EXTREMITIES

19

Peripheral Vascular Insufficiency: Surgical Goals and Methods

Christopher K. Zarins

Surgical procedures for peripheral vascular disease can be performed on an elective or emergency basis. Elective procedures correct chronic ischemia of the lower extremities, whereas emergency procedures respond to acute, severe life- and limb-threatening ischemia. Surgical considerations vary for these two types of conditions.

ELECTIVE SURGERY FOR PERIPHERAL VASCULAR INSUFFICIENCY

In general, patients undergoing elective vascular reconstruction for peripheral occlusive disease are elderly; most have a history of heavy smoking. Many have diabetes mellitus, hypertension, and significant coronary artery disease. Cerebrovascular disease, abnormally high plasma levels of lipids, and chronic obstructive pulmonary disease are also common. These considerations warrant careful preoperative assessment of cardiovascular, pulmonary, and renal func-

tion, plus careful monitoring during and after surgery.

Patients may undergo elective surgery for chronic peripheral occlusive disease for any of the following clinical conditions: (1) intermittent claudication, (2) ischemic rest pain, (3) ischemic ulceration, or (4) gangrene. Patients with claudication have symptoms on walking that are relieved by rest. Because limb loss is not imminent, reconstructive procedures for intermittent claudication are elective. Patients with rest pain, ulceration, and gangrene are at variable risk of imminent limb loss and may have severe, progressive ischemia. Under these circumstances, the need for reconstructive surgery may become more urgent.

Preoperative evaluation of the peripheral vascular system usually consists of noninvasive vascular tests, including determinations of systolic blood pressure at the level of the ankle by Doppler probe, and comparison of ankle and brachial systolic blood pressures. These tests not only help assess the severity of ischemia[1] and the urgency of revascularization[2] but also provide baseline values for evaluation of operative results.[3,4] The precise site of

317

obstructive arterial lesions is determined by angiography. Angiographic information is of great importance in planning the operative procedure. Antibiotics are usually given perioperatively to prevent graft infection.

Vascular reconstructive procedures are generally classified as either inflow or outflow reconstructive procedures. *Inflow* procedures bypass obstruction in the aortoiliac segment, whereas *outflow* procedures are performed distal to the inguinal ligament, to bypass femoropopliteal or distal obstruction.

Inflow Vascular Reconstruction

The most common reconstructive procedure performed to bypass obstruction in the aortoiliac segment is aortofemoral bypass.[5] Although direct aortoiliac thromboendarterectomy may be used occasionally, bypass is generally more satisfactory. Axillofemoral bypass, femorofemoral bypass, and thoracic aortofemoral bypass can also be used for inflow reconstruction under certain circumstances but incur lower patency rates than aortofemoral bypass procedures.[6-12] These procedures are discussed in Chapter 14.

Outflow Vascular Reconstruction

The most common vascular reconstructive procedure performed for occlusion beyond the inguinal ligament is the bypass graft that originates in the common femoral artery and extends to the popliteal or tibial artery, depending on preoperative angiographic evaluation of outflow vessels. These bypasses may be performed with reversed saphenous vein, in situ saphenous vein, or a prosthetic graft.[13] Each procedure involves different technical aspects of vessel dissection and exposure, anastomosis, and tunnelling.

Bypass Grafts for Outflow Vascular Reconstruction

The complexity of femoropopliteal and femorotibial bypass varies widely. The most appropriate site for distal anastomosis and the quality of outflow vessels are determined from preoperative angiography. Although saphenous vein appears to produce the best short- and long-term results,[14,15] use of this graft material requires longer operative time and greater technical expertise. The length and complexity of the operation are normally determined by the quality of the saphenous vein and the quality and size of the distal outflow vessels. Arteriography at the completion of surgery is usually required to assess the adequacy of the procedure. Although major blood loss and hemodynamic alterations do not in general occur in distal reconstruction, procedures may become lengthy. The anesthetist must anticipate this possibility by providing for drainage of the bladder by Foley catheter.

Reversed Saphenous Vein Bypass. In a reversed saphenous vein bypass (Fig. 19-1), the saphenous vein is dissected from its junction at the common femoral vein to the level of the distal anastomosis. All branches are ligated and divided, and the vein is excised and inspected. After exposure of the proximal and distal vessels, the saphenous vein is reversed in direction to permit blood flow in the direction of the valves and is tunnelled from the femoral artery to the appropriate distal vessel. The surgeon takes care not to damage, injure, or twist the vein. After completion of the proximal and distal anastomoses, the adequacy of flow is checked by the quality of the pulse and the character of intraoperative Doppler ultrasound signals. Adequacy of the distal anastomosis and outflow vessels are evaluated by angiography at the completion of surgery.

In Situ Saphenous Vein Bypass. In

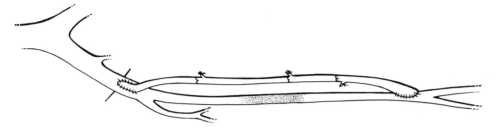

Fig. 19-1. Femoropopliteal bypass graft using saphenous vein that is reversed in direction to bypass an occluded superficial femoral artery.

in situ bypass (Fig. 19-2), the saphenous vein is not excised from its bed but merely exposed so that side branches can be ligated and valve locations identified. The proximal saphenous vein is sutured to the common femoral artery in an end-to-side fashion, and arterial blood flow is introduced into the saphenous vein. The valves that obstruct retrograde flow in the saphenous vein are lysed with a valvulotome (or some other comparable valve cutter) introduced through side branches. When all valves are rendered incompetent, blood should be seen flowing freely from the distal end of the vein. The end of the vein is then anastomosed to the appropriate distal artery. Again, patency is determined by pulse quality, Doppler ultrasonography, and angiography.

The in situ vein bypass has significant advantages over the reversed vein bypass. The large proximal saphenous vein is sutured to the large common femoral vein, and the small distal vein is sutured

to the small distal artery. The size match is particularly important for tibial artery bypass and permits the use of smaller saphenous veins previously thought unsuitable. In addition, because the vein is not removed from its bed, there is less trauma to the vein and less likelihood of twisting or kinking of the vein. These advantages have resulted in more frequent use of vein for grafting, plus improved patency rates.[16,17]

Prosthetic Graft Bypass.   Although human umbilical cord vein and Dacron have been used, polytetrafluoroethylene (PTFE; e.g., GORE-TEX) is the most commonly used prosthetic graft material. Prosthetic graft bypasses can be performed more quickly and require less dissection than saphenous vein graft bypasses, as multiple incisions do not have to be made for harvesting of the saphenous vein. However, prosthetic graft bypasses (particularly below the knee) incur significantly lower patency rates.[13] Inci-

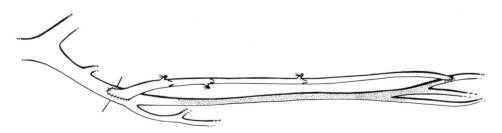

Fig. 19-2. Femoral-posterior tibial bypass using in situ saphenous vein. The vein is left in place, and valve lysis permits flow of blood in a retrograde direction in the vein.

sions expose the proximal and distal arteries, and a tunnelling instrument is used to tunnel the graft between the incisions. After completion of the proximal and distal anastomoses, intraoperative angiography is performed to ensure adequacy of the anastomoses and adequacy of runoff to the foot. During the procedure, the patient is usually given heparin, the effects of which are normally not reversed, as bleeding problems are rare.

Complications

Early complications include hemorrhage from the suture line or from a side branch of the saphenous vein. These can readily be controlled by suture repair. On completion of surgery, angiography is performed to detect graft thromboses, intimal flaps, and defects. These deficiencies are repaired before the patient is taken from the operating suite, to avoid early postoperative graft thrombosis. Graft patency is evaluated carefully in the postoperative recovery room. The patient's feet should be kept warm, and the patient should be well hydrated to prevent peripheral vasoconstriction, which may limit outflow from the graft. If graft thrombosis develops soon after surgery, the patient is returned promptly to the operating room for graft thrombectomy and for evaluation and correction of the cause of graft thrombosis. If a technical defect is found, it is repaired. One can expect blood loss that is occasionally sizable on flushing of the graft during graft thrombectomy.

EMERGENCY SURGERY FOR PERIPHERAL VASCULAR INSUFFICIENCY

Emergency surgery for peripheral vascular insufficiency is required when acute arterial occlusion produces severe ischemia and threatens limb viability. Immediate operation and restoration of blood flow are needed to avoid loss of the limb. Such patients are at high risk and require prompt, careful, and precise surgical and anesthetic management.

Causes, Symptoms, and Evaluation

Acute arterial occlusion can be caused by thrombosis of a stenotic or ulcerated atherosclerotic artery. It can also be caused by acute embolic occlusion in otherwise normal peripheral arteries. Such emboli usually originate from the heart, typically from patients with cardiac arrhythmias, recent myocardial infarctions, or ventricular aneurysms. However, 10 percent of patients with peripheral emboli have no demonstrable source of embolism.[18,19]

Acute arterial occlusion is manifested clinically by sudden onset of pain, coldness, numbness, and paresthesias. The extremity is pulseless and the patient may lose motor ability and sensation. The severity of ischemia and the urgency of surgery are best assessed by clinical examination. Viability of the lower extremities is best judged by evaluating motor ability and sensation. Abnormal sensation in the toes, feet, and legs in response to light touch, pin prick, and proprioception and loss of motor function in the feet and toes are hallmarks of acute ischemia and nonviability of the extremity. If ischemia is not reversed in a matter of hours, loss of the limb is probable. The length of time tissue can tolerate acute ischemia and recover after revascularization varies with the degree of ischemia and the adequacy of collateral vessels. Acute onset of symptoms with loss of motor ability and sensation in the feet requires the most immediate attention.

The cause of acute ischemia is an important determinant of the operative plan. If the source is arterial embolism, simple embolectomy with Fogarty catheters through a groin incision under local anesthesia may be sufficient (Fig. 19-3). However, if the cause is thrombosis of severely diseased atherosclerotic arteries, bypass reconstruction would be necessary. If time is sufficient, preoperative angiography may help to distinguish the two. However, sometimes the cause of acute ischemia is not discovered until surgery is under way. With acute ischemia, the surgeon and anesthetist must be prepared for not only the simple procedure but also the complex and lengthy procedure.

Surgery for Acute Arterial Ischemia

Because patients with acute ischemia are often very ill, optimal anesthetic management is critical. Use of a Foley catheter, monitoring of arterial and central blood pressures, and adequate fluid replacement are necessary. One can expect significant fluid losses in flushing of the artery during thrombectomy, as well as fluid losses sequestered in edematous revascularized tissue. Serum potassium levels can change quickly because of inevitable cell death and release of intracellular potassium into the circulation. High urinary output might be promoted, and alkalinization of the urine

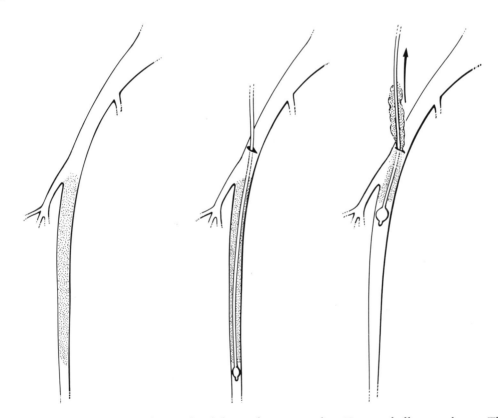

Fig. 19-3. Embolectomy of superficial femoral artery with a Fogarty balloon catheter. The deflated catheter is passed through and beyond the thrombus, and the balloon is inflated. Withdrawing the catheter then extracts the thrombus.

might be considered to prevent myoglobin deposition in the kidney. After revascularization of acutely ischemic muscle, cardiac dysrhythmias may occur, and the surgeon will be alert to the possibility of compartment syndrome (edema of the extremity that threatens distal circulation).

Surgery usually begins with a groin incision that exposes the femoral artery. Attempts are made to pass Fogarty catheters proximally and distally to establish blood flow and to extract thrombus. If simple femoral embolectomy is not successful in restoring flow, intraoperative angiography may be necessary to determine whether the primary problem is inadequate inflow or inadequate outflow. More complex reconstructive procedures such as aortofemoral, axillofemoral, or femoropopliteal bypass may be required depending on the clinical condition of the patient and intraoperative findings. Thus, surgical plans (and consequent anesthetic management) may change during surgery.

On restoring flow to the femoral artery, the surgeon may perform femoral venous drainage to avoid returning the initial venous effluent from an acutely ischemic extremity to the circulation. Drainage can entail significant blood loss, and good communication between the anesthetist and surgeon is beneficial. Mannitol may be administered because it is a free radical scavenger, and to promote urinary flow. Some clinicians stimulate high urinary output with alkaline urine to reduce pigment precipitation in renal tubules. After restoration of blood flow by either embolectomy or bypass graft, arteriography is frequently performed and fasciotomy may be required.[20]

SUMMARY

Anesthetic and operative management are much more complex and difficult for acute than for chronic arterial occlusion.

Appropriate anticipation of the problems of hyperkalemia, hypovolemia, cardiac dysrhythmias, myoglobinemia and myoglobinuria, renal failure, and compartment syndrome is helpful in attaining a successful outcome.

REFERENCES

1. Yao ST, Hobbs JT, Irvine WT: Ankle systolic pressure measurements in arterial disease affecting the lower extremities. Br J Surg 56:676–679, 1969
2. Bridges RA, Barnes RW: Segmental limb pressures. p. 79–92. In Kempczinski RF, Yao JST (eds): Practical Noninvasive Vascular Diagnosis. Year Book Medical Publishers, Chicago, 1982
3. Yao JST, O'Mara CS, Flinn WR et al: Postoperative evaluation of graft failure. p. 1–19. In Bernard VM, Towne JB (eds): Complications in Vascular Surgery. Grune & Stratton, Orlando, Fl, 1980
4. Bone GE, Hayes AC, Slaymaker EE, Barnes RW: Value of segmental limb blood pressures in predicting results of aortofemoral bypass. Am J Surg 132:733–738, 1976
5. Brewster DC, Darling RC: Optimal methods of aortoiliac reconstruction. Surgery 84:739–748, 1978
6. Mannick JA, Whittemore AD, Couch NP: Aortoiliac occlusive disease. p. 489–511. In Moore WS (ed): Vascular Surgery: A Comprehensive Review. 2nd. Ed. Grune & Stratton, Orlando, FL, 1986
7. Baird RJ, Johnston KW, Walker PM et al: Aortoiliofemoral occlusive disease. p. 344–352. In Wilson SE, Veith FJ, Hobson RW, II, Williams RA (eds): Vascular Surgery. Principles and Practice. McGraw-Hill, New York, 1987
8. Imparato AM, Sanoudos G, Epstein HY et al: Results in 96 aortoiliac reconstructive procedures: preoperative angiographic and functional classifications used as prognostic guides. Surgery 68:610–616, 1970
9. Moore WS, Cafferata HT, Hall AD, Blais-

dell FW: In defense of grafts across the inguinal ligament: an evaluation of early and late results of aorto-femoral bypass grafts. Ann Surg 168:207–214, 1968

10. Mannick JA, Williams LE, Nabseth DC: The late results of axillofemoral grafts. Surgery 68:1038–1043, 1970

11. Brief DK, Brener BJ: Extraanatomic bypasses. p. 414–424. In Wilson SE, Veith FJ, Hobson RW, II, Williams RA (eds): Vascular Surgery. Principles and Practice. McGraw-Hill, New York, 1987

12. Zarins CK, Kremser PC: Performance of thoracofemoral extraanatomic arterial bypass (videotape). 73rd Annual Clinical Congress Ciné Clinic, American College of Surgeons, 1987

13. Veith FJ, Gupta SK, Ascer E: Femoral, popliteal, and tibial occlusive disease. p. 353–375. In Wilson SE, Veith FJ, Hobson RW, II, Williams RA (eds): Vascular Surgery. Principles and Practice. McGraw-Hill, New York, 1987

14. Mannick JA, Jackson BT, Coffman JD, Hume DM: Success of bypass vein grafts in patients with isolated popliteal artery segments. Surgery 61:17–25, 1967

15. Reichle FA, Tyson RR: Comparison of long-term results of 364 femoropopliteal or femorotibial bypasses for revascularization of severely ischemic lower extremities. Ann Surg 182:449–455, 1975

16. Leather RP, Shah DM, Karmody AM: Infrapopliteal arterial bypass for limb salvage: increased patency and utilization of the saphenous vein used "in situ." Surgery 90:1000–1008, 1981

17. Buchbinder D, Singh JK, Karmody AM et al: Comparison of patency rate and structural changes of in situ and reversed vein arterial bypass. J Surg Res 30:213–222, 1981

18. Abbott WM, Maloney RD, McCabe CC et al: Arterial embolism: a 44 year perspective. Am J Surg 143:460–464, 1982

19. Connett MC, Murray DH, Jr., Wenneker WW: Peripheral arterial emboli. Am J Surg 148:14–19, 1984

20. Chin AK, Zimmerman JJ, Fogarty TJ: Acute arterial occlusion. p. 861–880. In Moore WS (ed): Vascular Surgery: A Comprehensive Review. 2nd Ed. Grune & Stratton, Orlando, FL, 1986

20

Anesthesia Goals for Surgery to Reduce Peripheral Vascular Insufficiency: One Approach at Loyola University Stritch School of Medicine

Neeraja B. Reddy
Tadikonda L. K. Rao

The primary goals for anesthesia for surgery to reduce peripheral vascular insufficiency consist of reducing surgical stress; providing perioperative analgesia, amnesia, and sedation; reducing intraoperative blood loss; and instituting sympathetic blockade. The last goal improves and increases distal runoff from the site of the operated vessel, thus maintaining patency of the vessel. Other goals for anesthesia include minimizing the metabolic and systemic disturbances that lead to perioperative morbidity and mortality, such as deep venous thrombosis and pulmonary embolism.

generalized process affecting the arteries of most organs (particularly the heart and brain), patients undergoing vascular reconstructive procedures also frequently have coronary artery or cerebrovascular disease. In one study of patients undergoing peripheral vascular operations, 50 percent had coronary artery disease; 60 percent had cerebrovascular lesions; 30 percent had hepatic disease; and 15 percent had renal artery disease.[1] The higher incidences of hypertension, diabetes mellitus, chronic obstructive pulmonary disease, and advanced age among these patients place them at greater risk of perioperative morbidity and mortality.

ASSOCIATED DISEASES

Atherosclerosis is the most common cause of peripheral vascular disease in the elderly. Because atherosclerosis is a

REGIONAL VERSUS GENERAL ANESTHESIA

Reconstructive vascular surgery of the lower extremity can be performed with general anesthesia or major conduction anesthesia, including subarachnoid block and epidural analgesia with or without intravenous sedation. For patients at high risk of postoperative complications who cannot tolerate major conduction blocks, regional nerve blocks of the sciatic, femoral, obturator, and femoral cutaneous nerves (the so-called "three-in-one" block) are also options.[2]

We believe that major conduction anesthesia in which the sensory level is limited to lower thoracic dermatomes produces the safest and most placid perioperative course, and the lowest mortality rate, for patients undergoing peripheral vascular surgery with concomitant cardiovascular, cerebrovascular, or respiratory disease. We base these beliefs on our own experiences and on data from other studies.

Vascular Complications

A retrospective study of 263 patients undergoing extrathoracic vascular surgery concluded that regional anesthesia was the technique of choice for 33 percent and that it was especially indicated for patients with intractable ischemic pain.[3] Nine percent of patients given regional anesthesia had vascular complications, and 3.4 percent had other complications. In contrast, 13.8 percent of patients given general anesthesia had vascular complications, and 6.9 percent had other complications.

Hemodynamic Stability

Other data suggest that regional anesthesia (with or without general anesthesia) provides greater hemodynamic stability for patients undergoing peripheral vascular surgery with cardiovascular, cerebrovascular, or respiratory disease than does general anesthesia by itself.

One report described a randomized prospective study of 18 American Society of Anesthesiologists (ASA) physical status III and IV patients undergoing aortofemoral bypass surgery.[4] The hemodynamic results of surgery under general anesthesia were compared with those for surgery under epidural anesthesia supplemented by nitrous oxide. Patients given general anesthesia had significant hypertension not specifically related to cross-clamping of the blood vessel and required administration of vasodilating drugs to reduce systemic vascular resistance. However, patients given regional and general anesthesia were more hemodynamically stable, provided optimal ventricular filling pressures were maintained. In that study, monitoring of pulmonary capillary wedge pressure and cardiac output by pulmonary artery catheter was beneficial in optimizing hemodynamic status and fluid therapy, especially during cross-clamping.[4]

In 1986, Christopherson[5] compared intraoperative events and deaths in patients undergoing peripheral vascular operations. She observed significant hemodynamic instability marked by frequent episodes of hypertension and tachycardia during surgery under general anesthesia. This hemodynamic instability may result in intraoperative or postoperative myocardial ischemia. In her hands, patients given regional anesthesia were perioperatively more hemodynamically stable. Christopherson concluded that regional anesthesia with adequate monitoring may be safer in patients with underlying major cardiovascular problems.

Sympathetic Blockade

Regional anesthesia for vascular operations of the lower extremity has theoretic advantages because it provides sympathetic blockade that increases circulation in the lower extremity and reduces the incidence of intravascular clotting. In the preoperative period, a lumbar epidural block effectively relieves ischemic "rest pain" to a better degree than any analgesic. Thus, a patient can undergo relatively pain-free angiographic studies to evaluate the possibility of operative correction of the obstruction.

Blood Flow

A conduction block initiated preoperatively can be extended through surgery and into the postoperative period by administration of local anesthetics through a catheter left in place in the epidural or subarachnoid space. Besides relieving pain, the block effectively interrupts the sympathetic outflow to the lower extremity that is responsible for maintaining the normal vasoconstrictive tone. Several events and conditions can increase vasomotor tone: intraoperative manipulation and injury to the vessels, heat loss caused by prolonged surgery, sympathetic stimulation because of light anesthesia, blood loss, and postoperative pain. The presence of a thrombus or plaque on the lining of a vessel produces a "reflex syndrome" mediated by the sympathetic chain.[6] Vasospasm of the involved artery and vasoconstriction of collateral circulation result, and blood flow to the lower extremity decreases. Therefore, inhibiting sympathetic outflow results in dilatation of the collateral vessels and an increase in the total blood flow in the extremity. Dilatation, in turn, increases runoff from the graft, thus facilitating blood flow through the graft. After sympathetic block, skin blood flow and temperature parallel the graft blood flow. Elevated skin temperature in the foot is an indication of improved perfusion and patency of the graft, provided environmental temperature is controlled.

Cousins and Wright[7] demonstrated that blood flow in the reconstructed graft in-creased approximately 51 percent after lumbar epidural block (Fig. 20-1) when mean arterial blood pressure did not change. This increase in blood flow was caused by a decrease in vascular resistance of the leg, as blood flow is directly proportional to arterial pressure and inversely proportional to vascular resistance. The increase in blood flow was approximately 500 ml/min after sympathetic block.

General anesthesia may not afford this important advantage. Sonnenfeld et al.[8] studied the hemodynamics of leg vessels exposed to halothane, enflurane, and neuroleptic drugs. All drugs increased vascular resistance in the leg; vascular resistance was almost twice as high with neuroleptic drugs as with inhalation agents. Furthermore, reducing sympathetic stimulation by replacing all blood lost during surgery with equal amounts of transfused blood significantly reduced vascular resistance in all three groups, especially those given neuroleptic drugs. We conclude that sympathetic stimulation under general anesthesia is to be avoided.

Increasing blood flow in the graft immediately after surgery may be an important factor affecting immediate patency of the graft, as a large number of grafts fail during this period. Graft failure may result from insufficient blood flow in the graft, spasm of collateral vessels, poor surgical technique, or diabetes mellitus. Increased blood viscosity secondary to polycythemia also decreases blood flow and contributes to graft failure.

Measuring intraoperative blood flow in vein grafts, Little et al.[9] concluded that 80 percent of graft failures resulted when blood flow in the graft was less than 60 ml/min and that 80 percent of grafts remained patent up to 3 months if blood flow exceeded 60 ml/min. Blood flows greater than 60 ml/min could be maintained as long as sympathetic block per-

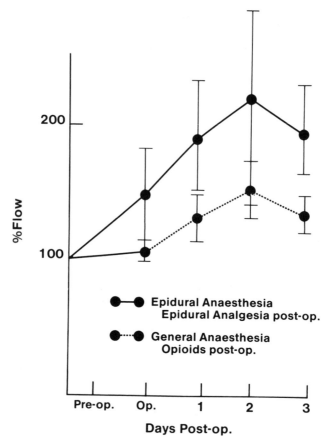

Fig. 20-1. Blood flow through the femoral artery grafts is higher in patients given epidural anesthesia for surgery followed by continuous epidural block for postoperative analgesia than in those given general anesthesia followed by opioids. Values are means ± standard error of the mean (SEM). (From Cousins and Wright[7] with permission.)

sisted. The longest sympathetic block studied lasted 72 hours.[9] Although the short-term benefits of sympathetic blockade have been demonstrated, the long-term benefits have not.

Another study of 10 patients compared lactate formation before and after lumbar sympathetic block to determine the effect of sympathectomy on blood flow to ischemic muscles.[10] During exercise, oxygen saturation was lower and lactate concentration higher in the femoral venous blood of patients with peripheral vascular disease. These changes in oxygen saturation and lactate concentration were caused by the inability of the atheroscle-

rotic leg to increase muscle blood flow to accommodate the degree of exercise. After sympathetic block, the values for venous blood lactate and oxygen saturation approached those for normal legs, suggesting improved nutritive blood flow to the lower limb.

Sympathetic constrictor tone is an important factor—but not the only factor—influencing blood flow. The sensory block produced by epidural analgesia abolishes pain reflexes that contribute to vasoconstriction and may influence vascular tone by other mechanisms. For example, 6 years after resection of the left abdominal sympathetic chain, a patient presented with signs of ischemic changes and severe pain in the left foot.[7] An epidural block relieved the pain and increased skin temperature. These effects suggest that other pathways for the mediation of this pain may exist.

The vasoconstrictive role of local sensory reflexes, motor nerves, and adrenal catecholamines released by afferent stimulation is not well understood. One explanation may be that synapses of sympathetic fibers are not confined to the ganglia of sympathetic chains but also exist in, or close to, the ventral roots, in "intermediary ganglia." These "extra-sympathetic" vasoconstrictive fibers take a course similar to that of motor fibers and may account for the occurrence of vasomotor reflexes after sympathectomy.[11]

Thromboembolic Complications

Another major advantage of regional (as opposed to general) anesthesia in vascular surgery is that the lower incidence of intravascular clotting and thromboembolic complications is significantly less.

Modig and co-workers[12] studied the effects of continuous lumbar epidural anesthesia and general anesthesia on the incidence of postoperative deep venous thrombosis and pulmonary embolism. Both complications occurred significantly less frequently after regional anesthesia than after general anesthesia (Fig. 20-2). Mortality rates at 4 weeks after surgery were also found to be lower with regional anesthesia.[13] The following factors may account for the advantages with regional anesthesia: an increased circulation in the lower extremity and rapid venous outflow from the lower extremity; decreased tendency for intravascular clotting; efficient fibrinolysis; a higher level of plasminogen activators; and decreased activation of factor VIII.

Addition of Vasoconstrictors

The addition of small doses of epinephrine to local anesthetics used for spinal or epidural block enhances the vasodilatory effect of vasomotor block (Fig. 20-3). β-adrenergic receptors have a lower threshold for stimulation with epinephrine than

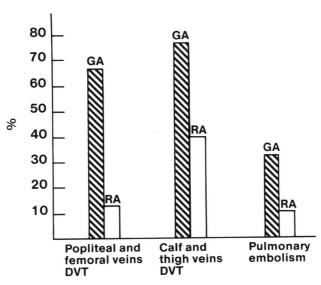

Fig. 20-2. After total hip replacement, deep venous thrombosis (DVT) and pulmonary embolus occur less frequently in patients given regional anesthesia (RA; specifically, epidural block) than in those given general anesthesia (GA). (From Modig et al.[12] with permission.)

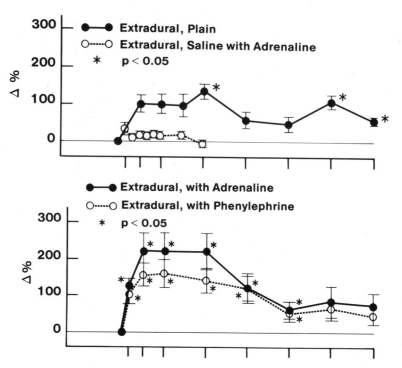

Fig. 20-3. Changes in blood flow in the leg after epidural injection of 20 ml of 2 percent lidocaine (**A**) by itself, and (**B**) with the addition of a vasoconstrictor, epinephrine (5 µg/ml) or phenylephrine (50 µg/ml). For comparison, part **B** also shows blood flow after epidural injection of saline containing epinephrine (5 µg/ml). Asterisks indicate significant ($P < 0.05$) changes from control. Values are mean ± SEM. (Redrawn from Stanton-Hicks[14] with permission.)

do α-adrenergic receptors. Thus, only a comparatively low concentration of epinephrine is necessary to activate β-adrenergic receptors. The epinephrine used to prolong a block may produce a secondary benefit, vasodilatation.[14]

The Endocrine and Metabolic Response to Surgery

Regional anesthesia can suppress or control the endocrine and metabolic response to surgery, both during and after surgery. That is, regional anesthesia suppresses surgery-induced increases in blood glucose, cortisol, catecholamines, antidiuretic hormone, renin, angiotensin,

aldosterone, and cyclic AMP. Whether perioperative suppression of increases in these hormones is beneficial or not is still controversial. However, for patients undergoing vascular operations, reduction of stress lowers catecholamine levels, thus presumably decreasing vascular resistance and increasing blood flow through the graft.

Blood Loss during Surgery

In general, regional anesthesia also incurs less intraoperative blood loss than does general anesthesia. This advantage may significantly decrease not only the amount of blood transfusion required during surgery but also the complications associated with transfusion.

Postoperative Mental Status

Patients undergoing major vascular surgery are usually elderly. After general anesthesia, the incidence of confusion is significantly higher in these patients. The incidence of postoperative confusion may be lower and the degree of mental alertness higher in these patients after regional anesthesia.

In conclusion, anesthetic goals for peripheral vascular operations in patients with multisystem diseases include reduction of myocardial work, increased leg and graft perfusion, and decreased thromboembolism. Presently available data indicate that these goals can be met by careful performance of a major conduction block and prudent intraoperative monitoring.

REFERENCES

1. Bohmert F, Horkenbach G: Spezielle anaesthesiologische probleme bei gesassoperationen. Anesthesiol Wiederbelebung 20:8–14, 1967
2. Giordano JM, Morales GA, Trout HH, DePalma RG: Regional nerve block for femoropopliteal and tibial arterial reconstructions. J Vasc Surg 4:351–354, 1986
3. Dercksen SJ: General and regional anesthesia for vascular surgery. Acta Anaesthesiol Belg 26:125, 1975
4. Rosseel P, Marichal P, Lauwers LF et al: A hemodynamic study of epidural versus intravenous anesthesia for aortofemoral bypass surgery. Acta Anaesthesiol Belg 36:345–363, 1985
5. Christopherson R: Hemodynamic stability and myocardial ischemia under general anesthesia and regional anesthesia. Eighth Annual Meeting, Society of Cardiovascular Anesthesiologists, Richmond, VA, 1986
6. Pratt GH: Anticoagulants and sympathetic nerve blocks in treatment of vascular lesions. Effective therapeutic combination. JAMA 152:903–905, 1953
7. Cousins MJ, Wright CJ: Graft, muscle, skin blood flow after epidural block in vascular surgical procedures. Surg Gynecol Obstet 133:59–64, 1971
8. Sonnenfeld T, Cronestrand R, von Euler C et al: Leg hemodynamics during different forms of anaesthesia in patients undergoing reconstructive vascular surgery. Acta Chir Scand 147:249–253, 1981
9. Little JM, Sheil AGR, Lowenthal J, Goodman AH: Prognostic value of intraoperative blood-flow measurements in femoropopliteal bypass vein-grafts. Lancet 2:648–651, 1968
10. Löfström B, Zetterquist S: The effect of lumbar sympathetic block upon the nutritive blood-flow capacity in intermittent claudication. A metabolic study. Acta Med Scand 182:23–39, 1967
11. Folkow B: Nervous control of the blood vessels. Physiol Rev 35:629–663, 1955
12. Modig J, Borg T, Karlström G et al: Thromboembolism after total hip replacement: role of epidural and general anesthesia. Anesth Analg 62:174–180, 1983
13. Modig J, Hjelmstedt Å, Sahlstedt B, Maripuu E: Comparative influences of epidural and general anaesthesia on deep venous thrombosis and pulmonary embolism after total hip replacement. Acta Chir Scand 147:125–130, 1981
14. Stanton-Hicks MA: Cardiovascular effects of extradural anaesthesia. Br J Anaesth 47:253–263, 1975

21

Anesthesia and Surgery for Peripheral Vascular Insufficiency of the Lower Extremities: One Approach at Emory University

Ira J. Isaacson

Anesthesia for the patient with peripheral vascular insufficiency of the lower extremities is a frequent challenge for the anesthetist. The anesthetic management of such patients varies not only from one locale to another, but often among anesthetists at the same institution. The following case report illustrates the anesthetic approach I use for patients with vascular insufficiency of the lower extremities.

A REPRESENTATIVE CASE REPORT

A 73-year-old man was referred to vascular surgeons at Emory because of increasing pain and occasional numbness of the right leg over 6 months; the patient's internist had diagnosed vascular insufficiency of the right leg. A vascular surgeon at Emory evaluated the patient com-

pletely, eliciting a history consistent with stable angina, non-insulin-dependent diabetes mellitus, mild chronic obstructive pulmonary disease (COPD), and long-standing hypertension. Therefore, the surgeon arranged for the patient to be admitted Monday morning for a full preoperative medical evaluation; femoropopliteal bypass surgery was scheduled for 2 days later. The vascular surgeon also alerted a cardiologist regarding the admission, so that a consultation could be made on arrival of the patient.

Logistically, this type of preoperative medical evaluation is an ongoing problem for us at Emory. Because we are a tertiary referral center, many of our patients live more than 100 miles away. It is difficult for the patient to see the vascular surgeon and all the other necessary consultants (e.g., cardiologists, endocrinologists, pulmonary specialists) in one clinic visit. Consequently, admission was scheduled for 48 hours before surgery to allow for the necessary medical evaluation.

Concomitant Cardiac Disease

When the patient arrived on Monday morning, the cardiologist saw him promptly. The patient gave a history consistent with increasing angina. Angina had occurred more frequently over the past few months, even though physical activity had been limited by leg pain. The patient said that as leg pain intensified, he became more emotionally unstable, which in turn seemed to trigger more frequent angina. The cardiologist placed the patient on a regimen that included a calcium channel antagonist and a nitroglycerin skin patch and scheduled a dipyridamole-thallium scan for the following morning for evaluation of unstable angina.

Dipyridamole-thallium imaging is part of our preoperative evaluation. In at least one study, thallium redistribution correlated with adverse cardiac events; it thus reliably identifies patients at high risk of postoperative ischemia before they undergo major vascular surgery.[1] Because of differing standards of practice, some cardiologists are more aggressive than others in evaluating patients preoperatively. Although not all vascular patients need invasive cardiac evaluations, the physicians involved could establish guidelines for assessing these patients regardless of which consultant sees the patient preoperatively. Figure 21-1 shows the algorithm that was created and is now used in my practice to assist in this standardization.

Some centers advocate routine preoperative cardiac catheterization for all patients undergoing surgery for vascular disease.[2] We realize that this practice is controversial and compromise by using the dipyridamole-thallium scan in patients who are either mildly symptomatic of coronary artery disease (CAD) or asymptomatic but who have abnormal electrocardiograms. For symptomatic patients, the results of the scan or cardiac catheterization determine the next step. If the patient has a correctable coronary disease, he or she is referred for coronary artery bypass grafting (CABG) or coronary artery angioplasty prior to vascular surgery. If there is no significant CAD, or if CAD is severe but inoperable, the necessary peripheral vascular surgery is undertaken.

Is this algorithm reasonable? Our ongoing collection of data regarding significant outcome variables (i.e., death, myocardial infarction, pulmonary edema, prolonged stay in the intensive care unit, cost of care) allows us to estimate continually whether such patients are receiving adequate preoperative evaluation. Our impression is that outcome depends in part on how carefully the patient is evaluated preoperatively and how well the patient's condition is optimized before the anesthetic is ever given.

On Tuesday afternoon, our patient underwent dipyridamole-thallium imaging. The scan revealed a perfusion defect, and redistribution was detected on delayed images; these conditions indicate active ischemia. The cardiologist strongly believed that the patient should undergo cardiac catheterization before elective peripheral vascular surgery. Therefore, the scheduled femoropopliteal bypass operation was postponed.

On Wednesday morning, the patient had cardiac catheterization, which showed 95 percent occlusion of the left anterior descending coronary artery; ejection fraction was 60 percent, and left ventricular filling pressures were normal. On Thursday, the patient successfully underwent balloon angioplasty of the coronary artery. Two days later, the patient was discharged from the hospital. Readmission for femoropopliteal bypass sur-

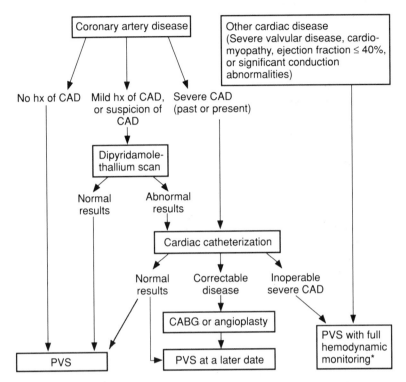

Fig. 21-1. Algorithm used at Emory for assessing the cardiac status of patients scheduled for peripheral vascular surgery. CABG = coronary artery bypass graft. *"Full hemodynamic monitoring" consists of use of an arterial line and a pulmonary artery catheter, as opposed to the usual monitoring commonly used in peripheral vascular surgery (two electrocardiographic leads; pulse oximeter; temperature monitoring; conversation with the patient, if regional anesthesia is chosen; noninvasive blood pressure monitor; and so forth).

gery was scheduled for 2 weeks. This delay allowed him to recuperate from angioplasty.

Peripheral Vascular Surgery

The patient returned in 2 weeks and was seen by his anesthesiologist the night before surgery. The anesthesiologist reviewed the previous admission, noted the thoroughness of the patient's cardiac evaluation and the optimization of car-

diac status, and obtained a history. The most important fact was that the patient had been free of angina since angioplasty. Current medications included a calcium entry blocker, an antihypertensive drug, a diuretic, and a bronchodilating drug. The patient controlled diabetes with diet alone. Thirty years earlier, he had had an uneventful cholecystectomy under what he thought was ether anesthesia. For the upcoming procedure, the anesthesiologist suggested spinal anesthesia for surgery and intrathecal administration of morphine for postoperative analgesia.

The anesthesiologist also discussed the need for invasive monitoring and a postoperative intensive care unit (ICU) stay of at least one night. The patient consented to this plan.

Preoperative Preparation

As is customary in my practice, the patient was brought to the anesthesia holding area prior to surgery. There, laboratory and radiographic data were reviewed. Blood glucose level was 187 mg/dl, and all other blood test results were normal. The chest radiograph (unchanged from previous chest radiographs) demonstrated changes consistent with COPD. A previously ordered screening pulmonary function study revealed an FEV_1 of 65 percent of predicted values with an actual value for FEV_1/FVC of 60 percent (FEV_1 = forced expiratory volume in 1 second; FVC = forced vital capacity). Blood pressure was 150/88 mmHg; systolic blood pressure ranged from 130 to 170 mmHg, and diastolic blood pressure ranged from 80 to 95 mmHg. The patient was given his usual morning medications with a small amount of water, plus 2 mg of midazolam intramuscularly as a premedicant. A peripheral intravenous line was started, and an arterial line was placed in the left radial artery. We started a 30- to 40-minute infusion of lactated Ringer's solution in preparation for the spinal anesthetic. A room air sample of arterial blood was analyzed to determine baseline blood gas levels.

Anesthesia and Intraoperative Care

In the operating room, an electrocardiogram (dual channel, leads II and V_5), a pulse oximeter, and a blood pressure monitor were all activated. We administered oxygen via nasal prongs at the rate of 3 L/min. The patient was then placed in the right lateral decubitus position for administration of the spinal anesthetic. This consisted of intrathecal injection of 0.75 mg (1.5 ml) of preservative-free morphine, followed by 13 mg of tetracaine with an equal volume of 10 percent dextrose in water, and 0.1 ml of 1:1,000 epinephrine. The patient was then turned supine. After 10 minutes, he had a T6 sensory level bilaterally, and at 20 minutes, a T4 sensory level bilaterally. He reported being comfortable, although heart rate had decreased from 82 to 58 beats/min. Likewise, blood pressure had decreased from 150/88 to 108/70 mmHg. The patient was given a supplemental 500-ml bolus of fluid intravenously. Additionally, 0.2 mg of glycopyrrolate was administered to increase heart rate to approximately 73 to 77 beats/min. Although blood pressure increased to 112/74 mmHg, this was still 20 percent lower than his normal range; therefore, a phenylephrine drip was begun (40 µg/ml) to increase systolic blood pressure to above 120 mmHg. This was accomplished easily and surgery proceeded uneventfully. Surgery lasted 3 hours, a period well within the range of effectiveness of the spinal anesthetic. The patient was given no additional analgesia but did receive a total of 1 mg of midazolam intraoperatively for sedation.

Postoperative Care

At the end of surgery, the patient was taken to the postanesthesia recovery room. Five hours after the spinal anesthesia, he could bend his knees and reported no pain; he then was discharged to the surgical intensive care unit (SICU). Because he had been given morphine intrathecally, the patient was monitored with an apnea monitor. No additional intravenous analgesics were required, as the patient reported no pain until the following morning. At that time, he reported tenderness of the incision, and oral analgesics were given. The patient was then discharged from the SICU.

At the postoperative visit by the anesthesiologist, the patient seemed pleased with the simplicity of the process and with the fact that he had experienced little pain.

DISCUSSION

Let us now discuss why a regional anesthetic was chosen, why the regional technique was a spinal anesthetic, and why intrathecal morphine was added. We will also discuss why a central venous catheter was not placed, and whether the postoperative stay in the ICU was necessary. Finally, did the patient receive both quality and cost-effective care?

The choice between regional and general anesthesia is based on the preferences of the anesthesiologist, the surgeon, and the patient. No prospective, randomized outcome studies have yet demonstrated that one technique is safer than another. A great deal of personal bias enters into the decision. Many physicians agree with us that avoidance of airway manipulation is prudent in the patient who has moderate COPD and is therefore at higher risk of postoperative pulmonary insufficiency.[3] However, the evidence for such avoidance is controversial. Also, many patients with COPD rely on their abdominal muscles for expiration and clearing of secretions. A spinal anesthetic to the T6 sensory level often weakens these muscles.

The length of surgery is another consideration. Because a single-shot spinal anesthetic may be inadequate if surgery is prolonged, some anesthetists prefer a continuous epidural technique. This preference involves another controversial issue. Should continuous epidural anesthesia be used if the patient is going to be given heparin intraoperatively, as our patient was? If an epidural technique is used and an epidural vein is entered inadvertently with the 17-gauge Tuohy needle or the epidural catheter, what actions should follow? Should surgery and heparinization continue, thereby risking the complications of epidural hematoma, or should surgery be postponed? This issue must be resolved before surgery starts. According to the protocol of Rao and El-Etr,[4] if an epidural vein is entered, surgery should be postponed 24 hours to reduce the risk of epidural hematoma formation after heparinization. Although the basis for this recommendation is admittedly very weak, Rao and El-Etr used these guidelines and had no complications with epidural anesthesia in patients subsequently given heparin.

My preference is to avoid the continuous epidural technique and, when regional anesthesia is chosen, to opt for a single-shot subarachnoid block with a 25- or 26-gauge needle. I believe that this approach retains the advantages of regional anesthesia and minimizes the risk of epidural hematoma.

Intrathecal injection of morphine, an easy adjunct to single-shot spinal anesthesia, is a routine part of the technique. In my practice, severe respiratory depression has not been a problem. However, other side effects (pruritus, urinary retention) are common but treatable with a low-dose (1 µg/kg/h) infusion of naloxone for 24 hours postoperatively. The benefits of intrathecal administration of local anesthetic and morphine include superb analgesia in most patients undergoing surgery of the lower extremities. Because postoperative pain is much less, the sympathetic response is less; therefore, hemodynamic variables are under better control. Patients are usually pleased with the results; most would definitely choose intrathecal injection of an opioid again if given the choice. Those patients who undergo general anesthesia can still benefit from intrathecal injection of morphine for postoperative analgesia.

Did our patient need invasive monitoring of central venous pressure? The thorough preoperative cardiac evaluation and the success of angioplasty gave us great confidence that his heart would be able to respond appropriately to the stresses associated with surgery. Although significant changes in ventricular end-diastolic pressure (preload) could occur with spinal anesthesia, we believed that his heart could now tolerate a fluid challenge. Because surgery did not involve aortic cross-clamping, large blood losses, or significant fluid shifts, anesthesia was provided without monitoring by central venous or pulmonary artery catheter.

Was the overnight stay in the ICU necessary? It is the current surgical policy at Emory that many patients undergoing major vascular surgery spend at least the first postoperative night in an ICU. We also believe that all patients given intrathecal administration of morphine require 24 hours of ICU stay with monitoring for apnea because of the risk of delayed respiratory depression.[5] If prospective studies of outcome data demonstrate that the incidence of critical postoperative events does not warrant an overnight stay in the ICU, this policy probably would change.

Finally, if the goal of the anesthesiologist in vascular surgery is to provide a safe and comfortable intraoperative course and to ensure an uneventful outcome, then our patient received quality care. Was the care cost-effective? One could argue that the patient did not need a cardiac evaluation on his first admission; that he could have just been taken to the operating room, given any one of several popular anesthetics, and that he would have done just as well—and for a lot less money. Frankly, only careful studies of outcome could determine which approach provides the most reasonable balance between the quality care patients deserve and the cost-effectiveness third-party payors demand. Unfortunately, such studies are not yet available.

REFERENCES

1. Boucher CA, Brewster DC, Darling RC et al: Determination of cardiac risk by dipyridamole-thallium imaging before peripheral vascular surgery. N Engl J Med 312:389–394, 1985
2. Hertzer NR, Beven EG, Young JR et al: Coronary artery disease in peripheral vascular patients. A classification of 1000 coronary angiograms and results of surgical management. Ann Surg 199:223–233, 1984
3. Tarhan S, Moffitt EA, Sessler AD et al: Risk of anesthesia in surgery in patients with chronic bronchitis and chronic obstructive pulmonary disease. Surgery 74:720–726, 1973
4. Rao TLK, El-Etr AA: Anticoagulation following placement of epidural and subarachnoid catheters: an evaluation of neurologic sequelae. Anesthesiology 55:618–620, 1981
5. Cousins MJ, Mather LE: Intrathecal and epidural administration of opioiods. Anesthesiology 61:276–310, 1984

22

Anesthesia for Vascular Surgery of the Lower Extremities: One Approach at Mount Sinai Hospital, New York

Mark A. Gettes
Joel A. Kaplan

At Mount Sinai Hospital in New York City, we provide anesthesia for approximately 300 vascular operations of the lower extremities a year. Our patients are typical of those undergoing vascular surgery around the country, in that the incidence of associated atherosclerotic coronary artery disease, hypertension, diabetes, and cigarette smoking is high.[1-3] Also, Mount Sinai has a large geriatric department, and a great number of its elderly patients are referred for surgery. The setting is a busy operative suite, with several vascular surgeons performing different types of bypass operations. We believe that optimal anesthetic management takes into account the patient's preoperative condition, the basic theoretic goals of anesthesia for peripheral vascular surgery, and the special demands of the specific procedure the patient is to undergo.

PREOPERATIVE ASSESSMENT

Proper anesthetic management of the patient begins with the preoperative assessment. Full discussion of preoperative management of the many disorders accompanying peripheral vascular disease is beyond the scope of this chapter and is well reviewed elsewhere.[4] In general, in the preoperative period, we use a "problem-oriented" approach to the patient. We believe that identifying specific problems simplifies the management of these often complex situations. Calling attention to a specific problem allows the anesthetist to direct preoperative interventions necessary to better prepare the patient for surgery. Furthermore, it allows the anesthetist to formulate a comprehensive anesthetic plan that follows

339

the patient's problem(s) throughout surgery.

We begin with a careful and complete history and physical examination. The availability of sophisticated technology for patient evaluation does not eliminate the need for these two preoperative assessments. One portion of the physical examination we emphasize is the taking of vital signs. We believe vital signs should be obtained with the patient both lying down and sitting, because the high incidences of hypertension and use of diuretics in these patients make hypovolemia very common. Although we try to recognize and correct hypovolemia in all patients, we pay particular attention to this condition if we are considering giving regional anesthesia.

Because of the high incidence of associated cardiac disease in these patients, the most important cause of morbidity and mortality after vascular surgery of the lower extremities is cardiac in nature. Therefore, preoperative assessment of the cardiovascular system is very important. Many studies have shown that the history is the most sensitive indicator of coronary artery disease.[1,5,6] The history and physical examination should evaluate the cardiovascular system thoroughly. We use the criteria of Goldman et al.,[7] with some modification, to estimate cardiac risk.[8] That is, we believe the presence of one or more of the following major risk factors indicates the need for further evaluation by the cardiology service: congestive heart failure, recent (within 6 months) myocardial infarction, heart rhythm other than sinus, more than five premature ventricular contractions per minute, severe or unstable angina, valvular disease, or ventricular dysfunction. We frequently use echocardiograms and radionuclide scans to do the following: (1) assess indices of ventricular function such as ejection fraction, cardiac output, and stroke volume; (2) identify areas of segmental wall motion abnormality, ventricular wall thickness, and chamber size; and (3) estimate valve cross-sectional area.[9]

We find it increasingly helpful to admit selected patients to the intensive care unit the day before surgery. At that time, we place pulmonary arterial and systemic arterial catheters and obtain hemodynamic data. We also construct a ventricular performance curve by measuring cardiac output at various filling pressures. We observe the effects of vasoactive medications and optimize hemodynamic status before transporting the patient to the operating room. In our opinion, the availability of such data before surgery has greatly enhanced our ability to manage these patients optimally during and after surgery.

Evaluation of the pulmonary system is also very important. When history or physical examination suggests significant pulmonary disease, bedside testing facilitates further evaluation. We frequently obtain preoperative arterial blood gases and have patients perform bedside spirometry. This information not only helps us decide between regional or general anesthesia but also provides baseline values for postoperative comparison.

Diabetic patients receive special attention regarding the degree of blood glucose control when coming to the operating room. Our aim is to avoid hypoglycemia and ketoacidosis and to keep glucose concentrations between 100 and 250 mg/dl. Studies on the effectiveness of the many regimens suggested for diabetic patients have shown that the choice of regimen is less important than frequent monitoring of glucose levels and appropriate adjustment of therapy.[10]

Finally, we believe obtaining a complete drug history is essential. Patients undergoing peripheral vascular surgery often take a variety of medications, including cardiac and antihypertensive drugs, that should be continued in the preoperative period. Knowledge of the patient's baseline medication is essential to avoid rebound phenomena and adverse drug interactions.

CHOICE OF REGIONAL OR GENERAL ANESTHESIA

Because the decision regarding regional or general anesthesia is crucial and controversial, we discuss the potential advantages and disadvantages of each technique (Table 22-1).

General Advantages and Disadvantages

Regional anesthesia offers the obvious advantage of avoiding airway manipulation, with its attendant potential for difficulty, trauma, and changes in cardiovascular stability. Fewer medications are given, thereby decreasing the possibility of adverse side effects and drug interactions. Hemodynamic changes occurring during regional anesthesia are more predictable and frequently easier to interpret than those occurring during general anesthesia. That is, the awake state may allow recognition of certain events that would be difficult to discern if general anesthesia were used (e.g., onset of hypoglycemia or angina). Another advantage is that regional anesthesia suppresses the endocrine and metabolic responses to surgery.[11,12] The incidence of postoperative pulmonary complications may also be lower with regional anesthesia.[13–16] Some evidence indicates that regional anesthesia produces fewer changes in mental state in elderly patients than does

Table 22-1. Advantages and Disadvantages of Regional and General Anesthetic

Anesthesia	Advantages	Disadvantages
Regional	Avoids airway problems and sequelae Fewer pulmonary complications Need for fewer medications Patient is awake Suppression of endocrine stress response Less blood loss (selected cases) Lower incidence of deep venous thrombosis (selected cases) Facilitates postoperative pain relief Hemodynamic stability Preferred by some patients	More difficult technically Potential for local anesthetic toxicity Potential for hypotension secondary to high block Higher incidence of hypothermia Fixed duration of action (spinal anesthesia) Potential for epidural hematoma Possibility of neurologic sequelae Airway not secured Unacceptable to some patients
General	High reliability Ease of administration Airway secured Hemodynamic stability (some techniques) Flexible duration of action Facilitates bronchopulmonary toilet Fewer changes in mental status Preferred by some patients	Potential for airway mismanagement Hemodynamic instability Variable patient response to drugs Drug interactions Inability to communicate with patient Potential for pulmonary complications Postoperative reflex depression Possibility of postoperative hypoventilation

general anesthesia, although this difference does not occur if intravenous sedation is given.[17,18] In certain conditions, regional anesthesia has specific advantages over general anesthesia: intraoperative blood loss is less in elective hip replacement and major pelvic surgery,[19-21] and the incidence of deep venous thrombosis is lower in total hip replacement.[22,23] Finally, regional anesthesia given by indwelling epidural catheters enables one to provide postoperative pain relief with either local anesthetics or epidural narcotics, with less sedation and fewer side effects.[24]

Regional anesthesia has several disadvantages. It is technically more difficult to administer. A 1985 study at a university hospital showed a 17 percent failure rate in administering spinal anesthesia.[25] The failure rate for epidural block may be even higher.[26] Performance of regional blocks frequently requires more time than induction of general anesthesia. Levels of regional anesthesia may be difficult to control, with high blocks leading to significant hypotension. Regional anesthesia also presents the possibility of local anesthetic toxicity, which is caused by high blood levels of the agent after accidental intravascular injection or systemic absorption of the drug. The potential for epidural hematoma also exists, and there is a small but definite risk of neurologic complications. Regional anesthesia is associated with a higher incidence of hypothermia, perhaps because of increased cutaneous blood flow and increased fluid requirements.[27] If the patient loses consciousness or has deficient airway reflexes, the airway is not protected. Finally, regional anesthesia is psychologically unacceptable to some patients.

Advantages of general anesthesia include its greater reliability and its relative ease of administration. To many patients, unconsciousness is a major advantage of general anesthesia. Also, certain techniques (i.e., high-dose fentanyl) are associated with great hemodynamic stability. Controlling the length of anesthesia is often easier with general anesthesia than with regional, particularly if inhalational techniques are used. For patients with severe pulmonary disease, controlled ventilation and the opportunity for bronchopulmonary toilet may be advantageous. Also, for those at risk of aspiration, the airway can be protected with an endotracheal tube.

A disadvantage of general anesthesia is its potential for major hemodynamic changes at certain times: during induction; during surgery, as the level of stimulation varies; and at emergence. Failure to manage the airway properly can be disastrous and is a leading cause of anesthesia-related deaths.[28] Pharmacodynamic and pharmacokinetic differences among patients can make it difficult to predict the degree and length of response to drugs. Depression of reflexes and respiratory drive may be significant postoperative problems.

Morbidity and Mortality for the Two Techniques

Regarding morbidity and mortality, is one technique superior for patients undergoing vascular surgery of the lower extremities? Unfortunately, studies directly addressing this question are rare. However, some studies have compared outcome for elderly patients having orthopedic surgery on the lower extremities under regional or general anesthesia. This patient group is roughly comparable to that undergoing lower extremity vascular surgery. The studies failed to show a significant difference between anesthetic techniques. Of seven prospective studies of mortality after surgery for hip fractures, five did not demonstrate a significant difference in mortality.[13,29–34] A more recent, much larger, randomized prospective study of 578 patients also failed to demonstrate a significant difference in 30-day mortality rates between spinal and general anesthesia (6 and 8 percent, respectively).[35]

Several recent studies have specifically compared regional and general anesthesia for vascular surgery of the lower extremities. One review of anesthesia records and charts showed no difference in mortality rate between regional and general anesthesia.[36] However, perioperative myocardial infarction and ischemia occurred more frequently with regional anesthesia. The investigators noted that patients were not randomly assigned to the two groups and that there may have been a tendency to give the sicker patients regional anesthesia (R. Christopherson, personal communication). The investigators also found that "intraoperative turbulence," as defined by large changes in blood pressure or heart rate, was significantly more common in the group given general anesthesia. An on-going follow-up study that randomly assigned patients to either regional or general anesthesia has initially shown a slightly higher incidence of myocardial ischemia in patients given general anesthesia (R. Christopherson, personal communication). In another recent study, hemodynamic variables were compared for patients undergoing femoropopliteal bypass surgery. More "hemodynamic turbulence" (hypertension) occurred in patients given general anesthesia.[37]

To date, there has been only one large-scale, prospective, randomized study comparing outcome after regional and general anesthesia in patients undergoing vascular surgery of the lower extremities.[38] This study of 101 patients found no difference in mortality rate between the two groups. Intraoperative hypotension occurred more frequently in the re-

gional (spinal) anesthesia group, whereas hypertension was more common in the general anesthesia group. Three percent of the patients given general anesthesia and none of the patients given spinal anesthesia had intraoperative changes in the ST segment. The incidences of changes in mental state were the same for both groups, although only a gross index was used. The major difference between groups was a higher incidence of postoperative pulmonary infection in patients given general anesthesia (35 versus 16 percent).

There is also no evidence that either regional or general anesthesia is superior regarding graft survival.[38,39] Although some studies have demonstrated increased graft blood flow under regional anesthesia in the early postoperative period,[40,41] no evidence exists that this effect translates into a higher rate of graft survival. Furthermore, in patients with fixed outflow obstruction distal to the graft, regional anesthesia may actually cause a "steal" of blood away from the graft by vasodilation of the opposite lower extremity, in a fashion analogous to an intracerebral steal.

In summary, the literature does not demonstrate the clinical superiority of either general or regional anesthesia for the patient undergoing vascular surgery of the lower extremities. When mortality and morbidity with general anesthesia is low, there is little advantage to be gained with regional anesthesia. The relatively healthy patient undergoing vascular surgery of the lower extremities is likely to do well with either technique.

Specific Patient Subgroups

Certain subgroups of patients, however, may benefit from one of the techniques. These patients may have composed a statistically insignificant percentage of the total number of patients in the studies discussed. Studies have not yet compared the relative anesthetic risk among patients in these subgroups. We believe that the choice between regional and general anesthesia is likely to be significant for several subgroups of patients.

We favor regional anesthesia for patients with severe obstructive or bronchospastic pulmonary disease. Regional anesthesia greatly simplifies patient care and does not involve endotracheal intubation, thereby decreasing morbidity. The deleterious effects of endotracheal intubation, cuff inflation,[42] certain general anesthetic agents,[43] and positive-pressure ventilation[44] on mucociliary function are well known, as is the drop in functional residual capacity that accompanies the onset of general anesthesia.[45] Also, the rate of complications is usually lower for patients with chronic obstructive pulmonary disease who are anesthetized with regional as opposed to general anesthesia.[12] On the other hand, endotracheal intubation can facilitate pulmonary toilet and has been used to treat pneumonia. In addition, abdominal relaxation may be greater with regional anesthesia than with general anesthesia, thus making recovery and coughing more difficult with regional anesthesia.

As previously noted, the one randomized, prospective study comparing regional and general anesthesia for lower extremity vascular surgery found a higher rate of pulmonary complications in the general anesthesia group. Patients who have difficult airway problems are also usually managed more easily with regional anesthesia. Although a variety of techniques are available for managing the difficult airway (e.g., fiberoptic intubation, awake intubation), use of regional anesthesia sidesteps this potentially difficult problem, thus simplifying patient care.

Another group of patients perhaps benefiting from regional anesthesia are those with "brittle" or poorly controlled 2 diabetes. Monitoring the state of consciousness of an awake patient can be invaluable in detecting impending hypoglycemia, the signs of which are difficult to discern during general anesthesia. We have seen several instances in which hypoglycemia was recognized and promptly treated because the patient became less arousable.

The optimal management of patients with cardiac disease is a complex and controversial topic. We believe that some cardiac patients are more easily managed under regional anesthesia. Patients with a history of angina can serve as their own "myocardial ischemia monitors" by remaining awake and reporting the onset of angina to the anesthetist. Unfortunately, many patients with coronary artery disease have "silent" ischemia and cannot report discomfort. Myocardial ischemia can be detected in the patient under general anesthesia by a variety of methods, including transesophageal echocardiography (the most sensitive of the three methods), monitoring of pulmonary artery wedge pressure, and monitoring of the electrocardiogram (ECG). However, two of these methods (echocardiography and pulmonary artery monitoring) are more complex and invasive, whereas electrocardiography is the least sensitive.[9] New computerized ST segment-monitoring systems may improve the sensitivity of the ECG in the operating room and allow for the detection of silent ischemia during anesthesia.

In some circumstances, we prefer general anesthesia to regional anesthesia. First, in our opinion, regional anesthesia should never be used if any of the following conditions exist: prior institution of full anticoagulant therapy, thrombocytopenia, platelet dysfunction, clotting factor deficiency or any other coagulopathy, increased intracranial pressure, and infection at the anticipated puncture site.[46] Second, some specific cardiovascular conditions are better managed with general anesthesia. For example, in aortic stenosis, the rapid profound vasodilation that regional anesthesia affords can cause coronary artery perfusion pressure to drop to unacceptably low levels, thus inducing myocardial ischemia. Patients with hypertrophic cardiomyopathy are also poor candidates for a regional block, as a decrease in afterload or left ventricular volume can increase obstruction of functional ventricular outflow. Finally, some patients are poor candidates for regional anesthesia from a psychological standpoint. In the absence of any other contraindications, we use general anesthesia for these patients.

Figure 22-1 shows the algorithm we use to decide which of our patients will be given general, epidural, or spinal anesthesia. We first note whether any of the absolute contraindications to regional anesthesia are present. If not, we determine whether the patient falls into any of the subgroups in which one technique is favored over the other, as discussed above. If the patient is not a member of one of these subgroups, then either general or regional anesthesia is acceptable. In this case (and, in reality, for all patients), the choice of anesthetic technique is made on the basis of the preferences of the patient and the individual anesthetist.

Length of Anesthesia

One of the major considerations in selecting regional or general anesthesia when either technique is equally acceptable—and in deciding between spinal or epidural anesthesia when a regional technique has been chosen—is the antici-

pated length of surgery. Chapter 19 reviews the different surgical approaches to vascular surgery of the lower extremities. Although these operations differ little in the physiologic stress presented to the patient, they differ widely in the length of time they require. At our institution, femoropopliteal bypass grafting with polytetrafluoroethylene (PTFE; GORE-TEX), usually to proximal portions of the lower extremity arterial tree, is a relatively short procedure. The typical operative time is 90 minutes or less. Procedures using reversed saphenous vein grafts usually take 2 to 2.5 hours. In situ, or nonreversed, saphenous vein grafts are used most frequently in patients requiring bypass distal to the popliteal artery. In situ grafting is typically a much longer procedure. Operative time is usually 3 to 3.5 hours, and 5 hours is not uncommon.

When general and regional anesthesia are equally acceptable, we give each type with approximately equal frequency for short and medium-length procedures. For the longer in situ procedures, our tendency is to choose general anesthesia. We find that these procedures last so long that some patients become restless and uncomfortable and require intravenous sedation. Many of the theoretical advantages of regional anesthesia are lost if the patient requires heavy sedation.

For regional anesthesia, we tend to choose spinal anesthesia for short and medium-length procedures. For us, spinal anesthesia is technically easier to administer than epidural anesthesia. Also, spinal anesthesia is associated with a lower failure rate and takes less time to achieve. This last factor is important in our busy operating rooms, because no preoperative block room is available. In terms of risk from epidural hematoma, spinal anesthesia offers a theoretical advantage over a continuous epidural technique, in which an epidural catheter is in place at the time of heparinization.

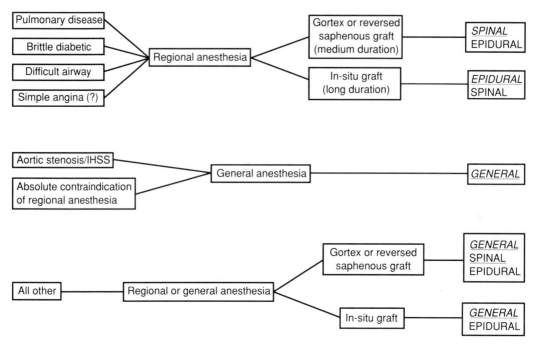

Fig. 22-1. The above algorithm shows the criteria we use to select general versus regional (and epidural versus spinal) anesthesia for subsets of patients undergoing vascular surgery of the lower extremities. The techniques more commonly chosen at our institution are set in italics IHSS = idiopathic hypertrophic subaortic stenosis; PTFE = polytetrafluoroethylene (GORE-TEX); "simple" angina = stable pain of low frequency, without evidence of left ventricular dysfunction.

For the longer in situ procedure done under regional anesthesia, however, we most frequently select epidural anesthesia over spinal anesthesia. Even with the addition of vasoconstrictors to the spinal anesthetic solution, the risk is high that the operation will outlast the block. Also, we tend not to add vasoconstrictors for diabetic patients. The ability to extend the epidural anesthesia to match the length of the operation is a major advantage. Another potential advantage of epidural anesthesia is that the level of the block can be built up slowly by administering incremental doses. This practice helps us avoid too rapid a change in cardiovascular function. That is, we can titrate administration of fluids to changes in preload. (Preload is affected because raising the level of block causes incremental changes in vasodilation). Should the patient need to be returned to the operating room for reexploration, the epidural catheter can be used for the second anesthetic.

Finally, it should be noted that all vascular surgery on the lower extremities can be done under local anesthesia if the patient is too ill to withstand regional or general anesthesia. Although some would say a regional or general anesthetic may result in less stress to the heart, the induction of anesthesia may cause significant cardiovascular changes, even if done meticulously. It is not common for us to use a local-anesthetic-only technique. We use this technique for particular procedures, for example, femorofemoral bypass, in which the shortness of the incision line makes it possible to obtain local anesthesia with only small quantities of drug. Simple embolectomies are also frequently performed with local anesthesia.

CONDUCT OF ANESTHESIA

Premedication

Ideally, the patient coming to the operating room for lower extremity vascular surgery should be free from anxiety and fully cooperative. Preoperative anxiety can cause hypertension and tachycardia, both of which increase myocardial oxygen demand and possibly induce myocardial ischemia, angina, or even myocardial infarction.[47] Given the high incidence of coronary artery disease in patients undergoing vascular surgery of the lower extremities, prevention of preoperative anxiety seems to us to be an important goal.

We believe that one of the best ways of preventing anxiety is to conduct a thorough preoperative visit. Our practice is to discuss the anesthetic plan, regional or general, with the patient and to describe the events that will transpire in the operating room before induction of anesthesia. Invasive procedures—whether placement of a venous or arterial cannula or performance of regional blocks—are discussed and the patient reassured that these can be accomplished in a largely pain-free manner. The preoperative visit is a time to establish rapport and gain the trust of the patient. This makes induction of anesthesia a safer and more pleasant experience for both the patient and anesthetist. Furthermore, the preoperative visit reveals which patients are likely to

be unduly anxious and thus require heavier than usual premedication.

Our patients are usually premedicated either with an oral dose of a benzodiazepine or with an intramuscular injection of a narcotic and an antiemetic. However, the choice and dosage of premedication are always tailored to the patient. Because elderly patients may be particularly sensitive to the depressant effects of both benzodiazepines and opiates, the drug dose is reduced.[48] Similarly, patients with pulmonary disease or reduced cardiac output may be more sensitive to these drugs, with resultant hypoventilation and hypoxia. In general, our policy is to premedicate our patients conservatively. Once the patient has arrived at the induction area, the premedication can be supplemented with rapidly acting intravenous drugs, with the patient under our direct observation. We believe that this procedure is preferable to incurring the risk of excessive premedication in the unattended, unobserved patient. Critically ill patients often are given no premedication at all.

We also believe that patients undergoing spinal or epidural anesthesia should not be premedicated excessively. The patient's ability to cooperate and communicate is important, both for performing the blocks and for evaluating the effectiveness and degree of anesthesia and possible side effects. Again, supplementation of premedication, both before and after the regional block, can be accomplished under direct observation by the anesthetist.

Occasionally, patients scheduled for vascular surgery of the lower extremities have ischemic pain. These patients are premedicated with analgesic drugs. Usually, they are already receiving intramuscular or intravenous narcotics, and the dose of premedication can be based on their response to the amount of medication they are already taking.

Monitoring

The safe management of patients under anesthesia requires frequent observation of many physiologic variables. Through diligent observation, deviations from normal ranges can be recognized quickly and corrective measures instituted. Because of the high incidence of associated diseases, patients scheduled for vascular surgery of the lower extremities may be less tolerant of such deviations than other, healthier patients. Optimal management of these patients requires meticulous and thorough monitoring.

At our institution, the standard of care for monitoring during either regional or general anesthesia for vascular surgery of the lower extremities consists of use of the following: continuous electrocardiographic display, manual or automatic blood pressure cuff, pulse oximeter, temperature probe, and precordial or esophageal stethoscope. Patients having general anesthesia are also monitored by means of a mass spectrometer. We use a modified electrocardiographic V_5 lead because it is the most sensitive for detection of myocardial ischemia.[49] The right arm lead is placed below the clavicle on the right shoulder, the left arm lead is in the V_5 position, and the left leg lead is in its usual position. Selecting lead I gives a modified V_5 lead, whereas lead II can be used for monitoring dysrhythmias and diagnosing ischemia of the inferior wall.[50] Whenever possible, the initial ECG is recorded on paper to serve as a baseline for intraoperative comparison.

Blood pressure is monitored by one of the automated noninvasive systems in many patients. Frequent determination of blood pressure is of great importance in these patients, who often have coronary and cerebrovascular disease. In our view, the pulse oximeter is tremendously valuable in monitoring patients under both general and regional anesthesia; we believe it is an excellent early warning system for ventilation and perfusion abnormalities and may warn of the development of hypoxia in the patient given sedative medication during regional anesthesia.

Temperature is monitored in all of these patients. During long procedures in which the entire lower extremity is exposed and incisions are long, patients often become hypothermic. We use esophageal temperature probes during general anesthesia and adhesive skin probes (placed in the axilla) during regional anesthesia.

Esophageal stethoscopes monitor heart and breath sounds in intubated patients, whereas precordial stethoscopes are used in patients under regional anesthesia. With general anesthesia, we use the mass spectrometer to measure the concentration of inhalation agent and the inspired end-tidal concentrations of carbon dioxide, nitrogen, and oxgyen. Measurement of the end-tidal concentration of carbon dioxide is helpful in maintaining normocarbia, which may be an important goal in patients with cerebrovascular disease.[51]

In many patients, we monitor blood pressure continuously via an arterial catheter. In addition to providing beat-to-beat determination of blood pressure, the arterial catheter provides additional indirect information derived from visual inspection of the pressure tracing—an estimate of pulse volume, myocardial contractility, and intravascular volume status. Additionally, the arterial catheter can be used for blood sampling; it thus facilitates monitoring of blood gases, electrolytes, glucose levels, and hematocrit. We consider the use of an arterial catheter for all patients but consider it most seriously for those with symptomatic cardiac disease, severe pulmonary disease, poorly controlled diabetes, or other metabolic disorders. We also seriously consider placing an arterial catheter in patients undergoing long procedures requiring intravenous administration of large volumes of fluids or blood.

Because large changes in intravascular volume are not common during vascular surgery of the lower extremities, we do not routinely monitor central venous pressure. The anesthetist has full access to the head and neck during surgery, and a central catheter can be inserted intraoperatively, if necessary.

Pulmonary artery pressure is also not monitored routinely. In procedures on the lower extremities, the need to monitor pulmonary artery pressure is more a function of the patient's condition than of the operation itself. The conditions we consider indications for placement of a pulmonary artery catheter are as follows: congestive heart failure, severe ventricular dysfunction with low ejection fraction, recent myocardial infarction, unstable angina, or severe valvular disease. Patients with poor renal function may also be candidates for preoperative placement of a pulmonary artery catheter.[52] As previously noted, we identify these patients preoperatively and place a pulmonary artery catheter the night before surgery while the patient is observed in the intensive care unit. A Foley catheter is usually used only when lengthy surgery is anticipated; we find that monitoring urinary output is often helpful in estimating the adequacy of volume replacement in lengthy procedures.

General Anesthesia

In our opinion, the goal of induction of general anesthesia in patients undergoing vascular surgery of the lower extremities should be a smooth transition from the awake state to surgical anesthesia and the maintenance of cardiovascular stability. We avoid not only excessive depression of hemodynamic status from a relative overdose of anesthetic but also sudden increases in sympathetic or parasympathetic tone from inadequate anesthesia during laryngoscopy and intubation. The key to safe induction is slow and gradual titration of induction drugs during close observation of hemodynamic status. We emphasize that although we are providing an induction scheme, in our opinion, the particular drugs administered are of less importance than the way in which they are used. In attempting to maintain hemodynamic stability, the anesthetist must be aware of the baseline range of hemodynamic values for that particular patient. Thus, systolic blood pressure of 100 mmHg is acceptable in a patient whose normal range is 90 to 120 mmHg but should probably be treated if the preoperative range was 160 to 190 mmHg.

After preoxygenation, we frequently begin induction of anesthesia with small incremental doses of an intravenous opioid, such as fentanyl citrate (1 to 2 µg/kg) until the patient begins to appear drowsy or the respiratory rate slows. It is essential that this phase of induction proceed in an unhurried manner, because the time to onset of action of intravenous drugs may be greater in a patient with low cardiac output. During this phase, we also administer a small dose of a nondepolarizing muscle relaxant to avoid narcotic-induced chest wall rigidity. Observation of the pulse oximeter is helpful during this phase, as oxygen saturation may begin to drop as respiratory rate decreases. At this point, we give thiopental in divided doses, 25 to 50 mg at a time, until unconsciousness occurs. Alternatively, if we believe ventricular function is so poor that the patient cannot tolerate the depressant effects of thiopental on myocardial contractility, we use a high-dose narotic technique (fentanyl, 10 to 30 µg/kg). Initially, we assist ventilation;

once unconscious, the patient is paralyzed and ventilation is controlled. Although muscle relaxation is not often necessary intraoperatively, in some instances it is given to facilitate intubation. In other situations, nondepolarizing relaxants are used, the specific drug being chosen on the basis of its cardiovascular effect. For example, pancuronium might be used if the heart rate has slowed substantially during induction; vecuronium might be chosen if the pulse rate is in the desired range. Use of nondepolarizing muscle relaxants offers the additional advantage of allowing adequate time for titration of additional drugs, if necessary, before intubation.

Once the patient is paralyzed and ventilation is controlled, we often estimate the readiness for endotracheal intubation by applying an electrical stimulus to test neuromuscular transmission. Placement of an oral airway or insertion of a Foley catheter at this stage is useful. If the patient responds to these maneuvers, we increase the depth of anesthesia before attempting intubation. Specifically, we administer a potent inhalation agent or additional doses of intravenous drugs such as fentanyl, thiopental, or lidocaine. After intubation, we confirm proper placement of the endotracheal tube, control ventilation with a mixture of oxygen and nitrous oxide (assuming oxygenation and blood pressure are adequate), and add a potent inhalational agent, if necessary. In the interval between induction and the start of surgery, stimulation of the patient is minimal, and it is not unusual for blood pressure to drop. If decreases of more than 20 percent from the desired level occur, we usually give small incremental doses of ephedrine.

After surgery begins, the anesthetist must continue to observe the patient and all monitored variables diligently. Depth of anesthesia may need to be adjusted as the level of surgical stimulation changes.

In general, once the incision is complete, the level of anesthesia needed for these procedures is not very deep compared with that needed for intra-abdominal or thoracic surgery. Muscle relaxation is also not required, although relaxants are often used in patients whose anesthesia is maintained with only nitrous oxide and narcotics. We frequently assess fluid status by vital signs, urinary output (if a Foley catheter is used), and inspection of the operative field, suction bottles, and sponges. In general, blood is transfused to keep hematocrit over 30 percent, so that the oxygen-carrying capacity of the blood will be optimal. It is important not to give too many red blood cells or inadequate amounts of crystalloid, as these practices would increase blood viscosity and the possibility of graft thrombosis. During long procedures involving significant blood loss, we find it helpful to obtain blood samples for determination of hematocrit, electrolyte levels, and blood gases.

Heat loss can be significant during surgery, especially in elderly patients, who often have a higher ratio of surface area to weight and a decreased vasoconstrictive response to cold.[53,54] Postoperative hypothermia may increase oxygen demand and myocardial work, potentially deleterious conditions for the patient with cardiac disease. Accordingly, we make every attempt to conserve heat during surgery. All fluids are passed through a warmer, a passive humidifier is placed in the breathing circuit proximal to the endotracheal tube,[55] and fresh gas flow is maintained at the rate of 3 L/min or less. We also wrap the patient's head, and any exposed area is covered with a blanket. Other institutions frequently use warming blankets and/or heated humidification of gases as well.

Intraoperative angiography is commonly performed during vascular surgery of the lower extremities and may be associated with changes in hemodynamic status. First, allergic reactions can occur. In one study, the incidence of adverse reactions to intravascularly injected contrast agents was 2.3 percent.[56] Second, intraoperative angiography may change the level of surgical stimulation. Blood pressure frequently decreases when surgical activity stops in preparation for angiography. Alternatively, blood pressure and heart rate occasionally increase dramatically when dye is injected, despite the appearance of adequate depth of anesthesia. Thus, the level of anesthesia may need to be adjusted at this time. Finally, repeat injection of contrast dye during multiple attempts at angiography may cause osmotic diuresis.

Unclamping of the femoral artery rarely affects hemodynamic status significantly. The lower extremity receives arterial blood through collateral blood vessels even when the femoral artery is occluded (as evidenced by the bleeding that occurs when the clamp is on); thus, the vascular bed of the leg is not empty when the clamp is removed. Furthermore, typical graft blood flow is not very high, usually being in the range of 100 to 200 ml/min.[39]

At the end of surgery, we make a decision regarding tracheal extubation based on standard criteria, including adequacy of ventilation, the degree of reversal of muscle relaxation, and the presence of protective airway reflexes. Temperature is also an important criterion. If patients have become hypothermic to 34°C or below, we sedate, ventilate, and actively warm them in the recovery room. The early postoperative period is a time of potential hemodynamic instability, with hypertension being very common.[37] Although we treat underlying causes (e.g., pain), we often need to control blood pressure with small, incremental doses of vasoactive medications. In our practice, labetalol, a rapidly-acting, mixed α- and β-adrenergic

antagonist, has proven very useful in this situation.[57] Labetalol lowers blood pressure as effectively as hydralazine but does not cause tachycardia, a condition that may be poorly tolerated by patients with cardiac disease.[58] Hypertensive episodes are most common at the beginning and end of the case, that is, at intubation and extubation (R. Christopherson, personal communication).[37] General anesthesia administered by mask, without intubation, may allow a smoother hemodynamic course by avoiding the stresses of intubation and extubation in selected patients. Although we routinely extubate the trachea during deep planes of anesthesia, others may extubate the trachea when their patients are less deeply anesthetized than ours.

Regional Anesthesia

Just as with general anesthesia, maintenance of cardiovascular stability is crucial during induction of spinal or epidural anesthesia. Hemodynamic studies performed during vascular surgery of the lower extremities show that the most common intraoperative cardiovascular complications of regional anesthesia are hypotension and bradycardia. Furthermore, in the largest of these studies, intraoperative hypotension seemed related to morbidity and mortality.[38] Therefore, the major goal of the anesthetist, in addition to achieving an adequate block, must be prevention of hypotension and bradycardia. To accomplish this, we carefully determine the drug dosage for regional anesthesia. To prevent or recognize an excessively high block, we closely observe the patient during onset of the anesthetic. We frequently monitor blood pressure and pulse rate and promptly treat deviations of 20 percent or more. Hypotension is treated with incremental doses of ephedrine, but incremental doses of phenylephrine (0.5 to 1 µg/kg) can be used in the patient with tachycardia. Because of the loss of sympathetic tone that accompanies a major conduction block, it is essential that the patient not be hypovolemic at the onset of anesthesia. For patients coming from the intensive care unit, one can easily determine volume status by measuring filling pressure. For other patients, we routinely check for postural hypotension. Although this check is part of the routine preoperative evaluation, patients can become hypovolemic in the interval between preoperative examination and arrival at the operating room. This occurs because of restriction of oral intake and intravascular injection of angiographic dyes for vascular studies. We advocate that intravenous hydration begin no later than the start of restriction of oral intake.

After establishment of appropriate monitoring devices, we insert a well-functioning 18-gauge or larger intravenous catheter and administer 500 to 1,000 ml of crystalloid before performing the block. This practice minimizes the hemodynamic effects of the sympathetic blockade that occur with the onset of the anesthetic. We then position the patient for the block. Although the sitting position can be used, we most frequently place the patient in the lateral decubitus position. Some theoretical advantage exists in having the patient lie with the operative side down. If the patient is kept in the lateral position during epidural anesthesia, the onset of sympathetic and sensory blockade is more rapid in the dependent side; we believe the sensory block may be denser and the length of the block on the dependent side substantially greater. Additionally, because the level will be higher on the dependent side, the total volume of anesthetic agent required and, hence, the degree of hypotension, will be less.[59] With spinal anesthesia, true unilateral anesthesia is difficult to achieve, even if the patient is kept on the operative side for 15 to 30 minutes. However, the block may be denser on the dependent side. Furthermore, even when true lateralization of the block is not achieved, the incidence of hypotension is lower and the time to onset of hypotension is longer than with conventional spinal anesthesia.[60] Our goal with both spinal and epidural anesthesia for procedures on the lower extremities is to produce a block to the T10 level. Although this level is slightly above the skin dermatome level necessary for the usual incisions (T12 to L1), sympathetic innervation of the lower extremity, which contains visceral afferent fibers, is believed to occur from T10 to L2.[46]

For *spinal anesthesia*, our choice of agent is usually 1 percent hyperbaric tetracaine. Procedures are rarely short enough that we are comfortable using lidocaine. The dose of tetracaine required to produce anesthesia to the T10 level in an average patient is usually 6 to 10 mg.[46,61] We typically use 8 mg of tetracaine and adjust for height. Age appears to affect the duration of spinal anesthesia but not the degree of spread.[62] We do not hesitate to add vasoconstrictors to the solution given to nondiabetic patients if a block of longer duration is desired. The safety of this practice has been demonstrated by numerous studies involving large numbers of patients.[61] Estimates of the effect of vasoconstrictors vary in the literature. A rough estimate that is consistent with our clinical experience is that adding 0.2 mg of epinephrine will increase the length of block 50 percent and that adding 5 mg of phenylephrine will increase the length of block 100 percent.[63–65]

Several other practical points are worth mentioning. First, a recent study demonstrating the high failure rate of spinal anesthesia at an academic institution emphasized the importance of having a free flow of cerebrospinal fluid (CSF) at the time of injection.[25] If CSF is not flowing freely, the needle should be repositioned. Second, performance of a subarachnoid block by a midline approach can be difficult in the elderly because of degenerative changes in the spine and decreased ability to flex the back. If difficulty is encountered, we do not persist for long periods but, instead, use a paramedian or lateral approach. Third, we believe it is helpful to give ephedrine prophylactically, either before the block is performed (25 mg intramuscularly) or immediately after the block is performed (5 mg intravenously), as opposed to waiting for the development of hypotension. Finally, the first 10 to 15 minutes after performance of the block is a critical time, during which we frequently and diligently monitor the spread of the block and the patient's vital signs.

When performing *epidural anesthesia*, one should remember that the elderly patient is more sensitive to the effects of local anesthetic agents. For example, the dose required to reach a given level of blockade is approximately 50 percent less in the 80-year-old.[66,67] To avoid an adverse reaction to local anesthetic, we reduce the maximum allowable dose by approximately the same amount in the elderly.

A variety of agents can be used for epidural anesthesia with satisfactory results. Despite its relatively short duration, chloroprocaine (3 percent) has the advantages of low systemic toxicity, rapid onset, and a high quality block. As the length of blockade increases in elderly patients, the frequency of redosing is not so common. Bupivacaine produces a long-lasting block requiring infrequent intraoperative reinjections and postoperative analgesia. Because its major disadvantage is cardiovascular toxicity, one must take meticulous care to avoid intravascular injection. Lidocaine (1.5 or 2 percent) offers

an advantageous combination of short onset time, moderate duration, and low cardiac toxicity. With the addition of epinephrine in a concentration of 1:200,000, the block is of higher quality and longer duration. Circulating levels of epinephrine are low, with a modest increase (10 to 20 percent) in heart rate, accompanied by lower peripheral vascular resistance, increased cardiac output, and normal or slightly lowered blood pressure.[68] Thus, addition of epinephrine is safe for most patients undergoing epidural anesthesia; however, we recognize the risk of tachycardia from both epinephrine and ephedrine.

For epidural anesthesia, we place a catheter at L4-5 or L3-4 and give all local anesthetic through the catheter. A test dose of 3 ml of 2 percent lidocaine with epinephrine (1:200,000) provides a check for both intravascular and subarachnoid injection. We never give more than 5 ml of drugs through the catheter at a time. As with spinal anesthesia, it is essential that the patient be monitored closely during onset of epidural anesthesia. This practice allows for accurate titration of the block level and prompt recognition and treatment of hypotension. Once blockade is achieved, repeat doses of one-half to one-third the initial dose may be necessary. The time interval to redosing can be estimated as 2 hours for bupivacaine, 1 hour for lidocaine with epinephrine, and 40 minutes for chloroprocaine.[68] Although we use this rough guide, we always examine the patient to ensure that the level of anesthesia is neither too high nor too low.

We administer supplemental oxygen via nasal cannula to all patients under regional anesthesia. The pulse oximeter is useful in ensuring adequate oxygenation. Administration of sedative medication is individualized to the needs of the patient. As noted, many of the theoretical advantages of regional anesthesia are lost as the dose of sedative medication is increased. Nonetheless, especially for longer procedures, many patients are more comfortable when sedated.

The use of regional anesthesia in patients undergoing intraoperative anticoagulation is still a controversial topic and is discussed fully in Chapter 20. Our feeling, based on studies with a large series of patients and low complication rates, is that regional anesthesia is safe for these patients.[69–72] The risk of performing regional anesthesia in patients taking aspirin or minidose heparin also seems to be quite low. Nevertheless, both on theoretical grounds and on the basis of case reports, there is reason for concern in these patients, and the practice remains controversial.[73–78] We therefore require a normal bleeding time for patients on aspirin, and a normal partial thromboplastin time for patients on minidose heparin, before proceeding with regional anesthesia. Furthermore, because the risks may be greater, the indications for regional anesthesia should be strong.

If attempted passage of the epidural catheter results in aspiration of frank blood, management is again controversial. Some advocate abandoning the technique and rescheduling the procedure the next day under general anesthesia.[69] Others abandon the continuous technique but proceed with the procedure under a single-shot technique or general anesthesia.[79] Our practice has been to remove the catheter and attempt to rethread it at a different level. We have not had a known complication using this technique. Once again, however, the perceived benefits of regional anesthesia should be weighed against the risks.

After surgery, our patients go to the recovery room. In general, pain seems to be well controlled with intramuscularly or intravenously administered narcotics as the block wears off. We do not routinely give epidural narcotics or repeated doses of local anesthetics. Neurologic function is followed closely in the recovery room, as delayed return of neurologic function may represent either an unusually long response to the local anesthetic or formation of an epidural hematoma. An epidural hematoma, although rare, is a potentially devastating complication and must be treated promptly to avoid permanent neurologic damage; therefore, high suspicion must be maintained. Case reports of epidural hematoma note that patients frequently complain of severe low back pain.[72,75,77] Any patient whose block does not seem to wear off completely and who complains of severe low back pain should be evaluated immediately for epidural hematoma. If we decide to use repeated doses of local anesthetics in the recovery room, we allow the block to regress partially between doses to ensure that neurologic function is intact. Epidural narcotics are not used routinely because of the rare potential danger of masking the symptoms of epidural hematoma. Finally, removal of the epidural catheter can in theory dislodge a clot that has sealed off an epidural vein; therefore, we believe the catheter should not be removed until the partial prothrombin time or activated clotting time has returned to normal.

Thus, our anesthetic management of patients undergoing lower extremity vascular procedures is tailored to the individual patient, taking into account preoperative status, the theoretical goals for perioperative management, and the special demands of the specific surgical procedure in question.

REFERENCES

1. Tomatis LA, Fierens EE, Verbrugge GP: Evaluation of surgical risk in peripheral vascular disease by coronary arteriog-

raphy: a series of 100 cases. Surgery 71:429–435, 1972

2. Cooperman M, Pflug B, Martin EW, Jr., Evans WE: Cardiovascular risk factors in patients with peripheral vascular disease. Surgery 84:505–509, 1978

3. Foëx P: Preoperative assessment of the patient with cardiovascular disease. Br J Anaesth 53:731–744, 1981

4. Roizen MF: Anesthetic implications of concurrent diseases. p. 255–357. In Miller RD (ed): Anesthesia. Vol. 1. 2nd Ed. Churchill Livingstone, New York, 1986

5. Hertzer NR, Beven EG, Young JR et al: Coronary artery disease in peripheral vascular patients. A classification of 1000 coronary angiograms and results of surgical management. Ann Surg 199:223–233, 1984

6. Benchimol A, Harris CL, Desser KB et al: Resting electrocardiogram in major coronary artery disease. JAMA 224:1489–1492, 1973

7. Goldman L, Caldera DL, Nussbaum SR et al: Multifactorial index of cardiac risk in noncardiac surgical procedures. N Engl J Med 297:845–850, 1977

8. Jeffrey CC, Kunsman J, Cullen DJ, Brewster DC: A prospective evaluation of cardiac risk index. Anesthesiology 58:462–464, 1983

9. Cahalan MK, Litt L, Botvinick EH, Schiller NB: Advances in noninvasive cardiovascular imaging: implications for the anesthesiologist. Anesthesiology 66:356–372, 1987

10. Walts LF, Miller J, Davidson MB, Brown J: Perioperative management of diabetes mellitus. Anesthesiology 55:104–109, 1981

11. Pflug AE, Murphy TM, Butler SH, Tucker GT: The effects of postoperative peridural analgesia on pulmonary therapy and pulmonary complications. Anesthesiology 41:8–17, 1974

12. Tarhan S, Moffitt EA, Sessler AD et al: Risk of anesthesia and surgery in patients with chronic bronchitis and chronic obstructive pulmonary disease. Surgery 74:720–726, 1973

13. McKenzie PJ, Wishart HY, Dewar KMS et al: Comparison of the effects of spinal anaesthesia and general anaesthesia on postoperative oxygenation and perioperative mortality. Br J Anaesth 52:49–54, 1980

14. Kehlet H: The modifying effect of general and regional anesthesia on the endocrine-metabolic response to surgery. Reg Anesth 7:538–548, 1982

15. Brandt MR, Fernandes A, Mordhorst R, Kehlet H: Epidural analgesia improves postoperative nitrogen balance. Br Med J 1:1106–1108, 1978

16. Covino BG: Reasons to preferentially select regional anesthesia. p. 61–65. IARS Review Course Lectures, 60th Congress. International Anesthesia Research Society, Cleveland, 1986

17. Hole A, Terjesen T, Breivik H: Epidural versus general anaesthesia for total hip arthroplasty in elderly patients. Acta Anaesthesiol Scand 24:279–287, 1980

18. Karhunen U, Jönn G: A comparison of memory function following local and general anaesthesia for extraction of senile cataract. Acta Anaesthesiol Scand 26:291–296, 1982

19. Modig J, Malmberg P: Pulmonary and circulatory reactions during total hip replacement surgery. Acta Anaesthesiol Scand 19:219–237, 1975

20. Ryan DW: Anaesthesia for cystectomy. A comparison of two anaesthetic techniques. Anaesthesia 37:554–560, 1982

21. Moir DD: Blood loss during major vaginal surgery. A statistical study of the influence of general anaesthesia and epidural analgesia. Br J Anaesth 40:233–240, 1968

22. Modig J, Borg T, Karlström G et al: Thromboembolism after total hip replacement: role of epidural and general anesthesia. Anesth Analg 62:174–180, 1983

23. Thorburn J, Louden JR, Vallance R: Spinal and general anaesthesia in total hip replacement: frequency of deep vein thrombosis. Br J Anaesth 52:1117–1121, 1980

24. Rawal N, Sjöstrand U, Christoffersson E et al: Comparison of intramuscular and epidural morphine for postoperative analgesia in the grossly obese: influence on postoperative ambulation and pulmonary function. Anesth Analg 63:583–592, 1984

25. Levy JH, Islas JA, Ghia JN, Turnbull C:

A retrospective study of the incidence and causes of failed spinal anesthetics in a university hospital. Anesth Analg 64:705–710, 1985

26. Mehta M, Salmon N: Extradural block. Confirmation of the injection site by X-ray monitoring. Anaesthesia 40:1009–1012, 1985

27. Carli F, Gabrielczyk M, Clark MM, Aber VR: An investigation of factors affecting postoperative rewarming of adult patients. Anaesthesia 41:363–369, 1986

28. Rosen M: Maternal mortality associated with anesthesia in England and Wales. p. 69–74. In Vickers MD, Lunn JN (eds): Mortality in Anaesthesia. (European Academy of Anaesthesiology. Vol. 3). Springer-Verlag, Berlin, 1983

29. Couderc E, Mauge F, Duvaldestin P, Desmonts JM: Résultats comparatifs de l'anesthésie générale et péridurale chez le grand vieillard dans la chirurgie de la hanche. Anesth Analg (Paris) 34:987–997, 1977

30. McLaren AD, Stockwell MC, Reid VT: Anaesthetic techniques for surgical correction of fractured neck of femur. A comparative study of spinal and general anaesthesia in the elderly. Anaesthesia 33:10–14, 1978

31. White IWC, Chappell WA: Anaesthesia for surgical correction of fractured femoral neck. A comparison of three techniques. Anaesthesia 35:1107–1110, 1980

32. Davis FM, Laurenson VG: Spinal anaesthesia or general anaesthesia for emergency hip surgery in elderly patients. Anaesth Intensive Care 9:352–358, 1981

33. Wickström I, Holmberg I, Stefánsson T: Survival of female geriatric patients after hip fracture surgery. A comparison of 5 anesthetic methods. Acta Anaesthesiol Scand 26:607–614, 1982

34. McKenzie PJ, Wishart HY, Smith G: Long-term outcome after repair of fractured neck of femur. Comparison of subarachnoid and general anaesthesia. Br J Anaesth 56:581–585, 1984

35. Valentin N, Lomholt B, Jensen JS et al: Spinal or general anaesthesia for surgery of the fractured hip? A prospective study of mortality in 578 patients. Br J Anaesth 58:284–291, 1986

36. Beattie C, Christopherson R, Manolio T, Pearson T: Myocardial ischemia may be more common with regional than with general anesthesia in high risk patients (abstract). Anesthesiology 64:A518, 1986

37. Damask MC, Weissman C, Barth A et al: General vs epidural—which is the better anesthetic technique for femoral-popliteal bypass surgery (abstract)? Anesth Analg 65:S39, 1986

38. Cook PT, Davies MJ, Cronin KD, Moran P: A prospective randomised trial comparing spinal anaesthesia using hyperbaric cinchocaine with general anaesthesia for lower limb vascular surgery. Anaesth Intensive Care 14:373–380, 1986

39. Mundth ED, Darling RC, Moran JM et al: Quantitative correlation of distal arterial outflow and patency of femoropopliteal reversed saphenous vein grafts with intraoperative flow and pressure measurements. Surgery 65:197–206, 1969

40. Cousins MJ, Wright CJ: Graft, muscle, skin blood flow after epidural block in vascular surgical procedures. Surg Gynecol Obstet 133:59–64, 1971

41. Terry HJ, Allan JS, Taylor GW: The effect of adding lumbar sympathectomy to reconstructive arterial surgery in the lower limb. Br J Surg 567:51–55, 1970

42. Sackner MA, Hirsch J, Epstein S: Effect of cuffed endotracheal tubes on tracheal mucous velocity. Chest 68:774–777, 1975

43. Forbes AR: Halothane depresses mucociliary flow in the trachea. Anesthesiology 45:59–63, 1976

44. Forbes AR, Gamsu G: Lung mucociliary clearance after anesthesia with spontaneous and controlled ventilation. Am Rev Respir Dis 120:857–862, 1979

45. Don H: The mechanical properties of the respiratory system during anesthesia. Int Anesthesiol Clin 15:113–136, 1977

46. Murphy TM: Spinal, epidural, and caudal anesthesia. p. 1061–1111. In Miller RD (ed): Anesthesia. Vol. 2. 2nd Ed. Churchill Livingstone, New York, 1986

47. Lunn JK, Stanley TH, Webster LR, Bidwai AV: Arterial blood-pressure and pulse-rate responses to pulmonary and radial arterial catheterization prior to cardiac and major vascular operations. Anesthesiology 51:265–269, 1979

48. Stanski DR, Watkins DW: Drug Disposition in Anesthesia. p. 137–191. Grune & Stratton, Orlando, FL, 1982

49. Blackburn H: The exercise electrocardiogram: technological, procedural, and conceptual development. pp. 220–258. In Blackburn H (ed): Measurement in Exercise Electrocardiography. Charles C Thomas, Springfield, IL, 1969

50. Kaplan JA, Thys DM: The electrocardiogram and anesthesia. p. 488–489. In Miller RD (ed): Anesthesia. Vol. 1. 2nd Ed. Churchill Livingstone, New York, 1986

51. Sørenson SC: Theoretical considerations on the potential hazards of hyperventilation during anaesthesia. Acta Anaesthesiol Scand, suppl., 67:106–110, 1978

52. Sladen RN: Can we prevent postoperative renal failure intraoperatively? ASA Refresher Course Lectures. Lecture 211. American Society of Anesthesiologists, Park Ridge, IL, 1982

53. Collins KJ, Exton-Smith AN, James MH, Oliver DJ: Functional changes in autonomic nervous responses with ageing. Age Aging 9:17–24, 1980

54. Vaughn MS, Vaughn RW, Cork RC: Postoperative hypothermia in adults: Relationship of age, anesthesia, and shivering to rewarming. Anesth Analg 60:746–751, 1981

55. Haslam KR, Nielsen CH: Do passive heat and moisture exchangers keep the patient warm? Anesthesiology 64:379–381, 1986

56. Shehadi WH: Adverse reactions to intravascularly administered contrast media. A comprehensive study based on a prospective study. Am J Roentgenol Radium Ther Nucl Med 124:145–152, 1975

57. Cummings AMM, Brown JJ, Lever AF et al: Treatment of severe hypertension by repeated bolus injections of labetalol. Br J Clin Pharmacol 8:199S–204S, 1979

58. Gabrielson G, Lingham R, Dimich I et al: Comparative study of labetalol and hydralazine in the treatment of postoperative hypertension (abstract). Anesth Analg 66:S63, 1987

59. Grundy EM, Rao LN, Winnie AP: Epidural anesthesia and the lateral position. Anesth Analg 57:95–97, 1978

60. Tanasichuk MA, Schultz EA, Matthews JH, Van Bergen FH: Spinal hemianalgesia: an evaluation of a method, its applicability, and influence on the incidence of hypotension. Anesthesiology 22:74–85, 1961

61. Bridenbaugh PO, Kennedy WF, Jr: Spinal, subarachnoid neural blockade. p. 149, 163. In Cousins MJ, Bridenbaugh PO (eds): Neural Blockade in Clinical Anesthesia and Management of Pain. JB Lippincott, Philadelphia, 1980

62. Greene NM: The Physiology of Spinal Anesthesia. 3rd Ed. p. 41–44. Williams & Wilkins, Baltimore, 1981

63. Park WY, Balingit PE, MacNamara TE: Effects of patient age, pH of cerebrospinal fluid, and vasopressors on onset and duration of spinal anesthesia. Anesth Analg 54:455–458, 1975

64. Concepcion M, Maddi R, Francis D et al: Vasoconstrictors in spinal anesthesia with tetracaine—a comparison of epinephrine and phenylephrine. Anesth Analg 63:134–138, 1984

65. Armstrong IR, Littlewood DG, Chambers WA: Spinal anesthesia with tetracaine—effect of added vasoconstrictors. Anesth Analg 62:793–795, 1983

66. Sharrock NE: Epidural anesthetic dose responses in patients 20 to 80 years old. Anesthesiology 49:425–428, 1978

67. Bromage PR: Ageing and epidural dose requirements. Segmental spread and predictability of epidural analgesia in youth and extreme age. Br J Anaesth 41:1016–1022, 1969

68. Cousins MJ: Epidural neural blockade. p. 200–211, 240, 255. In Cousins MJ, Bridenbaugh PO (eds): Neural Blockade in Clinical Anesthesia and Management of Pain. JB Lippincott, Philadelphia, 1980

69. Rao TKL, El-Etr AA: Anticoagulation following placement of epidural and subarachnoid catheters: an evaluation of neurologic sequelae. Anesthesiology 55:618–620, 1981

70. Odoom JA, Sih IL: Epidural analgesia and anticoagulant therapy. Experience with one thousand cases of continuous epidurals. Anaesthesia 38:254–259, 1983

71. Kane RE: Neurologic deficits following

epidural or spinal anesthesia. Anesth Analg 60:150–161, 1981

72. Owens EL, Kasten GW, Hessel EA, II: Spinal subarachnoid hematoma after lumbar puncture and heparinization: a case report, review of the literature, and discussion of anesthetic implications. Anesth Analg 65:1201–1207, 1986

73. Greensite FS, Katz J: Spinal subdural hematoma associated with attempted epidural anesthesia and subsequent continuous spinal anesthesia. Anesth Analg 59:72–73, 1980

74. Sahud MA, Cohen RJ: Aspirin-induced prolongation of the Ivy bleeding time. Its diagnostic usefulness. Calif Med 115:10–13, 1971

75. Helperin SW, Cohen DD: Hematoma following epidural anesthesia: report of a case. Anesthesiology 35:641–644, 1971

76. Locke GE, Giorgio AJ, Biggers SL, Jr et al: Acute spinal epidural hematoma secondary to aspirin-induced prolonged bleeding. Surg Neurol 5:293–296, 1976

77. Varkey GP, Brindle GF: Peridural anaesthesia and anti-coagulant therapy. Can Anaesth Soc J 21:106–109, 1974

78. De Angelis J: Hazards of subdural and epidural anesthesia during anticoagulant therapy: a case report and review. Anesth Analg 51:676–679, 1972

79. Stanley TH, Lunn JK: Anticoagulants and continuous epidural anesthesia (letter to editor). Anesth Analg 59:394–395, 1980

23

Anesthesia for Emergency Surgery for Peripheral Vascular Insufficiency

Michael F. Roizen

ACUTE PERIPHERAL VASCULAR OCCLUSION

The Need for Emergency Surgery

Four clinical conditions indicate the need for emergency surgery for chronic peripheral occlusive disease: (1) sudden development of a cold, pulseless leg; (2) sudden onset of severe ischemic pain that occurs even at rest; (3) sudden loss of sensation or motion in a leg, owing to vascular occlusion; and (4) gangrene. Patients with rest pain, ulceration, and/or gangrene may have severe progressive ischemia and are at variable risk of imminent limb loss. In the past, many of these patients simply would have had their leg placed in an ice bath. Such treatment is still an option for the very sick patient whose medical problem needs stabilization or optimization before surgery.

Emergency surgery for chronic peripheral vascular insufficiency becomes necessary when acute arterial occlusion causes severe ischemia and threatens viability of the limb. Immediate operation and restoration of blood flow are needed if limb loss is to be avoided. Depending on the cause of the occlusion, the patient may or may not be at high risk from other medical problems.

Acute arterial occlusion causes the extremity to suddenly become cold and pulseless. Patients usually complain of coldness, pain, numbness, and paresthesias and may lose motion and sensation in the leg. The severity of ischemia and the urgency of immediate operation can be assessed by evaluating the leg motion and sensation. Abnormal sensation in the toes, feet, and legs in response to light touch and pin prick, as well as abnormal proprioception and loss of motor function in the feet and toes, are hallmarks of acute ischemia and nonviability of the limb. If ischemia is not reversed in a matter of hours, loss of limb is probable.

Acute arterial occlusion may occur in patients who have preexisting peripheral occlusive or aneurysmal disease caused by thrombosis of a stenotic or ulcerated atherosclerotic artery. Acute arterial occlusion can also occur in normal periph-

359

eral arteries that contain emboli. When patients have cardiac arrhythmias, recent myocardial infarctions, or ventricular aneurysms, such emboli usually originate in the heart.[1,2]

Considerations When Planning the Operative Treatment

It is important to know the cause of acute arterial occlusion when planning operative treatment. If embolism has caused obstruction, Fogarty embolectomy through a groin incision under local anesthesia may suffice. However, if the cause is thrombosis of severely diseased atherosclerotic arteries, bypass reconstruction will be necessary. Preoperative angiography may be helpful in distinguishing the two; often the cause is not discovered until the vessel is opened. Thus, the anesthesiologist must be prepared for both a simple procedure and a complex, extended procedure.

Normally, peripheral vascular surgery does not entail major blood loss or hemodynamic changes. However, these procedures tend to be lengthy, making intraoperative urinary drainage advisable. Because the most important causes of morbidity and mortality in these procedures are cardiovascular in origin (with rates above 8 and 2 percent, respectively), the relatively "noninvasive" nature of peripheral vascular surgery and the absence of major hemodynamic alterations should not lull the anesthesiologist into a too-casual attitude.[3–5] Patients with acute ischemia may be very ill. Significant fluid losses may be anticipated when the artery is flushed during thrombectomy, and fluid may be sequestered in edematous revascularized tissue. Serum potassium levels can change quickly, as cell death and release of intracellular potassium into the circulation are likely to occur.

Myoglobin may also be released into the circulation, and the development of a compartment syndrome (increased tissue pressure leading to decreased blood flow, ischemia, and neural dysfunction) is possible.

An incision in the groin is usually made for exposure of the femoral artery. Attempts to pass Fogarty catheters proximally and distally are made in the effort to establish flow and extract the thrombus. If flow is not restored in this manner, more complex reconstructive procedures such as aortofemoral, axillofemoral, or femoropopliteal bypass may be required. Femoral venous drainage on restoration of flow to the femoral artery can aid in management by disposing of the initial venous effluent from an acutely ischemic extremity. This process may entail significant blood loss.

Patients undergoing peripheral vascular disease may have some of the many disorders associated with vascular disease in general, such as diabetes, smoking and its sequelae, chronic pulmonary disease, hypertension, and ischemic heart disease. Other sources discuss the management of concurrent diseases in detail.[6] Perhaps the most important aspect of planning perioperative management of concurrent diseases is understanding and searching for the end-organ effects of these conditions and applying the appropriate drug therapy. Although emergency surgery requires that such effects be assessed quickly, attempts at rapid control of blood pressure or electrolyte levels may be more hazardous than not treating the condition or trying to control the abnormality slowly. At our institution, the exception to this general rule of avoiding attempts at rapid control pertains to diabetic ketoacidosis. That is, we first treat this condition and then wait for evidence of progress toward normal acid-base status before initiating emergency peripheral vascularization.

Another consideration when dealing with concurrent disease is that patients with limb ischemia may be so sick that they have forgotten or neglected to take their chronic medications. Because discontinuing a drug may be more hazardous than continuing drug therapy and being cognizant of its effects, when such neglect comes to our attention, we administer the missing drug intravenously or intramuscularly at the time of surgery.

EMERGENCY PERIPHERAL VASCULAR SURGERY: ANESTHESIA GOALS AND MANAGEMENT

There is perhaps no other disease entity about which the anesthesiologist can be so easily misled as peripheral vascular occlusion. Even experienced vascular surgeons and anesthesiologists can greatly underestimate the potential dangers associated with peripheral vascular procedures.

Acute peripheral vascular occlusion must be attended to quickly. Although this problem appears to be localized in the extremity, it is vitally important to remember that the occluding material may originate in the heart or major arteries. Therefore, peripheral vascular occlusion may result from a more serious cardiovascular problem. In fact, some of the sickest patients I have ever anesthetized were patients who had peripheral vascular occlusion. As evidence, morbidity and mortality following these distal operations approach those following infra-aortic reconstruction; these complications are mainly cardiac in origin. Thus, while I tend to use epidural anesthesia and epidural narcotics for pain relief, I believe that attention to body temperature, oxygen delivery, and hemodynamic

stability should be just as intense for peripheral vascular procedures as for aortic procedures, which involve much greater hemodynamic fluctuations.

Monitoring

The devices and the concerns described for surgery for visceral ischemia (Ch. 10) and abdominal aortic reconstruction (Ch. 18) also apply to surgery for acute peripheral vascular occlusion, with special attention to the postoperative period. For example, my monitoring practice stresses preservation of myocardial, pulmonary, and renal function as well as intravascular volume. Although I rarely insert an arterial catheter for peripheral vascular surgery, I frequently monitor urinary output and some form of ventricular filling pressure, the latter usually via pulmonary artery catheter. This catheter allows monitoring of systemic vascular resistance, cardiac output, and pulmonary capillary wedge pressure. I prefer the external jugular route for insertion, although many anesthetists use the internal jugular or subclavian route. Except for patients who have demonstrated myocardial ischemia in areas other than the anterior myocardial wall, I use a modified chest lead V_5 to monitor the electrocardiogram (ECG) during surgery.

In addition, I almost always monitor body temperature and maintain it meticulously by warming all fluids, starting before surgery. Also, the patient is placed on heating mattresses on the operating room table. This attempt to maintain body heat is especially valuable for postoperative limb perfusion, because limb blood flow decreases in the cold patient who is trying to preserve heat. Many surgeons believe that this decrease in blood flow reduces flow rates through the graft and increases the chance of vascular occlusion in the freshly revascularized limb. If necessary, anesthetic gases are humidified.

I have found two-dimensional transesophageal echocardiography (2D TEE) to be an invaluable tool for monitoring myocardial function during general anesthesia (see Ch. 28). A short-axis cross-sectional view of the left ventricle provides an excellent qualitative assessment of left ventricular filling volume, global ventricular contractility, and regional ventricular function.[7] When a discrepancy has existed between pulmonary capillary filling pressures obtained by pulmonary artery catheters and filling pressures obtained by 2D TEE, I have found the latter to be more reliable and useful.[7–9] Because of the size of the transducer and the oral route of insertion, I do not use 2D TEE during regional anesthesia not accompanied by general anesthesia and tracheal intubation. Instead, during regional anesthesia, I rely on the patient's condition and on changes in pulmonary capillary wedge pressures to guide fluid therapy.

Several variables can be used to assess perfusion of the organs. For the heart, I evaluate myocardial contractility, as judged by global and regional wall motion on the two-dimensional transesophageal echocardiogram[7,10,11]; changes in the ST segment on the modified chest lead V_5 of the ECG; and cardiac output. For the kidney, I use urinary output as my guide to perfusion (I believe that 20 to 30 ml of urine per 0.5 hour per 70 kg of body weight is adequate in this operation, as opposed to less in other vascular operations; see Ch. 10).

Protecting the Heart

As in aortic reconstruction (see Ch. 10), I protect the heart by trying to keep hemodynamic variables within the range of preoperative values.[6] Without evidence to the contrary, I must assume that a little

hypertension is just as harmful as a little hypotension. For example, in extreme cases, I may let systolic blood pressure fall to as low as 90 mmHg or rise to as high as 190 mmHg if the preoperative range is 110 to 170 mmHg.

The following contingency plan would go into effect if values approached or exceeded the limits of the normal preoperative range. If blood pressure reaches 150 mmHg, the amount of anesthetic would be increased; at approximately 160 mmHg, nitroprusside would be infused; at 165 or 175 mmHg, the table would be tilted. If systolic blood pressure drops to 110 mmHg, the anesthetic would be decreased and the possible causes of hypotension reviewed. At 105 mmHg, I would decrease the amount of anesthetic even more and would place the patient in a head-down position. At 100 mmHg, more fluid would be infused, and the patient would be tilted in a steeper head-down position. The possible causes of hypotension would be reviewed again, and, if possible, the cause corrected. At 90 mmHg, I would start a dilute drip infusion of phenylephrine (10 mg in 500 ml of saline or 5 percent dextrose in water, infused at a rate that increases systolic blood pressure to approximately 100 mmHg).

For heart rate, I again set a range of acceptable intraoperative values based on preoperative determinations. For example, if the preoperative range were 60 to 90 beats/min, treatment would be initiated if intraoperative values exceeded those limits. Here, however, I assume that tachycardia is of greater concern than bradycardia and avoid it more aggressively. At 95 beats/min, I might increase the anesthetic, give more narcotic, or add an intravenous drip of a β-adrenergic receptor-blocking drug. At 100 beats/min, I would give a bolus injection or begin an intravenous drip of a β-adrenergic receptor-blocking drug, assuming values for intravascular fluid volume were acceptable. At 45 beats/min, I might decrease the anesthetic or administer a dilute solution of dopamine (200 mg in 500 ml of saline or 5 percent dextrose in water) to keep heart rate within the acceptable range.

Again, I emphasize that I tend to tolerate bradycardia more than tachycardia during these operations, because I believe that minimizing myocardial oxygen demand should be of primary importance. Use of 2D TEE gives some latitude in the range of acceptable values before intervention. However, I do not allow pulmonary artery pressures to remain abnormal (that is, below 5 or above 15 mmHg) during this procedure, assuming that these values are confirmed by echocardiographic values. I aggressively treat increases in pulmonary artery pressure by administering nitroglycerin or nitroprusside, depending on whether the suspected cause is an increase in preload or an increase in afterload.[12,13]

For low pressures, I infuse more fluid. If at all possible, I try to avoid administering exogenous vasoconstrictors. Although coronary and cerebral vessels are not as densely innervated as some other parts of the body, administration of α_1- and α_2-adrenergic agents can still induce cerebral vasoconstriction. In addition, α-adrenergic vasoconstriction may cause an adverse effect on the myocardium. Some believe this effect occurs because of the important role α-adrenergic vasoconstrictors play in maintaining an appropriate distribution of blood flow between the outer and inner myocardium.[14] These agents induce myocardial dilation and perhaps myocardial ischemia (the problem of a stretched, dilated myocardium).[15] In any regard, the incidence of myocardial ischemia is more than twice as high in patients who are deeply anesthetized and whose systemic pressure is maintained with an infusion of phenylephrine than in patients whose blood

pressure is maintained with only light anesthesia and endogenous vasoconstrictors.[15]

Protecting the Kidneys

Intraoperative urinary output does not predict postoperative renal function.[16] However, because of the release of myoglobin and potassium from dead or dying muscle in the extremity, emergency peripheral vascular surgery is one operation for which I induce diuresis. I try to do this without dilating the heart or overloading the vascular tree, as such fluid volume often complicates postoperative care.

Postoperative Care

It is during the postoperative period that most cardiac problems arise and that pain relief and correction of hemodynamic and fluid disequilibrium are most likely to be needed. Care must be taken, I believe, not to allow overhydration to occur intraoperatively in support of blood pressure, as this condition can cause congestive heart failure as epidural sympathectomy fades. As for surgery for aortic disease, I routinely tilt the patient head down (while monitoring gas exchange closely) for the last hour of the operation. Dye loads given for completion angiography also contribute to fluid shifts, and I consider monitoring of left ventricular filling volume important for successful outcome for these patients.

The surgeons' concerns for patients with peripheral vascular insufficiency include not only those involving the cardiovascular system but also specific problems related to operative repair. Graft patency is evaluated carefully in the recovery room. Most surgeons believe that the patient's feet should be kept warm and that the patient should be well hydrated so that peripheral vasoconstriction, which may limit outflow from the new graft, does not occur. If graft thrombosis develops soon after surgery, the patient is returned promptly to the operating room for graft thrombectomy and for evaluation and correction of the cause of thrombosis.

ONE PLAN FOR PROVIDING ANESTHESIA FOR EMERGENCY PERIPHERAL VASCULAR SURGERY

The following describes my usual practice when providing anesthesia for emergency peripheral vascular surgery.

Anticoagulants are commonly administered to patients suspected of having peripheral vascular occlusion. If a patient has already been given anticoagulants, the appropriateness of using a major conduction block (subarachnoid or epidural block with or without placement of a catheter) is controversial (see Ch. 24). Some believe this is a safe practice. Cunningham et al.[17] reported no hematomas after continuous epidural anesthesia in 100 patients undergoing resection of abdominal aortic aneurysms and operations for aortoiliac occlusion. Another group described continuous epidural anesthesia in 3,168 patients and continuous subarachnoid anesthesia in 841 patients undergoing peripheral vascular surgery of the lower extremities.[18] Patients who had already been given anticoagulants or who had leukemia, thrombocytopenia, hemophilia, or traumatic insertion of the catheter were given general anesthesia. No hematomas or neurologic sequelae were evident. However, my practice is to avoid major conduction block anesthesia in patients given anticoagulants who then must undergo emergency surgery for acute peripheral vascular occlusion. This practice is based on anecdotal case reports of epidural hematoma that caused paraplegia under such circumstances.[19-21]

If general anesthesia is chosen and the patient is judged to have a full stomach, I administer metoclopramide (10 mg/70 kg of body weight, intravenously) as early as possible. Then, preoxygenation is followed by rapid-sequence induction: administration of small doses of fentanyl or sufentanil, small-to-moderate doses of thiopental (0.5 to 5 mg/kg, depending on the response to the test dose of thiopental), and a rapid-acting muscle relaxant; application of cricoid pressure; and endotracheal intubation. To blunt the hemodynamic effects of laryngeal visualization and endotracheal intubation, one may administer an intravenous bolus of lidocaine, sodium nitroprusside, nitroglycerin, esmolol, or additional fentanyl, sufentanil, or thiopental.

If hypotension occurs after induction, I administer 100 percent oxygen, elevate the patient's legs, and rapidly administer blood and fluids. If these measures fail to produce adequate blood pressure and perfusion, I infuse phenylephrine or dopamine until blood pressure returns toward normal.

For patients who are believed not to have a full stomach, a gentle, slow titration of volatile agents or narcotics, combined with 50 percent nitrous oxide, is administered. In my experience, any hemodynamic instability that has occurred in these patients has usually been caused by acid-base or electrolyte disturbances. As mentioned earlier, these patients often have hyperkalemia and acidosis, which arise from ischemic extremities; such ischemia may cause release of myoglobin into the circulation. Although the surgical procedure may be only a peripheral one, cardiac problems, generalized atherosclerosis, fluid shifts, and disturbances in electrolyte levels and acid-base balance, as well as the high morbidity and mortality associated with these procedures, can take the overly casual anesthesiologist by surprise. In fact, I often monitor blood gases, acid-base status, and electrolyte values two or three times more frequently during this form of peripheral vascular surgery than during even elective thoracoabdominal aortic reconstruction. Skill and intensive care as meticulous as that given patients with visceral ischemia may benefit those with peripheral vascular insufficiency as well. I also believe that care of the patient should be just as meticulous immediately after surgery as during surgery.

CONCLUSION

Surgery for acute peripheral occlusion does not incur the great hemodynamic changes accompanying occlusion of the aorta. However, this advantage should not lull the anesthesiologist into believing that vigilance about myocardial well-being will not be rewarded when caring for patients undergoing emergency peripheral vascular surgery. These patients often have hyperkalemia and acidosis that arise from ischemic extremities; such ischemia also may cause release of myoglobin into the circulation. Although the surgical procedure may be only a peripheral one, cardiac problems, generalized atherosclerosis, fluid shifts, and disturbances in electrolyte levels and acid-base balance, as well as the high morbidity and mortality associated with these procedures, can surprise the overly casual anesthesiologist. In addition, meticulous attention to beneficial practices such as prehydration and use of warming mattresses is probably more important to patient outcome than is the occasional stroke of therapeutic brilliance. Finally,

it is most important to remember that the best patient results probably are achieved when the great vigilance shown during surgery is also applied before surgery (albeit quickly) and especially after surgery.

REFERENCES

1. Abbott WM, Maloney RD, McCabe CC et al: Arterial embolism: a 44 year perspective. Am J Surg 143:460–464, 1982
2. Connett MC, Murray DH, Jr., Denneker WW: Peripheral arterial emboli. Am J Surg 148:14–19, 1984
3. Veith FJ, Gupta SK, Ascer E: Femoral, popliteal, and tibial occlusive disease. p. 353–375. In Wilson SE, Veith FJ, Hobson RW, III, Williams RA (eds): Vascular Surgery. Principles and Practice. McGraw-Hill, New York, 1987
4. Mannick JA, Jackson BT, Coffman JD, Hume DM: Success of bypass vein grafts in patients with isolated popliteal artery segments. Surgery 61:17–25, 1967
5. Reichle FA, Tyson RR: Comparison of long-term results of 364 femoropopliteal or femorotibial bypasses for revascularization of severely ischemic lower extremities. Ann Surg 182:449–455, 1975
6. Roizen MF: Anesthetic implications of concurrent diseases. p. 255–357. In Miller RD (ed): Anesthesia. Vol 1. 2nd Ed. Churchill Livingstone, New York, 1986
7. Roizen MF, Beaupre PN, Alpert RA et al: Monitoring with two-dimensional transesophageal echocardiography. Comparison of myocardial function in patients undergoing supraceliac, suprarenal-infraceliac, or infrarenal aortic occlusion. J Vasc Surg 1:300–305, 1984
8. Kalman PG, Wellwood MR, Weisel RD et al: Cardiac dysfunction during abdominal aortic operation: the limitations of pulmonary wedge pressures. J Vasc Surg 3:773–781, 1986
9. Beaupre PN, Cahalan MK, Kremer PF et al: Does pulmonary artery occlusion pressure adequately reflect left ventricular

filling during anesthesia and surgery (abstract)? Anesthesiology 59:A3, 1983

10. Smith JS, Cahalan MK, Benefiel DJ et al: Intraoperative detection of myocardial ischemia in high-risk patients: electrocardiography versus two-dimensional transesophageal echocardiography. Circulation 72:1015–1021, 1985

11. Pandian NG, Kerber RE: Two-dimensional echocardiography in experimental coronary stenosis. I. Sensitivity and specificity in detecting transient myocardial dyskinesis: comparison with sonomicrometers. Circulation 66:597–602, 1982

12. Flaherty JT, Magee PA, Gardner TL et al: Comparison of intravenous nitroglycerin and sodium nitroprusside for treatment of acute hypertension developing after coronary artery bypass surgery. Circulation 65:1072–1077, 1982

13. Gerson JI, Allen FB, Seltzer JL et al: Arterial and venous dilation by nitroprusside and nitroglycerin—is there a difference? Anesth Analg 61:256–260, 1982

14. Feigl EO: The paradox of adrenergic coronary vasoconstriction. Circulation 76:737–745, 1987

15. Smith JS, Roizen MF, Cahalan MK et al: Does anesthetic technique make a difference? Augmentation of systolic blood pressure during carotid endarterectomy: effects of phenylephrine versus light anesthesia and of isoflurane versus halothane on the incidence of myocardial ischemia. Anesthesiology 69:846–853, 1988

16. Alpert RA, Roizen MF, Hamilton WK et al: Intraoperative urinary output does not predict postoperative renal function in patients undergoing abdominal aortic revascularization. Surgery 95:707–711, 1984

17. Cunningham FO, Egan JM, Inahara T: Continuous epidural anesthesia in abdominal vascular surgery. A review of 100 consecutive cases. Am J Surg 139:624–627, 1980

18. Rao TLK, EL-Etr AA: Anticoagulation following placement of epidural and subarachnoid catheters: an evaluation of neurologic sequelae. Anesthesiology 55:618–620, 1981

19. Brem SS, Hafler DA, Van Uitert RL et al: Spinal subarachnoid hematoma: a hazard of lumbar puncture resulting in reversible paraplegia. N Engl J Med 304:1020–1021, 1981

20. De Angelis J: Hazards of subdural and epidural anesthesia during anticoagulant therapy: a case report and review. Anesth Analg 51:676–679, 1972

21. Edelson RN, Chernik NL, Posner JB: Spinal subdural hematomas complicating lumbar puncture. Arch Neurol 31:134–137, 1974

CONTROVERSIES
AND OTHER
ISSUES

24

Regional Anesthesia for Vascular Surgery of the Lower Extremities: Considerations Regarding Anticoagulation

Neeraja B. Reddy
Tadikonda L. K. Rao

Most investigations have concluded that regional anesthesia is the anesthetic of choice for vascular surgery of the lower extremities. Besides providing perioperative anesthesia and analgesia, major conduction anesthesia blocks sympathetic outflow, thereby preventing vasoconstriction, which may be enhanced by manipulation and injury to vessels during surgery, heat loss from prolonged exposure, and post operative pain. Regional anesthesia also maximally vasodilates the collateral vessels in the surgical area.

Patients undergoing peripheral vascular surgery often have been given, or will be given, anticoagulant drugs. This chapter briefly reviews the anticoagulants commonly used for patients undergoing vascular surgery of the lower extremities under regional anesthesia. It also discusses the safety of instituting regional anesthesia if anticoagulants are to be given during surgery.

ANTICOAGULANT TREATMENT

Heparin

Heparin prevents blood from coagulating by binding with antithrombin III to neutralize factors XIIa, XIa, IXa, Xa, and thrombin itself. The mean values for the half-life of 100, 200, and 400 international units of heparin per kilogram of body weight injected intravenously in humans are 56, 96, and 152 minutes, respectively.[1] Thus, we believe heparin should be discontinued 5 to 6 hours before surgery, and we ensure that coagulation indices (prothrombin time [PT] and partial thromboplastin time [PTT]) are normal before instituting regional anesthesia.

Subcutaneous administration of low doses of heparin prevents thrombus formation (and thus deep venous thrombosis) in susceptible patients by neutralizing thrombin precursors as they are generated. Although PT and PTT tests remain normal because the systemic coagulation mechanism does not change, thrombin time may increase. This regimen can be continued during the perioperative period.

Warfarin

The major therapeutic use of warfarin is to continue anticoagulation treatment started with heparin. Warfarin produces a rapid decrease in factor VII, an event that can cause bleeding without providing protection against thrombosis. Patients who metabolize warfarin slowly have a rapid increase in PT within 24 hours; on discontinuation of warfarin, PT tests may be abnormal for as long as 7 days. Patients who metabolize warfarin rapidly can reverse its effects within 2 to 3 days of discontinuation of the drug. We discontinue warfarin at least 3 to 7 days before surgery; if anticoagulation is required, depending on the cause and necessity, we institute intravenous heparin. In emergency cases, administration of vitamin K could be expected to reverse the effect of warfarin within 7 to 11 hours. If PT does not normalize, fresh frozen plasma can be administered.

Antiplatelet Drug Therapy

Aspirin and dipyridamole inhibit platelet function by interfering with the synthesis of cyclic endoperoxidase and thromboxane A_2 from arachidonic acid in platelet membrane. Platelets are acetylated irreversibly by aspirin, the effect lasting the whole life of the platelet, approximately 5 days. Therefore, patients on antiplatelet drug therapy should discontinue medication at least 1 week before surgery. However, in an emergency, a one-unit platelet transfusion will normalize function of the acetylated proteins by starting the aggregation reaction.

Dextran

Dextrans are polymolecular glucose polysaccharides. Two forms, described by molecular weight, are currently available for intravenous use: dextran 40 and dextran 70. Dextrans exert an antithrombotic effect by a combination of mechanisms: (1) they expand blood volume and decrease the viscosity of blood; (2) they coat surfaces, reducing the interface between vessel wall and blood elements; (3) they coat platelets, reducing their adhesiveness and ability to aggregate; and (4) they interfere with the polymerization of fibrin and thus increase fibrinolysis.

SAFETY OF MAJOR CONDUCTION ANESTHESIA WITH ANTICOAGULATION TREATMENT

The Controversy

To prevent clotting during surgery and to reduce perioperative thrombotic and thromboembolic complications, patients undergoing vascular reconstructive procedures often receive anticoagulant therapy at some time during the perioperative period. We believe epidural and subarachnoid blocks are contraindicated in patients concurrently receiving anticoagulant therapy, as bleeding into the peridural or subarachnoid space may occur if the needle traumatizes one of the blood vessels.[2] However, controversy exists as to whether epidural or subarachnoid catheters should be placed in patients before anticoagulation therapy.

Occasional case reports have documented the occurrence of peridural hematomas leading to transient or permanent neurologic damage in patients given anticoagulants after catheterization of the epidural space[3-7]; however, the incidence of this major complication is unknown.

Spinal epidural or subarachnoid hematoma can occur either spontaneously or after anticoagulation therapy without trauma. Twenty-five percent of spontaneous spinal epidural hematomas are associated with anticoagulation therapy.[8] In the published case reports of hematoma formation after insertion of catheters for continuous epidural anesthesia in patients subsequently given anticoagulants, clotting time was usually not monitored.[4-6] Even when clotting time was monitored, heparin was administered without regard to clotting time.[5] Because of these case reports, controversy exists regarding the safety of using continuous epidural or subarachnoid block for patients who might later be given anticoagulation drugs during surgery.

Experience at Loyola University

In 1981, Rao and El-Etr[9] reported the incidence of neurologic complications arising from anticoagulant therapy given after placement of epidural or subarachnoid catheters in 4,011 patients undergoing vascular surgery of the lower extremities. The study involved 3,164 patients given continuous epidural anesthesia and 847 patients given continuous spinal anesthesia at two hospitals over a 5-year period (1973 to 1978). All patients had a clinical neurologic examination (including evaluation of cranial nerves) by an anesthetist, plus laboratory hematologic screening prior to surgery. Hematologic screening included determination of he-moglobin level, hematocrit, platelet count, PT, and PTT. The following describes the procedures and results of that study.

Continuous Regional Anesthesia

A 17-gauge Tuohy needle was used to reach either the peridural or subarachnoid space. After proper identification of the space, a catheter was threaded 1 to 2 cm beyond the tip of the needle. If blood was aspirated at any time during the procedure, the technique was abandoned and the patient was rescheduled for surgery under general anesthesia on the following day. In four instances, regional anesthesia had to be abandoned because of aspiration of blood.

The local anesthetic used for peridural block and the addition of epinephrine (1:200,000) varied according to the preference of the anesthetist. All subarachnoid blocks were obtained with 0.5 percent hyperbaric tetracaine without addition of epinephrine.

Heparin Administration and Clotting Time

Prior to anticoagulation therapy, baseline activated clotting time was measured (78 ± 28 seconds, mean ± SEM). Approximately 50 to 60 minutes after performance of the regional block, heparin was administered in 500-unit incremental doses every 3 minutes to keep activated clotting time at approximately twice the baseline value (174 ± 30 seconds, mean ± SEM). The heparin dose (2,600 ± 400 units, mean ± SEM) was repeated every 6 hours, following measurement of the activated clotting time, throughout the period of anticoagulation therapy.

At the end of surgery, patients were transferred to the recovery room with the catheters in place, to be used as needed for pain relief, sympathetic blockade, or anesthesia for reexploration of blood vessels. At 24 hours after insertion, the catheters were removed; 1 hour later, patients were given their maintenance dose of heparin. The patients were evaluated by the anesthetist for neurologic complications.

Postoperative Neurologic Complications

None of the four patients in whom regional anesthesia had to be abandoned had postoperative neurologic complications after general anesthesia. Four patients given epidural anesthesia had paresthesias of the thigh and leg 3 to 4 days after removal of the catheter; these complications resolved within 3 weeks. One patient given spinal anesthesia had numbness on the anterolateral aspect of the thigh on the third day after operation; examination revealed loss of sensation to touch and pinprick. This effect did not resolve until 6 months after surgery. Fifteen patients (nine given epidural anesthesia and six given subarachnoid anesthesia) complained of low backache on the third or fourth day after operation; backache resolved completely after analgesic therapy. No patient had any sign or symptom of epidural or subarachnoid spinal cord compression.

Practices Decreasing the Incidence of Hematoma

Two factors may account for the absence of peridural hematoma in this series. First, patients with a history of leukemia, thrombocytopenia, or hemophilia and those undergoing anticoagulant therapy were not given continuous regional anesthesia. Second, administration of heparin was monitored throughout the perioperative period by assessment of activated clotting time. Thus, administration of excessive heparin was avoided. For peripheral vascular procedures, only lower levels of anticoagulants (activated clotting time of 130 to 150 seconds) are needed.[10] Because the levels of antithrombin III

vary with the individual, heparin requirements also vary with the individual and can be predicted correctly only by monitoring the activated clotting time.[11]

Another important consideration may be the timing of catheter removal. If the catheter is removed within 1 hour before administration of the next dose of heparin, circulating levels of heparin should be relatively low, thus minimizing the chance of bleeding into the epidural space.

Minor self-limiting neurologic complications such as paresthesias and residual postoperative anesthesia of the lower extremity, as occurred in five of our patients, may be caused by direct trauma to nerve roots by the catheter, the needle, or surgery itself. Similar complications have been reported in a large series of epidural anesthetics, but complete recovery usually occurred within a few weeks to months.[12] Patients who complain of backache should be observed closely, as backache may signal the onset of peridural hematoma.[4,8,12,13] Other possible causes of neurologic deficit include arachnoiditis, trauma, and inadvertent injection of toxic material.

In conclusion, we believe that the need to give anticoagulants intraoperatively should not be, in itself, a contraindication to the use of regional anesthesia. We also believe that proper patient selection, atraumatic technique, monitoring of anticoagulant activity, and removal of the catheter when the circulating level of heparin is low are practices that minimize the incidence of spinal, epidural, or subarachnoid hematoma after anticoagulant therapy in patients who have peridural or subarachnoid catheters in place.

REFERENCES

1. Olsson P, Lagergren H, Ek S: The elimination from plasma of intravenous heparin. An experimental study on dogs and

humans. Acta Med Scand 173:619–630, 1963

2. Bromage PR: Epidural Analgesia. p. 231, 232, 467. WB Saunders, Philadelphia, 1978

3. Gingrich TF: Spinal epidural hematoma following continuous epidural anesthesia. Anesthesiology 29:162–163, 1968

4. Butler AB, Green CD: Hematoma following epidural anaesthesia. Can Anaesth Soc J 17:635–639, 1970

5. Helperin SW, Cohen DD: Hematoma following epidural anesthesia: report of a case. Anesthesiology 35:641–644, 1971

6. Janis KM: Epidural hematoma following postoperative epidural analgesia: a case report. Anesth Analg 51:689–692, 1972

7. Varkey GP, Brindle GF: Peridural anaesthesia and anti-coagulant therapy. Can Anaesth Soc J 21:106–109, 1974

8. Spurny OM, Rubin S, Wolf JW, Wu WQ: Spinal epidural hematoma during anti-

coagulant therapy. Report of two cases. Arch Intern Med 114:103–107, 1964

9. Rao TLK, El-Etr AA: Anticoagulation following placement of epidural and subarachnoid catheters: an evaluation of neurologic sequelae. Anesthesiology 55:618–620, 1981

10. Vitez TS: Intraoperative anticoagulant management. Contemp Surg 13 (Sept):29–42, 1978

11. Williams JW, Bentler E, Ersler AJ: Part IV (Hemostasis). pp. 997–1263. In Williams WJ (ed): Hematology. McGraw-Hill, New York, 1972

12. Gutterman P: Acute spinal subdural hematoma following lumbar puncture. Surg Neurol 7:355–356, 1977

13. Messer HD, Forshan VR, Brust JCM, Hughes JEO: Transient paraplegia from hematoma after lumbar puncture. A consequence of anticoagulant therapy. JAMA 235:529–530, 1976

Monitoring of the Electroencephalogram during Carotid Endarterectomy

Michael T. McCaffrey

Carotid endarterectomy is currently the subject of much discussion in the literature. Investigators disagree over the extent to which this procedure offers advantages over the best medical treatment, and whether intraoperative techniques such as shunting and electrophysiologic monitoring reduce the morbidity and mortality associated with the operation. Functioning of the two organs most responsible for morbidity and mortality—the heart and the brain—can be monitored intraoperatively. Although few serious questions have arisen about the value of monitoring the heart during carotid endarterectomy, no consensus exists regarding the value of monitoring the brain. This chapter briefly reviews the techniques and issues involved in electroencephalographic monitoring during carotid endarterectomy.

THE ELECTROENCEPHALOGRAM

The scalp-recorded electroencephalogram (EEG) reflects the electrical activity of the underlying cerebral cortex. The most important contributors are postsynaptic potentials—both excitatory and inhibitory—arising from the dendrites and cell bodies of cortical neurons. These postsynaptic potentials result from both intracortical and extracortical influences. Both corticocortical connections and projections from thalamic and brain stem sources appear to be involved in generation of the EEG. Action potentials contribute comparatively little to the EEG. Their rapid time course and relative asynchrony and the small currents involved in the generation of action potentials are unfavorable for detection at the scalp. Because electrical currents are attenuated by passage through resistive tissues such as the meninges, skull, and skin, potentials arising in the vicinity of the recording electrodes (i.e., those nearer the surface of the brain) contribute more to the activity recorded from those electrodes than do potentials arising at more distant locations (i.e., deeper in the brain). However, high-amplitude activity may be detected at a considerable distance.

The EEG is recorded from electrodes, two per channel of the EEG, placed on the scalp. The two-electrode leads are connected to the inputs of a differential amplifier. The output of this type of amplifier is proportional to the voltage difference between the two inputs. The human central nervous system produces electrical activity ranging from below 1 Hz to over 1,000 Hz in frequency. The frequency range to be examined depends on the type of information desired. For most applications in the operating room, it is sufficient to examine the spontaneously generated frequencies below 20 to 30 Hz. The use of frequency filters reduces the contribution of extraneous (nonneural) electrical activity such as that arising from muscle, the electrocardiograph, and nonbiologic sources.

When recorded in this manner, the EEG produces a voltage value for each moment in time for each channel, often 16 or more channels. Electroencephalographic analysis then consists of assessing the amplitude and frequency of the signals recorded at many locations on the scalp. Disturbances in the underlying cerebral cortex manifest as changes in the amplitude and frequency of electroencephalographic signals recorded over these areas.

Unfortunately, proper interpretation of the conventionally displayed EEG in the operating room is unwieldy. The encephalographer must extract the features (amplitude, frequency, symmetry) from the EEG and monitor changes during the procedure.

Display of Data

As a result, various methods have been developed that enable a computer to recognize and extract the pertinent features. Thus, a portion of the interpretation process can be mechanized. It is then a relatively simple process to monitor the changes in these variables during surgery. A number of mathematical descriptors of the EEG have been proposed.[1] Probably the most common transform of the EEG in the operating room involves Fourier analysis of the waveforms to index the frequency of the signals. This process takes discrete epochs of the EEG, analyzes them, and returns a description of the epoch in terms of power as a function of frequency. A common display for the results of this type of analysis is the compressed spectral array,[2] which displays the results of the analysis of successive epochs in any easy-to-understand format. Commercially available machines for use in the operating room typically offer two channels of data analysis. During carotid endarterectomy, these two channels are recorded from electrodes placed on the scalp over brain areas supplied by the ipsilateral internal carotid artery.

Several techniques for the topographic display of electroencephalographic features have recently been developed. These techniques involve recording the EEG from multiple channels (20 or more), analyzing the data, and interpolating values for the variables for scalp locations between the electrodes. The data are then displayed as a map of the scalp that is shaded or colored to represent different values of the variables. Variables that may be mapped in this manner include power in specified frequency bands. Some users have expressed concerns about normalization and other statistical issues; however, these issues reflect difficulties in comparing maps between patients. In the operating room, the most meaningful comparison is that between states within the same patient, that is, before and after clamping, or right side versus left side. It is not necessary to determine whether the patient's EEG is normal or abnormal when compared with some normal population, but rather, whether it has changed from previous measures. Thus, each patient serves as his or her own control. Topographic display of electroencephalographic data may be useful in the operating room as equipment costs decrease and familiarity with the technique and its limitations increases.

Factors Affecting the Electroencephalogram

Cerebral Blood Flow

For electrical activity of the brain to exist, as manifested by the amplitude and frequency of electroencephalographic signals, cerebral blood flow (CBF) must be at least 15 to 20 ml/100 g/min. This dependence is referred to as the flow threshold for electrical failure. One study analyzed 1,145 consecutive carotid endarterectomies monitored with intraoperative EEG and measurement of CBF (using intra-arterial injection of xenon 133).[3] Blood flow was manipulated during anesthesia to maintain a normal EEG, that is, to avoid excessive depth of anesthesia. The blood flow required to achieve this goal was 15 ml/100 g/min. This level was approximately 30 percent of normal flow. Other studies produced similar values.[4,5] The flow threshold for electrical failure is somewhat higher than the flow threshold for cell death, which is approximately 10 to 15 ml/100 g/min.[6–8] Thus, electrical failure occurs at a higher flow rate than cell death. It is likely that the degree of reduction of CBF is inversely related to the length of time ischemia can be tolerated without infarction.[7,9] Thus, mild ischemia will be tolerated for a longer time than severe ischemia.

The fact that some areas of the brain may have CBF that is below the threshold for electrical failure but above the threshold for metabolic failure (i.e., they lie in an "ischemic penumbra") has two important implications. First, the EEG can only report the higher threshold; therefore, the occurrence of changes on EEG without accompanying deficits cannot be regarded as false-positive results. In other words, it is possible for the EEG to change without an observable neurologic deficit, because CBF can fall below the flow threshold for electrical failure but remain above the flow threshold for cell death. On the other hand, keeping CBF above the threshold for EEG changes should be sufficient to prevent ischemic damage. Second, if tissue is in the ischemic penumbra, it cannot be monitored by the EEG because it is electrically silent. Such tissue may exist in patients with recent or evolving strokes. In some reports, such patients undergo carotid endarterectomy as soon as 1 day after the development of maximal, stable neurologic deficit.[10] Comparison of changes on EEG from baseline may not be an adequate monitor of the risk of new neurologic deficit in these patients.

Anesthetic Agents

Correct interpretation of electroencephalographic changes during surgery depends on knowledge of the EEG effects of anesthetic and physiologic manipulations. All clinically useful concentrations of general anesthetics affect the EEG. Narcotics used in balanced techniques, such as fentanyl and alfentanil, also affect the EEG. In one study, an infusion of fentanyl (150 μg/min) or alfentanil (1,500 μg/min) given to unpremedicated patients produced progressive slowing of frequency and increases in amplitude as the serum concentration of narcotic increased.[11] These changes on EEG lagged behind the serum concentrations by several minutes, the lag being greater with fentanyl than with alfentanil. The EEG is also changed by administration of volatile anesthetics. For example, both enflurane[12,13] and halothane[13,14] produce high-frequency activity during light anesthesia, followed by slowing of the EEG as anesthesia deepens. Similar changes occur with other volatile anesthetic agents.[15]

Physiologic Variables

Physiologic variables such as temperature and blood pressure also produce effects on the EEG. For example, changes in temperature and blood pressure may change the amplitude and frequency of signals. An EEG recorded during rewarming of patients after cardiopulmonary bypass showed that total power and peak power frequency correlated linearly with temperature.[16] The mean ($\pm$ SEM) magnitude of change per degree Celsius was $1,215 \pm 150 \ \mu V^2$ for total power and 0.39 ± 0.04 Hz for peak power. Hypotension can also change the EEG. Although autoregulation of CBF usually occurs at systemic pressures from approximately 50 to 150 mmHg, impairment of autoregulatory mechanisms during pressure alterations in this range may significantly reduce CBF. In addition, hypoxia, hypercarbia, and hypocarbia can modify the EEG.[16]

Clinical Considerations

The fact that changes in concentrations of anesthetic agents and in physiologic variables can produce electroencephalographic effects similar to those produced by cerebral ischemia (namely, reductions in power and changes in frequency) has two important implications. First, if the EEG is to be monitored in the operating room, changes in the amount and kind of anesthetics administered, as well as changes in the values of relevant physiologic variables, should be minimized before the occurrence of critical surgical manipulations such as clamping of the internal carotid artery. If, for example, an increase in the concentration of a volatile agent or a bolus of a narcotic is given at about the same time as the artery is clamped, it would not be possible to determine the cause of the resulting change on EEG. Also, if the anesthetist is not monitoring the EEG, he or she must communicate with the person who is monitoring the EEG. Such communication can benefit both parties: there is much electroencephalographic information of interest to the anesthetist, and interpretation of effects on EEG is facilitated by knowledge of changes in anesthetic concentrations and physiologic variables.

MONITORING OF THE ELECTROENCEPHALOGRAM DURING CAROTID ENDARTERECTOMY

The linkage of CBF and the electrical activity of the brain has led to use of the EEG to monitor the adequacy of cerebral perfusion during surgery that possibly compromises CBF. Probably the most common application of intraoperative monitoring of the EEG is in assessing CBF during carotid endarterectomy. Significant electroencephalographic changes on clamping of the artery are believed to indicate cerebral ischemia and the need for corrective measures. "Significant" changes on EEG consist of reductions in amplitude of 50 percent or more or marked slowing of the EEG. Also, any changes of this sort that occur on the EEG for the operated side but not the unoperated side are considered significant.

New Neurologic Deficits after Carotid Endarterectomy

Postoperative neurologic deficits after carotid endarterectomy appear to be caused by embolization, postoperative thrombosis of the operative site, cerebral reperfusion injury, or flow-related ischemia. Neurologic deficit from carotid endarterectomy is usually caused by the first three conditions. However, a few patients have cerebral ischemia on interruption of blood flow of the internal carotid artery. One study of 345 patients undergoing 359 elective carotid endarterectomies under local anesthesia reported a low incidence of permanent (1.7 percent) and transient (4.3 percent) neurologic deficit.[17] Of six instances of intraoperative deficit, three occurred during dissection, two on release of the clamp, and one during carotid occlusion. An additional 15 patients had transient or permanent deficit within the first 4 days of surgery. All of these deficits except the one during clamping were probably caused by thromboembolism. In this study, then, one-sixth of the intraoperative deficits apparently resulted from flow-related ischemia. This study and other investigations indicate that while thromboembolism is the chief cause of postoperative neurologic deficit, cerebral ischemia does occasionally occur after interruption of flow in one internal carotid artery. These are the patients who may benefit from intraoperative monitoring of the EEG.

Experience at the University of Chicago

The University of Chicago has used the continuous and/or Fourier-transformed EEG to monitor carotid endarterectomies since 1984.[18–20] Two channels of the EEG (left and right centroparietal leads) were analyzed by a Berg-Fourier analyzer (OTE Biomedica) to show the power in six frequency bands. Comparison of conventional displays (voltage versus time) and processed displays (e.g., power versus frequency) demonstrates

that the latter provides faster and more sensitive indication of change.[21,22]

In a series of 105 consecutive endarterectomies under general (usually inhalational) anesthesia at the University of Chicago, the Fourier-transformed EEGs of all patients were analyzed retrospectively to show the power in three frequency bands: low (0.25 to 6.0 Hz), middle (6.0 to 10.5 Hz), and high (10.5 to 16.0 Hz).[19] Investigators saw three patterns of electroencephalographic responses to cross-clamping of the carotid. Mild or no power reduction (<50 percent power reduction in any frequency band) occurred in 82 patients (78 percent). Marked power reduction (>50 percent power reduction in one or two frequency bands) occurred in 12 patients (11 percent). Global power reduction (power reduction >50 percent in all three frequency bands) occurred in 11 patients (11 percent). Although these changes usually manifested on the operated side, slowing and reduction in amplitude were occasionally noted bilaterally. Contralateral changes did not occur without ipsilateral changes.

At the University of Chicago, preoperative criteria for placement of a temporary indwelling shunt include recent (within 6 weeks) stroke, occlusion of the contralateral carotid artery, or the existence of intracranial stenosis. Intraoperative criteria for shunt placement include significant changes on the EEG at the time of temporary clamping. In the series just described, 34 patients (32 percent) had placement of a temporary indwelling shunt.[19] In 19 patients (18 percent), shunts were placed on the basis of preoperative criteria alone. Of the 12 patients with *marked* power reduction, five had placement of shunts on the basis of preoperative criteria. The other seven patients in this group did not undergo placement of shunts. No immediate postoperative deficit was observed in this group.

Of 11 patients with *global* power reduction, 10 had shunts placed. Although placement of the shunt was usually followed by reversal of electroencephalographic changes within a few minutes, sometimes attenuation of high-frequency activity persisted. No immediate postoperative deficit occurred in this group. For one patient with global power reduction, technical reasons prevented shunting of carotid blood flow. The EEG remained suppressed for the 45 minutes of occlusion. On awakening, this patient had hemiparesis contralateral to the operated carotid and a dense homonymous hemianopia. Real-time imaging confirmed patency of the operated carotid. The neurologic deficits resolved within approximately 24 hours.

The investigators concluded that CBF should be shunted if activity on the EEG decreases more than 50 percent in all frequency bands on the operated side after clamping of the internal carotid artery. However, such a conclusion assumes that some of these patients would have had neurologic deficit without placement of a shunt. Although this assumption is logical, it has not been demonstrated in a controlled study. The issue of shunt placement in patients manifesting marked (as opposed to global) power reduction is less clear. Although no postoperative deficit occurred in this group, almost half of these patients had placement of a shunt based on preoperative criteria. Thus, some of the patients manifesting power reduction on EEG may have been at risk of cerebral ischemia after clamping of the internal carotid artery.

Evaluating the Usefulness of Monitoring the EEG

Some believe that neither placement of indwelling shunts nor monitoring of the EEG is needed to reduce the incidence of neurologic deficit resulting from car-

otid endarterectomy. The value of placing an indwelling shunt, like the value of carotid endarterectomy itself, has yet to be rigorously established. Differences in surgical techniques and selection criteria make it difficult to compare series of carotid endarterectomies and the associated deficit rates. However, some large series of carotid endarterectomies not using indwelling shunts have had low values for morbidity and mortality.[23,24] Review of the literature indicates that similar morbidity and mortality are observed whether shunts are used routinely, selectively, or not at all.[25]

Several studies have raised the question of whether monitoring of the EEG is useful in carotid endarterectomy. For example, one study described 176 consecutive patients undergoing carotid endarterectomy without shunt but with monitoring of the EEG. Although most clamp-associated changes on EEG related to reductions in regional CBF, postoperative deficits were usually caused by embolism.[26] Other studies have yielded similar results.[27]

Other authors are more optimistic about the use of electroencephalographic monitoring to indicate cerebral well-being during carotid endarterectomy. In one series, 1,145 carotid endarterectomies were monitored with an EEG and measurements of CBF using xenon. All new neurologic deficits on awakening from anesthesia had been predicted by changes on the EEG.[3] In another study, 111 carotid endarterectomies were monitored using a single channel of the EEG, analyzed in real time to produce a density spectral array.[28] Among patients with no preoperative neurologic deficit, new postoperative deficits appeared in only those patients ($n = 7$) who had ischemic electroencephalographic events lasting at least 10 minutes. However, the EEG was not predictive in patients with preoperative neurologic deficit. One such patient without intraoperative changes on EEG had a new postoperative deficit; another patient who had changes lasting 13 minutes had no demonstrable new postoperative deficit.

The need for caution when monitoring patients with preexisting neurologic deficit was emphasized in a report of 125 patients who had had stroke or reversible ischemic neurologic deficit before undergoing carotid endarterectomy.[29] Both stump pressure and the EEG were believed to be unreliable indicators of cerebral perfusion in these patients. The authors of this paper believe that after a stroke or a reversible ischemic neurologic deficit, a zone of ischemic brain exists. In theory, this zone is more vulnerable to diminished perfusion during carotid endarterectomy than normal brain tissue would be. In this series, EEG and stump pressure were apparently not sufficiently sensitive indicators of perfusion to such areas.

Many have found the EEG to be a reliable monitoring tool during cross-clamping of the carotid artery. Monitoring of the EEG can be used to determine how long cross-clamping can be tolerated without placement of a shunt. Cross-clamping for more than 15 minutes during significant changes on EEG is a potentially dangerous practice.[30] Monitoring of the EEG has also been used to indicate the need for an indwelling shunt by surgeons who wish to shunt selectively or to limit the use of shunts in their patients.[31,32] In addition, the EEG can be used to determine the effects of changes in blood pressure or cardiac rhythm on cerebral blood flow.[31] In a report of 172 carotid endarterectomies, the EEG was monitored in only the last 93 endarterectomies.[33] Its use was associated with a reduction in the placement of indwelling shunts (from 49 to 12 percent) and with a reduction in the combined major neurologic morbidity and mortality (from 2.3 to

1.1 percent). In summary, monitoring the EEG may provide several advantages.[34] It allows one to safely dispense with a shunt in instances in which one might have placed a shunt because of preoperative or intraoperative criteria (such as low stump pressure). It may also allow one to decrease afterload in the patient at risk of myocardial ischemic events. It permits an unhurried, technically superior endarterectomy. Finally, EEG monitoring not only identifies delayed ischemia but also aids in detecting other problems such as shunt malfunction.

Other issues that have been raised in evaluating the appropriateness of EEG monitoring during carotid endarterectomy include the occurrence of false-positive and false-negative results and cost-effectiveness. Intraoperative false-positive results (i.e., changes on the EEG not supported by a demonstrable neurologic deficit) may result from several factors. First, the brain can tolerate brief periods of ischemia without the occurrence of infarction. Thus, temporary, reversible changes on the EEG usually do not incur postoperative neurologic deficit. Second, the EEG is a sensitive but nonspecific measure. The EEG can be affected by many influences other than cerebral ischemia (e.g., anesthesia and changes in temperature and blood pressure). Third, the blood flow threshold for electrical failure is higher than the flow threshold for metabolic failure. Therefore, although the EEG may be an "early warning system" for cerebral ischemia, not all changes on the EEG necessarily indicate that infarction is taking place. Fourth, focal embolic events are not always detected by EEG. Except as noted above (i.e., in patients with preexisting neurologic deficit; strokes in evolution; or recent, reversible ischemic neurologic deficits), there are relatively few reports of false-negative results. In general, patients who do not have intraoperative changes on EEG do not awaken with new neurologic deficits. Because most neurologic deficits after carotid endarterectomy do not result from flow-related ischemia, detection of changes on EEG does not guarantee that placement of a shunt will reverse the deficit. In fact, placement of a shunt is associated with a low but definite risk of embolism.[3]

Cost-Effectiveness

To evaluate the cost-effectiveness of electroencephalographic monitoring, one can compare the cost of monitoring with the cost of the deficits that monitoring prevents. For example, let us assume that 80,000 carotid endarterectomies are performed each year, that the deficit rate is 3 percent per year (2,400 new deficits), and that monitoring prevents one-sixth of these deficits (400 deficits a year).[17] Let us also assume that 10 percent more patients would be given carotid shunts because of changes on EEG and that 0.7 percent would have neurologic deficits.[3] The result would be an additional 56 deficits related to the monitoring and 344 deficits preventable by the monitoring. If each deficit costs approximately $100,000 in medical care, lost wages, and productivity, the deficits preventable by monitoring would represent $34,400,000 a year. The break-even point for monitoring costs would be $432 per patient. At that price, the cost of monitoring would equal the cost of the deficits that monitoring would prevent. That is, if monitoring could be provided for less than that amount, it would be considered cost-effective. This analysis neglects the benefit that electroencephalographic monitoring may have in preserving myocardial function. It also neglects factors to which no dollar amount can be assigned, such as human suffering.

Changing the cost per deficit, the per-

centage of deficits preventable by monitoring, and the deficit rate would of course change the break-even point. However, as long as the percentage of deficits preventable by monitoring is not zero, the break-even point would also not be zero. The implication is that there is some cost below which monitoring is cost-effective for large-scale application. However, whether such monitoring is cost-effective at any given institution depends on other factors.

It seems likely that carotid endarterectomy will continue to be used to reduce the risk of thromboembolism and ischemia secondary to carotid occlusive disease, even in the absence of convincing evidence that it does so to a greater degree than the best medical treatment. Plans are under way for a randomized study (similar to the extracranial-intracranial bypass study[35]) that should help answer the question. However, if morbidity and mortality of carotid endarterectomy can be held to essentially zero, the risk-benefit ratio would improve significantly. The demonstration that some patients have significant ischemic symptoms on clamping of the internal carotid artery means that some form of cerebral monitoring sensitive to ischemia-induced changes may help reduce perioperative deficits to zero. Monitoring of the EEG appears to be a convenient, relatively risk-free, sensitive technique that can be used to make carotid endarterectomy a safer procedure.

SUMMARY

The scalp-recorded EEG reflects the electrical activity of the underlying cortical tissue. Conventional recording methods produce huge amounts of information—a voltage value at each instant in time for each pair (16 or more) of electrodes. The interpretation of this type of information is unwieldy in the operating room. Data reduction methods describe the EEG in terms of various calculated variables and chart the changes in these variables over time.

Various physiologic and anesthetic manipulations affect the EEG. Reductions in CBF, changes in temperature, the occurrence of hypotension, and administration of anesthetic agents have characteristic effects on the EEG. The proper interpretation of electroencephalographic changes during surgery depends on a knowledge of the effects of the commonly used anesthetic agents on the EEG.

Because the electrical activity of the brain depends on the adequacy of CBF, the EEG has been used to monitor cerebral perfusion during procedures in which CBF may be reduced (e.g., carotid endarterectomy). The most common intraoperative use of the EEG is to indicate the adequacy of cerebral perfusion after clamping of the internal carotid artery for endarterectomy. Frequently, changes on EEG are used to indicate the need for placement of an indwelling shunt during clamping. Differences of opinion exist as to the usefulness of the EEG (and the shunt itself) in this application. Issues that have been raised in this context include the occurrence of false-positive and false-negative results, the value of the EEG in preserving both brain and myocardium, and the cost-effectiveness of monitoring the EEG.

REFERENCES

1. Matthis P, Scheffner D, Benninger C: Spectral analysis of the EEG: comparison of various spectral parameters. EEG Clin Neurophysiol 52:218–221, 1981
2. Bickford RG, Billinger TW, Fleming NI et al: The compressed spectral array (CSA)—a pictorial EEG. Proc San Diego Biomed Symp 11:365–370, 1972
3. Sundt TM, Jr., Sharbrough FW, Piepgras DG et al: Correlation of cerebral blood flow and electroencephalographic changes during carotid endarterectomy. With results of surgery and hemodynamics of cerebral ischemia. Mayo Clin Proc 56:533–543, 1981
4. Trojaborg W, Boysen G: Relation between EEG, regional cerebral blood flow and internal carotid artery pressure during carotid endarterectomy. EEG Clin Neurophysiol 34:61–69, 1973
5. Sharbrough FW, Messick JM, Jr., Sundt TM Jr: Correlation of continuous electroencephalograms with cerebral blood flow measurements during carotid endarterectomy. Stroke 4:674–683, 1973
6. Jones TH, Morawetz RB, Crowell RM et al: Thresholds of focal cerebral ischemia in awake monkeys. J Neurosurg 54:773–782, 1981
7. Astrup J, Siesjö BK, Symon L: Thresholds in cerebral ischemia—the ischemic penumbra (editorial). Stroke 12:723–725, 1981
8. Symon L, Brierley JB: Morphological changes in cerebral blood vessels in chronic ischemic infarction; flow correlation obtained by the hydrogen clearance method. In Cervós-Navarro J et al. (ed): The Cerebral Vessel Wall. Raven Press, New York, 1976
9. Carter LP, Yamagata S, Erspamer R: Time limits of reversible cortical ischemia. Neurosurgery 12:620–623, 1983
10. Pritz MB: Carotid endarterectomy after recent stroke: preliminary observations in patients undergoing early operation. Neurosurgery 19:604–609, 1986
11. Scott JC, Ponganis KV, Stanski DR: EEG quantitation of narcotic effect: the comparative pharmacodynamics of fentanyl and alfentanil. Anesthesiology 62:234–241, 1985
12. Levy WJ: Power spectrum correlates of changes in consciousness during anesthetic induction with enflurane. Anesthesiology 64:688–693, 1986
13. Pichlmayr I, Lips U, Kunkel H: The Elec-

troencephalogram in Anesthesiology: Fundamentals, Practical Applications, Examples. Springer-Verlag, New York, 1984

14. Wark KJ, Sebel PS, Verghese C et al: The effect of halothane on cerebral electrical activity. An assessment using the cerebral function analysing monitor (CFAM). Anaesthesia 41:390–394, 1986
15. Bart AJ, Homi J, Linde HW: Changes in power spectra of electroencephalograms during anesthesia with fluroxene, methoxyflurane and Éthrane. Anesth Analg 50:53–63, 1971,
16. Grundy BL: EEG monitoring in the operating room and critical care unit. If, when, and what machine? Anesthesiol Rev 12(5):73–80, 1985
17. Steed DL, Peitzman AB, Grundy BL, Webster MW: Causes of stroke in carotid endarterectomy. Surgery 92:634–641, 1982
18. Graham AM, Gewertz BL, Zarins CK: Predicting cerebral ischemia during carotid endarterectomy. Arch Surg 121:595–598, 1986
19. Ivanovic LV, Rosenberg RS, Towle VL et al: Spectral analysis of EEG during carotid endarterectomy. Ann Vasc Surg 1:112–117, 1986
20. Gewertz BL, McCaffrey M: Intraoperative monitoring during carotid endarterectomy. Curr Prob Surg 24:475–532, 1987
21. Chiappa KH, Burke SR, Young RR: Results of electroencephalographic monitoring during 367 carotid endarterectomies. Use of a dedicated minicomputer. Stroke 10:381–388, 1979
22. Grundy BL, Sanderson AC, Webster MW et al: Hemiparesis following endarterectomy: comparison of monitoring methods. Anesthesiology 55:462–466, 1981
23. Whitney DG, Kahn EM, Estes JW, Jones CE: Carotid artery surgery without a temporary indwelling shunt. 1,917 consecutive procedures. Arch Surg 115:1393–1399, 1980
24. Baker WH, Dorner DB, Barnes RW: Carotid endarterectomy: is an indwelling shunt necessary? Surgery 82:321–326, 1977

25. Ferguson GG: Intra-operative monitoring and internal shunts: are they necessary in carotid endarterectomy? Stroke 13:287–289, 1982
26. Blume WT, Ferguson GG, McNeil DK: Significance of EEG changes at carotid endarterectomy. Stroke 17:891–897, 1986
27. Morawetz RB, Zeiger HE, McDowell HA, Jr et al: Correlation of cerebral blood flow and EEG during carotid occlusion for endarterectomy (without shunting) and neurologic outcome. Surgery 96:184–189, 1984
28. Rampil IJ, Holzer JA, Quest DO et al: Prognostic value of computerized EEG analysis during carotid endarterectomy. Anesth Analg 62:186–192, 1983
29. Rosenthal D, Stanton PE, Jr., Lamis PA: Carotid endarterectomy. The unreliability of intraoperative monitoring in patients having had stroke or reversible ischemic neurologic deficit. Arch Surg 116:1569–1575, 1981
30. Collice M, Arena O, Fontana RA et al: Role of EEG monitoring and cross-clamping duration in carotid endarterectomy. J Neurosurg 65:815–819, 1986
31. Phillips MR, Johnson WC, Scott RM et al: Carotid endarterectomy in the presence of contralateral carotid occlusion. The role of EEG and intraluminal shunting. Arch Surg 114:1232–1239, 1979
32. Whittemore AD, Kauffman JL, Kohler TR, Mannick JA: Routine electroencephalographic (EEG) monitoring during carotid endarterectomy. Ann Surg 197:707–713, 1983
33. Cho I, Smullens SN, Streletz LJ, Fariello RG: The value of intraoperative EEG monitoring during carotid endarterectomy. Ann Neurol 20:508–512, 1986
34. Blackshear WM, Jr., Di Carlo V, Seifert KB, Connar R: Advantages of continuous electroencephalographic monitoring during carotid artery surgery. J Cardiovasc Surg 27:146–153, 1986
35. The EC/IC Bypass Study Group: Failure of extracranial-intracranial arterial bypass to reduce the risk of ischemic stroke. Results of an international randomized trial. N Engl J Med 313:1191–1200, 1985

Monitoring and Predictive Value of Somatosensory and Motor Evoked Potentials for Peripheral Vascular Surgery

Michael T. McCaffrey

SIGNALS (EVOKED POTENTIALS) VERSUS "NOISE"

Monitoring of cortical evoked potentials allows one to assess the integrity of the spinal cord and its central connections during surgery. It does this by separating the electrical activity of the brain that is related to a specific stimulus (the signals) from the spontaneous electrical activity of the brain that is not related to the stimulus (the "noise"). The neural activity evoked by such stimuli has been studied extensively by using various sensory stimuli. Flashes of light produce visual evoked potentials (VEPs), clicks in the ear produce auditory (AEPs) or brain stem auditory evoked potentials (BAEPs), and electrical stimuli to various peripheral nerves produce somatosensory evoked potentials (SSEPs).

The primary problem is an unfavorable signal-to-noise ratio. The neural potentials evoked by any sensory stimulus are much smaller than the spontaneous electrical activity recorded at the same time. When recorded noninvasively from the scalp, evoked signals range in amplitude from a few tenths of a microvolt (after auditory stimulation) to a few microvolts (after electrical stimulation of an appropriate peripheral nerve) to 10 or so microvolts (after visual stimulation). In contrast, the spontaneous electrical activity of the brain (that is, the noise) can be 100 μV or more in amplitude when recorded from the scalp.

The circumstance that enables one to separate the signal from the noise is that the signal always occurs at a certain time after the stimulus, whereas the noise bears no temporal relationship to the stimulus. That is, the evoked potential has a known latency. By giving repeated stimuli and summing (or averaging) the resulting responses, one can "average out" the noise. At a latency following stimulation during which no signal directly related to stimulation is present, the expected value of the average of many trials will be zero, because some trials

383

will record negative voltages, whereas other trials will record positive voltages, randomly distributed around zero. At a latency where a signal (either positive or negative) is present, the expected value of the average will be something other than zero. Therefore, a zero value of the average at a certain latency indicates no stimulus-related activity at that latency, whereas a nonzero value of the average indicates the presence of stimulus-related activity at that latency. It can be shown mathematically that the degree of improvement in the signal-to-noise ratio is proportional to the square root of the number of trials averaged. Thus, averaging 100 trials will improve the signal-to-noise ratio by a factor of 10, but doubling the number of trials to 200 will improve the ratio by only a factor of 14.

SOMATOSENSORY EVOKED POTENTIALS

The most frequently used evoked potential in vascular procedures is the somatosensory evoked potential. The SSEP is usually elicited by electrical stimulation of a peripheral nerve at an intensity sufficient to produce a twitch of the muscle supplied by that nerve. The resulting afferent activity may be recorded from more cephalad portions of the nerve, the spinal cord and brain stem, and thalamocortical projections. The most important variables relating to evoked potentials are the latency and amplitude of the afferent volley recorded at successively higher levels of the nervous system. Latency indicates the conduction velocity characteristics of the pathway; and amplitude indicates the number and synchrony of the conducting fibers in the pathway. Damage to the pathways mediating these responses manifests as changes in these two variables.

Sites of Stimulation and Recording

SSEPs may be elicited from nerves in the upper or lower extremities. Because the median nerve yields larger evoked potentials than do other nerves in the upper extremity, it is the upper extremity nerve most commonly used for intraoperative recordings. The radial or ulnar nerves can also be used. Common recording sites include the skin over the nerve at the elbow; the brachial plexus (Erb's point); the second, fifth, or seventh cervical vertebra; and the scalp over cortical somatosensory receiving areas. The posterior tibial nerve in the lower extremity (and also the peroneal nerve) is commonly used when the injury is likely to occur much below C6–C7. More invasive recording techniques, such as recording from the epidural space or interspinous ligaments, have been described.[1] The peripheral recording sites (popliteal fossa and lumbar or thoracic spinous processes) are used to assess adequacy of stimulation and proper functioning of the recording apparatus. The recordings made from the cervical spine reflect activity generated in subcortical locations. These recordings are more resistant to the effects of anesthesia than those made from the scalp.

Neural Pathways and Changes in Latency and Amplitude

The peripheral fibers that are activated by the type of electrical stimulation used to evoke potentials (i.e., transcutaneous stimulation at, or slightly above, the motor threshold) are the large, myelinated fibers in the nerve. The central course of these fibers is important in localizing the site of damage. After stimulation of the posterior tibial or median nerve, the afferent volley propagates itself along ipsilateral first-order neurons (after upper and lower extremity stimulation) and second-order neurons (after lower extremity stimulation) to synapse in the nuclei gracilis and cuneatus and other brain stem nuclei. The brain stem nuclei project to contralateral thalamic nuclei, which in turn project to cortical somatosensory receiving areas via the thalamocortical radiations.[2] The spinal pathways are located in the dorsal columns and the dorsal part of the lateral fasciculus and are thus physically distinct from the more laterally and anteriorly located motor pathways. In addition, the pathways responsible for mediating the SSEP may have a different vascular supply (dorsal) than do most of the spinal pathways mediating locomotion (ventral). These two facts mean that the motor and sensory pathways have a different susceptibility to both trauma and ischemia, and may account for some of the false-positive and false-negative results observed when the SSEP is used to predict motor function.

The effects of lesions along the pathway mediating the response manifest as changes in the response at recording sites cephalad to the lesion. These changes usually consist of decreases in amplitude and increases in latency. Anesthesia also affects the latency and amplitude of SSEPs. Volatile anesthetic agents increase the latency and depress the amplitude of SSEPs.[3] Concentrations of 0.5 to 1.0 minimum alveolar concentration (MAC) of halothane, enflurane, or isoflurane produce changes in SSEPs that are very similar to those caused by spinal cord damage. Nitrous oxide potentiates these changes. Also, one study found that clinically useful doses of thiopental or fentanyl produced only modest amplitude depression and latency increases in short-latency components of the upper extremity SSEP.[4] Etomidate increased the latency but also increased the amplitude of the early cortical components of the SSEP. Another study reported that during fentanyl-based anesthesia, administration of 0.25 to 1.0 percent enflurane or isoflurane resulted in less alteration of the SSEP than did 50 percent nitrous oxide.[5] These studies were conducted in neurologically intact patients and used stable concentrations of anesthetic gases.

In fact, many patients who could benefit from monitoring are not neurologically intact. The injured pathway may be more susceptible to the effects of anesthetic agents than the intact pathway. In addition, the peripheral vasodilatory effects of volatile anesthetic agents are often used to control blood pressure; therefore, stable concentrations may not be achieved. The foregoing indicates that the anesthetic most compatible with monitoring of SSEPs in the operating room may be an oxygen-narcotic technique in which the inhaled agent is held at a low (0.25 to 0.50 percent), unchanging concentration and blood pressure is controlled by administration of a pure vasoactive, intravenous agent such as nitroprusside.

Effectiveness of SSEPs as a Monitoring Technique and Predictor of Outcome

Cerebral Blood Flow During Carotid Endarterectomy

SSEPs may be used in the operating room to assess the adequacy of cerebral blood flow (CBF) during carotid endarterectomy. Global cerebral ischemia alters the latency and amplitude of evoked potentials. At a CBF of approximately 15 ml/100 g/min, cortical evoked potentials are abolished; at higher flows, the amplitude of the response changes more than the latency.[6] Other studies cite similar values.[7,8] However, this topic has not been investigated as completely as have the changes in spontaneous electroencephalographic activity produced by alterations in CBF.

The SSEP may be a sensitive indicator of ischemia during carotid endarterectomy. One case report described a 69-year-old woman undergoing carotid endarterectomy during general anesthesia without placement of a temporary indwelling shunt.[9] The median nerve was stimulated, and the resulting afferent activity was recorded from a cervical spinous process and the scalp over the cortical somatosensory receiving area in the parietal cortex. The time between the appearance of activity at the two recording sites indicated the central conduction time of the afferent volley. The cortical evoked potential disappeared immediately after temporary occlusion of the carotid artery, although the potential recorded from the nape of the neck persisted. The cortical potentials were abnormal for 15 minutes after removal of the clamp. Immediately after awakening from anesthesia, the patient had paresis and hypoesthesia of the contralateral arm, conditions that resolved within 24 hours.

Another report describes 25 carotid endarterectomies performed under general anesthesia without the use of an intraluminal shunt and with monitoring of SSEPs.[10] Two patients had electrical unresponsiveness after temporary carotid occlusion, one bilaterally and one unilaterally. The patient with the unilateral changes had a perioperative stroke, the only one in this series.

Others who have monitored SSEPs during carotid endarterectomy with both cervical plexus block and general anesthesia report that the SSEP is a sensitive measure of cerebral ischemia and of the need for a shunt.[11,12] The incidence of placement of a shunt based on SSEP criteria was roughly the same as the incidence of selective placement of shunt based on electroencephalographic criteria—approximately 10 percent.

The absence of complications on awakening in this series limits the conclusions that can be drawn concerning the predictive value of the SSEP in carotid endarterectomy. Although the experience with SSEP monitoring during carotid endarterectomy is relatively small compared with that for electroencephalographic monitoring, the observed results are encouraging. In general, the electroencephalogram (EEG) is easier to collect, it is a continuous measure, and it appears to be less prone to technical mishaps than SSEPs. Until more data accumulate comparing the EEG and SSEP during carotid endarterectomy, I believe monitoring of the EEG is preferable to monitoring of SSEPs during this procedure.

Spinal Cord Ischemia during Repair of the Aorta

Surgical procedures that interrupt blood flow through the thoracic aorta are associated with significant postoperative neurologic deficit, the incidence being as high as 15 percent. Lower extremity neurologic deficit relates to preoperative rupture of an aneurysm, reattachment of large intercostal and lumbar arteries, clamp time, aortic dissection, the extent of the aneurysm, and the age of the patient.[13] The fact that the lower extremity SSEP is mediated by an end organ at risk during repair of aortic aneurysms has led to the proposal that the SSEP be used to monitor spinal cord integrity during such procedures.

Among 22 consecutive patients undergoing surgical correction of an aortic coarctation, temporary occlusion of the aorta changed the evoked potentials in 9 (41 percent).[14] These changes were rapid in three patients and delayed (18 to 21 minutes) in six. The rapid alterations of the evoked potential signals were related to poor collateral circulation, as evidenced by a retrospective review of the preoperative aortogram. Loss of the evoked potential for more than 14 minutes was associated with postoperative neurologic deficit. Another study monitored seven patients undergoing surgical repair of aortic coarctation ($n = 1$), thoracic aneurysm ($n = 5$), or thoracoabdominal aneurysm ($n = 1$).[15] When ischemic changes were detected by changes in the SSEP signals, increasing distal circulation by use of shunts, femorofemoral bypass, or reimplantation of intercostal arteries reversed these changes. No discernible postoperative neurologic deficit occurred in that series.

Postoperative Motor Function

Such studies indicate that the SSEP may be a sensitive indicator of spinal cord ischemia during aortic cross-clamping in operations to repair the aorta. In addition, the length of time that the SSEP is absent may predict postoperative motor function. One case report of a patient undergoing removal of a dissecting thoracic aortic aneurysm illustrates this point.[16] SSEPs were unobtainable in this patient for about 40 minutes. The SSEPs returned to approximately baseline amplitude by the end of the procedure, although a small increase in latency remained. On awakening from anesthesia, the patient was paraplegic. Therefore, reversible changes in the SSEP may be associated with postoperative motor deficit; the length of time the signals are absent appears to be the relevant variable.

False-Negative Results

Because the SSEP is mediated by spinal pathways that are physically distinct from motor pathways in both location and vascular supply, the use of the SSEP to predict postoperative motor function rests on an assumption: good predictions can only be expected if the anticipated injury is likely to affect dorsal and ventral cord similarly. This assumption may be valid for the two vascular procedures discussed above, carotid endarterectomy and aortic procedures involving cross-clamping of the upper thoracic aorta. For other procedures, however (e.g., posterior spinal fusions with Harrington-type instrumentation, tumor resections, and laminectomies), disturbing incidents of false-negative results have been reported.[17–19] Such results were caused by failure to monitor the pathway at risk, failure to interpret the evoked potentials correctly, and development of the deficits after termination of monitoring.[20] This uncertainty concerning false-negative results and the relevant variables involved in the interpretation of the SSEPs has been, in part, the impetus for the development of motor evoked potentials.

MOTOR EVOKED POTENTIALS

Motor evoked potentials (MEPs) differ from SSEPs in that the MEP tests efferent, motor pathways, whereas the SSEP tests afferent, sensory pathways. Although several methods for eliciting MEPs have been proposed, these differ only in details of the stimulation and recording techniques.[21–23] The general idea is to stimulate the motor pathways at their origin in the cerebral cortex and to record the resulting efferent neural activity in the spinal cord, peripheral nerve, or muscles. The first attempts to elicit MEPs used electrical stimulation. However, to be generally applicable in the operating room and in other clinical applications, such stimulation must be effective through the closed skull. Electrical stimulation through the closed skull requires voltages that can cause significant discomfort.

The MEP technique monitors motor pathways directly, whereas the use of the SSEP to predict motor function is an indirect monitor. Therefore, use of MEPs to monitor pathways should produce significantly fewer false-positive and false-negative results than would the use of SSEPs for the same purpose. Animal work indicates that this expectation is realistic. The MEP in cats appears to be more sensitive to weight-drop injury than the SSEP, as lower levels of weight-drop injury are required to produce changes in the MEP signal than in the SSEP signal.[24] The MEP also appears to be a better predictor of the return of motor function following weight-drop injury in the cat than does the SSEP.[25] In the dog, the MEP is sensitive to the effects of global ischemia induced by cardiac fibrillation.[26] Although experience with the MEP in humans undergoing surgery is limited, initial reports have been encouraging. Evaluation of MEPs as a monitoring technique during carotid endarterectomy has begun.[27] During occlusion of the middle cerebral artery in cats, the MEP shows changes within minutes of cessation of blood flow.[28]

An even newer technique uses pulsed magnetic fields to stimulate human nervous tissue noninvasively.[29] This technique is painless and allows assessment of the central motor pathways in awake patients. No part of the stimulator touches the patient. The usefulness of this technique in the operating room has yet to be reported.

led to the use of various electrophysiologic tests to assess the functional integrity of the CNS in the operating room. The two most common approaches involve measuring the spontaneous activity of the CNS using an EEG or measuring the responses of the CNS to various stimuli by using evoked cortical potentials.

Evoked potentials may be obtained by stimulating sensory (SSEPs) or motor (MEPs) systems. SSEP and MEP testing are techniques that can be applied to monitor the integrity of the spinal cord and its central connections during surgery. The SSEP has been used extensively in the operating room and clinic, with the result that some of its shortcomings have become apparent. False-positive and false-negative results have been reported when the SSEP is used to predict postoperative motor function after procedures in which dissociation of the motor and sensory pathways in the spinal cord is possible (i.e., tumor resections and operative correction of scoliosis using Harrington-type instrumentation). The SSEP appears to be a somewhat more accurate indicator when the most likely complication is a transverse lesion of the spinal cord, as in interruption of blood flow through the thoracic aorta. A newer technique, monitoring of the MEP, uses electrical or magnetic stimulation to assess efferent motor pathways directly. It thus promises to be a clinically useful indicator of the functional integrity of the motor pathways in humans. Much more experience is needed to define the uses and limitations of the MEP in vascular surgery.

SUMMARY

The human central nervous system (CNS) is very sensitive to the ischemia that can be induced during vascular surgery involving the blood supply to the brain or spinal cord. This sensitivity has

REFERENCES

1. Dinner DS, Lüders H, Lesser RP, Morris HH: Invasive methods of somatosensory evoked potential monitoring. J Clin Neurophysiol 3:113–130, 1986

2. York DH: Somatosensory evoked potentials in man: differentiation of spinal pathways responsible for conduction from the forelimb vs hindlimb. Prog Neurobiol 25:1–25, 1985

3. Peteson DO, Drummond JC, Todd MM: Effects of halothane, enflurane, isoflurane, and nitrous oxide on somatosensory evoked potentials in humans. Anesthesiology 65:35–40, 1986

4. McPherson RW, Sell B, Traystman RJ: Effects of thiopental, fentanyl, and etomidate on upper extremity somatosensory evoked potentials in humans. Anesthesiology 65:584–589, 1986

5. McPherson RW, Mahla M, Johnson R, Traystman RJ: Effects of enflurane, isoflurane, and nitrous oxide on somatosensory evoked potentials during fentanyl anesthesia. Anesthesiology 62:626–633, 1985

6. Prior PF: EEG monitoring and evoked potentials in brain ischaemia. Br J Anaesth 57:63–81, 1985

7. Ropper AH: Evoked potentials in cerebral ischemia. Stroke 17:3–5, 1986

8. Branston NM, Symon N: Cortical EP, blood flow, and potassium changes in experimental ischemia. p. 527–530. In Barber C (ed): Evoked Potentials. University Park Press, Baltimore, 1978

9. Russ W, Fraedrich G: Intraoperative detection of cerebral ischemia with somatosensory cortical evoked potentials during carotid endarterectomy—presentation of a new method. Thorac Cardiovasc Surg 32:124–126, 1984

10. Jacobs JA, Brinkman SD, Morrell RM et al: Long-latency somatosensory evoked potentials during carotid endarterectomy. Am Surg 49:338–344, 1983

11. Markland ON, Dilley RS, Moorthy SS, Warren C, Jr: Monitoring of somatosensory evoked responses during carotid endarterectomy. Arch Neurol 41:375–378, 1984

12. Moorthy SS, Markand ON, Dilley RS et al: Somatosensory-evoked responses during carotid endarterectomy. Anesth Analg 61:879–883, 1982

13. Crawford ES, Crawford JL, Safi JH et al: Thoracoabdominal aortic aneurysms: preoperative and intraoperative factors determining immediate and long-term results of operations in 605 patients. J Vasc Surg 3:389–404, 1986

14. Kaplan BJ, Friedman WA, Alexander JA, Hampson SR: Somatosensory evoked potential monitoring of spinal cord ischemia during aortic operations. Neurosurgery 19:82–90, 1986

15. Cunningham JN, Jr., Laschinger JC, Merkin HA et al: Measurement of spinal cord ischemia during operations upon the thoracic aorta. Initial clinical experience. Ann Surg 196:285–296, 1982

16. Takaki O, Okumura F: Application and limitation of somatosensory evoked potential monitoring during thoracic aortic aneurysm surgery: a case report. Anesthesiology 63:700–703, 1985

17. Dinner DS, Lüders H, Lesser RP et al: Intraoperative spinal somatosensory evoked potential monitoring. J Neurosurg 65:807–814, 1986

18. Ginsburg HH, Shetter AG, Raudzens PA: Post-operative paraplegia with preserved intraoperative somatosensory evoked potentials. J Neurosurg 63:296–300, 1985

19. Lesser RP, Raudzens P, Lüders H et al: Postoperative neurological deficits may occur despite unchanged intraoperative somatosensory evoked potentials. Ann Neurol 19:22–25, 1986

20. Friedman WA, Grundy BL: Monitoring of sensory evoked potentials is highly reliable and helpful in the operating room. J Clin Monit 3:38–47, 1987

21. Levy WJ, McCaffrey M, York DH, Tanzer F: Motor evoked potentials from transcranial stimulation of the motor cortex in cats. Neurosurgery 15:214–227, 1984

22. Merton PA, Morton HB: Stimulation of the cerebral cortex in the intact human subject (letter to editor). Nature 285:227, 1980

23. Rossini PM, Marciani MG, Caramia M et al: Nervous propagation along "central" motor pathways in intact man: characteristics of motor responses to "bifocal" and "unifocal" spine and scalp non-invasive stimulation. EEG Clin Neurophysiol 61:272–286, 1985

24. Levy WJ, McCaffrey M, York D: The

motor evoked potential in cats with acute spinal cord injury. Neurosurgery 19:9–19, 1986

25. Levy WJ, McCaffrey M, Hagichi S: The motor evoked potential as a predictor of recovery in chronic spinal cord injury. Neurosurgery 20:138–142, 1987

26. Konrad PE, Tacker WA, Levy WJ et al: Motor evoked potentials in the dog: effects of global ischemia on spinal cord and peripheral nerve signals. Neurosurgery 20:117–124, 1987

27. Levy WJ, Jr: Clinical experience with motor and cerebellar evoked potential monitoring. Neurosurgery 20:169–182, 1987

28. Oro J, Levy WJ: Motor evoked potential as a monitor of middle cerebral artery ischemia and stroke. Neurosurgery 20:192–193, 1987

29. Barker AT, Freeston IL, Jalinous R, Jarratt A: Clinical evaluation of conduction time in central motor pathways using magnetic stimulation of human brain (letter). Lancet 1:1325–1326, 1986

The Appropriateness of Swan-Ganz Catheterization in Patients Undergoing Vascular Surgery

Nathan L. Pace

Until 1970, assessment of hemodynamic status in the operating room depended on auscultation of blood pressure and heart rate, manometric determination of central venous pressure, and clinical observations by the anesthetist. Although clinical observations never lose their value, the art and science of monitoring have changed dramatically. In 1970, Swan et al.[1] described their use of a balloon flotation pulmonary arterial catheter (BFPAC) in 100 patients, thus presenting the Swan-Ganz catheter* as a practical, bedside method of catheterizing the right side of the heart. Since then, anesthetists have become adept at invasive monitoring using both intra-arterial and pulmonary arterial catheters.

A vast number and variety of bedside physiologic monitors are now available to

transduce and display the pressures of the heart and vascular system electronically. A variety of Swan-Ganz catheters not only measure blood pressure but also allow intermittent determination of cardiac output (thermodilution technique) and continuous display of mixed venous oxygen saturation. Standarized approaches for access to the central circulation and for flotation of the catheter are widely accepted.[2-5] BFPACs truly do meet the three design criteria set forth by Swan and colleagues: (1) they provide a reliable, prompt passage of the catheter to the pulmonary artery; (2) their placement causes only minimal dysrhythmias; and (3) they can be placed without the need for fluoroscopic guidance.

The widespread use of Swan-Ganz catheters by the hundreds of thousands each year has troubled some observers.[6,7] A prominent academic pulmonologist recently denounced the overuse of such devices. He labeled their popularity a type of faddish medical cultism and imputed motives of monetary gain to the manufacturers and to the "Swanning" physi-

---

* Throughout this chapter, the editor has used the more familiar "Swan-Ganz catheter" instead of "BFPAC".

cians.[8,9] Can the anesthetist justify the use of Swan-Ganz catheters in the operating room?

The question of whether or not Swan-Ganz catheters should be used in patients undergoing vascular surgery consists of two parts. (1) How reliably and accurately do such catheters provide data? (2) Which of these data actually help to decrease the morbidity of patients undergoing vascular surgery? This chapter addresses these two questions and then discusses the role I believe Swan-Ganz catheters should play now and in the future.

INFORMATION PROVIDED BY SWAN-GANZ CATHETERS

Cardiac Output

Addition of a thermistor in the tip of the catheter occurred very soon after introduction of the basic catheter.[10] Using the Stuart Hamilton equation, a bedside microprocessor unit integrates temperature changes in pulmonary artery blood after rapid injection of a bolus of cold fluid into the right atrium. This process allows estimation of cardiac output, which is the average volume of blood pumped over several heart beats, expressed in liters per minute. Most users make three measurements over a few minutes and take the average to be cardiac output. To standardize the effects of changes in intrathoracic pressure, each bolus is injected at the same point in the respiratory cycle (see Ch. 3). By following these and a few other simple guidelines, one can make reproducible and interpretable flow measurements in almost all patients. Little controversy exists concerning the validity of estimates of cardiac output provided by Swan-Ganz catheters and the thermodilution technique.

Mixed Venous Oxygen Saturation

By 1972, modification of the Swan-Ganz catheter enabled one to measure the in vivo oxygen saturation of hemoglobin in mixed venous blood ($S\bar{v}O_2$).[11] This process involves the intermittent transmission of several different wavelengths of infrared light to the catheter tip by a fiberoptic channel. The blood then absorbs, refracts, and reflects the light. The relative intensities of the reflected light at the different frequencies allow the derivation of $S\bar{v}O_2$. These early oximetric Swan-Ganz catheters were fragile and unreliable and were soon abandoned. Two new currently available oximetric catheters have greater ruggedness and longevity.[12] Both rely on reflectance spectrophotometry and use either two or three wavelengths of light. Unfortunately, the calibration of the two-wavelength system drifts excessively over 6 to 10 hours; the difference between true and measured saturation values ranges from 5 to 31 percent.[12] These large errors are clinically important and discourage the clinical use of the two-wavelength system.

Many anesthetists believe that values for in vivo oxygen saturation indicate whole body tissue oxygenation and thus reflect tissue perfusion. Such interpretations use arguments concerning the equilibrium of venous and tissue oxygen. These interpretations ignore the nature of mixed venous blood: $S\bar{v}O_2$ is the result of the mixing of venous blood from various organs, each of which has its own blood flow, oxygen extraction, and tissue oxygen tension.[13] Therefore, $S\bar{v}O_2$ is a weighted average of the body's mix of venous oxygen saturations for various organs. In both normal and abnormal physiologic states, blood flow can be redistributed between and within organs, and organ uptake of oxygen can change. This redistribution of organ blood flow and change in oxygen uptake are usually not accessible to measurement. Thus, measurements of $S\bar{v}O_2$ do not accurately reflect oxygen delivery and tissue oxygenation of specific organs.

Rearranging the terms of the Fick equation shows that $S\bar{v}O_2$ may be considered the ratio of oxygen consumption to cardiac output:

$$S\bar{v}O_2 \ \alpha \ C\bar{v}O_2 = CaO_2 - \dot{V}O_2/\dot{Q}$$

where $C\bar{v}O_2$ is mixed venous oxygen content, CaO_2 is arterial oxygen content, $\dot{V}O_2$ is oxygen consumption per minute (STPD), and $\dot{Q}$ is cardiac output. The use of $S\bar{v}O_2$ to estimate this ratio depends on the steady-state constancy of arterial oxygen content, hemoglobin concentration, blood flow, oxygen extraction, and blood transit time at the time of measurement.[14] Although $S\bar{v}O_2$ has been advocated as an early warning of insufficient cardiac output, the accuracy of this application has not been validated.[15] Others have advocated using continuous oximetry to titrate therapeutic maneuvers such as the infusion of inotropic drugs, but this practice also has not been validated.[16] In any case, the higher cost of oximetric Swan-Ganz catheters has discouraged their widespread use. Few clinical research reports have evaluated the merits of these oximetric devices.

"Wedge" Pressures

The concept of using a "wedge" pressure in the pulmonary artery vasculature to estimate pulmonary capillary, pulmonary venous, and left atrial pressures originates in the cardiac catheterization laboratory.[17] Under fluoroscopic guidance, a hollow cannula having a patent tip is advanced manually into the pulmonary artery until the tip lodges in a small branch. If the tip of the catheter totally occludes the artery, all blood flow would cease beyond the catheter in the subsegment nourished by the blocked artery. Although the blood vessel beyond the tip of the catheter bifurcates repeatedly, eventually becoming capillaries and recombining into pulmonary veins, conceptually and functionally, the motionless blood beyond the tip of the catheter becomes an extension of the fluid column of the catheter lumen. This stationary column of blood ends where the pulmonary veins of the "wedged" lung region meet the small pulmonary veins (which contain flowing blood) from adjacent lung regions. If the patency of the fluid path from the catheter tip to the pulmonary veins is ensured, the pressure in the tip of the catheter must be in equilibrium with the pressure in the pulmonary veins of the adjacent lung subsegments (Fig. 27-1).

Pressure Tracings: Technical Considerations

The pressure waveforms of Swan-Ganz catheters are viewed after electronic transduction. The accuracy of transmission of the waveform depends on the fidelity of the catheter itself, the connecting tubing, and the transducer system (see Ch. 3).[18] The transducer is set to zero pressure at the level of the left atrium; the fourth intercostal space in the midaxillary line serves well as a reference mark of the left atrium, regardless of body position. Pressure at the catheter tip during occlusion should be independent of tip position within the pulmonary vasculature, as long as the vascular path between artery and vein is patent.

By convention, pulmonary capillary wedge pressure (PCWP) should be read at the end of expiration. In the anesthetized patient, it is almost always possible to create a period of apnea sufficiently long to obtain a reliable PCWP reading. In the patient who is breathing spontaneously, large fluctuations in respiratory pressure can create artifactual changes in

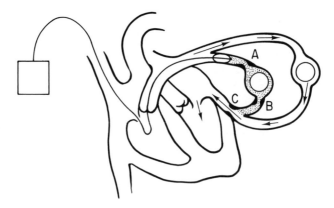

Fig. 27-1. Principles of measuring PAOP. During occlusion of the pulmonary artery by the balloon, blood flow ceases from the tip of the catheter to the confluence of veins from occluded and nonoccluded lung subsegments. Narrowing of the static column (dotted area) at the arterioles (A), the pulmonary capillaries (alveoli), or the venules (B) does not affect PAOP, whereas similar narrowing of the flowing columns (the pulmonary veins, C) will cause PAOP to overestimate left atrial pressure. (Modified from O'Quin and Marini,[27] with permission.)

the pressure tracing.[19] It can be difficult or impossible to distinguish the moment of end-expiration on the PCWP tracing. Accurate determination of PCWP may require an analog recording of the pressure tracing on a strip chart recorder (see Ch. 3).[20]

Other types of technical problems are possible regarding PCWP readings. Overinflation of the balloon can occlude the tip of the catheter. If the lumen is occluded and the continuous flushing device continues to infuse fluid, an easily recognized nonpulsatile, increasing pressure tracing results. Partial occlusion of the pulmonary artery is more difficult to detect; it probably occurs when an eccentric balloon inflation does not totally occlude the vessel lumen or when the balloon is straddling a vessel bifurcation. The pressure measured during partial occlusion is higher than during full occlusion. Such artifactual PCWPs are common in patients monitored invasively for critical illness.[21] No study has systematically investigated the frequency of artifactual partial wedging during operating room monitoring. When the validity of a

PCWP measurement is in question, three criteria must be met.[21] First, the phasic contour of the pulmonary artery waveform should change on occlusion. Second, mean pulmonary arterial pressure should decrease on occlusion. Third, the oxygen partial pressure or saturation of blood withdrawn from the wedged Swan-Ganz catheter should be higher than that of arterial blood.

"Wedge" Pressures and PAOP

The advantage of using a balloon-tipped catheter is that one can wedge and unwedge the catheter tip repeatedly without manipulating the catheter. As the balloon is inflated (usual volume, 1.0 to 1.5 ml), the onrushing blood "floats" the balloon and pulls the catheter farther into the pulmonary vascular tree until a branch of the pulmonary artery is occluded. Because the cross-sectional area of catheter tip is an order of magnitude larger when the balloon is inflated than when it is not, a larger branch of the pulmonary artery is blocked by the inflated balloon than by the manually advanced and wedged catheter tip. Thus, the region of lung in which blood flow ceases is much greater. For this reason, many prefer to call a wedge pressure measurement made by an inflated balloon-tipped catheter the "pulmonary artery occlusion pressure" (PAOP). Wedge readings and PAOP seem to give similar values[1]; occasionally, the identifying of PAOP with wedge pressure measurements has been questioned.[22,23] However, in most other chapters of this book, PCWP is assumed to be PAOP.

PAOP as an Estimate of Pulmonary Capillary Pressure

Hydrostatic pressure is the major force determining the net movement of fluid from the pulmonary capillaries into the lung parenchyma. Under normal conditions, this hydrostatic pressure in the pulmonary capillaries is approximately midway between pulmonary artery and pulmonary venous pressure (PVP). Although PAOP is used to estimate capillary pressure, even under normal conditions, PAOP clearly underestimates capillary pressure, as PAOP equilibrates with pulmonary venous pressure. In abnormal states such as acute respiratory failure, the gradient between pulmonary arterial and pulmonary venous pressures is often higher. In addition, since the distribution of vascular resistance along the vascular path between the pulmonary arteries and veins is unknown, the degree of underestimation of pulmonary capillary pressure by PAOP after lung injury is probably even greater.

Some believe that the decrease in pressure measured at the catheter tip after occlusion of the pulmonary artery consists of a fast and a slow phase. The pressure at the inflection point between these phases of pressure decline seems to be a good estimate of capillary filtration pressure.[24,25] Whether this method can be commonly and reliably used in the operating room and critical care environment has not been established. Even if

such an estimate of capillary pressure could be obtained, it is uncertain whether clinical decision-making concerning infusion of intravenous fluids and vasoactive drugs would differ significantly from that currently resulting when PAOP is used to estimate capillary pressure.

PAOP as an Estimate of Pulmonary Venous Pressure

Because the flaccid pulmonary capillaries collapse when extravascular pressure exceeds intraluminal pressure, PAOP equals PVP only when PVP exceeds alveolar pressure. Such a condition is represented by zone III of the lung described by West et al.[26] (Fig. 27-2).[27] If alveolar pressure exceeds PVP (zone II), then during pulmonary artery occlusion, the runoff of pressure at the catheter tip stops when the alveolar pressure collapses the capillary, keeping PAOP higher than PVP. This phenomenon is known as the "alveolar waterfall effect." The presence or absence of a discrepancy between PAOP and PVP depends on the complex interaction of the following factors: (1) the height of the catheter tip in relationship to the left atrial plane during occlusion; (2) left atrial pressure (LAP); and (3) the level of alveolar pressure (especially as influenced by the use of positive end-expiratory pressure [PEEP]).

Because the catheter tip follows blood flow, and because the patient is usually supine, a position that minimizes the vertical height of the lung, the catheter tip usually migrates into zone III during pulmonary artery occlusion. However, the addition of PEEP, the occurrence of hypovolemia, unexpected changes in body position, and the chance displacement of the catheter tip above the level of the left atrium can all produce an artifactual elevation in PAOP. These conditions convert the segment of the lung the catheter tip has occluded, or will occlude, from having zone III characteristics to having

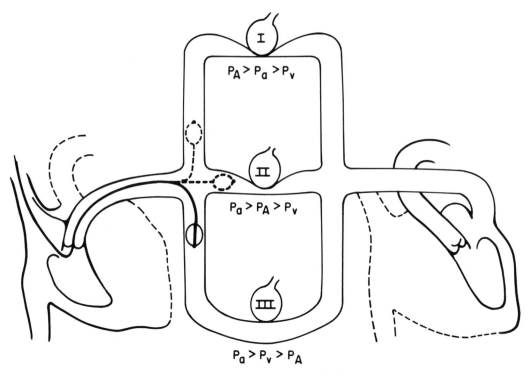

Fig. 27-2. Pulmonary artery occlusion pressure (PAOP) and the three functional zones of the lung (described by West et al.[26]) in which different hemodynamic conditions govern blood flow. The location of the tip of the catheter in relation to the left atrial plane affects the relationship of PAOP to other pressure measurements. That is, if the tip of the catheter is in zone II, PAOP reflects alveolar pressure (P_A). If the tip of the catheter is in zone III, PAOP approximates pulmonary venous pressure (P_v). The tip of the catheter is not likely to float into zone I, because zone I has no perfusion (i.e., P_A exceeds pulmonary arterial pressure [P_a]). (Modified from O'Quin and Marini,[27] with permission.)

zone II or zone I characteristics. If, during the addition or removal of PEEP, there is a concomitant increase or decrease in PAOP of less than half the change in PEEP, then the catheter tip is likely, but not certainly, to be in zone III.[27] Ultimately, the presence or absence of discrepancy between PAOP and PVP is not discernible unless PVP or LAP can be measured independently (see Ch. 3 for another view and explanation of this phenomenon).

Pulmonary venous pressure may differ from LAP if there is obstruction of the pulmonary veins. This large vein obstruction can result from tumors, vasculitis, fibrosis, and use of surgical clamps. Experimentally, a waterfall effect has been demonstrated at the exit of pulmonary veins from the lung; its clinical importance is unknown. Under these unusual circumstances of pulmonary vein obstruction, PVP will be higher than LAP.

A discrepancy between LAP and left ventricular end-diastolic pressure (LVEDF) is especially characteristic of mitral valve stenosis. With decreases in left ventricular distensibility (myocardial infarction, hypertrophy), atrial contraction plays a more important role in ventricular filling. Under these conditions, atrial contraction raises LVEDP as much as 10 mmHg higher than LAP just at the time of mitral valve closure. Left atrial pressure and PAOP now reflect not LVEDP but left ventricular diastolic pressure before atrial contraction. The importance of left atrial contraction for left ventricular filling is enhanced when left ventricular compliance decreases.

PAOP as an Estimate of Left Ventricular Filling (Preload)

The use of PAOP to estimate left ventricular filling pressure (preload) assumes that PAOP, PVP, LAP, and are equal. Although these entities are generally equal, disease and medical therapies can disturb their relationship and lead to invalid interpretation of monitoring data.[27,28]

The actual filling pressure of the left ventricle is the transmural distending pressure (i.e., the pressure inside the ventricle minus the pressure outside the ventricle). The inside pressure is called LVEDP and is estimated by PAOP or LAP; the outside pressure is called the pericardial or juxtacardiac pressure. Juxtacardiac pressure is similar, but not identical, to either intrapleural or esophageal pressure. Attempts to measure juxtacardiac pressure directly or indirectly by measuring intrapleural or esophageal pressure are fraught with technical difficulties, and this has not become a common clinical practice.

During quiet breathing, juxtacardiac pressure is slightly below atmospheric pressure. Under such conditions, PAOP, LAP, or LVEDP (measured relative to atmospheric pressure in the usual fashion) is a reasonable estimate of transmural pressure. When airway pressure is elevated by PEEP or by mechanical ventilation in patients with obstruction of airflow, variable amounts of airway pressure may be transmitted through the lung parenchyma, thus raising intrapleural, juxtacardiac, and intravascular pressures to different degrees. Therefore, PAOP,

LAP, and LVEDP would overestimate transmural filling pressure.

Measurement of PAOP during a brief period of removal of PEEP can be done but may reflect a hemodynamic state different than that occurring during PEEP. Also, some patients are likely to become hypoxemic during measurements of PAOP if the fractional concentration of inspired oxygen (FIO_2) is not increased momentarily. At present, there is no practical way of measuring transmural pressure during PEEP.

THE LEFT VENTRICULAR PRESSURE-VOLUME RELATIONSHIP

Characteristics of Left Ventricular Filling (Preload)

Even if PAOP reflected LVEDP perfectly, there would be inherent limitations in using blood pressure to estimate filling. In 1915, Starling[29] said that "the energy of contraction, however measured, is a function of the length of the muscle fibre" prior to muscle contraction. Known today as "Starling's law of the heart," it is usually reformulated to read that at any given functional state of the myocardium, the force of ventricular contraction depends on its end-diastolic wall tension and stretch or its end-diastolic volume. To use any pressure measurements—be it LAP or PAOP or LVEDP—to estimate left ventricular end-diastolic volume (LVEDV), one must understand the concept of chamber compliance.[30] Chamber compliance is the change in diastolic volume that occurs with change in diastolic pressure ($\Delta V/\Delta P$). Both intrinsic factors (muscle stiffness and chamber geometry) and extrinsic factors (interactions between the pericardium and ven-

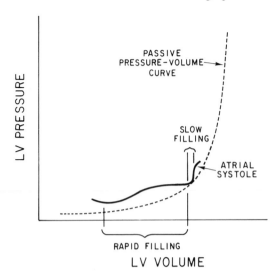

Fig. 27-3. This idealized representation of left ventricular (LV) diastolic filling shows that left ventricular diastolic pressure is greater than that predicted from the passive pressure-volume curve except during slow diastolic filling.

tricle) determine the relationship between pressure and volume.

Diastolic ventricular filling consists of three phases. The initial phase is one of rapid ventricular filling immediately after opening of the mitral valve. This phase is followed by a long period of slow ventricular filling. Then, at the end of diastole, ventricular volume and pressure increase briefly and rapidly during atrial systole.

Figure 27-3 shows graphically the relationship between pressure and volume during filling of the left ventricle. This relationship is curvilinear; that is, pressure increases slowly at low volumes but rapidly at high volumes. Compliance is not constant along such a curve, being high at low pressures and volumes and less at high pressures and volumes. Compliance ($\Delta V/\Delta P$) can be made constant by using a semilogarithmic plot. This curve may be modified in either position (intercept) or shape (change in slope). The

characteristics of chamber compliance are thus specified by two constants, the slope and the intercept.

Determinants of Chamber Compliance

One variable that does affect the characteristics of chamber compliance is the stiffness of myocardial muscle. Chamber compliance decreases (i.e., the curve becomes steeper) as muscle stiffness increases.

During the slow filling phase of diastole, the pressure-volume relationship of the ventricle is described by this passive pressure-volume curve. During rapid atrial filling and during atrial systole, pressure and volume within the left ventricle deviate from the passive pressure-volume curve; ventricular pressure is higher than would be predicted from the passive relationship. Several intrinsic determinants of diastolic function account for this discrepancy: (1) inadequate time for isovolumic relaxation prior to opening of the mitral valve, (2) the phenomenon of ventricular suction during the very early portion of diastole, (3) viscous resistance to stretch, and (4) greater end-systolic volume. Increases in factors 1,3, and 4 tend to raise pressure; increases in factor 2 lower pressure.[30]

Several extrinsic factors also influence compliance characteristics of the left ventricle. The presence of an intact pericardium lowers the compliance (i.e., the pressure-volume curve is steeper) for all cardiac chambers, including the left ventricle. The right ventricle may act as an outside force on the left ventricle. If the right ventricle distends, the interventricular septum is displaced to the left and compresses the left ventricle; this is called "ventricular interaction." Ventricular interaction is magnified considerably by the presence of an intact pericardium.

A variety of clinical circumstances affect left ventricular stiffness. Cardiomyopathies and use of vasodilating drugs (nitroglycerin and nitroprusside) increase compliance. Relief of ischemia also increases compliance. In contrast, ischemia or infarction, right ventricular overload, hemorrhagic and septic shock, and use of PEEP or inotropic drugs (dopamine) decrease compliance. The mechanisms of action involve the intrinsic and extrinsic factors described above.

Consequences of Variations in Chamber Compliance Characteristics

Several consequences arise from variations in compliance characteristics of the left ventricle during diastole. First, both left ventricular systolic dysfunction (decreased contractility) and left ventricular diastolic dysfunction (decreased compliance) can cause pulmonary venous hypertension. This condition increases pulmonary capillary pressure, which in turn increases pulmonary extravascular water. As a result, lung function and gas exchange are impaired, and dyspnea occurs.

Second, interpretation of data may be inaccurate if one does not take into consideration variations in compliance characteristics. To interpret hemodynamic data, one usually plots cardiac output or left ventricular stroke work against left ventricular filling pressure (usually PAOP). Pulmonary artery occlusion pressure is used when determinations of LVEDV are not clinically available. One then compares the result with a band of "normal" or expected responses that has been determined empirically. If the observations lie below the normal band, myocardial contractility is usually assumed to be impaired. However, a proper appreciation of diastolic function reveals that there is a fundamental ambiguity in interpretation. Specifically, both depressed systolic function and reduced left ventricular chamber compliance are factors that could account for the existence of data points below the normal band.

FACTORS DETERMINING THE POTENTIAL BENEFIT OF USING SWAN-GANZ CATHETERS

The Swan-Ganz catheter has been used in extremely diverse clinical situations. Commonly accepted indications for its use include (1) complicated myocardial infarction, (2) acute respiratory failure, (3) severe cardiovascular dysfunction, and (4) the use of complicated anesthetic or surgical procedures. Monitoring with Swan-Ganz catheters aims to provide data helpful in assessing the adequacy of perfusion; managing intravenous fluid therapy; diagnosing myocardial ischemia; and evaluating ventilatory therapies, vasoactive drugs, hemodialysis, and assisted circulation. However, no controlled clinical trial has yet demonstrated that using these devices reduces morbidity or mortality for any disease.[31] Arguments for its use must be made on the grounds of plausibility of benefit. Before choosing to use a Swan-Ganz catheter for an anesthetic procedure, the following factors should be assessed.

The Stress of Surgery on Homeostasis

Vascular surgery procedures consist of two distinct groups: those involving and those not involving the aorta. Resection and grafting of abdominal aortic aneurysms, aortoiliac bypass grafts, and surgery to correct visceral ischemia incur large blood losses and important systemic changes in blood flow and vascular resistance. In contrast, procedures to correct cerebral ischemia and peripheral vascular insufficiency usually involve only clinically insignificant blood loss and only localized changes in blood flow. As a result, use of the Swan-Ganz catheter is usually limited to surgery involving the aorta.

The consensus in both the anesthesia and surgical literatures is that the Swan-Ganz catheter is useful in at least some patients undergoing aortic reconstruction. Differences of opinion remain, however, regarding whether all such patients, or only those with certain associated diseases, should be monitored. As mentioned before, such recommendations are not based on controlled clinical trials. Also, the anesthesia and surgical literatures differ in their emphasis: anesthetists tend to use the Swan-Ganz catheter to recognize and control intraoperative and postoperative hemodynamic status,[32] whereas surgeons focus on the preoperative use of these catheters to assess volume status and cardiac reserve, and to monitor fluid loading.[33,34]

Review of elective surgery for abdominal aortic aneurysm shows a dramatic reduction in morbidity and mortality over the last 40 years. This increased safety has been attributed in part to the common[35] or universal[36] use of Swan-Ganz catheters for perioperative monitoring. However, other improvements have also decreased morbidity and mortality to various degrees: the early institution of aggressive surgical intervention, more liberal preoperative and intraoperative administration of fluids, universal use of intra-arterial monitoring, and the availability of postoperative assisted ventilation. With so many changes in medical care occurring simultaneously, one can only be skeptical about conclusions regarding the unique importance of Swan-Ganz catheters. For example, the importance of the liberal use of crystalloid solutions was well recognized before invention of the BFPAC.[37]

The Ability of Data Obtained by the Swan-Ganz Catheter to Improve Perioperative Care

Although cardiac and pulmonary diseases often occur in patients with non-aortic disease, they are especially prevalent in patients undergoing aortic surgery. Regardless of the anticipated surgery, does the presence of cardiac or pulmonary disease, in and of itself, warrant the routine use of a Swan-Ganz catheter? Currently available reports do not answer this question with certainty. Although my practice is to use these catheters liberally in such patients, I am not able to say whether more frequent or less frequent use of these devices is right or wrong.

One disease for which considerable data are available is myocardial infarction. Earlier (1973 to 1976) epidemiologic surveys reported the rate of reinfarction in patients with a history of myocardial infarction who were undergoing noncardiac surgery. At that time, the rate of reinfarction was at least 25 percent if surgery occurred within 3 months of a myocardial infarction.[38] However, an update (1977 to 1982) showed that this rate had decreased to approximately 6 percent.[38] Differences in patient care between these two experiences included wider use of invasive hemodynamic monitoring (both Swan-Ganz and intra-arterial catheters), β-adrenergic receptor-blocking drugs, and vasodilating drugs. Also, preoperative medical management had become more fastidious. The authors of this report were properly hesitant in speculating about which of these changes contributed to the reduction in the rate of reinfarction.

Again, the anesthesia and surgical literatures differ in emphasis. Anesthesia reports emphasize intraoperative use. Surgical reports, such as that by Del Guercio and Cohn,[39] describe the routine preoperative use of Swan-Ganz catheters in elderly patients to assess their fitness for surgery. Shoemaker et al.[40] described a randomized trial of Swan-Ganz catheter use during and after surgery in high-risk patients. The authors claimed that use of the catheter to maintain a hyperdynamic circulatory state improved survival. If this report is confirmed, reasonable proof of the benefit of the Swan-Ganz catheter during and after high-risk surgery would finally be available.

The Reliability of PAOP as an Estimate of Left Ventricular Filling

The concern that changes in left ventricular compliance make PAOP an inaccurate measure of left ventricular filling (preload) are not merely theoretical. Investigators have shown that at the following times, little or no correlation exists between PAOP and LVEDV: during severe sepsis and acute cardiac disease,[41] immediately after cardiopulmonary bypass for coronary artery bypass grafting,[42] and several hours after coronary artery bypass grafting.[43]

Many studies have investigated hemodynamic status before, during, and after aortic surgery.[44,45] Such studies usually measure cardiac output and PAOP and calculate cardiac index. However, more recent studies have used more direct methods of measuring ventricular volumes during aortic surgery; these reports show an inconstant relationship between PAOP and LVEDV, both during[46] and after[47] clamping of the aorta.

Complications Associated with the Use of Swan-Ganz Catheters

Anecdotal reports of complications appeared soon after the widespread clinical use of Swan-Ganz catheters. The most serious included sudden death from dysrhythmias and exsanguinating, asphyxiating pulmonary hemorrhage from pulmonary artery rupture. Evaluation of the relative risk of using these devices is now possible because of a prospective study of over 6,000 operative patients in whom a Swan-Ganz catheter was placed.[48] Of these patients, only one died from a direct complication related to use of the catheter. In general, the complications were mostly transient and self-limiting; the incidence of morbidity and mortality associated with the use of a Swan-Ganz catheter was low. (However, complications from misinterpretation of the waveform and numbers generated from the catheter were not included in these totals and are perhaps the most frequent and most serious.)

CONCLUSION

The reservations I expressed a decade ago[49] regarding the interpretation of PAOP seem to be worth considering even today. For one thing, PAOP is an unreliable estimate of LVEDV. During high or fluctuating pleural pressure, PAOP is likely to reflect alveolar pressure. Furthermore, if left ventricular compliance changes, no measurement of pressure adequately tracks left ventricular filling. Also, during lung injury and pulmonary arterial hypertension, PAOP may underestimate the hydrostatic pressure in pulmonary capillaries.

Have anesthetists and surgeons been deluding themselves for over 15 years about the real merits of data obtained by Swan-Ganz catheterization of patients undergoing aortic surgery? Possibly. On the other hand, one can speculate that PAOP and cardiac output data are being used, or are capable of being used, in a more sophisticated manner. For example, a sudden large increase in PAOP may indicate either left ventricular dysfunction from a change in contractility or compliance or intravascular volume overload. Serial determinations of cardiac output help assess the results of remedial changes in left ventricular afterload, depth of anesthesia, and intravenous administration of fluids.

One is still left with the uncertainty of the real value of the Swan-Ganz catheter. Clearly, PAOP data are not the specific measures of left ventricular filling, as originally hoped. However, many researchers and clinicians have used these catheters extensively to monitor aortic surgery. They have also developed rules of thumb for data interpretation and have vouched for the efficacy of the device. The most likely resolution for this dilemma is the advent of new methods of measuring cardiovascular variables.[50,51] One new method is transesophageal echocardiography, a technique that provides direct observation of the cross-sectional area and wall motion of the left ventricle. Abnormalities in segmental left ventricular wall motion appear to be a very early sign of myocardial ischemia. If this new technique can be made less expensive, and if real-time quantitation of volume and motion can be developed, transesophageal echocardiography will probably supplement or even replace the Swan-Ganz catheter during aortic surgery.

REFERENCES

1. Swan HJC, Ganz W, Forrester J, et al: Catheterization of the heart in man with the use of a flow-directed balloon-tipped catheter. N Engl J Med 283:447–451, 1970

2. Gore JM, Alpert JS: Handbook of Hemodynamic Monitoring. Little, Brown, Boston, 1984

3. Keefer JR, Barash PG: Pulmonary artery catheterization. p. 177–228. In Blitt CD (ed): Monitoring in Anesthesia and Critical Care Medicine. Churchill Livingstone, New York, 1985

4. Sprung CL (ed): The Pulmonary Artery Catheter: Methodology and Clinical Applications. University Park Press, Baltimore, 1983

5. Whalley DG: Haemodynamic monitoring: pulmonary artery catheterization. Can Anaesth Soc J 32:299–305, 1985

6. Puri VK, Kyff J: Pulmonary artery catheterization—uses and abuses. Int J Clin Monit Comput 3:107–115, 1986

7. Schwartz AJ: Pulmonary artery catheters: there are still concerns with their routine use. J Cardiothorac Anesth 1:7–9, 1987

8. Robin ED: The cult of the Swan-Ganz catheter. Overuse and abuse of pulmonary flow catheters. Ann Intern Med 103:445–449, 1985

9. Robin ED: Overuse and abuse of Swan-Ganz catheters. Int J Clin Monit Comput 4:5–9, 1987

10. Ganz W, Donoso R, Marcus HS et al: A new technique for measurement of cardiac output by thermodilution in man. Am J Cardiol 27:392–396, 1971

11. Cole JS, Martin WE, Cheung PW, Johnson CC: Clinical studies with a solid state fiberoptic oximeter. Am J Cardiol 29:383–388, 1972

12. Gettinger A, DeTraglia MC, Glass DD: In vivo comparison of two mixed venous saturation catheters. Anesthesiology 66:373–375, 1987

13. Miller MJ: Tissue oxygenation in clinical medicine: an historical review. Anesth Analg 61:527–535, 1982

14. Zierler KL: Theory of the use of arteriovenous concentration differences for measuring metabolism in steady and nonsteady states. J Clin Invest 40:2111–2125, 1961

15. Schmidt CR, Frank LP, Forsythe SB, Estafanous FG: Continuous $S\bar{V}O_2$ measurement and oxygen transport patterns in car-

diac surgery patients. Crit Care Med 12:523–527, 1984

16. Hassan E, Roffman DS, Applefeld MM: The value of mixed venous oxygen saturation as a therapeutic indicator in the treatment of advanced congestive heart failure. Am Heart J 113:743–749, 1987

17. Rapaport E, Dexter L: Pulmonary "capillary" pressure. Methods Med Res 7:85–93, 1958

18. Gardner RM: Direct blood pressure measurement—dynamic response requirements. Anesthesiology 54:227–236, 1981

19. Schmitt EA, Brantigan CO: Common artifacts of pulmonary artery and pulmonary artery wedge pressures: recognition and interpretation. J Clin Monit 2:44–52, 1986

20. Maran AG: Variables in pulmonary capillary wedge pressure: variation with intrathoracic pressure, graphic and digital recorders. Crit Care Med 8:102–105, 1980

21. Morris AH, Chapman RH, Gardner RM: Frequency of technical problems encountered in the measurement of pulmonary artery wedge pressure. Crit Care Med 12:164–170, 1984

22. Royster RL, Johnson JC, Prough DS et al: Differences in pulmonary artery wedge pressures obtained by balloon inflation *versus* impaction techniques. Anesthesiology 61:339–341, 1984

23. Zidulka A, Hakim TS: Wedge pressure in large vs. small pulmonary arteries to detect pulmonary venoconstriction. J Appl Physiol 59:1329–1332, 1985

24. Cope DK, Allison RC, Parmentier JL et al: Measurement of effective pulmonary capillary pressure using the pressure profile after pulmonary artery occlusion. Crit Care Med 14:16–22, 1986

25. Collee GG, Lynch KE, Hill RD, Zapol WM: Bedside measurement of pulmonary capillary pressure in patients with acute respiratory failure. Anesthesiology 66:614–620, 1987

26. West JB, Dollery CT, Naimark A: Distribution of blood flow in isolated lung; relation to vascular and alveolar pressures. J Appl Physiol 19:713–724, 1964

27. O'Quin R, Marini JJ: Pulmonary artery occlusion pressure: clinical physiology, measurement, and interpretation. Am Rev Respir Dis 128:319–326, 1983

28. Raper R, Sibbald WJ: Misled by the wedge? The Swan-Ganz catheter and left ventricular preload. Chest 89:427–434, 1986

29. Starling EH: The Linacre lecture on the law of the heart. Given at Cambridge, 1915. Longmans, Green & Co., London, 1918

30. LeWinter MM: Diastolic function and the hypertrophied ventricle. p. 200–212. In Utley JR (ed): Perioperative Cardiac Dysfunction. Cardiothoracic Surgery Series. Vol. 3. Williams & Wilkins, Baltimore, 1985

31. Pace NL: But what does monitoring do to patient outcome? Int J Clin Monit Comput 1:197–200, 1985

32. Attia RR, Murphy JD, Snider M, et al: Myocardial ischemia due to infrarenal aortic cross-clamping during aortic surgery in patients with severe coronary artery disease. Circulation 53:961–965, 1976

33. Grant KC: Utility and application of pulmonary artery catheterization in aortic and aortoiliac disease. Can J Surg 29:256–258, 1986

34. Bush HL, Jr., LoGerfo FW, Weisel RD et al: Assessment of myocardial performance and optimal volume loading during elective abdominal aortic aneurysm resection. Arch Surg 112:1301–1306, 1977

35. Darling RC, Brewster DC: Elective treatment of abdominal aortic aneurysms. World J Surg 4:661–667, 1980

36. Whittemore AD, Clowes AW, Hechtman HB, Mannick JA: Aortic aneurysm repair. Reduced operative mortality associated with maintenance of optimal cardiac performance. Ann Surg 192:414–421, 1980

37. Thompson JE, Vollman RW, Austin DJ, Kartchner MM: Prevention of hypotensive and renal complications of aortic surgery using balanced salt solution: thirteen-year experience with 670 cases. Ann Surg 167:767–778, 1968

38. Rao TLK, Jacobs KH, El-Etr AA: Reinfarction following anesthesia in patients with myocardial infarction. Anesthesiology 59:499–505, 1983

39. Del Guercio LRM, Cohn JD: Monitoring operative risk in the elderly. JAMA 243:1350–1355, 1980

40. Shoemaker WC, Appel PL, Kram HB et al: Prospective trial of supranormal values of survivors as therapeutic goals in high-risk surgical patients. Chest 94:1176–1186, 1988

41. Calvin JE, Driedger AA, Sibbald WJ: Does the pulmonary capillary wedge pressure predict left ventricular preload in critically ill patients? Crit Care Med 9:437–443, 1981

42. Ellis RJ, Mangano DT, VanDyke DC: Relationship of wedge pressure to end-diastolic volume in patients undergoing myocardial revascularization. J Thorac Cardiovasc Surg 78:605–613, 1979

43. Hansen RM, Viquerat CE, Matthay MA et al: Poor correlation between pulmonary arterial wedge pressure and left ventricular end-diastolic volume after coronary artery bypass graft surgery. Anesthesiology 64:764–770, 1986

44. Gooding JM, Archie JP, Jr., McDowell H: Hemodynamic response to infrarenal aortic cross-clamping in patients with and without coronary artery disease. Crit Care Med 8:382–385, 1980

45. Walker PM, Johnston KW: Changes in cardiac output during major vascular surgery. Am J Surg 140:603–605, 1980

46. Roizen MF, Beaupre PN, Alpert RA et al: Monitoring with two-dimensional transesophageal echocardiography. J Vasc Surg 1:300–305, 1984

47. Kalman PG, Wellwood MR, Weisel RD et al: Cardiac dysfunction during abdominal aortic operation: the limitations of pulmonary wedge pressures. J Vasc Surg 3:773–781, 1986

48. Shah KB, Rao TLK, Laughlin S, El-Etr AA: A review of pulmonary artery catheterization in 6,245 patients. Anesthesiology 61:271–275, 1984

49. Pace NL: A critique of flow-directed pulmonary arterial catheterization. Anesthesiology 47:455–465, 1977

50. Cahalan MK, Litt L, Botvinick EH, Schiller NB: Advances in noninvasive cardiovascular imaging: implications for the anesthesiologist. Anesthesiology 66:356–372, 1987

51. Clements FM, de Bruijn NP: Perioperative evaluation of regional wall motion by transesophageal two-dimensional echocardiography. Anesth Analg 66:249–261, 1987

28

Role of Two-Dimensional Transesophageal Echocardiography during Anesthesia for Vascular Surgery

John E. Ellis
David J. Benefiel
Michael F. Roizen

Transesophageal echocardiography (TEE) is a well-established technique that is being used at an increasing number of medical centers in the United States. It is used in the operating room, the intensive care unit (ICU), and the echocardiographic laboratory to diagnose acute and preexisting cardiac disease. Most of the published work regarding intraoperative TEE has described patients undergoing cardiac surgery.[1–5] However, we believe that use of TEE in patients who have heart disease but are undergoing noncardiac surgery (particularly vascular surgery) is the area in which TEE has the greatest promise, both as a special research tool and as an important *routinely used* clinical monitor.

As a routinely used clinical monitor, TEE would provide information regarding myocardial ischemia, intravascular volume status, and contractile perfor-mance. Regional myocardial ischemia would be detected when new segmental wall motion abnormalities occur. In ad-dition, structural cardiac defects, both preexisting and acute, could be detected. For this application, TEE overcomes the limitations of two-dimensional precordial echocardiography: the incompatibility of the technique with surgical positioning, the need to position the transducer within the sterile field, the difficulty of main-taining precise orientation with tight skin contact, and frequent interference with the sound beam by lung tissue during controlled ventilation in the supine po-sition.[6]

Transesophageal echocardiography is also becoming increasingly popular in the echocardiography lab, where its ad-vantages over precordial echocardiogra-phy allow superior diagnosis of cardiac disease.[7,8] Other uses include calculation

405

of stroke volume, perfusion scanning of the myocardium, intraoperative assessment of the repair of structural cardiac defects, and detection of air and thromboemboli. In the future, characterization of myocardial, renal, and hepatic blood flow may be possible; contrast echocardiography has the potential of revealing the cause of myocardial ischemia during vascular surgery.

HOW TRANSESOPHAGEAL ECHOCARDIOGRAPHIC VIEWS ARE OBTAINED

The transducer used for TEE is functionally the same as that used in precordial echocardiography but is miniaturized for insertion into the esophagus. Typically, a transducer is mounted at the tip of an endoscope (Fig. 28-1). The tip is passed into the esophagus and is thus posterior to the heart and great vessels. The image obtained depends on the depth of insertion, the rotation of the body of the endoscope, and, to a limited degree, manipulation of the tilt control of the endoscope. Once the desired image plane has been found, the controls can be locked and the image monitored continuously without constant attention to the transducer. Because no layer of air obstructs the view (as in precordial echocardiography), the quality of the image is generally excellent. In addition, the proximity of the esophagus to the heart allows use of transducers having higher frequency, shorter range, and better resolution than those used for precordial echocardiography. The views, however, are limited to those lying in an axial plane originating at the esophagus.

As the transducer moves down the esophagus, the trachea blocks the anterior image toward the heart and great ves-

sels. When the transducer passes the carina, however, the ascending aorta can be seen (Fig. 28-2). The quality of this view depends on the location of the carina relative to the aforementioned structures. As the transducer passes inferior to the pulmonary artery, the left atrium becomes the structure closest to the esophagus, and the aortic valve can be visualized (Fig. 28-3). Moving more distally produces a tangential four-chamber view through the left atrium (Fig. 28-4). Below the atrioventricular groove, TEE obtains short-axis views of the left ventricle. Passage of the transducer distally first produces images of the base of the heart and the mitral valve, then the papillary muscles (Fig. 28-5), and finally an apical short-axis view of the heart. These echocardiographic cross-sections have been verified through direct anatomic comparisons.[9,10] Although TEE involves some potential for injury to the esophagus, no complications have occurred at our two institutions in well over 2000 uses.

ECHOCARDIOGRAPHY IN ISCHEMIC HEART DISEASE

Acute myocardial ischemia rapidly decreases myocardial performance. Various human models (including the brief total ischemia that accompanies percutaneous coronary angioplasty[11-13] and ergonovine challenge in patients with variant angina[14]) have been used to define the stages of ischemia-induced dysfunction. Changes in diastolic function (decreased compliance) usually precede decrements in systolic function (segmental wall motion abnormality, SWMA); electrocardiographic abnormalities and angina occur later, if at all. Therefore, because it can detect both decreased compliance and decrements in systolic function, echocar-

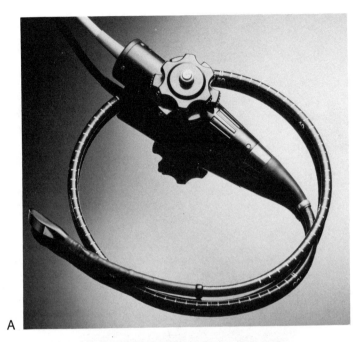

A

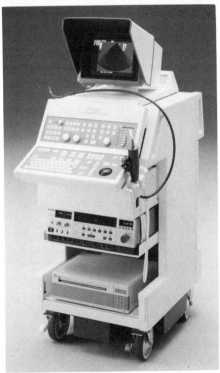

B

Fig. 28-1. In transesophageal echocardiography, (**A**) a transducer is mounted on the end of a gastroscope. (**B**) The transducer is attached to an echocardiographic machine. (Courtesy of General Electric, Waukesha, Wisc.)

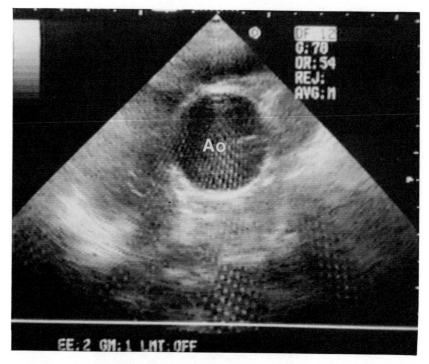

Fig. 28-2. Transesophageal echocardiographic short-axis view of the ascending aorta (Ao). Areas that are filled with blood appear dark. When the actual "on-line" echocardiographic images are viewed in the operating room, aortic pulsations can be seen to enlarge the aorta.

diography is an excellent intraoperative technique for early detection of myocardial ischemia. During graded regional myocardial ischemia, the ischemic region rapidly develops an SWMA that progresses from abnormal relaxation during diastole[15] to dysfunction during systole, that is, hypokinesia, akinesia, and finally dyskinesia.[16,17]

The acoustic properties of normal myocardium, ischemic myocardium, and infarcted myocardium differ quantitatively, making differentiation of these regions possible on that basis rather than on the basis of segmental wall motion. Computer-assisted analysis of echo character may simplify and increase the reliability with which myocardial ischemia is detected.[18] Ultimately, automated detection systems could reduce the amount of observer training required for detection of ischemia, making wider use of TEE more feasible.

Measurements of cavity length and muscle thickening from echocardiograms closely correspond with measurements made with other accepted techniques such as direct measurement[9] or use of sonomicrometers.[19,20] The ventricular wall normally thickens during systole: experiments in dogs show that the degree of wall thickening during systole (as measured on echocardiograms) is a precise indicator of contractility.[21] Precordial echocardiography is already known to produce reliable and reproducible measurements of cardiac function and wall motion abnormalities,[22–25] and interobserver comparison studies have shown that wall motion abnormalities can be

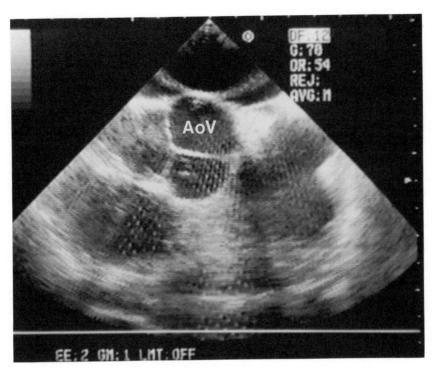

Fig. 28-3. Transesophageal echocardiographic short-axis view of the aortic valve (AoV).

identified reliably by anesthetists using TEE, even after little training.[26]

The appearance of a new intraoperative SWMA that persists throughout surgery predicts postoperative myocardial infarction (MI). Cahalan et al.[27] showed that SWMA could be detected reliably during surgery in 43 high-risk surgical patients. Seven of these patients had unresolved SWMAs; five of those seven had MIs. No patient without a persistent SWMA had an MI. Among patients who had MIs, the area of the persistent SWMA detected by TEE during surgery corresponded to the area of infarction indicated on the postoperative electrocardiogram (ECG). The two patients who had new persistent SWMAs without MIs may have had prolonged postischemic myocardial dysfunction.[28]

Smith et al.[29] demonstrated the superiority of two-dimensional transesopha-geal echocardiography (2D TEE) over electrocardiography (six limb leads and lead V$_5$ were used) for the intraoperative detection of myocardial ischemia. Of 50 high-risk patients undergoing aortic or coronary surgery, 24 had new intraoperative SWMAs, whereas only 6 had electrocardiographic changes in the ST segment. All six patients with changes in the ST segment also had new SWMAs. All three patients who had perioperative MIs also had persistent intraoperative SWMAs; in contrast, only one patient had changes in the ST segment. The control group of 10 healthy patients undergoing noncardiovascular surgery had no SWMAs, changes in the ST segment, or MIs. Smith and co-workers also confirmed the observation of Cahalan and colleagues[27] that when new SWMAs persist, myocardial infarction is likely to have occurred. In another study, the ap-

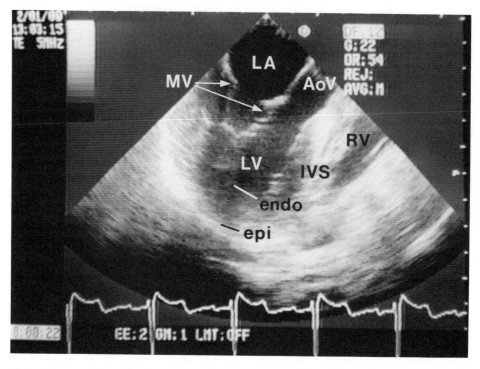

Fig. 28-4. Transesophageal echocardiographic view of the four chambers of the heart through the left atrium (LA). MV = mitral valve leaflets; AoV = aortic outflow tract and aortic valve; IVS = interventricular septum; LV = left ventricle; RV = right ventricle; endo = endocardial border; and epi = epicardial border. (Usually, actual structures are easier to visualize using the moving pictures seen in the operating room rather than these "still" images.)

pearance of new intraoperative SWMAs that persisted until skin closure were predictive of myocardial infarction.[30]

Monitoring with TEE has shown that myocardial dysfunction improves immediately after coronary revascularization. Topol et al.[31] used TEE to demonstrate immediate improvement of dysfunctional myocardial segments in patients undergoing coronary revascularization. The segments demonstrating the most severe dysfunction before bypass were those most likely to show sustained improvement after revascularization. In addition, precordial echocardiograms obtained 1 week after surgery showed a high degree of correlation between SWMA seen immediately after bypass and that

seen 1 week later. Therefore, TEE appears to be able not only to diagnose intraoperative myocardial ischemia but also to document long-standing improvement in myocardial performance.

Two-dimensional echocardiography has been used to reliably diagnose acute MI and to predict complications in the post-MI period.[32–35] Therefore, persistent intraoperative SWMAs detected with TEE indicate a high likelihood of MI and identify patients at high risk of postoperative complications. Thus, TEE may allow segregation of patients needing more intensive postoperative care. Monitoring with TEE in the postoperative period has been able to identify patients at risk of complications after coronary artery

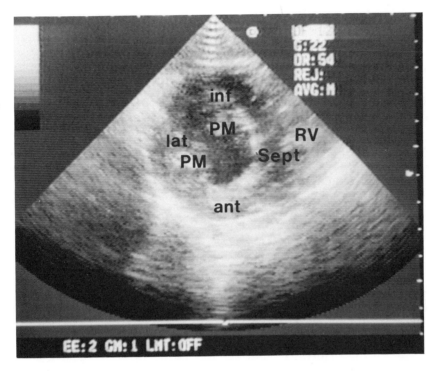

Fig. 28-5. Transesophageal echocardiographic short-axis view of the left ventricle at the level of the papillary muscles. RV = right ventricle; Sept = interventricular septum; Ant = anterior wall of the left ventricle; lat = lateral wall of the left ventricle; inf = inferior/posterior wall of the left ventricle; and PM = papillary muscles.

bypass graft (CABG) surgery. Leung et al.[36] described 40 patients monitored with TEE immediately after induction of anesthesia through 4 hours in the ICU. Of the 40 patients, 20 (50 percent) had SWMA at some point during the study period; *these episodes occurred most frequently after bypass and in the ICU.* The new occurrence of SWMA after bypass was particularly ominous: of 16 such patients, 6 had major complications (cardiac death or MI). Of the 24 patients who did not have SWMA after bypass, none had major complications. This study highlights not only the necessity for continued vigilance in the postoperative period but also the discovery that abnormalities immediately after bypass probably indicate new infarction during the attempted sur-

gical revascularization and a high likelihood of morbidity.

USE OF TEE IN MANAGING PATIENTS UNDERGOING VASCULAR SURGERY

Because atherosclerosis is a systemic disease, patients undergoing vascular surgery often have significant coronary artery disease.[37] Several investigators have used TEE to improve detection of myocardial ischemia during vascular surgery. Half of the patients studied by Smith et al.[29] were undergoing aortic reconstruction. Roizen et al.[38] studied patients who had aortic occlusion (clamping) at various levels during aortic reconstruction. Of patients undergoing occlusion at the supraceliac level, 92 percent had some type of wall motion abnormality (i.e., global hypokinesis or SWMAs), 44 percent had SWMAs, and 8 percent had MIs. Of patients undergoing occlusion at the suprarenal level, 33 percent had global hypokinesis and 17 percent had new SWMAs; no patient had an MI. No patient undergoing occlusion at the infrarenal level had SWMAs or MIs.

Gewertz et al.[39] studied 49 high-risk patients who had 50 major vascular procedures. Twelve patients (24 percent) had SWMAs at baseline, probably representing old areas of infarction. Fourteen patients (28 percent) had new SWMAs during surgery. Of these 14 patients, 10 were treated successfully, as wall motion was normalized; none of these patients had an MI. However, persistent SWMAs were associated with increased morbidity and mortality: of the four patients with persistent SWMA, one patient had intraoperative cardiac arrest and died, and another had a subendocardial MI. In a similar patient population, Ellis et al.[40] demonstrated that TEE detected twice as many instances of intraoperative ischemia as did monitoring of the six limb leads and the V_5 lead of the ECG.

Given this experience with TEE during vascular surgery, we aggressively treat new SWMAs with antianginal agents (nitrates and β-adrenergic receptor-blocking agents) while maintaining filling volumes and pressures at a level low enough to maintain blood pressure and organ perfusion (e.g., urinary output greater than 0.125 ml/kg/h[41]).

Transesophageal echocardiography has been used in research to evaluate anesthetic practice in carotid surgery. Smith et al.[42] examined the echocardiographic effects of two methods of raising blood

pressure at the time of carotid occlusion during halothane-N_2O or isoflurane-N_2O anesthesia. In two groups, blood pressure was increased by administering a "light" general anesthetic (0.46 to 0.49 minimum alveolar concentration [MAC] of volatile anesthetic in 50 percent N_2O). In two other groups, blood pressure was increased 20 percent above the preoperative range by administering 0.9 MAC of volatile anesthetic in 50 percent N_2O and then infusing phenylephrine. No difference existed between the isoflurane and halothane groups regarding myocardial ischemia detected by TEE or electrocardiography. However, the use of phenylephrine was associated with an increased incidence of new SWMAs: new SWMAs occurred in 13 of 29 patients given phenylephrine but in only 5 of 31 patients given "light" anesthesia ($P < 0.05$). Also, systolic wall stress was higher and the rate-corrected velocity of circumferential shortening was lower in patients given phenylephrine. These last two changes are not surprising, given the addition of the effects of the vasoconstrictor phenylephrine to the myocardial depressant effects of the volatile anesthetics.

Based on the results of this study, we avoid the routine use of vasoconstrictors during carotid surgery but, instead, decrease the anesthetic to allow blood pressure to rise. Although inotropes may be more effective than vasoconstrictors in increasing blood pressure and cardiac output without increasing wall stress or the incidence of SWMA, this hypothesis remains to be proved. In our practice, we prefer to allow blood pressure to remain within the preoperative range and to monitor the transesophageal echocardiogram for myocardial ischemia and the electroencephalogram (EEG) for adequacy of cerebral perfusion. As long as the EEG does not indicate ischemia, we may well use vasodilators to reduce afterload and stress on the heart. It is our belief, although unsubstantiated, that by using these two monitors, we can keep blood pressure adequate for cerebral and myocardial perfusion without placing undue strain on the heart. This "ideal blood pressure" is likely to differ for every patient, as blood flow past an obstruction in the cerebral or myocardial circulation may be pressure dependent,[43] and the relative degree of cerebral and coronary stenosis and collateralization may vary among patients.

Transesophageal echocardiography has also been used to evaluate the effects of preoperative normovolemic hemodilution on left ventricular function in patients undergoing aortic reconstruction. Although normovolemic hemodilution allows the clinician to decrease the risk of disease associated with transfusion, concerns have persisted that the decreased oxygen-carrying capacity of the blood might exacerbate the potential for intraoperative myocardial ischemia. Van der Linden et al.[44] studied 15 patients undergoing aortic surgery during normovolemic hemodilution. All patients had ejection fractions greater than 50 percent but demonstrated reperfusion defects (hypoperfused viable myocardium) on preoperative thallium scanning.[45] Before induction of anesthesia, patients were monitored with electrocardiographic lead CM_5, a pulmonary artery catheter, and TEE (the short-axis view of the left ventricle at the mid-papillary muscle level). After induction of anesthesia, blood was withdrawn to produce a hematocrit of 30 percent, and intravascular volume was restored with colloid infusion. No increase in cardiac index occurred after normovolemic hemodilution; pulmonary capillary wedge pressure (PCWP) and left ventricular end-diastolic area (LVEDA) also did not change. Systemic oxygen consumption did not change; mixed venous oxygen content decreased, reflecting a compensatory in-

crease in oxygen extraction. Most important, no new SWMAs occurred, nor was there electrocardiographic evidence of myocardial ischemia. Although this study does not address whether or not normovolemic hemodilution is accompanied by a similar safety during the hemodynamic stresses of surgery, preoperative hemodilution appears to be a safe practice. Using TEE to document myocardial wellbeing is reassuring, given the greater sensitivity of TEE (compared with electrocardiography) in detecting intraoperative myocardial ischemia.[29,40]

MYOCARDIAL CONTRAST ECHOCARDIOGRAPHY

Some investigators have injected ultrasonic contrast agents into the cardiovascular circulation to characterize myocardial blood flow.[46] This technique has been used in the catheterization laboratory[47] and in the operating room[48] to document restoration of coronary blood flow after percutaneous coronary angioplasty and CABG surgery. Contrast echocardiography may allow real-time visualization of regional myocardial blood flow. The microbubbles of air in the contrast agent reflect ultrasound to a greater degree than do tissue or blood, thus creating white images on the echocardiogram. Currently used contrast agents include sonicated meglumine diaztrizoate (Renografin-76), hand-agitated saline, and hydrogen peroxide.[49] The recent introduction of stable, prepared solutions of albumin microbubbles (2 to 8 μm in size) makes available a standard echo contrast agent that does not require acute preparation; this characteristic permits repeated studies. Microbubbles of this size are small enough to mimic red blood cells and to pass unhindered through the microcirculation.[50] Their ability to pass through the pulmonary circulation[51] allows injection of contrast agents from peripheral venous sites, making the technique less invasive. Initial studies have revealed these microbubbles to be free of neurologic or hemodynamic side effects.[52] At present, computer processing is required to document the changes in grey levels resulting from the entry of microbubbles into the myocardium. Currently, the only way to visualize myocardial perfusion in real time is to inject contrast agent into the aortic root or the coronary arteries.[53] Still, the technique holds promise for the intraoperative characterization of myocardial blood flow.

Thus, TEE has a current place in our practice. It more sensitive than electrocardiography in detecting myocardial ischemia. It also helps guide treatment of intraoperative myocardial ischemia, assessment of fluid therapy, and identification of patients according to risk. If perfusion echocardiography becomes a practical reality in that microbubbles can be injected into a peripheral vein, the role of TEE may be enhanced by its direct use to assess myocardial perfusion.

USE OF 2D TEE TO DETECT ABNORMALITIES IN CARDIAC FUNCTION

The use of 2D TEE in assessing cardiac performance is well established.[54,55] Likewise, TEE has been shown to be valuable in assessing cardiac performance both intraoperatively[42,56–59] and in the nonsurgical setting.[60,61]

The advent of 2D TEE has improved the ability to quantify cardiac function. Cardiac volumes and ejection fraction measured by echocardiography correlate with values determined by angiography,[62,63] radionuclide studies,[64] and in vitro measurement.[65] Beaupre et al.[66]

studied the relationship between PCWP and LVEDA determined by TEE. Transesophageal echocardiography was superior to PCWP for measuring preload. In another study of 12 patients with good left ventricular function who were undergoing CABG surgery, the short-axis view of LVEDA was a better predictor of cardiac output (and, hence, a "better index of left ventricular preload").[67]

Others have used radionuclide techniques to show that PCWP is a poor predictor of left ventricular end-diastolic volume after bypass[68,69] and after aortic reconstruction.[70] In the one study, Kalman et al.[70] demonstrated that left ventricular compliance decreased after removal of the aortic cross-clamp. In our experience, filling pressures and LVEDA usually do not increase after reperfusion, perhaps suggesting that Kalman and colleagues were seeing myocardial ischemia. Our practice of using TEE to guide volume therapy before and during temporary aortic occlusion may minimize myocardial stretch and thus reduce the frequency of such changes in compliance after reperfusion. For this reason, after reperfusion we attempt to keep LVEDA at baseline levels; if PCWP increases out of proportion to LVEDA, we consider the possibility of myocardial ischemia. In either case (myocardial ischemia and/or altered compliance), TEE helps to guide aggressive vasodilator therapy.

Cronnelly and co-workers studied altered left ventricular compliance by examining the effects of general anesthetics[71] and volume loading[72] on hemodynamic and TEE variables during renal transplantation surgery. Because patients undergoing renal transplantation depend on intravascular volume for control of blood pressure and often have coronary artery disease, their hemodynamic responses mimic those of vascular patients undergoing stressful stimuli. Cronnelly and colleagues[71,72] found that induction of general anesthesia with isoflurane reduced LVEDA to below awake baseline levels, whereas halothane and enflurane produced no significant changes in ventricular size. Administration of 1 L of lactated Ringer's solution did not change LVEDA but did increase filling pressures, suggesting poor ventricular compliance. We believe this study highlights the importance of avoiding fluid overload in patients undergoing vascular surgery, as the stiff ventricles of hypertensive patients may easily develop diastolic failure that produces pulmonary edema.

Sudden changes in systemic vascular resistance are also detected readily by TEE. Roizen et al.[73] were assisted by TEE in the anesthetic management of patients undergoing surgical resection of pheochromocytoma, a procedure incurring sudden dramatic changes in systemic vascular resistance and contractility. Beaupre et al.[74] observed decreased left ventricular preload and afterload in a patient being monitored with TEE who had an anaphylactic reaction to cefazolin sodium. We frequently see a similar echocardiographic pattern (small, hypercontractile left ventricle and tachycardia) during the mesenteric retraction phase of transabdominal aortic reconstruction. If hemodynamic changes are threatening and do not resolve quickly after the surgeons reduce retraction, some anesthetists (for example, coauthor J. Ellis but not M. Roizen) administer an α-adrenergic agonist, based on the presumption that the heart is empty because of excessive vasodilation caused by release of prostacyclin.[75,76]

Transesophageal echocardiography is also useful in evaluating right ventricular function. Ellis et al.[77] reported right ventricular dilatation following air embolism and thromboembolism in patients undergoing liver transplantation. In this study, right ventricular dilatation affected

left ventricular filling. This pattern of septal encroachment on left ventricular filling caused by pulmonary hypertension and right ventricular failure has been documented with echocardiography in patients with pulmonary emboli[78] and with chronic obstructive pulmonary disease (COPD).[79] Echocardiography has also detected cor pulmonale (pulmonary hypertension and right ventricular hypertrophy and/or enlargement) with twice the sensitivity of clinical methods such as the physical examination, electrocardiography, and chest radiographs.[80] Because cigarette smoking and COPD are common in patients undergoing vascular surgery, we often assess right ventricular function as well with TEE during vascular procedures. In patients with cor pulmonale detected by TEE, we are more likely to place a pulmonary artery catheter for the assessment of biventricular function in the perioperative period; central venous pressure is likely to be a poor predictor of left ventricular filling. If right ventricular failure is sufficient to produce septal shift, PCWP also may rise, despite a small left ventricle; in this case, PCWP would wrongly predict left ventricular distension. Thus, in such patients, TEE can help clarify both left and right ventricular compliances and guide specific therapy. Although right ventricular failure is notoriously difficult to treat,[81] its recognition may be useful in improving patient outcome.

Key in our management of vascular surgery patients is our use of TEE as a guide to ventricular filling. *We are careful not to distend the heart with excessive fluid administration.* Our concern is that an elevated left ventricular end-diastolic pressure will diminish subendocardial perfusion,[82] presumably predisposing the heart to left ventricular ischemia. Whether or not this rationale is correct, our experience leads us to believe that left ventricular distension causes myocardial ischemia. In addition, such hypervolemia may predispose the heart to congestive heart failure when mechanical ventilation is discontinued at the end of surgery.

Lemaire et al.[83] recently highlighted the deleterious effects of hypervolemia in 15 ICU patients with COPD and presumed coronary artery disease. Despite adequate respiratory mechanics, attempts to discontinue mechanical ventilation were not successful in these patients. Radionuclide scans demonstrated acute biventricular dysfunction, while tachycardia, diaphragm fatigue, and elevated serum levels of catecholamines accompanied spontaneous ventilation. After a week of vigorous diuresis, mechanical ventilation, and nutritional support, attempts to discontinue mechanical ventilation were successful in most of these patients.

Some controversy exists about the role of nitrous oxide in exacerbating coronary insufficiency during surgery. Although experimental studies have provided evidence of nitrous oxide-induced regional ischemia,[84] two clinical studies using TEE to evaluate regional wall motion in patients undergoing CABG surgery showed no increase in SWMA after addition of nitrous oxide to a narcotic anesthetic.[85,86] However, both investigations studied only a small number of patients. In the last report, one of the seven patients studied had increases in pulmonary and systemic vascular resistances and global hypokinesis on TEE after exposure to nitrous oxide. Although the ability of nitrous oxide to cause sympathetic stimulation[87] and to elevate systemic[88] and pulmonary vascular[89] resistances is well documented, TEE has not completely resolved the issue of the safety of nitrous oxide in patients with coronary artery disease. One of the authors of this chapter (J. Ellis) avoids the use of nitrous oxide in patients with ischemic heart disease, whereas another coauthor (M. Roizen) uses it routinely.

USE OF 2D TEE TO DETECT STRUCTURAL DEFECTS

Precordial echocardiography is a principal method of assessing structural cardiac defects and, in some instances, supplants angiography.[90] Transesophageal echocardiography has become an important means of detecting cardiac and noncardiac vascular and mass lesions near the esophagus.[91–100] Transesophageal echocardiography is especially useful in diagnosing atrial[8] and valvular abnormalities, including mitral valve prolapse,[7] and has also been used to diagnose and aid in the intraoperative removal of an intercardiac tumor.[101]

Using a transesophageal echocardiographic probe with an integral pulsed Doppler transducer, Schlüter et al.[102] were able to determine blood flow across the mitral valve in patients with mitral insufficiency. Other investigators have employed Doppler TEE to assess the mitral valve[103] and congenital structural cardiac defects in children.

Doppler TEE has also been helpful in calculating cardiac output by integrating the transmitral diastolic velocity profile. This integral, when multiplied by the cross-sectional area of the mitral valve, yields an approximation of stroke volume.[104] Correlation coefficients reported for cardiac output determined in this fashion with thermodilution cardiac output vary from 0.71[105] to 0.95.[106] The ability to quantitate cardiac output potentially extends the efficacy of intraoperative TEE.

The effectiveness of TEE in assessing the repair of congenital cardiac lesions with the resulting changes in shunt flow is presently under investigation, as a pediatric Doppler transesophageal echo probe has recently become available.[103] "Color-flow" Doppler is also now available.[104] Such devices provide rapid Doppler interrogation of the entire two-dimensional echocardiogram and display the direction and velocity of blood flow as color superimposed on the two-dimensional echocardiogram. Some report that "on-heart" color-flow Doppler echocardiography facilitates and alters anesthetic and surgical management of pediatric patients undergoing repair of congenital heart defects.[107] In this method, the transducer is placed directly on the heart during surgery.

When color-flow Doppler is not available, contrast echocardiography may be used to evaluate intracardiac blood flow. Valvular regurgitation may be documented with this technique, using microbubbles as a contrast medium.[108] This technique has been combined with TEE to detect ostium secundum atrial septal defects during surgery.[109] With the use of contrast, TEE has identified patent foramen ovale during posterior fossa craniotomy in the sitting position.[110] Carrying this technique further, Guggiari et al.[111] described the effectiveness of preoperative contrast echocardiography, in conjunction with coughing and Valsalva maneuvers, in identifying patients at risk of paradoxical air embolization during craniotomy in the sitting position. Seven patients were found to have patent foramen ovale, and four patients had echocardiograms that were uninterpretable (because of technical reasons). Therefore, these 11 patients did not undergo neurosurgery in the sitting position. None of the remaining 44 patients undergoing procedures in the sitting position had evidence of paradoxical air embolization.

USE OF TEE TO DETECT UNWANTED INTRAVASCULAR AIR

The precordial Doppler transducer technique has been the principal method of detecting air embolism during surgery.

However, in this application, TEE is at least as sensitive and probably more sensitive.[112–118] Transesophageal echocardiography easily detects air entering the systemic circulation after cardiopulmonary bypass, thereby providing guidance in the elimination of this potential source of organ damage.[119–121] Two-dimensional echocardiograms obtained by placing the transducer directly on the heart in the surgical wound have also been used for detection of cardiac air retained after bypass.[122] However, this technique is inferior to TEE, as monitoring for air during this period requires interruption of surgery.

FUTURE USES OF TEE

Transesophageal echocardiography is an important experimental and clinical tool. What remains to be determined is how widespread its use will be in the near future. Will it complement or supplant pulmonary artery catheterization, and, if so, under what circumstances? The size and contractility of the heart and the nature of regional wall motion are more useful information to the clinician than are filling pressures obtained by pulmonary artery catheter. One advantage of the pulmonary artery catheter is that it provides an easy method of measuring cardiac output, which TEE at present does not. In addition, a pulmonary artery catheter provides pulmonary venous pressures—helpful information in diagnosing and preventing pulmonary venous congestion and pulmonary edema. Finally, the pulmonary artery catheter is easy to continue to use in the postoperative period after tracheal extubation. We now use TEE to assess biventricular function when placement of a central venous pressure or pulmonary artery catheter is being considered during surgery. If both right and left ventricular functions are normal, we believe that a central venous pressure catheter normally suffices for postoperative management.

The issue of the cost-effectiveness of TEE has not been resolved. At present, the echocardiograph and probe cost approximately as much as a standard precordial system. In our experience, the probes can be used about one hundred times without repair. As use of the equipment increases, the cost may decrease. We believe that TEE could eventually be comparable in cost to monitoring techniques widely used at present. As with any monitoring technique, the usefulness of TEE depends on the skill and interpretive ability of the operator. Diversion of attention from the patient and misinterpretation of data that results in erroneous treatment are potential hazards of TEE. As echocardiography is more thoroughly integrated into the undergraduate medical curriculum, its increased use in the operating room will follow naturally. The application of contrast echocardiography to describe coronary, renal, and hepatic perfusion will begin, we believe, in the next 5 years and will grant the anesthetist more power to understand the benefits and risks of therapeutic maneuvers.

REFERENCES

1. Cahalan MK, Litt L, Botvinick EH, Schiller NB: Advances in noninvasive cardiovascular imaging: implications for the anesthesiologist. Anesthesiology 66:356–372, 1987
2. Clements FM, de Bruijn NP: Perioperative evaluation of regional wall motion by transesophageal two-dimensional echocardiography. Anesth Analg 66:249–261, 1987
3. Seward JB, Khandheria BK, Oh JK et al: Transesophageal echocardiography: Technique, anatomic correlations, implementation, and clinical applications. Mayo Clin Proc 63:649–680, 1988
4. Schlüter M, Hanrath P: The clinical application of transesophageal echocardiography. Echocardiography 1:427–442, 1984
5. Visser CA, Koolen JJ, van Wezeel HB, Dunning AJ: Transesophageal echocardiography: technique and clinical applications. J Cardiothorac Anesth 2:74–91, 1988
6. Popp RL, Rubenson DS, Tucker CR, French JW: Echocardiography: M-mode and two-dimensional methods. Ann Intern Med 93:844–856, 1980
7. Zenker G, Erbel R, Krämer G et al: Transesophageal two-dimensional echocardiography in young patients with cerebral ischemic events. Stroke 19:345–348, 1988
8. Gussenhoven EJ, Taams MA, Roelandt JRTC et al: Transesophageal two-dimensional echocardiography: its role in solving clinical problems. J Am Coll Cardiol 8:975–979, 1986
9. Schlüter M, Hinrichs A, Thier W et al: Transesophageal two-dimensional echocardiography: comparison of ultrasonic and anatomic sections. Am J Cardiol 53:1173–1178, 1984
10. Hinrichs A, Schlüter M, Kremer P et al: Zweidimensionale transösophageale Echokardiographie: Vergleich echokardiographischer und anatomischer Schnittbilder [English abstract: 2-Dimensional transesophageal echocardiography: comparison of echocardiographic and anatomic section pictures]. Ultraschall Med 4:243–247, 1983
11. Wohlgelernter D, Jaffe CC, Cabin HS et al: Silent ischemia during coronary occlusion produced by balloon inflation: relation to regional myocardial dysfunction. J Am Coll Cardiol 10:491–498, 1987
12. Visser CA, David GK, Kan G et al: Two-dimensional echocardiography during percutaneous transluminal coronary angioplasty. Am Heart J 111:1035–1041, 1986
13. Labovitz AJ, Lewen MK, Kern M et al: Evaluation of left ventricular systolic and diastolic dysfunction during tran-

sient myocardial ischemia produced by angioplasty. J Am Coll Cardiol 10:748–755, 1987

14. Picano E, Distante A, Masini M et al: Echocardiographic documentation of myocardial ischemia in presence of angina pectoris without ST-T changes. Can J Cardiol, Suppl. A:67A–70A, 1986

15. Serruys PW, Jaski B, Wijns W et al: Early changes in wall motion and wall thickness during percutaneous transluminal coronary angioplasty in man. Can J Cardiol, Suppl. A:221A–232A, 1986

16. Tennant R, Wiggers CJ: Effect of coronary occlusion on myocardial contraction. Am J Physiol 112:351–361, 1935

17. Forrester JS, Wyatt HL, da Luz PL et al: Functional significance of regional ischemic contraction abnormalities. Circulation 54:64–70, 1976

18. Aylward PE, McPherson DD, Kerber RE et al: Ultrasonic tissue characterization in coronary artery disease. p. 509–531. In Kerber RE (ed): Echocardiography in Coronary Artery Disease. Futura Publishing, Mount Kisco, NY, 1988

19. Pandian NG, Kerber RE: Two-dimensional echocardiography in experimental coronary stenosis. I. Sensitivity and specificity in detecting transient myocardial dyskinesis: comparison with sonomicrometers. Circulation 66:597–602, 1982

20. Pandian NG, Kieso RA, Kerber RE: Two-dimensional echocardiography in experimental coronary stenosis. II. Relationship between systolic wall thinning and regional myocardial perfusion in severe coronary stenosis. Circulation 66:603–611, 1982

21. O'Boyle JE, Parisi AF, Nieminen M et al: Quantitative detection of regional left ventricular contraction abnormalities by 2-dimensional echocardiography. Comparison of myocardial thickening and thinning and endocardial motion in a canine model. Am J Cardiol 51:1732–1738, 1983

22. Heng MK, Wyatt HL, Meerbaum S et al: An analysis of the reproducibility of 2-dimensional echocardiographic measurements (abstract). Am J Cardiol 41:390, 1978

23. Sahn DJ, DeMaria A, Kisslo J, Weyman A: Inter-observer variability in the quantitative evaluation of M-mode echocardiograms: survey and recommendations (abstract). Am J Cardiol 41:390, 1978

24. Moynihan PF, Parisi AF, Feldman CL: Quantitative detection of regional left ventricular contraction abnormalities by two-dimensional echocardiography. I. Analysis of methods. Circulation 63:752–760, 1981

25. Parisi AF, Moynihan PF, Folland ED et al: Quantitative detection of regional left ventricular contraction abnormalities by two-dimensional echocardiography. II. Accuracy in coronary artery disease. Circulation 63:761–767, 1981

26. Abel MD, Nishimura RA, Callahan MJ et al: Evaluation of intraoperative transesophageal echocardiography. Anesthesiology 66:64–68, 1987

27. Cahalan MK, Kremer PF, Beaupre PN et al: Intraoperative myocardial ischemia detected by transesophageal 2-dimensional echocardiography (abstract). Anesthesiology 59:A164, 1983

28. Braunwald E, Kloner RA: The stunned myocardium: prolonged, postischemic ventricular dysfunction. Circulation 66:1146–1149, 1982

29. Smith JS, Cahalan MK, Benefiel DJ et al: Intraoperative detection of myocardial ischemia in high-risk patients: electrocardiography versus two-dimensional transesophageal echocardiography. Circulation 72:1015–1021, 1985

30. Shively B, Watters T, Benefiel D et al: The intraoperative detection of myocardial infarction by transesophageal echocardiography (abstract). J Am Coll Cardiol 7:2A, 1986

31. Topol EJ, Weiss JL, Guzman PA et al: Immediate improvement of dysfunctional myocardial segments after coronary revascularization: detection by intraoperative transesophageal echocardiography. J Am Coll Cardiol 4:1123–1134, 1984

32. Horowitz RS, Morganroth J: Immediate detection of early high-risk patients with acute myocardial infarction using two-

dimensional echocardiographic evaluation of left ventricular regional wall motion abnormalities. Am Heart J 103:814–822, 1982

33. Gibson RS, Bishop HL, Stamm RB et al: Value of early two-dimensional echocardiography in patients with acute myocardial infarction. Am J Cardiol 49:1110–1119, 1982

34. Horowitz RS, Morganroth J, Parrotto C et al: Immediate diagnosis of acute myocardial infarction by two-dimensional echocardiography. Circulation 65:323–329, 1982

35. Eaton LW, Weiss JL, Bulkley BH et al: Regional cardiac dilatation after acute myocardial infarction. Recognition by two-dimensional echocardiography. N Engl J Med 300:57–62, 1979

36. Leung J, O'Kelly B, Tubau J et al: Prognostic importance of regional wall motion abnormalities in patients undergoing coronary artery bypass grafting (abstract). Anesthesiology 69:A913, 1988

37. Hertzer NR, Beven EG, Young JR et al: Coronary artery disease in peripheral vascular patients. A classification of 1000 coronary angiograms and results of surgical management. Ann Surg 199:223–233, 1984

38. Roizen MF, Beaupre PN, Alpert RA et al: Monitoring with two-dimensional transesophageal echocardiography. Comparison of myocardial function in patients undergoing supraceliac, suprarenal-infraceliac, or infrarenal aortic occlusion. J Vasc Surg 1:300–305, 1984

39. Gewertz BL, Kremser PC, Zarins CK et al: Transesophageal echocardiographic monitoring of myocardial ischemia during vascular surgery. J Vasc Surg 5:607–613, 1987

40. Ellis JE, Roizen MF, Aronson S et al: Comparison of two automated ST-segment analysis systems, EKG (including T wave inversion analysis), and transesophageal echocardiography for the diagnosis of intraoperative myocardial ischemia (abstract). Anesthesiology 69:A5, 1988

41. Alpert RA, Roizen MF, Hamilton WK et al: Intraoperative urinary output does not predict postoperative renal function in patients undergoing abdominal aortic revascularization. Surgery 95:707–711, 1984

42. Smith JS, Roizen MF, Cahalan MK et al: Does anesthetic technique make a difference? Augmentation of systolic blood pressure during carotid endarterectomy: effects of phenylephrine *versus* light anesthesia and of isoflurane *versus* halothane on the incidence of myocardial ischemia. Anesthesiology 69:846–853, 1988

43. DeBoer LWV, Rude RE, Davis RF et al: Extension of myocardial necrosis into normal epicardium following hypotension during experimental coronary occlusion. Cardiovasc Res 16:423–427, 1982

44. Van der Linden P, Baron JF, Philip I et al: Normovolemic hemodilution in anesthetized patients with coronary artery disease: effects of hemodynamic and LV function (abstract). Anesthesiology 67:A135, 1987

45. Boucher CA, Brewster DC, Darling RC et al: Determination of cardiac risk by dipyridamole-thallium imaging before peripheral vascular surgery. N Engl J Med 312:389–394, 1985

46. Feinstein SB, Ten Cate FJ, Zwehl W et al: Two-dimensional contrast echocardiography. I. In vitro development and quantitative analysis of echo contrast agents. J Am Coll Cardiol 3:14–20, 1984

47. Feinstein SB, Lang RM, Dick C et al: Contrast echocardiographic perfusion studies in humans. Am J Cardiac Imag 1:29–37, 1986

48. Smith JS, Feinstein SB, Kapelanski D et al: Intraoperative determination of myocardial perfusion using contrast echocardiography (abstract). Anesthesiology 65:A27, 1986

49. Kemper AJ, O'Boyle JE, Sharma S et al: Hydrogen peroxide contrast-enhanced two-dimensional echocardiography: real-time in vivo delineation of regional myocardial perfusion. Circulation 68:603–611, 1983

50. Feinstein SB, Shah PM, Bing RJ et al: Microbubble dynamics visualized in the

intact capillary circulation. J Am Coll Cardiol 4:595–600, 1984

51. Keller MW, Feinstein SB, Watson DD: Successful left ventricular opacification following peripheral venous injection of sonicated contrast agent: an experimental evaluation. Am Heart J 114:570–575, 1987

52. Keller MW, Feinstein SB: New developments in contrast echocardiography. p. 443–465. In Kerber RE (ed): Echocardiography in Coronary Artery Disease. Futura Publishing, Mount Kisco, NY, 1988

53. Lang RM, Borow KM, Neumann A et al: Effect of intracoronary injections of sonicated microbubbles on left ventricular contractility. Am J Cardiol 60:166–171, 1987

54. Quinones MA, Gaasch WH, Alexander JK: Influence of acute changes in preload, afterload, contractile state and heart rate on ejection and isovolumic indices of myocardial contractility in man. Circulation 53:293–302, 1976

55. Ruschhaupt DG, Sodt PC, Hutcheon NA, Arcilla RA: Estimation of circumferential fiber shortening velocity by echocardiography. J Am Coll Cardiol 2:77–84, 1983

56. Beaupre PN, Cahalan MK, Kremer PF et al: Isoflurane, halothane, and enflurane depress myocardial contractility in patients undergoing surgery (abstract). Anesthesiology 59:A59, 1983

57. Roizen MF, Alpert RA, Beaupre PN et al: Transesophageal echocardiography: cardiovascular function after various levels of aortic occlusion (abstract). Anesthesiology 59:A163, 1983

58. Matsumoto M, Oka Y, Strom J et al: Application of transesophageal echocardiography to continuous intraoperative monitoring of left ventricular performance. Am J Cardiol 46:95–105, 1980

59. Smith JS, Cahalan MK, Benefiel DJ et al: Fentanyl versus fentanyl and isoflurane in patients with impaired left ventricular function (abstract). Anesthesiology 63:A18, 1985

60. Terai C, Uenishi M, Sugimoto H et al: Transesophageal echocardiographic di-

mensional analysis of four cardiac chambers during positive end-expiratory pressure. Anesthesiology 63:640–646, 1985

61. Clements FM, de Bruijn NP, Kisslo JA: Transesophageal echocardiographic observations in a patient undergoing closed-chest massage. Anesthesiology 64:826–828, 1986

62. Folland ED, Parisi AF, Moynihan PF et al: Assessment of left ventricular ejection fraction and volumes by real-time, two-dimensional echocardiography. A comparison of cineangiographic and radionuclide techniques. Circulation 60:760–766, 1979

63. Schiller NB, Acquatella H, Ports TA et al: Left ventricular volume from paired biplane two-dimensional echocardiography. Circulation 60:547–555, 1979

64. Clements FM, Harpole D, McCann R et al: Transesophageal echocardiography and first pass radionuclide angiography: a comparison of ejection fractions, areas, and volumes (abstract). Society of Cardiovascular Anesthesiologists, New Orleans, April 1988

65. Helak JW, Reichek N: Quantitation of human left ventricular mass and volume by two-dimensional echocardiography. In vitro anatomic validation. Circulation 63:1398–1407, 1981

66. Beaupre PN, Cahalan MK, Kremer PF et al: Does pulmonary artery occlusion pressure adequately reflect left ventricular filling during anesthesia and surgery (abstract)? Anesthesiology 59:A3, 1983

67. Thys DM, Hillel Z, Goldman ME et al: A comparison of hemodynamic indices derived by invasive monitoring and two-dimensional echocardiography. Anesthesiology 67:630–634, 1987

68. Hansen RM, Viquerat CE, Matthay MA et al: Poor correlation between pulmonary arterial wedge pressure and left ventricular end-diastolic volume after coronary artery bypass graft surgery. Anesthesiology 64:764–770, 1986

69. Ellis RJ, Mangano DT, VanDyke DC: Relationship of wedge pressure to end-diastolic volume in patients undergoing myocardial revascularization. J Thorac Cardiovasc Surg 78:605–613, 1979

70. Kalman PG, Wellwood MR, Weisel RD et al: Cardiac dysfunction during abdominal aortic operation: the limitations of pulmonary wedge pressures. J Vasc Surg 3:773–781, 1986

71. Cronnelly R, Kremer PF, Beaupre PN et al: Hemodynamic response to anesthesia in patients with end-stage renal disease (abstract). Anesthesiology 59:A47, 1983

72. Cronnelly R, Kremer PF, Beaupre P et al: Hemodynamic response to fluid challenge in anesthetized patients with end-stage renal disease (abstract). Anesthesiology 59:A49, 1983

73. Roizen MF, Hunt TK, Beaupre PN et al: The effect of alpha-adrenergic blockade on cardiac performance and tissue oxygen delivery during excision of pheochromocytoma. Surgery 94:941–945, 1983

74. Beaupre PN, Roizen MF, Cahalan MK et al: Hemodynamic and two-dimensional transesophageal echocardiographic analysis of an anaphylactic reaction in a human. Anesthesiology 60:482–484, 1984

75. Hudson JC, Wurm WH, O'Donnell TF, Jr et al: Hemodynamics and prostacyclin release in the early phases of aortic surgery: comparison of transabdominal and retroperitoneal approaches. J Vasc Surg 7:190–198, 1988

76. Seltzer JL, Goldberg ME, Larijani GE et al: Prostacyclin mediation of vasodilation following mesenteric traction. Anesthesiology 68:514–518, 1988

77. Ellis JE, Lichtor JL, Chung MR et al: Mechanism of myocardial dysfunction during liver transplantation: the role of isolated left ventricular failure (abstract). Anesthesiology 67:A82, 1987

78. Jardin F, Dubourg O, Guéret P et al: Quantitative two-dimensional echocardiography in massive pulmonary embolism: emphasis on ventricular interdependence and leftward septal displacement. J Am Coll Cardiol 10:1201–1206, 1987

79. Jardin F, Gueret P, Prost J-F et al: Two-dimensional echocardiographic assessment of left ventricular function in chronic obstructive pulmonary disease. Am Rev Respir Dis 129:135–142, 1984

80. Himelman RB, Struve SN, Brown JK et al: Improved recognition of cor pulmonale in patients with severe chronic obstructive pulmonary disease. Am J Med 84:891–898, 1988

81. Burrows FA, Klinck JR, Rabinovitch M, Bohn DJ: Pulmonary hypertension in children: perioperative management. Can Anaesth Soc J 33:606–628, 1986

82. Bache RJ, Vrobel TR, Ring WS et al: Regional myocardial blood flow during exercise in dogs with chronic left ventricular hypertrophy. Circ Res 48:76–87, 1981

83. Lemaire F, Teboul J-L, Cinotti L et al: Acute left ventricular dysfunction during unsuccessful weaning from mechanical ventilation. Anesthesiology 69:171–179, 1988

84. Leone BJ, Philbin DM, Lehot J-J et al: Gradual or abrupt nitrous oxide administration in a canine model of critical coronary stenosis induces regional myocardial dysfunction that is worsened by halothane. Anesth Analg 67:814–822, 1988

85. Cahalan MK, Prakash O, Rulf ENR et al: Addition of nitrous oxide to fentanyl anesthesia does not induce myocardial ischemia in patients with ischemic heart disease. Anesthesiology 67:925–929, 1987

86. Slavik JR, LaMantia KR, Kopriva CJ et al: Does nitrous oxide cause regional wall motion abnormalities in patients with coronary artery disease? An evaluation by two-dimensional transesophageal echocardiography. Anesth Analg 67:695–700, 1988

87. Fukunaga AF, Epstein RM: Sympathetic excitation during nitrous oxide-halothane anesthesia in the cat. Anesthesiology 39:23–36, 1973

88. Wong KC, Martin WE, Hornbein TF et al: The cardiovascular effects of morphine sulfate with oxygen and with nitrous oxide in man. Anesthesiology 38:542–549, 1973

89. Schulte-Sasse U, Hess W, Tarnow J: Pulmonary vascular responses to nitrous oxide in patients with normal and high pulmonary vascular resistance. Anesthesiology 57:9–13, 1982

90. Weyman A: Cross-Sectional Echocardiography. p. 137–491. Lea & Febiger, Philadelphia, 1982

91. Nellessen U, Daniel WG, Lichtlen PR: Bedeutung der transösophagealen Echokardiographie in der Diagnostikkardialer und parakardialer raumfordernder Prozesse [English abstract: Importance of transesophageal echocardiography in the diagnosis of cardiac and paracardiac space-occupying processes]. Z Kardiol 75:91–98, 1986

92. Aschenberg W, Schlüter M, Kremer P et al: Transesophageal two-dimensional echocardiography for the detection of left atrial appendage thrombus. J Am Coll Cardiol 7:163–166, 1986

93. Stern H, Erbel R, Börner N et al: Spontaner Echokontrast, registriert mittels transösophagealer Echokardiographie bei Aortendissektion Typ III (English abstract: Spontaneous echocontrast, recorded by transesophageal echocardiography in type III aortic dissection]. Z Kardiol 74:480–481, 1985

94. Schreiner G, Erbel R, Mohr-Kahaly S et al: Nachweis von Aneurysmen des Vorhofseptums mit Hilfe der transösophagealen Echokardiographie [English abstract: Detection of aneurysms of the atrial septum using transesophageal echocardiography]. Z Kardiol 74:440–444, 1985

95. Nellessen U, Daniel WG, Matheis G et al: Impending paradoxical embolism from atrial thrombus: correct diagnosis by transesophageal echocardiography and prevention by surgery. J Am Coll Cardiol 5:1002–1004, 1985

96. Börner N, Erbel R, Braun B et al: Diagnosis of aortic dissection by transesophageal echocardiography. Am J Cardiol 54:1157–1158, 1984

97. Isaji F: [English abstract: Diagnosis of atrial septal defect (secundum type) with transesophageal echocardiography: special reference to size and type of ASD.] Nippon Kyobu Geka Gakkai Zasshi 32:37–49, 1984

98. Thier W, Schlüter M, Kremer P et al: Transösophageale zweidimensionale Echokardiographie: bessere Darstellung intraatrialer Strukturen [English abstract: Two-dimensional transesophageal echocardiography: a better presentation of intra-atrial structures]. Dtsch Med Wochenschr 108:1903–1907, 1983

99. Schlüter M, Langenstein BA, Thier W et al: Transesophageal two-dimensional echocardiography in the diagnosis of cor triatriatum in the adult. J Am Coll Cardiol 2:1011–1015, 1983

100. Kajita M, Nishiyama M, Tengan I et al: [English abstract: Transesophageal echocardiography for the diagnosis of lung cancer with left atrial involvement.] Kyobu Geka 36:122–126, 1983

101. Topol EJ, Biern RO, Reitz BA: Cardiac papillary fibroelastoma and stroke. Echocardiographic diagnosis and guide to excision. Am J Med 80:129–132, 1986

102. Schlüter M, Langenstein BA, Hanrath P et al: Assessment of transesophageal pulsed Doppler echocardiography in the detection of mitral regurgitation. Circulation 66:784–789, 1982

103. Shively B, Cahalan M, Benefiel D, Schiller N: Intraoperative assessment of mitral valve regurgitation by transesophageal Doppler echocardiography (abstract). J Am Coll Cardiol 7:228A, 1986

104. Feigenbaum H: Echocardiography. 4th Ed. p. 41, 188–204. Lea & Febiger, Philadelphia, 1986

105. Ellis JE, Runyon-Hass A, Lichtor JL et al: Can Doppler ultrasound, targeted by two dimensional transesophageal echocardiography, be used to measure cardiac output (abstract)? Anesthesiology 67:A638, 1987

106. Roewer N, Bednarz F, Dziadzka A, Schulte am Esch J: Intraoperative cardiac output determination from transmitral and pulmonary blood flow measurements using transesophageal pulsed Doppler echocardiography (abstract). Anesthesiology 67:A639, 1987

107. Greeley WJ, Ungerleider RM, Stanley T, Kisslo JA: Intraoperative echocardiography and color flow imaging during pediatric cardiovascular anesthesia and surgery (abstract). Society of Cardiovascular Anesthesiologists, New Orleans, April 1988

108. Goldman ME, Mindich BP: Intraoperative two-dimensional echocardiography: new application of an old technique. J Am Coll Cardiol 7:374–382, 1986

109. Hanrath P, Schlüter M, Langenstein BA et al: Detection of ostium secundum atrial septal defects by transoesophageal cross-sectional echocardiography. Br Heart J 49:350–358, 1983

110. Cucchiara RF, Seward JB, Nishimura RA et al: Identification of patent foramen ovale during sitting position craniotomy by transesophageal echocardiography with positive airway pressure. Anesthesiology 63:107–109, 1985

111. Guggiari M, Lechat PH, Garen C et al: Prevention of paradoxical air embolism by 2-D contrast echocardiography in neurosurgical patients in the seated position (abstract). Anesthesiology 63:A425, 1985

112. Furuya H, Suzuki T, Okumura F et al. Detection of air embolism by transesophageal echocardiography. Anesthesiology 58:124–129, 1983

113. Cucchiara RF, Nugent M, Seward J, Messick JM: Detection of air embolism in upright neurosurgical patients by 2-D transesophageal echocardiography (abstract). Anesthesiology 59:A388, 1983

114. Glenski JA, Cucchiara RF: Transcutaneous O_2 and CO_2 monitoring of neurosurgical patients: detection of air embolism. Anesthesiology 64:546–550, 1986

115. Glenski JA, Cucchiara RF, Michenfelder JD: Transesophageal echocardiography and transcutaneous O_2 and CO_2 monitoring for detection of venous air embolism. Anesthesiology 64:541–545, 1986

116. Roewer N, Beck H, Kochs E et al: Nachweis venöser Embolien wahrend intraoperativer Uberwachung mittels transoesophagealer zweidimensionaler Echokardiographie [English abstract: Detection of venous embolism during intraoperative monitoring by two-dimensional transesophageal echocardiography]. Anasth Intensivther Notfallmed 20:200–205, 1985

117. Furuya H, Okumura F: Detection of paradoxical air embolism by transesophageal echocardiography. Anesthesiology 60:374–377, 1984

118. Cucchiara RF, Nugent M, Seward JB, Messick JM: Air embolism in upright neurosurgical patients: detection and localization by two-dimensional transesophageal echocardiography. Anesthesiology 60:353–355, 1984

119. Oka Y, Inoue T, Hong Y et al: Retained intracardiac air. Transesophageal echocardiography for definition of incidence and monitoring removal by improved techniques. J Thorac Cardiovasc Surg 91:329–338, 1986

120. Oka Y, Moriwaki KM, Hong Y et al: Detection of air emboli in the left heart by M-mode transesophageal echocardiography following cardiopulmonary bypass. Anesthesiology 63:109–113, 1985

121. Topol EJ, Humphrey LS, Borkon AM et al: Value of intraoperative left ventricular microbubbles detected by transesophageal two-dimensional echocardiography in predicting neurologic outcome after cardiac operations. Am J Cardiol 56:773–775, 1985

122. Rodigas PC, Meyer FJ, Haasler GB et al: Intraoperative 2-dimensional echocardiography: ejection of microbubbles from the left ventricle after cardiac surgery. Am J Cardiol 50:1130–1132, 1982

29

Management of Immediate Problems after Abdominal Aortic Surgery

David J. Cullen

Patients undergoing abdominal aortic surgery often have many preexisting problems that require special perioperative management.[1] Many of these patients have hypertension and/or serious coronary, cerebral, or renal vascular disease. Most have a long history of smoking and often have coexisting chronic lung disease, bronchospastic disorders, and the many varieties of lung dysfunction. Renal dysfunction is also common, owing either to concomitant diabetes or to congenital or acquired disease of the renal arteries.

Given this extensive potential for disease, let us consider the technique of prophylactic continuation of mechanical ventilation immediately after surgery, the merits of supportive respiratory care for such patients, and the relationship of this technique to many of the complications that so commonly occur immediately after surgery.

RESIDUAL ANESTHESIA

Narcotics

Narcotics are among the most important and useful drugs in providing intraoperative analgesia for patients undergoing abdominal vascular surgery, particularly those with unstable cardiovascular function. To keep hemodynamic variables relatively stable in patients undergoing abdominal vascular surgery who also have severe coronary disease or poor left ventricular function, one may need to give the same large doses of narcotics one would give patients undergoing cardiac surgery. In patients with good left ventricular function, with or without coronary disease, narcotics may provide more satisfactory analgesia and stability than inhalation anesthesia.[2]

Even though smaller doses of narcotics are needed when such drugs are supplemented with volatile anesthetics, the residual effects of narcotics may result in postoperative somnolence, respiratory depression, and residual analgesia. Fentanyl, supposedly a short-acting narcotic, has, in fact, a long duration of action that contributes to respiratory depression when it is given in large doses or in incremental doses over time[3–7] (Fig. 29-1). Of course, narcotics such as morphine (which has an excretion half-life similar to that of fentanyl) and meperidine will produce residual effects well into the postoperative period. Because of the high

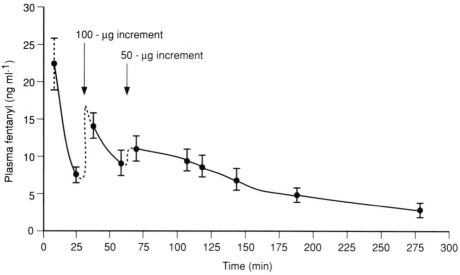

Plasma fentanyl concentrations (means ± SEM) in the 10 patients in group B (increment group).

Fig. 29-1. The rate of fall of mean (± standard error of the mean) concentrations of fentanyl citrate in plasma decreased in 10 patients as incremental doses of fentanyl citrate were administered. (From McQuay et al.,[6] with permission.)

incidence and severity of cardiac disease in patients undergoing abdominal vascular surgery, a rapid, uncontrolled emergence from anesthesia with resulting hypertension and tachycardia can produce devastating complications by itself, let alone if accompanied by hypoxia and/or hypercarbia from inadequate respiratory function. Therefore, many patients would benefit by a slow, smooth emergence from anesthesia, that is, a gradual awakening that allows physiologic functions to stabilize in the presence of adequate oxygenation and ventilation.

At the end of surgery, many clinicians reverse narcotic depression with naloxone, a potent narcotic antagonist. In patients undergoing abdominal surgery, this practice may be particularly risky for several reasons: the short duration of action of naloxone[8]; the possibility of induced nausea and vomiting[9]; the hypertension and tachycardia caused by narcotic antagonism[10]; the possibility of myocardial ischemia[11] and pulmonary

edema[12]; and the difficulty of managing patients who have multiple dressings, tubes, and catheters in place when residual narcotic analgesia is suddenly reversed. I believe that patients who have residual narcotic analgesia after abdominal aortic surgery should not be given naloxone; instead, intubation and mechanical ventilation should continue as the narcotic effect wears off spontaneously and the patient awakens gradually.

Inhalation Anesthetics

Inhalation anesthetics are often the mainstay of anesthesia for abdominal vascular surgery, particularly in patients with good left ventricular function. The use of inhalation anesthetics allows administration of high concentrations of oxygen, rapid onset and termination of effect for easier control of blood pressure during widely varying stimuli, and the ability to provide not just analgesia but complete anesthesia. However, the effects of inhalation anesthesia also persist well into the postoperative period. In addition to depressing the ventilatory response to carbon dioxide,[13,14] inhalation anesthetics severely reduce or obliterate the ventilatory response to hypoxia, even when the alveolar concentration of anesthetic is extremely low[15-18] (Fig. 29-2). Halothane, enflurane, and isoflurane are all potent respiratory depressants that interefere with or abolish the ventilatory re-

sponse to hypoxia in healthy patients. Extrapolating these data to sick, elderly patients undergoing the stress of abdominal vascular surgery, one could predict that their ability to respond to hypoxia would be minimal or nonexistent.

The fastest way to eliminate volatile anesthetics from the body after discontinuing their administration is to continue mechanical ventilation into the postoperative period, thereby maintaining alveolar ventilation and reducing the alveolar partial pressure of anesthetic.[19] Were these patients to breathe spontaneously, they would probably hypoventilate; thus, the rate of excretion of volatile anesthetic would be lower[19] and the likelihood of hypercarbia and hypoxia higher with spontaneous respiration than with mechanical ventilation.

Nondepolarizing Muscle Relaxants

Abdominal aortic surgery usually requires administration of large doses of nondepolarizing muscle relaxants; reversal of the effects of these drugs can be

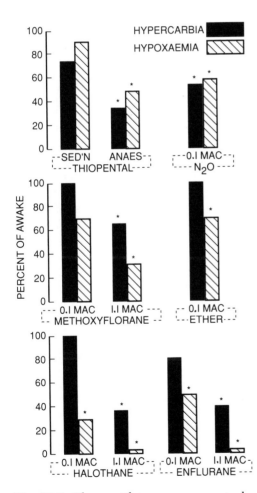

pressed as percentages of values for the awake state. The response to hypercarbia was defined as being the slope of the ventilation-PCO_2 relationship. The response to hypoxemia was defined as being the values for "ΔV_{I45}," i.e., the measured increment in instantaneous ventilation from hyperoxia to an end-tidal carbon dioxide partial pressure of 45 mmHg. Sed'n = sedation; * = significant difference from awake. (From Knill and Clement,[17] with permission [thiopental data from Knill RL, Bright S, Manninen P: Hypoxic ventilatory responses during thiopentone sedation and anaesthesia in man. Can Anaesth Soc J 25:366–372, 1978; enflurane data from Knill RL, Manninen PH, Clement JL: Ventilation and chemoreflexes during enflurane sedation and anaesthesia in man. Can Anaesth Soc J 26:353–360, 1979; halothane data from Knill and Gelb.[16])

Fig. 29-2. The ventilatory responses to hypercarbia and to hypoxemia are profoundly depressed by enflurane and halothane. Heights of bars depict mean responses, ex-

problematic. For one thing, such drugs can cause undesirable side effects: bradycardia, excessive salivation, bronchospasm, and bowel hypermotility (with neostigmine, edrophonium, or pyridostigmine) and tachycardia and dysrhythmias (with atropine or glycopyrrolate).[20] Also, even though large doses of these antagonists are usually needed to accomplish complete reversal, in many instances even large doses do not reverse neuromuscular blockade completely. Finally, neuromuscular blockade is potentiated by volatile anesthetics. In one study, for example, the concentration of enflurane was reduced abruptly. It took approximately 41 minutes for a new steady state of neuromuscular blockade to occur.[21] Thus, expecting complete reversal and motor strength sufficiently vigorous for adequate breathing and coughing and for sustaining oxygenation and ventilation immediately after aortic reconstructive surgery may be unrealistic and may expose the patient to increased risk.

Thus, I believe that residual anesthesia is desirable in the immediate postoperative period and that attempts to awaken and reverse analgesia and neuromuscular blockade rapidly may be hazardous. The patient who undergoes aortic reconstruction may best be served by not eliminating residual anesthesia, which can gradually wear off as other physiologic variables return to normal over the subsequent few hours.

PHYSIOLOGIC INSTABILITY AFTER ABDOMINAL AORTIC SURGERY

The prophylactic use of mechanical ventilation after abdominal aortic surgery must be tailored to the many physiologic abnormalities that occur after this surgi-cal procedure. These physiologic dysfunctions are usually unavoidable, and some are present in all patients recovering from abdominal aortic surgery.

Hypertension

Hypertension occurs in many patients after abdominal vascular surgery. For one thing, most of these patients are hypothermic and therefore undergo peripheral vasoconstriction. Also, if nitrous oxide is given intraoperatively, its concentration in the alveoli is very low by the time the patient enters the postoperative recovery room or intensive care unit.[19] The alveolar concentration of the potent inhalation anesthetics is also low enough to allow hypertension to occur. In addition, many patients can perceive pain even if they cannot consciously demonstrate that perception. Although hormonal sources of hypertension have been investigated, the results are inconclusive. Some suggest that a reflex or renal-mediated release of renin that results from altered renal blood flow occurs during suprarenal and even infrarenal aortic occlusion.[22] Others have not demonstrated such effects, and the basis for postoperative hypertension remains obscure.[23,24]

Hypertension also may occur if too much time has elapsed since the patient took any antihypertensive medications that were being taken preoperatively, even if such medication was taken the morning of surgery.

The dangers of hypertension in the immediate postoperative period concern the increase in pressure at vascular anastomoses, the possibility of intracranial hemorrhage, and, most important, the possible occurrence of myocardial ischemia in these susceptible patients. Often, hypertension is accompanied by tachycardia or at least the absence of reflex bradycardia. Therefore, myocardial oxygen demand is higher because impedance to ejection increases while diastolic filling time decreases. Under these conditions, the addition of inadequate ventilation and/or hypoxia would be devastating, because both hypercarbia and hypoxia can stimulate further hypertension. More important, these conditions can increase myocardial ischemia,[25] the susceptibility to ventricular dysrhythmias, and the likelihood of myocardial infarction.

If patients are not in obvious pain, therapy for postoperative hypertension is fairly straightforward. Rather than deepening anesthesia in the intensive care unit, one tries to reduce vascular resistance. Many approaches have been successful. First, moderately long acting vasodilators such as hydralazine (with or without propranolol) or labetalol (an α- and β-adrenergic receptor-blocking drug) can be administered to patients before discharge from the operating room.[26] If β-adrenergic receptor-blocking drugs are given before surgery, their use should be resumed as hypertension develops, unless the patient is bradycardic. Intravenous propranolol or our current preference, labetalol, beginning with small intravenous doses, will establish some baseline level of antihypertensive effect that can be continued postoperatively.

Alternatively, one can titrate short-acting intravenous drugs such as nitroglycerin, nitroprusside, or trimethaphan to achieve the desire blood pressure. Advantages of this approach include tight control and easy reversibility if and when hypotension develops. Disadvantages include too much reduction in blood pressure, an event that occurs quite commonly in patients whose hypertension is caused by peripheral vasoconstriction, yet who may still be hypovolemic; the possibility that difficulties with the infusion devices, tubing, and delivery system will lead to variable amounts of drug administered; and finally, an antiplatelet

effect of nitroglycerin[27] and sodium nitroprusside[28] (but not labetalol[29] or trimethaphan[30]).

Specifically, labetalol can be administered as an intravenous bolus beginning with 5 mg. The dose is then increased incrementally to 10, 20, and, if necessary, 40 mg after waiting an appropriate length of time to determine the effect of each dose (15 to 30 minutes).

If hypertension is extreme, an infusion of drugs such as nitroglycerin and/or nitroprusside may be necessary to control hypertension until the patient warms and blood volume is redistributed. We usually begin treatment with very small doses of nitroglycerin or nitroprusside, 10 to 15 μg/min, titrating the dose to effect. Blood pressure is optimally kept within some reasonable range of the normal preoperative values for that patient.

Patient responses are extremely variable. Easy control of hypertension may be obtained within 60 seconds of using 5 mg of labetalol. In other instances, however, one may need to give 800 to 1,000 μg/min of both nitroglycerin and nitroprusside plus administration of β-adrenergic receptor-blocking drugs and diuretics. Hypertension is often more severe in patients who were hypertensive preoperatively or who had renal artery stenosis. In an unusual situation, severe rebound hypertension occurs after discontinuation of clonidine.[31] Intravenous administration of α-methyldopa is an effective substitute, although some hours are required before adequate levels are achieved.

Hypothermia

Unless special precautions are taken to maintain normothermia in the operating room, most patients undergoing abdominal vascular surgery will be hypothermic at the end of surgery. Hypothermia is caused by air conditioning in the operating room, the high turnover of room air, the openness of the abdomen and peritoneal surface, and administration of less than completely warmed blood and fluids. Even when all means are taken to prevent hypothermia (e.g., use of blood warmers, keeping room temperatures above 20°C, and use of heated humidifiers in the anesthesia circuit), most patients undergoing abdominal vascular surgery will still experience at least a mild degree of hypothermia.[32] As a consequence, drug metabolism is slowed, emergence is prolonged, and reversal of neuromuscular blockade may be delayed.[33,34] Although blood volume may be abnormally low, hypovolemia does not become apparent until rewarming and vasodilation have occurred. Many patients will undergo peripheral vasoconstriction, with a shift of blood volume to the central vascular compartment and high left and right atrial filling pressures. Rapid warming is not necessarily appropriate, as it may lead to shivering, increased oxygen consumption and carbon dioxide production,[35] and precipitous decreases in blood pressure. Allowing hypothermia to continue is also not desirable. Slow warming of the patient with surface-warming devices and residual drug effects to reduce shivering produces a slow increase in oxygen consumption and carbon dioxide production while physiologic variables continue to approach normal values.

Hypotension and Hypovolemia

Hypotension rarely occurs immediately after surgery unless the patient is actively losing blood. In most cases, hypotension occurs after rewarming and vasodilation have revealed the presence of hypovolemia. Most commonly, these patients were not given sufficient intra-operative volume replacement because blood pressure and filling pressures were adequate as surgery concluded. Often, the chest roentgenogram taken immediately after surgery (Fig. 29-3) shows unusually clear lung fields and small, transparent pulmonary vessels. These conditions are not normal after major abdominal vascular surgery involving large shifts in blood and fluids, use of intra-abdominal retractors, blood transfusion, and so forth. Therefore, a clear chest film indicates relative hypovolemia that usually manifests as hypotension when the patient warms. Thus, to prevent the decrease in blood pressure that so commonly occurs, one should anticipate the need to replace intravascular volume as hypertension recedes.

Hypokalemia

After abdominal vascular surgery, patients are often hypokalemic. First, many of these patients have been chronically depleted of potassium by preoperative diuretic therapy. Then, in the operating room, massive transfusion may result in more uptake of potassium by red blood cells than can be provided by the high potassium content of the transfused packed cells. Furthermore, mannitol and/or "loop diuretics" (i.e., those acting primarily in the loop of Henle) are often used prophylactically before temporary aortic occlusion, to maintain urinary output; such treatments further deplete serum potassium. In the presence of a varying physiologic state on emergence from anesthesia (which includes patient warming and shifting of intravascular fluid from central to peripheral vasculature), hypokalemia is more likely to induce ventricular irritability than it would under normal conditions. We therefore believe that one should treat hypokalemia occurring at this time. Hypokalemia

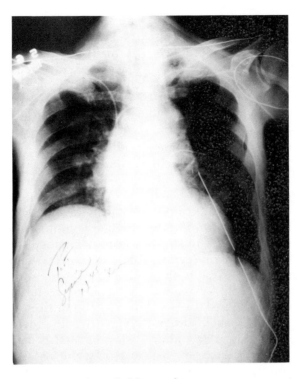

Fig. 29-3. The exceedingly clear lung fields on chest roentgenogram immediately after resection of an aortic aneurysm, an 18-hour procedure requiring massive transfusion, are inappropriate and suggest hypovolemia. In this instance, hypovolemia was apparent clinically as well. The immediate postoperative chest roentgenogram is also useful in determining proper placement of the pulmonary artery catheter, central venous pressure catheter, endotracheal tube, and chest tube. A gastrostomy tube would not be visible on the roentgenogram.

is particularly worrisome in patients who are chronically taking digitalis: when hypokalemia exists, digitalis toxicity may occur at levels of digoxin usually normal for the patient. We attempt to keep serum potassium levels above 3.5 mEq/L by carefully infusing concentrated solutions of potassium chloride through central venous catheters. Some physicians may question the wisdom of this policy in light of the documented hazards of intravenous potassium therapy.

Oliguria

Oliguria is a symptom of hypoperfusion of the kidney, which, if severe, can lead to renal dysfunction. Thus, after abdominal vascular surgery, the cause of oliguria must be sought immediately.

Many patients arrive at the operating room already at risk of renal dysfunction because of dehydration from chronic use of diuretic drugs, poor nutrition prior to surgery, and angiographic dye studies. In the last instance, dye not only promotes further diuresis in potentially dehydrated patients but also has renal tubular toxicity of its own.[36] Also, preexisting renal dysfunction caused by renal artery stenosis (congenital or acquired) or diabetic nephropathy is common in patients undergoing abdominal vascular surgery. After all oral intake has been restricted for 8 hours, these patients are brought to the operating room, where invasive monitoring is instituted, usually before anesthesia begins. Institution of monitoring may further increase stress and reduce renal blood flow and urinary output. This potential hypovolemia is one reason we hydrate the patient intravenously as soon as oral intake is restricted. Induction of anesthesia is often accompanied by hypotension caused by contracted volume status and myocardial depression; such hypotension also decreases renal blood flow. Surgical stimulus increases catecholamine levels, which may in turn reduce renal blood flow even more. If the patient is taking nonsteroidal anti-inflammatory drugs for other medical problems, renal risk is even greater.[37,38] That is, the normal oscillation of renal vascular tone—vasoconstriction followed by vasodilation—is ablated by such drugs through their inhibition of prostaglandin synthetase, an action that prevents synthesis of prostaglandin E_2. Therefore, patients taking nonsteroidal anti-inflammatory drugs should be considered at extremely high risk of renal dysfunction, and all measures should be intensified to protect renal blood flow.

Intraoperatively, the kidney is severely stressed because hypotension is unavoidable at times, for example, during bowel traction, sudden blood loss, or the institution of deeper anesthesia than anticipated. Infrarenal aortic cross-clamping changes blood flow and its distribution within the kidney.[39–41] Because suprarenal aortic cross-clamping abolishes renal blood flow altogether, clamp time should be minimal. To avoid prolonged renal ischemia during especially difficult surgical procedures on the aorta and renal artery, one may need to employ specific techniques for renal preservation. The human kidney can tolerate approximately 30 to 60 minutes of complete ischemia before irreversible renal dysfunction occurs.[42,43] To avoid intrarenal blood clotting, communication between surgeon and anesthetist must ensure that heparin is administered before aortic occlusion.

Finally, atheromatous emboli can be released inadvertently when an aortic cross-clamp is applied, thereby distributing atheromatous debris throughout the kidney; widespread distribution of such material can lead to irreversible renal failure.[44]

Many clinicians give mannitol and/or loop diuretics prior to aortic cross-clamping to provide solute for excretion, the rationale being that intrinsic renal vasoconstriction is minimized when renal blood flow is maintained and solute excretion is high. However, if patients are primed with volume administration prior to temporary aortic occlusion, no benefit seems to result from this practice of giving diuretic drugs to prevent renal failure.[45]

Several studies have compared the effects of various forms of anesthesia on renal blood flow. One hypothesis was that sympathectomy from epidural anesthesia preserved renal blood flow to a greater degree than did general anesthesia, in which sympathetic tone is somewhat preserved.[40,46] Because this hypothesis was not confirmed, no advantage appears to exist in selecting epidural over general anesthesia for this purpose.[46]

Hypotension often occurs immediately after aortic blood flow is restored and further stresses the kidney already at significant risk of ischemic damage. Thus, with the many causes of renal dysfunction apparent in the context of abdominal aortic surgery, postoperative oliguria must be taken extremely seriously. I believe that preventive measures to improve renal blood flow are paramount to the outcome of renal function. Almost always, hypovolemia is at least a major, if not the only, cause of postoperative oliguria and is easily treated with intravascular volume therapy. Continued cardiovascular monitoring is exceedingly important when oliguria occurs, as the cause of oliguria can usually be determined with proper hemodynamic monitoring. In the absence of pulmonary vascular measurements, a low central venous pressure soon after surgery almost always indicates hypovolemia. If a pulmonary artery catheter is in place, low values for pulmonary capillary wedge pressure, cardiac output, and stroke volume—together with high or normal values for peripheral vascular resistance—are extremely useful data for alerting the clinician to the need for intravascular volume therapy for oliguria. Once volume loading has been accomplished and filling pressures are as high as appropriate (usually 12 to 15 mmHg for patients who previously had normal filling pressures), and once stroke volume has improved with volume therapy, continuing oliguria should be treated with low doses of dopamine, which has both renal vasodilating and natriuretic properties.[47]

Oliguria relates to the prophylactic continuation of mechanical ventilation because preservation of renal function is of far greater importance than discontinuing the patient from mechanical ventilation and extubating the trachea. Maintaining adequate renal perfusion may require giving intravascular volume therapy to the point of even decreasing respiratory function to some extent.[48] For this reason, mechanical ventilation should be maintained until renal function is stable. The small adverse effect of positive-pressure ventilation, with or without positive end-expiratory pressure (PEEP), on renal function[49–51] can be eliminated easily by infusion of fluids and/or administration of low doses of dopamine.[52,53] Once again, maintenance of normal homeostasis of oxygenation and ventilation while other organ system functions are being addressed is crucial, I believe, to optimal care after abdominal aortic surgery.

SPECIFIC REASONS FOR PROPHYLACTIC POSTOPERATIVE CONTINUATION OF MECHANICAL VENTILATION

Although no data demonstrate a beneficial effect of prophylactic continuation of mechanical ventilation after abdominal aortic surgery,[54] it seems reasonable to assume that many of these patients would not be ready for tracheal extubation in the operating room, that is, they would not be able to provide their own ventilation and oxygenation immediately after surgery. For such patients, postoperative ventilation should continue until recovery from anesthesia, muscle relaxation, and hypothermia have been demonstrated and until analgesia is sufficient without the accompaniment of excessive respiratory depression. On the other hand, early removal of the endotracheal tube may lessen analgesic requirements and reduce the need for vasoactive substances. Patients should not have significant abdominal distension from peritoneal and bowel edema or have intraperitoneal or retroperitoneal hemorrhage. Because these patients have been given heparin intraoperatively, some surgeons wish to reverse its effects with protamine at the end of the procedure; others prefer to keep the blood in a slight state of anticoagulation. The use of heparin and other practices and conditions increase the potential for clotting abnormalities. Such practices and conditions include massive transfusion, to which many of these patients may be subjected; previous hypotension, which may cause vascular stasis; and the leeching out of platelets on prosthetic grafts.

Monitoring of a distal pulse may be very important because loss of a pulse distal to the vascular anastomosis sometimes indicates the need for angiography and/ or vascular reexploration. Good communication between surgeon and anesthetist or intensivist is essential so that the patient is not weaned from mechanical ventilation and the trachea extubated only to find that he or she must be prepared for return to the operating room.

Gastrointestinal function does not return to normal immediately after surgery, and the presence of a nasogastric tube can be quite irritating. Many surgeons place a gastrostomy tube for gravity drainage intraoperatively. This practice reduces the incidence of postoperative nausea and vomiting. The nasogastric tube can be removed before patients experience discomfort from prolonged nasogastric intubation. Bloody diarrhea soon after surgery may indicate colon ischemia in the distribution of the inferior mesenteric artery, an extremely serious problem.[55,56]

WEANING FROM MECHANICAL VENTILATION

When all of the above considerations have been carefully scrutinized and the patient is apparently stable in all nonrespiratory systems, weaning from mechanical ventilation[57,58] and tracheal extubation usually proceed quite rapidly. Often, enough time has elapsed that reversal of neuromuscular blocking drugs given in the operating room is no longer necessary. However, if neuromuscular blockade has been allowed to diminish spontaneously, the time course is unpredictable, and reversal with drugs should be considered. In a study of 10 patients undergoing major abdominal surgery whose muscle relaxants were allowed to diminish spontaneously, "recovery" was defined as being 70 percent recovery of the train-of-four response.

With this definition, recovery of neuromuscular function required at least 2 hours and as much as 10 hours.[59] No factor correlated with the length of time between the last dose of muscle relaxant and 70 percent recovery of the train-of-four response. Thus, the clinician should be guided by the clinical signs of neuromuscular recovery (head lift, hand grasping, tongue protrusion, eye opening, vital capacity, and inspiratory force), as well as by monitoring of the train-of-four response. Slowing the rate of mechanical ventilation by using intermittent mandatory ventilation has been well tolerated by most patients and eases the task of the nursing staff.[60,61] Using this technique, the patient increases minute ventilation incrementally until gas exchange is acceptable with no ventilatory support. Under the circumstances of a large abdominal incision and known decreases in functional residual capacity (FRC) as a result of anesthesia[62] and surgery in the supine position, we routinely use low levels of PEEP (approximately 5 cm of water) during ventilation and weaning to continuous positive airway pressure (CPAP).

After patients have demonstrated satisfactory oxygenation, stability of $PaCO_2$ and pH, and adequate mechanics of ventilation by simple tests (vital capacity of 10 to 15 ml/kg and inspiratory force of at least -25 cm of H_2O), most patients can be transferred to CPAP quickly and the trachea can be extubated.[58,63] Some advocates of intermittent mandatory ventilation believe that a patient's ability to keep arterial pH at or above 7.35 is a better predictor of success in weaning from mechanical ventilation than the traditional criteria regarding inspiratory force and vital capacity.[64] No advantages result from instituting a trial period on a T-piece without PEEP, because mean airway pressures decrease and more alveolar collapse may occur if patients breathe through an endotracheal tube without

PEEP than if they breathe spontaneously after tracheal extubation.[65,66] We individualize the process of weaning from ventilation and extubating the trachea based on the rate at which a patient awakens, the rate the patient maintains or develops the mechanics of ventilation, and the status of the other nonrespiratory factors discussed earlier. As the mechanical ventilatory rate decreases, cardiovascular and renal effects of positive-pressure ventilation also become less pronounced.[67] If venous return improves, cardiac output and blood pressure are usually more stable; theoretically, renal blood flow will increase slightly as well. Except in the rare patient with severe chronic pulmonary disease, weaning from mechanical ventilation and tracheal extubation are easily accomplished as long as cardiovascular variables are stable.

MASSIVE INTRA-ABDOMINAL HEMORRHAGE

On rare occasion, massive intra-abdominal bleeding and/or massive intraperitoneal and bowel edema occur to such an extent that diaphragmatic motion and respiration become severely compromised. As intra-abdominal tension increases, the diaphragm cannot descend to facilitate normal lung excursion, and spontaneous breathing becomes more difficult.

I assess intra-abdominal pressure crudely and simply by measuring the height of a water column with a nasogastric or gastrostomy tube or bladder catheter. Using this method, I have found massive increases in intra-abdominal pressure (i.e., from 40 to 80 cm of water, normal being zero or less) after abdominal aortic surgery. The widespread effects of this increased intra-

abdominal pressure necessitate extreme support.[68–70]

For example, several conditions associated with high intra-abdominal pressure can cause renal dysfunction: hypotension and inadequate cardiac output and stroke volume; compression of the renal cortex by the surrounding intra-abdominal pressure; and high renal venous pressure that narrows the renal perfusion pressure gradient.[71] Relief of massively increased intra-abdominal pressure may reverse oliguria and renal dysfunction.[72]

Increased intra-abdominal pressure greatly compromises respiratory function and necessitates the use of positive-pressure ventilation with increasing amounts of PEEP to preserve FRC and gas exchange. Even with increased PEEP, at extremely high levels of intra-abdominal pressure, the lungs become difficult to ventilate.[69,70] Compliance and gas exchange deteriorate rapidly, and the inability to ventilate satisfactorily may become life-threatening.

Cardiovascular function is also severely compromised as intra-abdominal pressure rises. The heart is compressed between the lungs (which are being ventilated with high peak airway pressures and with PEEP) and the diaphragm (which is being pushed cephalad, thus preventing the heart from expanding caudad). High left and right atrial filling pressures are accompanied by low stroke volume and usually tachycardia. Radioisotopic imaging of myocardial function in such situations (i.e., gated pool scans) demonstrate that the heart is not failing but behaving as if in tamponade: ventricular volumes are small or normal in the presence of very high filling pressures, and left ventricular ejection fraction is usually high.[69] Supportive therapy is necessary to keep the patient alive until the patient's situation either improves or a decision is made to return the patient to the operating room. In the operating room, the patient would undergo abdominal decompression to enable ventilation, circulation, and renal function to return. Such patients have often been given massive transfusion in an attempt to maintain systemic blood pressure and cardiac output. These patients usually have a coagulopathy and will undoubtedly need more blood products and intravascular volume expansion during surgery for abdominal decompression; thus, intraoperative management can be extremely complex and hazardous. However, decompression may be lifesaving in the patient with declining gas exchange and high intra-abdominal pressure.

SUMMARY

Patients undergoing abdominal aortic reconstructive surgery are subject to many preoperative, intraoperative, and postoperative problems. In many instances, prophylactic continuation of mechanical ventilation provides oxygenation and ventilation until other organ systems stabilize, at which time weaning from mechanical ventilation and tracheal extubation can usually be undertaken quickly, efficiently, and safely.

REFERENCES

1. Young AE, Sandberg GW, Couch NP: The reduction of mortality of abdominal aortic aneurysm resection. Am J Surg 134:585–590, 1977
2. Benefiel DJ, Roizen MF, Lampe GH et al: Morbidity after aortic surgery with sufentanil vs isoflurane anesthesia (abstract). Anesthesiology 65:A516, 1986
3. Becker LD, Paulson BA, Miller RD et al: Biphasic respiratory depression after fentanyl-droperidol or fentanyl alone used to supplement nitrous oxide anesthesia. Anesthesiology 44:291–296, 1976
4. Bentley JB, Borel JD, Nenad RE, Jr., Gillespie TJ: Age and fentanyl pharmacokinetics. Anesth Analg 61:968–971, 1982
5. Harper MH, Hickey RF, Cromwell TH, Linwood S: The magnitude and duration of respiratory depression produced by fentanyl and fentanyl plus droperidol in man. J Pharmacol Exp Ther 199:464–468, 1976
6. McQuay HJ, Moore RA, Paterson GMC, Adams AP: Plasma fentanyl concentrations and clinical observations during and after operation. Br J Anaesth 51:543–550, 1979
7. Stoeckel H, Schüttler J, Magnussen H, Hengstmann JH: Plasma fentanyl concentrations and the occurrence of respiratory depression in volunteers. Br J Anaesth 54:1087–1095, 1982
8. Ngai SH, Berkowitz BA, Yang JC et al: Pharmacokinetics of naloxone in rats and in man: basis for its potency and short duration of action. Anesthesiology 44:398–401, 1976
9. Longnecker DE, Grazis PA, Eggers GWN, Jr: Naloxone for antagonism of morphine-induced respiratory depression. Anesth Analg 52:447–453, 1973
10. Tanaka GY: Hypertensive reaction to naloxone (letter to editor). JAMA 228:25–26, 1974
11. Patschke D, Eberlein HJ, Hess W et al: Antagonism of morphine with naloxone in dogs: cardiovascular effects with special reference to the coronary circulation. Br J Anaesth 49:525–533, 1977
12. Flacke JW, Flacke WE, Williams GD: Acute pulmonary edema following naloxone reversal of high-dose morphine anesthesia. Anesthesiology 47:376–378, 1977
13. Munson ES, Larson CP, Jr., Babad AA et al: The effects of halothane, fluroxene and cyclopropane on ventilation: a comparative study in man. Anesthesiology 27:716–728, 1966
14. Fourcade HE, Stevens WC, Larson CP, Jr et al: The ventilatory effects of Forane, a new inhaled anesthetic. Anesthesiology 35:26–31, 1971

15. Gelb AW, Knill RL: Subanaesthetic halothane: its effect on regulation of ventilation and relevance to the recovery room. Can Anaesth Soc J 25:488–494, 1978

16. Knill RL, Gelb AW: Ventilatory responses to hypoxia and hypercapnia during halothane sedation and anesthesia in man. Anesthesiology 49:244–251, 1978

17. Knill RL, Clement JL: Variable effects of anaesthetics on the ventilatory response to hypoxaemia in man. Can Anaesth Soc J 29:93–99, 1982

18. Knill RL, Kieraszewicz HT, Dodgson BG, Clement JL: Chemical regulation of ventilation during isoflurane sedation and anaesthesia in humans. Can Anaesth Soc J 30:607–614, 1983

19. Stoelting RK, Eger EI, II: The effects of ventilation and anesthetic solubility on recovery from anesthesia: an *in vivo* and analog analysis before and after equilibration. Anesthesiology 30:290–296, 1969

20. Flacke WE, Flacke JW: Cholinergic and anticholinergic agents. p. 169–170. In Smith NT, Corbascio AN (eds): Drug Interactions in Anesthesia. 2nd Ed. Lea and Febiger, Philadelphia, 1986

21. Gencarelli PJ, Miller RD, Eger EI II, Newfield P: Decreasing enflurane concentrations in *d*-tubocurarine neuromuscular blockade. Anesthesiology 56:192–194, 1982

22. Gal TJ, Cooperman LH, Berkowitz HD: Plasma renin activity in patients undergoing surgery of the abdominal aorta. Ann Surg 179:65–69, 1974

23. Grant RP, Jenkins LC: Modification by preoperative beta-blockade of the renin response to infrarenal aortic cross-clamping. Can Anaesth Soc J 30:480–486, 1983

24. Grindlinger GA, Vegas AM, Williams GH et al: Independence of renin production and hypertension in abdominal aortic aneurysmectomy. Am J Surg 141:472–477, 1981

25. Powers ER, Powell WJ, Jr: Effect of arterial hypoxia on myocardial oxygen consumption. Circ Res 33:749–756, 1973

26. Koch G: Haemodynamic effects of combined α- and β-adrenoceptor blockade after intravenous labetalol in hypertensive patients at rest and during exercise.

Br J Clin Pharmacol, 3: suppl. 3, 725–728, 1976

27. Lichtenthal PR, Rossi EC, Louis G et al: Bleeding time and platelet aggregation following nitroglycerin (abstract). Anesthesiology 55:A17, 1981

28. Saxon A: Inhibition of platelet function by nitroprusside (letter to editor). N Engl J Med 295:281–282, 1976

29. Hines R, Barash PG: Labetalol: vasodilation without platelet dysfunction (abstract). Anesthesiology 65:A35, 1986

30. Hines R, Barash PG: Trimethaphan: does it alter platelet function? (abstract). Anesthesiology 65:A573, 1986

31. Brodsky JB, Bravo JJ: Acute postoperative clonidine withdrawal syndrome. Anesthesiology 44:519–520, 1976

32. Vaughan MS, Vaughan RW, Cork RC: Postoperative hypothermia in adults: relationship of age, anesthesia, and shivering to rewarming. Anesth Analg 60:746–751, 1981

33. Ham J, Miller RD, Benet LZ, et al: Pharmacokinetics and pharmacodynamics of *d*-tubocurarine during hypothermia in the cat. Anesthesiology 49:324–329, 1978

34. Miller RD, Agoston S, van der Pol F et al: Hypothermia and the pharmacokinetics and pharmacodynamics of pancuronium in the cat. J Pharmacol Exp Ther 207:532–538, 1978

35. Rodriguez JL, Weissman C, Damask MC et al: Physiologic requirements during rewarming: suppression of the shivering response. Crit Care Med 11:490–497, 1983

36. Coggins CH, Fang LS-T: Acute renal failure associated with antibiotics, anesthetic agents, and radiographic contrast agents. p. 283. In Brenner BM, Lazarus JM (eds): Acute Renal Failure. WB Saunders, Philadelphia, 1983

37. Fox DA, Jick H: Nonsteroidal anti-inflammatory drugs and renal disease. JAMA 251:1299–1300, 1984

38. Terragno NA, Terragno DA, McGiff JC: Contribution of prostaglandins to the renal circulation in conscious, anesthetized, and laparotomized dogs. Circ Res 40:590–595, 1977

39. Abbott WM, Austen WG: The reversal of renal cortical ischemia during aortic oc-

clusion by mannitol. J Surg Res 16:482–489, 1974

40. Gamulin Z, Forster A, Morel D et al: Effects of infrarenal aortic cross-clamping on renal hemodynamics in humans. Anesthesiology 61:394–399, 1984

41. Gelman S, Patel K, Bishop SP et al: Renal and splanchnic circulation during infrarenal aortic cross-clamping. Arch Surg 119:1394–1399, 1984

42. Arendshorst WJ, Finn WF, Gottschalk CW: Pathogenesis of acute renal failure following temporary renal ischemia in the rat. Circ Res 37:558–568, 1975

43. Donohoe JF, Venkatachalam MA, Bernard DB, Levinsky NG: Tubular leakage and obstruction after renal ischemia: structural-functional correlations. Kidney Int 13:208–222, 1978

44. Thurlbeck WM, Castleman B: Atheromatous emboli to the kidneys after aortic surgery. N Engl J Med 257:442–447, 1957

45. Alpert RA, Roizen MF, Hamilton WK et al: Intraoperative urinary output does not predict postoperative renal function in patients undergoing abdominal aortic revascularization. Surgery 95:707–711, 1984

46. Gamulin Z, Forster A, Simonet F et al: Absence of protective renal effects of epidural anesthesia in patients undergoing aortic abdominal surgery (abstract). Anesthesiology 61:A185, 1984

47. Hilberman M, Maseda J, Stinson EB et al: The diuretic properties of dopamine in patients after open-heart operation. Anesthesiology 61:489–494, 1984

48. Cullen DJ: Acute renal failure: pathophysiology and prevention. pp. 2229–2251. In Miller RD (ed): Anesthesia. Vol. 3. 2nd Ed. Churchill Livingstone, New York, 1986

49. Priebe H-J, Heimann JC, Hedley-Whyte J: Mechanisms of renal dysfunction during positive end-expiratory pressure ventilation. J Appl Physiol 50:643–649, 1981

50. Priebe H-J, Hedley-Whyte J: Respiratory support and renal function. Int Anesthesiol Clin 22:203–226, 1984

51. Venus B, Mathru M, Smith RA et al: Renal function during application of positive end-expiratory pressure in swine: effects of hydration. Anesthesiology 62:765–769, 1985

52. Qvist J, Pontoppidan H, Wilson RS et al: Hemodynamic responses to mechanical ventilation with PEEP: the effect of hypervolemia. Anesthesiology 42:45–55, 1975

53. Hemmer M, Suter PM: Treatment of cardiac and renal effects of PEEP with dopamine in patients with acute respiratory failure. Anesthesiology 50:399–403, 1979

54. Shackford SR, Virgilio RW, Peters RM: Early extubation versus prophylactic ventilation in the high risk patient: a comparison of postoperative management in the prevention of respiratory complications. Anesth Analg 60:76–80, 1981

55. Johnson WC, Nabseth DC: Visceral infarction following aortic surgery. Ann Surg 180:312–318, 1974

56. Ottinger LW, Darling RC, Nathan MJ, Linton RR: Left colon ischemia complicating aorto-iliac reconstruction. Causes, diagnosis, management, and prevention. Arch Surg 105:841–846, 1972

57. Pontoppidan H, Laver MB, Geffin B: Acute respiratory failure in the surgical patient. Adv Surg 4:163–254, 1970

58. Schmidt GB: Prophylaxis of pulmonary complications following abdominal surgery, including atelectasis, ARDS, and pulmonary embolism. Surg Annu 9:29–73, 1977

59. Brand JB, Cullen DJ, Wilson NE, Ali HH: Spontaneous recovery from nondepolarizing neuromuscular blockade: correlation between clinical and evoked responses. Anesth Analg 56:55–58, 1977

60. Downs JB, Douglas ME: Intermittent mandatory ventilation: why the controversy (editorial)? Crit Care Med 9:622–623, 1981

61. Downs JB, Klein EF, Jr., Desautels D et al: Intermittent mandatory ventilation: a new approach to weaning patients from mechanical ventilators. Chest 64:331–335, 1973

62. Hedenstierna G, Strandberg Å, Brismar B et al: Functional residual capacity, thoracoabdominal dimensions, and central blood volume during general anesthesia with muscle paralysis and mechanical ventilation. Anesthesiology 62:247–254, 1985

63. Browne AGR, Pontoppidan H, Chiang H et al: Physiological criteria for weaning patients from prolonged artificial ventilation. Abstracts of Scientific Papers. p. 69. Annual Meeting of the American Society of Anesthesiologists, 1972

64. Millbern SM, Downs JB, Jumper LC, Modell JH: Evaluation of criteria for discontinuing mechanical ventilatory support. Arch Surg 113:1441–1443, 1978

65. Annest SJ, Gottlieb M, Paloski WH et al: Detrimental effects of removing end-expiratory pressure prior to endotracheal extubation. Ann Surg 191:539–545, 1980

66. Khan FA, Mukherji R, Chitkara R et al: Positive airway pressure in patients receiving intermittent mandatory ventilation at zero rate. The role of weaning in chronic obstructive pulmonary disease. Chest 84:436–438, 1983

67. Steinhoff H, Falke K, Schwarzoff W: Enhanced renal function associated with intermittent mandatory ventilation in acute respiratory failure. Intensive Care Med 8:69–74, 1982

68. Kashtan J, Green JF, Parsons EQ, Holcroft JW: Hemodynamic effects of increased abdominal pressure. J Surg Res 30:249–255, 1981

69. Coyle JP, Cullen DJ, Teplick R et al: Cardiovascular, pulmonary, and renal effects of massively increased intra-abdominal pressure in critically ill patients. Crit Care Med 17:118–121, 1989

70. Richardson JD, Trinkle JK: Hemodynamic and respiratory alterations with increased intra-abdominal pressure. J Surg Res 20:401–404, 1976

71. Richards WO, Scovill W, Shin B, Reed W: Acute renal failure associated with increased intra-abdominal pressure. Ann Surg 197:183–187, 1983

72. Smith JH, Merrell RC, Raffin TA: Reversal of postoperative anuria by decompressive celiotomy. Arch Intern Med 145:553–554, 1985

30

Blood Transfusion Therapy for Vascular Surgery

Michael F. O'Connor
Steven Roth
Michael F. Roizen

Stored, packed red blood cells (pRBCs) are used routinely instead of whole blood for patients requiring transfusion during vascular surgery. This chapter examines the evidence documenting the safety and relative effectiveness of this practice, and of the commonly used techniques for avoiding transfusion of homologous blood, during vascular surgery.

Blood was the first human tissue to be transplanted, and its components remain the most frequently transplanted human tissue today.[1] Scientific understanding of the mechanisms of blood rejection (transfusion reaction) has made blood by far the safest human tissue to transplant and constitutes the foundation of modern transplant immunology. Over the past 20 years, the patterns of therapy with blood products have changed—and continue to change. Several developments are responsible: the ability to separate blood into its various components, the rising cost of these components, and the grow-ing awareness of the infectious complications of transfusion therapy.

The modern practice is to use specific components to correct specific clinical defects—pRBCs for anemia, platelets for thrombocytopenia, cryoprecipitate for factor VIII defects, and fresh frozen plasma (FFP) for generalized depletion of clotting factors. All of these products are used with variable frequency in vascular surgery. Furthermore, several techniques devised to avoid transfusion of homologous blood are commonly used in vascular surgery: autologous predeposit of blood, acute preoperative hemodilution, and intraoperative salvage of blood from the surgical field (autotransfusion).

Several issues deserve careful consideration by anesthetists. Do any medical or economic conditions still remain that warrant therapy with whole blood for vascular surgery? What blood products other than red blood cells are vascular surgery patients likely to need? What are the risks and benefits of each of the various methods of avoiding transfusion of homologous blood?

Acute massive hemorrhage is still considered by many to be an indication for therapy with whole blood.[2–6] A wide variety of guidelines and justifications have been offered. Miller and Brzica[2] give whole blood when blood loss exceeds 1,500 ml/70 kg of body weight. Sheldon et al.[3] transfuse fresh whole blood when blood loss exceeds 10 units/70 kg in 12 hours, aiming both to provide immediately functioning components and to avoid complications from lactic acidosis, hyperkalemia, citrate intoxication, and dilutional thrombocytopenia. Isbister[4] recommends the use of fresh whole blood in patients who lose more than 50 percent of their blood volume in a controlled setting and the use of ultrafresh (less than 4 hours old) whole blood in patients who lose more than 100 percent of their blood volume in 4 hours or less. Schmidt[5] argues that all patients given more than four units of blood should be transfused with whole blood to provide adequate platelets and coagulation factors, to minimize exposure to hepatitis (because of multiple donors), and to minimize the cost of blood products to the patient. Counts et al.[6] recommend that patients who require both red cells and volume replacement be transfused with whole blood or modified whole blood to maintain adequate hemostasis; however, they give no guidelines about when this should be done. None of these investigators describes a well-controlled clinical trial supporting their recommendations, leaving the wary reader in a quandry.

For the purpose of our discussion, "moderate blood loss" is defined as being loss of 50 to 100 percent of blood volume (5 to 10 units in the average 70-kg adult) in less than 24 hours; "massive hemorrhage" describes blood loss greater than this. Patients undergoing vascular surgery often undergo moderate hemorrhage and, occasionally, massive hemorrhage.

SAFETY OF PACKED RED BLOOD CELLS IN MODERATE HEMORRHAGE

The safety and effectiveness of using small quantities of pRBCs instead of whole blood was documented in a large, prospective study by Robertson and Polk in 1975.[7] A total of 294 patients whose blood was being cross-matched for elective surgery were randomly assigned to receive either whole blood or pRBCs. Eighty-one patients were given an average of 1.3 units of blood. No difference occurred between patients given pRBCs and those given whole blood with respect to morbidity, mortality, amount of blood lost, or length of hospital stay.

Patterns of blood product utilization have changed dramatically since Robertson and Polk performed their study, presumably because of the increased cost of blood products and the growing awareness of the possible infectious complications. For example, the amounts of blood given to patients by Robertson and Polk were very small (average, 1.3 units). Only 2 of 81 patients who were transfused received more than three units of blood. The Transfusion Transmitted Viruses Study, a more recent (1981) study of transfusion practices at four major urban medical centers, reported that the average recipient of blood transfusions received 3.7 units.[8] As another example of changing patterns in blood therapy, the ratio of cross-matched units of blood to transfused units of blood was high (6:1) in the 1975 study, compared with the current ratio of approximately 2:1. Thus, although Robertson and Polk documented the safety and efficacy of transfusing small quantities of pRBCs instead of whole blood, changes in transfusion practices limit the application of their conclusions to current practices.

In what we judge to be the most thorough comparison of pRBCs and whole blood to date, Shackford et al.[9] documented the safety and effectiveness of using pRBCs instead of whole blood for moderate blood loss. They randomly allocated 28 patients undergoing aortic reconstruction to receive either whole blood or pRBCs reconstituted with lactated Ringer's solution. Additional fluids were infused during surgery and for 3 days after surgery to keep pulmonary capillary wedge pressure (PCWP) within 2 mmHg of its preoperative value. No statistically significant differences existed between groups regarding the amount of blood transfused (average, 6.5 units), morbidity, mortality, or coagulation profiles. Although colloid osmotic pressure was significantly lower in patients given pRBCs reconstituted with lactated Ringer's solution, intrapulmonary shunt did not differ significantly between groups.

It is interesting that the average amount of blood lost by these patients exceeded the criteria set by three studies advocating therapy with whole blood (Miller and Brzica,[2] Isbister,[4] and Schmidt[5]). None of the patients in this study had any of the complications commonly associated with massive transfusion (thrombocytopenia, bleeding diathesis, disseminated intravascular coagulation, or pulmonary edema).

POTENTIAL BENEFIT OF PROVIDING THE PLATELETS, CLOTTING FACTORS, AND COLLOID PRESENT IN WHOLE BLOOD

Platelets

Arguments for using whole blood instead of pRBCs include (1) provision of platelets to avoid dilutional and functional thrombocytopenia; (2) provision of clotting factors, particularly factors V and VIII, to avoid factor deficiencies; and (3) provision of colloid to avoid hypovolemia and the pulmonary edema associated with massive electrolyte infusion. Are moderately or massively hemorrhaging patients at risk of any of these complications? Would they benefit from the availability of these products in whole blood?

Thrombocytopenia (platelet count of less than 150,000 cells/mm^3) is probably the most common consequence of massive transfusion.[6,10,11] Patients with thrombocytopenia may have a bleeding diathesis. Petechiae, ecchymoses, and hematuria occur, as does oozing of blood from venipuncture sites and cut surfaces. Serum fibrinogen levels are usually normal. Thrombocytopenia from massive transfusion has two components: a decrease in the absolute number of platelets and a decrease in the function (thrombocytopathy) and viability of remaining platelets. All of these conditions contribute to the coagulation abnormalities associated with massive transfusion.

Miller et al.[10] correlated the risk of coagulopathy with decreasing platelet counts in Vietnam War casualties. Patients with platelet counts less than 65,000 cells/mm^3 were at increased risk of hemorrhagic diathesis. Other investigators have reported similar observations (Figs. 30-1 and 30-2).[6,11] These observations are remarkably different from those for patients with chronic thrombocytopenia, who may maintain adequate hemostasis with platelet counts as low as 10,000 cells/mm^3.

Clinical studies have documented abnormal platelet function in massively bleeding patients. Lim et al.[12] associated bleeding diathesis in massively transfused patients with abnormal platelet function (as measured by adenosine diphosphate- and epinephrine-stimulated aggregation), not absolute platelet count.

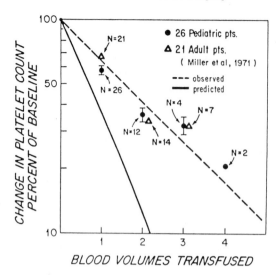

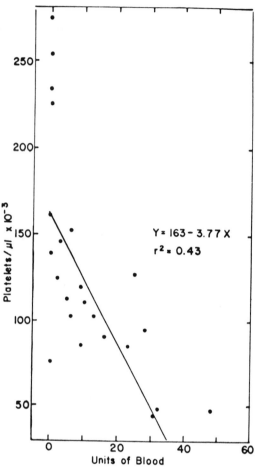

Fig. 30-1. This figure compares the changes in platelet concentration during massive blood transfusion in pediatric patients (Coté et al.[11]) and adult Vietnam War trauma victims (Miller et al.[10]). The broken line represents the observed changes; the solid line, the expected changes. If one assumes in the adult study that 10 units (5 L) of whole blood is equivalent to one blood volume and then plots the percentage change from baseline, the values for adults agree closely with those for pediatric patients. Thus, changes in platelet concentration during blood transfusion are similar in pediatric and adult patients when all data are correlated with estimated *blood volumes transfused.* Assuming a 70-kg vascular patient begins with a platelet count of 200,000/mm³ and that bleeding from thrombocytopenia does not occur until fewer than 75,000 platelets/mm³ are available, these data would lead one to expect a need for platelets until after the 20th unit of pRCBs has been given. (Reprinted from Coté et al.,[11] with permission.)

Clearly, most patients undergoing major vascular surgery will not experience hemorrhage of this magnitude. Nevertheless, a significant number will. When should they be transfused with platelets? Could such transfusion be avoided or minimized by using fresh whole blood?

Platelets, no matter how prepared or

Fig. 30-2. Platelet count is plotted against the number of units of blood transfused to the patient before blood sampling. No platelet transfusions had been given to any of the patients represented in this graph. Again, assuming normal coagulation in the vascular patient until platelet count is 75,000/mm³, these data would lead one to believe that this would occur at approximately 16 units of transfusion in the vascular patient. (Reprinted from Counts et al.,[6] with permission.)

stored, rapidly lose viability and function. Platelets stored at 4°C quickly lose their viability, whereas platelets stored at 22°C quickly lose their function.[13–17] The platelets in stored whole blood or stored pRBCs are best viewed as clinically functionless. To maximize the clinical benefit derived from them, one must store platelets at room temperature for no longer than 5 days.

Platelet transfusion is the common remedy for thrombocytopenia caused by massive transfusion. Despite the diminished function and viability of stored platelets, several reports describe resolution of intraoperative bleeding diathesis after transfusion of platelets.[6,10,11] In these reports, patients who had an intraoperative bleeding diathesis were given platelets, and the efficacy of the transfusion was evaluated by subjective observers. Although these were not well-controlled, double-blinded prospective studies, their observations are probably valid, as each patient acted as his or her own control. Miller and Brzica[2] recommend transfusing platelets to keep the platelet count higher than 75,000 cells/mm^3 in surgical patients. This action usually becomes necessary after a patient has been given 15 to 20 units of whole blood.[2] Penner[18] advocates keeping the platelet count above 100,000 cells/mm^3 in surgical patients. Tomasulo[19] transfuses platelets only when patients have a bleeding diathesis. Although this more conservative approach avoids unnecessary transfusion of platelets, coagulopathy must become clinically apparent before the patient even begins to receive therapy for platelet deficiencies.

Drawbacks to this strategy include intraoperative delay in obtaining platelets, delay in arrest of bleeding, and increased requirement for blood transfusions before effective hemostasis is restored. Nevertheless, we believe this conservative approach may be a good guideline for patients undergoing vascular surgery, because only a few massively hemorrhaging patients have a bleeding diathesis, and because platelet transfusions in themselves incur some risk for the patient.

Platelet transfusions have long-term side effects that argue for conservative transfusion regimens. Platelet transfusions are not routinely cross-matched or HLA (human leukocyte group A)-matched. Thus, most platelet transfusions are HLA-mismatched. Transfusion of uncross-matched, HLA-mismatched platelets may result in inoculation and sensitization of patients to other blood groups and HLA antigens.[20] More than 70 percent of medical patients given multiple platelet transfusions over an extended period (up to 7 months) do not benefit from further platelet transfusion.[21] Platelet antigen systems mediating these immune phenomena are poorly understood.[22] Similar studies have not been conducted in surgical patients but might reveal the existence of a similar phenomenon.

Post-transfusion purpura, an acute autoimmune thrombocytopenia, is now a well-recognized complication of transfusion.[22] Furthermore, female patients of childbearing age (or younger) may be exposed to Rh(D) and HLA antigens through platelet transfusions, predisposing their children to hemolytic disease of the newborn and neonatal alloimmune thrombocytopenic purpura.[20,22] Although this is not likely to be a consideration in the vast majority of patients undergoing vascular surgery, some vascular patients (for example, female patients who have fibromuscular dysplasia) do fall into this category. Platelet transfusion carries the risk of infection from viruses such as non-A, non-B hepatitis (now called hepatitis C); hepatitis B virus (HBV); and human immunodeficiency virus (HIV), specifically, human T-lymphotropic virus type III (HTLV-III), as well as the risk of infection from as yet unrecognized infectious agents. Clearly, sensitive tests of platelet count and function would be very useful in guiding platelet therapy.

Template bleeding time and thromboelastography provide clinical information about the adequacy of platelet count and function that absolute platelet count alone does not provide. Template bleeding time, which involves lancing an arm or leg and actually measuring bleeding time, is not commonly used (although it has been) for intraoperative assessment of platelet status.[6,11] Surprisingly, Miller et al.[10] and Counts et al.[6] found bleeding time to be a poor predictor of coagulation abnormalities in massively transfused patients.

Thromboelastography has been reported to provide a sensitive measure of platelet count and function and requires only 2 ml of freshly drawn blood.[23,24] It therefore may prove to be a useful adjunct to the platelet count in determining the cause of difficult-to-control surgical bleeding.[23] Kang et al.[25] described liver transplantation procedures during which hemotherapy was guided by thromboelastography. Substantially more platelets and cryoprecipitate and less fluids and fresh frozen plasma were given to these patients than to historical controls. Unfortunately, no prospective studies have documented the use of thromboelastography in liver transplantation or its application in other settings involving moderate or massive hemorrhage. Guidelines for its application in vascular surgery and assessment of its cost-effectiveness or benefit-risk ratio are therefore difficult to assess or discuss at present. Obviously, vascular surgery patients rarely bleed as much as liver transplant recipients. Furthermore, vascular patients almost always have normal liver function and therefore have fewer derangements in hemostasis than do liver transplant recipients. It is therefore unlikely that thromboelastography would be cost-effective at institutions not also using this technology for guiding hemotherapy during liver transplantation.

There are substantial differences between stored blood and fresh whole blood in the availability of functioning platelets. Because platelets stored in pRBCs or whole blood at 4°C quickly lose their viability, both should be considered platelet-poor blood products capable of contributing to thrombocytopenia in massively transfused patients.[13] Platelets in fresh whole blood retain their function and viability; therefore, using fresh whole blood may significantly decrease the risk of dilutional thrombocytopenia and thrombocytopathy in patients given massive transfusions. Vascular surgery patients at risk of massive hemorrhage and dilutional thrombocytopenia would clearly benefit from receiving fresh whole blood, if available.

Clotting Factors

Concern about provision of clotting factors with whole blood has focused on factors V and VIII.[2] However, depletion of factors V and VIII has been difficult to document as a cause of altered hemostasis in massive transfusion. Miller et al.[10] found that although factors V and VIII were depleted in the stored blood they administered, depletion of these factors was not associated with clinically significant bleeding. Counts et al.[6] found a weak correlation between depletion of factor VIII (to levels as low as 30 percent of normal) and clinically significant bleeding, possibly contradicting Miller's conclusions about the level of factor VIII necessary for hemostasis (Figs. 30-3 to 30-4).

Some of the difference between the two studies may be attributable to the fact that Miller and co-workers studied trauma patients in Vietnam, whereas Counts and colleagues studied patients admitted to a trauma unit in Seattle, Washington. Furthermore, Counts and colleagues used "modified whole blood," which had 85 percent of platelets and 60 percent of factor VIII removed at the time of preparation.[6] Nevertheless, fresh whole blood contains more factor VIII

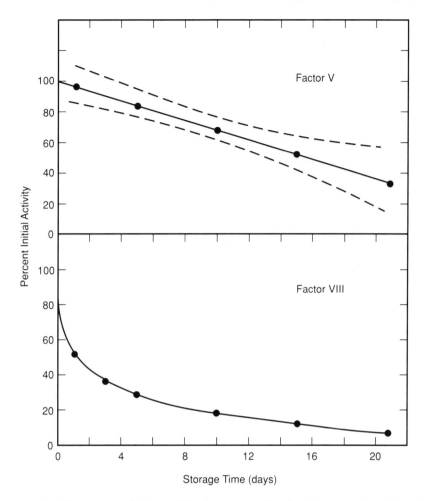

Fig. 30-3. Levels of factors V and VIII in blood anticoagulated with citrate phosphate dextrose and stored at 4°C. Least-squares regression lines for factor V were calculated from assays of 10 units of blood from normal, random donors. The 95 percent confidence limits are given for factor V. For factor VIII, the initial half-time was 24 hours. (Reprinted from Counts et al.,[6] with permission.)

than stored whole blood; and both, because they contain more plasma, contain more factor VIII than pRBCs or modified whole blood.

We conclude that little evidence supports the idea that correcting apparent factor V and factor VIII deficits is of benefit to massively transfused patients. Also, no evidence indicates that the increased factors available in whole blood are of clinical benefit to patients given transfusions. Clearly, patients undergoing sur-

gical bleeding almost never have deficiencies in clotting factors and therefore almost never require transfusion of blood products to replete those factors.

Colloid versus Crystalloid

The presence or absence of colloid in transfused blood may be important in the development of pulmonary edema and the aggravation of adult respiratory dis-

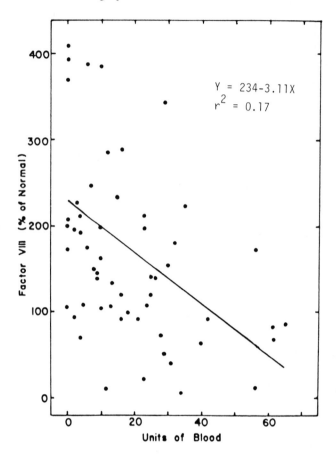

Fig. 30-4. Factor VIII levels are plotted against the number of units transfused prior to blood sampling. The regression was statistically significant: F = 11.68; 1.56 df; P = 0.001. Thus, adequate amounts of this factor for clotting should be present in the vast majority of vascular patients until well over 20 units of stored pRBCs have been administered. However, the wide variation in factor levels means that no absolute rules can be made. (Reprinted from Counts et al.,[6] with permission.)

tress syndrome (ARDS); hence, the difference between whole blood and pRBCs may be quite substantial in this regard. The basis for this concern is application of the Starling equation to the clinical setting. The Starling equation predicts that infusion of large quantities of crystalloid will lower colloid osmotic pressure (COP) substantially, allowing a high-pressure pulmonary edema to occur at low PCWP. Lowering COP may also aggravate any preexisting ARDS or pulmonary capillary leakage. Therefore, because of this effect, patients given large

quantities of crystalloid are hypothesized to be at increased risk of pulmonary edema from any cause. As a high percentage of vascular surgery patients have concomitant heart disease and congestive heart failure, this issue is especially important to them. Surprisingly, studies in animals have yielded conflicting evidence regarding the reality of this hypothesized effect.[26–29] The clinical evidence for this effect in humans is scant, and the literature is filled with conflicting reports.

Numerous case reports associate pul-

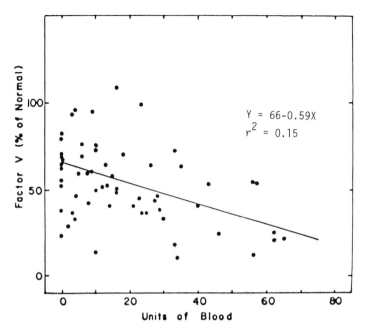

Fig. 30-5.   Factor V levels are plotted against the number of units of blood transfused prior to blood sampling. The regression was statistically significant: $F = 14.92$; 1.58 df; $P = 0.001$. Please note that although the correlation was statistically significant, there was significant scatter in the data. (Reprinted from Counts et al.,[6] with permission.)

monary edema with infusion of large quantities of crystalloid.[30,31] In addition, three clinical studies comparing crystalloid with colloid found either some advantage to the use of colloid or some disadvantage to the use of crystalloid (Table 30-1).[32–34] Skillman et al.[32] randomly assigned 16 patients undergoing aortic surgery to receive either lactated Ringer's solution or 5 percent albumin in saline during surgery as a supplement to whole blood. Patients given colloid had significantly higher intravascular volume, less pulmonary shunt, less weight gain, and higher COP than patients given crystalloid. In the second study, Boutros et al.[34] randomly assigned 24 patients recovering from major aortic surgery to receive 2.5 percent albumin, 0.45 normal saline, or lactated Ringer's solution in the first 48 hours of recovery. Fluids were infused until PCWP reached its preoperative levels. Intrapulmonary shunt increased in

patients given lactated Ringer's solution but not in patients given normal saline or albumin. In the third study, Jelenko et al.[33] randomly assigned 19 burn patients to receive lactated Ringer's solution, hypertonic saline, or hypertonic saline with 1.25 percent albumin during resuscitation. Fluids were infused to keep mean arterial blood pressure from 60 to 110 mmHg and urine output above 30 to 50 ml/h. Several benefits accrued to patients given hypertonic colloid: they were resuscitated more quickly, required less fluid for resuscitation, had a lower incidence of ARDS, required shorter periods of mechanical ventilation, and gained less weight than patients given either of the other two fluid regimens.

Generalization of these three study results is limited by several factors. The number of patients assigned to each treatment group (five to eight) was small compared with other studies in the literature.

Table 30-1. Pulmonary Edema: Summary of Studies Comparing Crystalloid and Colloid Transfusions

| | | Transfusion | | |
| | | Lactated Ringer's Solution | Albumin-Containing Solution | |
Study	Patients[a] (n)	(L)	(L)	Outcome[b]
Skillman et al.[32]	16	4.2 ± 0.6	2.5 ± 0.3	+ Colloid
Jelenko et al.[33]	19	23.5 ± 6	7 ± 3	+ Colloid
Boutros et al.[34]	24	6.2	7.4	+ Colloid
Virgilio et al.[35]	29	11.3 ± 0.8	6.2 ± 0.4	No difference
Shires et al.[38]	18	8.4 ± 0.2	4.8 ± 0.3	No difference
Lowe et al.[36]	141	5.4 ± 3.4	5.9 ± 3.1	No difference
Metildi et al.[37]	46	12.5 ± 11.3	9.4 ± 3.0	No difference
Goodwin et al.[39]	50	13.1	8.5	+ Crystalloid

[a] Total number of patients in the study.
[b] "Outcome" refers to the possible development of pulmonary edema or possible aggravation of adult respiratory distress syndrome. + Colloid = an advantage accrued to the transfusion of colloid (albumin-containing solution); + crystalloid = an advantage accrued to the transfusion of crystalloid (lactated Ringer's solution).

Also, the studies by Skillman and co-workers[32] and Boutros and colleagues[34] are not pure comparisons of crystalloid with colloid. For example, both groups in Skillman's study received whole blood during surgery and colloid after surgery. Similarly, all patients studied by Boutros and co-workers received whole blood intraoperatively. Skillman et al. do not describe the specific guidelines they used for fluid therapy, a shortcoming that introduces the possibility of systematic bias in their study. Because Jelenko et al.[33] used small quantities of colloid in hypertonic saline, their results are difficult to compare with other study results in the literature. Finally, although these three studies associate increased intrapulmonary shunt with infusion of crystalloid, none documents an associated difference in morbidity or mortality.

In contrast, four other clinical studies have shown no difference between colloid and crystalloid (Table 30-1). Virgilio et al.[35] randomly assigned 29 patients undergoing major aortic operations to receive either lactated Ringer's solution or 5 percent albumin in lactated Ringer's solution intraoperatively and during a 3-day recovery period. Fluids were infused to keep PCWP and cardiac output at preoperative levels and to produce a urine output of at least 50 ml/h. Although fluid requirements were higher and COP substantially lower in patients given lactated Ringer's solution, no differences seemed to exist between the two groups with respect to intrapulmonary shunt or outcome.

In a study by Lowe et al.,[36] 141 patients undergoing laparotomy for trauma were randomly assigned to receive either lactated Ringer's solution or 4 percent albumin in lactated Ringer's solution during both initial resuscitation and surgery. Fluids were infused to normalize heart rate and blood pressure and to keep urine output above 50 ml/h. No significant differences in outcome, incidence of pulmonary failure, or postoperative pulmonary function occurred between the two groups.

Metildi et al.[37] randomly assigned 46 patients admitted to a surgical intensive care unit with signs of pulmonary edema (intrapulmonary shunt exceeding 20 percent) to receive either crystalloid or colloid fluids during the first 2 days of treatment. Fluids were administered to maintain adequate PCWP and cardiac output, as judged by arterial pH, base deficit, and mixed venous oxygenation. Although, after 48 hours, intrapulmonary shunt was higher with crystalloid, no difference in COP or outcome existed between the two groups.

In the fourth study, Shires et al.[38] randomly assigned 18 patients undergoing aortic operations to receive either lactated Ringer's solution or Plasmanate (human plasma protein fraction) during surgery and for 18 hours after surgery. Fluids were infused to keep cardiac output and PCWP at preoperative levels and to produce a urine output of more than 30 ml/h. Patients given crystalloid had increased fluid requirements and decreased COP; however, the two groups did not differ in intrapulmonary shunt or outcome.

The studies finding no benefit to colloid administration are larger and less flawed than the three studies more favorable to use of colloids. The study by Virgilio and co-workers[35] fails to describe guidelines for blood transfusion but is otherwise well designed. Generalization of the conclusions of Lowe and co-workers[36] are limited by several factors. Because these investigators do not describe a specific endpoint for resuscitation prior to operation, systematic differences may have existed between the two groups. Furthermore, a significant number of patients did not receive large quantities of fluid, as reflected in both the average amount of fluid transfused (approximately 5 L) and the average amount of blood transfused (1.5 units). The comparison of crystalloid with colloid in patients with pulmonary edema by Metildi and co-workers[37] is probably the boldest clinical trial to date. Its principal weakness is poorly specified guidelines

for fluid therapy. The study by Shires and colleagues[38] confirmed the results of Virgilio and co-workers.[35] Taken together, these studies suggest that the use of crystalloid rather than colloid does not increase intrapulmonary shunt (except in patients who already have pulmonary edema), morbidity, or mortality.

One last study reported an advantage to using crystalloid. Goodwin et al.[39] randomly assigned 50 burn patients to receive either lactated Ringer's solution or 2.5 percent albumin in lactated Ringer's solution during initial resuscitation. Fluids were administered to stabilize vital signs and to produce a urine output of 30 to 50 ml/h. Patients given crystalloid required more fluid and had longer times before normalization of cardiac output. Surprisingly, patients given colloid had significantly more lung water (on postburn days 2 through 7). The weakness in the design of this study is the same as that for previously described studies on trauma or burn patients—the therapeutic endpoints of resuscitation are poorly specified.

The weight of the evidence in these studies suggests that no difference exists between crystalloid and colloid in the setting of moderate hemorrhage. The larger, well-designed studies of Virgilio and co-workers[35] and Shires and colleagues[38] offer the most convincing evidence supporting this conclusion. However, in the absence of clinical studies comparing crystalloid with colloid for massive hemorrhage, the extrapolation of this conclusion to vascular surgery patients, if it is to be done at all, requires careful consideration. Although vascular surgery patients may benefit from the colloid available in whole blood, information about when such a benefit would begin, or how important it is, is not available at this time. Large volumes of crystalloid have been used safely in prospective studies involving moderate hemorrhage in the setting of vascular surgery.

ACUTE COMPLICATIONS OF MASSIVE TRANSFUSION

The most frequent acute complications of massive transfusion are hypervolemia and hypovolemia, transfusion reactions, citrate intoxication, hypothermia, and microaggregate-induced ARDS. Some of these are of documented clinical importance, whereas others have been elusive or impossible to document as clinically important. Does the use of pRBCs instead of whole blood alter the risk or severity of these complications in vascular surgery?

Massive hemorrhage increases the risk of the kinds of clerical errors that cause most transfusion reactions today.[40,41] No precautions beyond the usual should be necessary to avoid this complication. Because transfusion reaction is mediated by antigens on the red blood cell membrane, and because pRBCs and whole blood contain the same amount of red blood cells, no difference probably exists between the two with respect to risk or severity of transfusion reactions. Any measure that reduces a patient's exposure to blood originating from the blood bank (such as intraoperative scavenging and reinfusion of autologous blood) would clearly reduce the risk of transfusion reaction.

Citrate toxicity (depletion of serum ionized calcium) has been difficult to implicate as a complication of massive transfusion. Rapid infusion of citrate may produce sequestration of serum calcium, resulting in decreased myocardial contractility, low cardiac output, and hypotension.[2] In their review of the literature, Miller and Brzica[2] concluded that citrate toxicity is rare and probably occurs only in functionally anhepatic patients or at very high rates of blood infusion (above 150 ml/70/kg/min). Others have reached similar conclusions.[42–44] The clinical im-

portance of citrate toxicity in liver transplant recipients was documented by Borland et al.,[45] who used very rapid (10-minute) determination of serum ionized calcium to guide calcium replacement in pediatric liver transplant recipients. These patients required multiple doses of calcium chloride (15 mg/kg) to maintain adequate levels of serum ionized calcium.[45] Because vascular surgery patients usually have normal liver function and rarely experience hemorrhage of this magnitude, citrate toxicity and hypocalcemia almost never occur in vascular surgery if blood flow to the liver has not been interrupted. (Chapter 10 discusses the problem of citrate intoxication when mesenteric blood flow is interrupted.)

Hypothermia (body temperature of less than 30°C) in the surgical patient may increase ventricular irritability and predispose the patient to cardiac arrest.[46] A major potential cause of hypothermia in the surgical patient, especially one who is massively transfused, is infusion of unwarmed (4°C) blood.[46] This complication can be avoided by using commercially available blood warmers and should therefore be a rare problem in vascular surgery patients requiring transfusion.[46] Warmed blood has the added advantage of being able to be infused more quickly. The hypothermia associated with major operations is probably aggravated by infusion of room temperature crystalloid solutions (which have 40 percent of the cooling capacity of blood at 4°C) and can be prevented by warming the crystalloids. Because all fluids infused intraoperatively can be warmed, pRBCs and whole blood should not differ in their propensity to cause hypothermia. Thus, unintentional hypothermia can be almost totally avoided during vascular surgery.

Massive transfusion has been associated with ARDS since the Vietnam War. The explanation for this association has been difficult to elucidate. By itself, massive transfusion (i.e., more than 22 units within 12 hours) has only recently been shown to be a significant risk factor for ARDS.[47] That is, retrospective and prospective studies have previously failed to demonstrate an association between massive hemorrhage and ARDS.[48,49]

Clinical investigations have focused on the role of microaggregates in the development of transfusion-related pulmonary edema. Microaggregates have been difficult to document as a possible cause of such edema. There is no question that microaggregates are present in stored blood products,[50] nor is there any question that some of these microaggregates are not filtered by standard 180-μm filters.[50] Clinical studies by Reul et al.[51] and Barrett et al.[52] demonstrated an apparent benefit from using micropore (40-μm) filters to remove these particles from transfused blood. As Miller and Brzica[2] pointed out, problems with the design of these studies make it difficult to accept their results or conclusions. In fact, the results of these two studies are quite surprising: the 40-μm filters removed at best only 12 percent of the microaggregates in infused blood; furthermore, they generated more microaggregates than they removed when more than 10 units of blood were filtered through them.[50]

Durtschi et al.[50] and Snyder et al.[53] conducted well-designed randomized studies comparing the effectiveness of microfilters as a supplement to the standard 160- to 265-μm and 260-μm filters. Both groups found no benefit from using micropore filters. Microfilters have the disadvantage of removing most of the platelets from the blood passing through the filter, potentially contributing to any thrombocytopenia a patient may later have.[54–56] For this reason, micropore filtration of blood is not a wise practice. No data document any difference in the size or number of microaggregates in whole blood and pRBCs. We therefore cannot compare the two with respect to their propensity to cause this complication.

COST AND RISK OF INFECTION FOR PACKED RED BLOOD CELLS VERSUS WHOLE BLOOD

Infection from syphilis; HIV (HTLV-III); HBV; or non-A, non-B (NANB or hepatitis C) hepatitis are all long-term risks of transfusion with any blood product. Administration of any blood product—whole blood, platelets, FFP, factor VIII, or cryoprecipitate—incurs risk of infection. Relatively sensitive and inexpensive screening tests exist for syphilis, HIV (HTLV-III), and HBV. As a result, new infections with these agents occur only rarely and are attributable to either logistical error or screening test failure (e.g., such as occurs because of the lack of production of antibody for up to 6 months after HIV infection). At present, the only screening test for NANB hepatitis is elevated levels of serum alanine aminotransferase in donor blood.[57] A screening test for hepatitis C (the newest name for NANB) has been announced by CETUS in the Wall St. Journal, but has yet to be documented in the medical literature. Although this test is relatively sensitive, it is not very specific; therefore, patients given blood products remain at significant risk of NANB hepatitis. Risk of infection with NANB hepatitis increases as exposure to different donors increases (Table 30-2). Transfusion of a single unit of whole blood, pRBCs, platelets, FFP, or cryoprecipitate exposes the recipient to a single donor, whereas transfusion of commercially available factor VIII exposes recipients to a very large number of donors (approximately 600).[19] Does using pRBCs instead of whole blood change a patient's risk of infection with NANB hepatitis?

Packed red blood cells might increase the risk of NANB hepatitis by increasing requirements for other blood products. Unfortunately, no clinical studies have specifically addressed this question.

Table 30-2.   Relationship Betweem Volume of Transfusion and Incidence of Non-A, Non-B Hepatitis

Units Transfused	Incidence of Non-A, Non-B Hepatitis (% of Patients)				
	All TTVS Centers	NY	Barnes	Houston	UCLA
1	6.9	2.9	1.7	11.5	8.8
2–3	10.5	6.4	3.1	19.5	11.8
4–5	11.0	8.3	6.4	22.2	22.9
6–15	12.0	14.0	4.9	24.0	21.1

TTVS Centers = Transfusion Transmitted Viruses Study centers; NY = New York; Barnes = Washington University, St. Louis, MO; and UCLA = University of California, Los Angeles. (Data from Hollinger et al.[8])

Nevertheless, evidence from studies discussed earlier in this paper indicates that using pRBCs should not increase requirements for platelets, FFP, and cryoprecipitate during moderate blood loss. All stored blood is deficient in platelets. Thus, patients given pRBCs for either moderate or massive hemorrhage should not have higher requirements for platelet transfusion than patients given stored whole blood. Patients undergoing moderate hemorrhage who have normal livers do not require the clotting factors available in FFP or cyroprecipitate, nor do they benefit from the colloid available in FFP. Therefore, patients given transfusions of pRBCs for moderate hemorrhage should not have higher requirements for either FFP or cyroprecipitate than patients given stored whole blood.[58–60] Similarly, massively hemorrhaging patients do not require the clotting factors available in either FFP or cryoprecipitate, although they may benefit from the colloid available in FFP. Therefore, the use of pRBCs instead of whole blood may not increase a patient's requirements for other blood products during massive hemorrhage, either.

The occurrence of liver failure constitutes the important exception to the above conclusions. Patients with liver failure may benefit from the colloid and clotting factors in whole blood and FFP and may require cryoprecipitate to maintain adequate levels of factor VIII. Transfusing these patients with each of these components separately entails exposure to an excessively large number of donors.

In one study, liver transplantation recipients whose hemotherapy was guided by thromboelastography received an average of 17 units of pRBCs, 18.3 units of FFP, 20.8 units of platelets, and 12.2 units of cryoprecipitate during transplantation (68.3 units total).[25] The most direct way of providing these patients with the blood products they need is to transfuse fresh whole blood. This provides a larger quantity of functional components than transfusions of specific components and minimizes the exposure of recipients to different donors. Therefore, the use of fresh whole blood instead of pRBCs or stored whole blood in massively hemorrhaging patients has three advantages: (1) it provides the largest quantity of functioning, viable platelets; (2) it minimizes exposure to different donors; and (3) it is probably less expensive than using costly prepared components (pRBCs or modified whole blood, platelets, FFP, and cryoprecipitate). Stored whole blood probably offers no advantage over pRBCs in moderate or massive hemorrhage. Fresh whole blood may be the blood product of choice for massively hemorrhaging patients. It is therefore unlikely that the vast majority of patients undergoing vascular surgery would benefit from receiving either stored whole blood or fresh whole blood, as these patients only rarely sustain hemorrhage great enough to cause thrombocytopenia.

TECHNIQUES TO MINIMIZE TRANSFUSION OF HOMOLOGOUS BLOOD

Autologous predeposit of blood, acute preoperative hemodilution, and salvage of autologous blood from the surgical field are all techniques devised to minimize transfusion of homologous blood and the subsequent exposure to infectious disease. What are the risks and benefits of each of these techniques in the setting of vascular surgery?

Autologous Predeposit of Blood

Autologous predeposit of blood has been commonly practiced for over 20 years.[61] Nevertheless, no published report specifically addresses the use of this technique for vascular surgery. Its use promotes conservation of resources, a practice that has gained wide acceptance in the blood banking community.[62,63] The limitations of this technique are the patient's ability to regenerate red blood cells and to tolerate the anemia incurred by the phlebotomy necessary for deposit. Storage practices also limit the usefulness of autologous predeposit of blood.

Most blood banks use a hematocrit of 34 percent as the lower limit required for predeposit of autologous blood. The ability of vascular surgery patients to tolerate this degree of anemia and to regenerate the red cell mass donated must be assessed on an individual basis by their physicians. As a group, such patients tend to tolerate anemia much less well than their younger counterparts, the patient group for whom most autologous predeposit programs were designed.[64] Oral iron supplementation helps these patients recover from the anemia caused by autologous predeposit of blood.[65,66] Iron supplementation or the soon-to-be-released genetically engineered erythropoietic factors also allow patients to arrive at surgery in a state of maximal erythropoiesis.[67] Such a state would allow them to quickly generate the red blood cells they need to resolve any anemia that remains after surgery. Unfortunately, autologously predeposited blood has on occasion been mislabeled and transfused, causing severe hemolytic transfusion reactions.[68] For this reason, patients who are to receive predeposited blood usually have their blood cross-matched before receipt of autologous blood. Vascular surgery patients who are able to regenerate the blood they predeposit can be expected to avoid transfusion of that amount of homologous blood. In most cases, this will amount to one to four units of pRBCs.

Salvage of Autologous Blood from the Surgical Field

Intraoperative salvage and reinfusion of autologous blood has been reviewed extensively.[67,69–73] Most devices in use today are based on the semicontinuous flow centrifugation and cell-washing technique first described by Wilson and co-workers.[74,75] Unfortunately, it is difficult to judge the safety and efficacy of this practice for vascular surgery on the basis of published reports.[76–86] There are no randomized, prospective studies in the literature. Most reports involve a small number of patients who are compared with historical controls. Also, the studies having larger patient populations reach further back in time to obtain their historical controls.

In what we judge to be the best study to date, Hallett et al.[86] compared 50 patients undergoing aortic vascular surgery with 50 historical controls (patients who had surgery in the 6 months before the study). Hallett and colleagues were able to avoid transfusion of homologous blood in 68 percent of their patients. The remaining 32 percent required pRBCs to maintain their hematocrit, FFP in amounts comparable to that received by controls, and twice as many platelets as received by controls. Overall, exposure to different donors was reduced by at least 25 percent and possibly as much as 57 percent (depending on whether the platelet packs were pooled from many donors or obtained from only one). No difference in morbidity or mortality occurred between the two groups.

Autologous blood transfusion has not been proved safe or efficacious in a large, prospective, randomized study. Nevertheless, the published clinical literature to date demonstrates that disaster does not ensue when autologous blood is transfused and that the exposure of recipients to different donors may be significantly lower.

Acute Preoperative Hemodilution

Hemodilution consists of reducing the hematocrit by means of an isovolemic exchange of blood for crystalloid or colloid solution. In practice, the hematocrit is generally reduced to 20 to 30 percent and, on rare occasion, to less than 20 percent. Blood is removed using a central venous or arterial catheter either immediately before or after induction of anesthesia. Because of hemodilution, blood lost from the site of surgery contains a lower concentration of red blood cells. Thus, the effective loss of red cells as well as other components is reduced. Autologous blood is reinfused at a later time, in reverse order from its removal (so as to reinfuse the blood richest in red blood cells and clotting factors at the latest time), ideally after surgical hemostasis has been achieved.

The physiologic effects of hemodilution have been investigated extensively in anesthetized dogs subjected to isovolemic exchange of blood with crystalloids or with colloids such as dextran or plasma.[87] During this situation of acutely induced anemia, which represents a decrease in tissue oxygen delivery, physiologic responses consist of increases in cardiac output and tissue oxygen extraction. Oxygen uptake increases approximately 5 to 10 percent, owing mostly to increased oxygen uptake by myocardial and skeletal muscle. Changes in cardiac output relate to several factors. Because of a decrease in blood viscosity, peripheral vascular resistance decreases according to the relationship $R = nZ$, where R = total peripheral resistance, n = viscosity, and Z = total vascular hindrance.[88,89] As a result, at a given hematocrit, cardiac output increases to a greater extent when the hemodilutent is low-molecular-weight (38,000) dextran than when it is high-molecular-weight (460,000) dextran.[90] The decrease in total peripheral resistance during hemodilution results in an increase in cardiac output because of reduced afterload and increased venous return.

Furthermore, redistribution of blood volume from peripheral to central compartments increases during hemodilution.[91] Distribution of blood flow changes, with decreases in blood flow (vasoconstriction) in the liver, intestine, spleen and kidney, and increases in blood flow in the heart and brain.[90] These increases in blood flow in the heart and brain are disproportionate to the increase in cardiac output, indicating an important adaptive response by which limited oxygen supply is diverted to vital areas. Activation of the sympathetic nervous system increases venomotor tone and stimulation of cardiac sympathetic nerves, which maintain or augment myocardial contractility.[92]

Hemodilution has been used to decrease blood transfusion requirements for various surgical procedures, including general, thoracic, open heart, orthopedic, and vascular surgery.[93] In one study, use of hemodilution and retransfusion during vascular operations on the distal aorta and lower extremities appeared to reduce blood transfusion requirements from 3.8 ± 1.8 units (± one standard deviation) to 0.5 ± 0.9 units, with no apparent adverse patient outcome.[94] To avoid the use of homologous blood entirely in vascular surgical patients, Cutler[95] combined autotransfusion, hemodilution, and surgical techniques reported to decrease unnecessary dissection and blood loss in 138 aortic reconstructions. Hemodilution below a hematocrit of 30 percent was not permitted in patients having positive results on preoperative stress tests. Cutler was able to avoid blood transfusion entirely in 43 percent of elective procedures and in 8 percent of emergency procedures. Again, no adverse outcome was attributable to hemodilution. This combined technique was also cost-effective, producing an average savings of $260 per patient.

Because of the high prevalence of coronary artery disease in vascular surgical patients, the greatest risk associated with hemodilution relates to the possibility of myocardial ischemia during periods of increased myocardial oxygen requirement or decreased myocardial oxygen delivery. The major benefits consist of decreased viscosity and the resulting improved flow characteristics of blood.

Studies of the effects of hemodilution on the myocardial energy balance during hemodilution have produced ambiguous results. Two factors have been responsible: (1) differences in technique (i.e., use of an animal model, comparison of crystalloid versus colloid, comparison of awake versus anesthetized subjects), and (2) associated systemic effects of hemodilution (i.e., increased sympathetic discharge, increased heart rate and contractility).

Various studies have shown that these associated systemic effects of hemodilution can themselves affect myocardial oxygen blood supply and demand. Jan and Chien[96] subjected dogs to isovolumetric exchange of blood with plasma and found that myocardial oxygen consumption remained constant when hematocrit was 20 to 60 percent. Interestingly, the range of optimum hematocrit for systemic oxgen transport was narrower (hematocrit, 40 to 60 percent). Holtz et al.[97] performed hemodilution in conscious dogs using 6 percent dextran. At a hematocrit of 13 percent, and after release of a temporary circumflex coronary artery occlusion, coronary blood flow increased, mainly in the subepicardium as opposed to the subendocardium. This occurrence indicates a limited dilatory capacity in the subendocardium during hemodilution. Most et al.[98] demonstrated in pigs subjected to hemodilution with saline and albumin (hematocrit, 17 percent) that with 85 to 90 percent stenosis of the left anterior descending artery, maximal oxygen delivery distal to the stenosis decreased in both the endocardium and epicardium. Again, this points out the limited vasodilatory capacity in the myocardium during hemodilution. In another study, Crystal and Salem[99] studied the direct effects of hemodilution on regional coronary hemodynamics using a selectively perfused left anterior descending artery preparation. With perfusion pressure reduced 50 percent (a situation simulating coronary insufficiency) and at a hematocrit of 17 percent, both myocardial oxygen consumption and myocardial contractility decreased, suggesting compromised myocardial oxygenation and contractile function. One study in patients with coronary artery disease undergoing abdominal aortic surgery used only modest hemodilution (hematocrit, 30 percent) and found that cardiac index was not higher than in nonhemodiluted patients.[100] Although systemic oxygen transport decreased in hemodiluted patients, oxygen consumption decreased as well.

Considering the results of these studies, one could theorize that hemodilution to extremely low hematocrits (less than 20 percent) may be associated with myocardial ischemia if myocardial oxygen requirement increases or myocardial oxygen supply decreases. Insufficient data are available regarding the safety of more moderate degrees of hemodilution (hematocrit, 20 to 30 percent) in anesthetized animals or patients with coronary artery stenosis.

Hemodilution may also affect coagulation. Laks et al.[101] performed hemodilution with Plasmanate in surgical patients and demonstrated a decrease in platelet count, dilution of coagulation factors, and prolonged bleeding time. All of the changes were reversed after reinfusion of the patients' blood, with no increase in blood loss during the surgical procedure. Rosberg[102] demonstrated similar changes induced during hemodilution with dextran, again without increases in blood loss during surgery.

In summary, hemodilution may be an acceptable way of reducing blood transfusion requirements in selected patients undergoing vascular surgery. Until further data are available, however, reductions in hematocrit below 30 percent in patients with demonstrated coronary artery disease might be approached with caution after careful assessment of the risk-benefit ratio.

SUMMARY

There is no evidence that infusion of stored whole blood is more beneficial to massively hemorrhaging patients (blood loss exceeding 10 units 70 kg of body weight) than infusion of pRBCs. Although such patients may benefit from the colloid that stored blood provides, no studies document this effect. Substantial evidence indicates that pRBCs diluted with lactated Ringer's solution or normal saline are adequate blood replacement for moderate hemorrhage (blood loss of 5 to 10 units/70 kg). Many questions must be answered before scientifically sound conclusions can be made about the relative effectiveness and safety of using pRBCs rather than whole blood for massive hemorrhage. Studies that remain to be done include a "blind" study of the efficacy of platelet transfusion; a randomized trial of fresh whole blood versus pRBCs in liver transplantation (pRBCs reconstituted with normal saline before being brought to the anesthetist), trauma surgery, vascular surgery, and burn surgery; and a long-term study of alloimmunization in surgical patients given platelet and blood transfusions.

The literature does allow some conclusions and recommendations to be made. Massively hemorrhaging patients are likely to require platelet transfusions to reverse the dilutional thrombocytopenia and thrombocytopathy accompanying massive hemorrhage. Hemorrhaging patients with abnormal liver function (from hemophilia, drug effects, liver failure) may require the clotting factors and colloid available in FFP and may benefit from the factor VIII available in cryoprecipitate. No other circumstances probably exist that warrant use of FFP or cryoprecipitate for surgery. Fresh whole blood may reduce the high cost and exposure of recipients to different donors that massive transfusion usually entails and therefore may still be the blood product of choice in this setting. Although autotransfusion and/or hemodilution may be useful in reducing blood transfusion requirements in vascular surgical patients, further research is needed regarding the safety of hemodilution in patients with coronary artery disease.

REFERENCES

1. Wilson RF, Mammen E, Walt AJ: Eight years of experience with massive blood transfusions. J Trauma 11:275–285, 1971
2. Miller RD, Brzica SM, Jr: Blood, blood components, colloids and autotransfusion therapy, p. 1329–1367. In Miller RD (ed): Anesthesia. Vol. 2. 2nd Ed. Churchill Livingstone, New York, 1986
3. Sheldon GF, Lim RC, Jr., Blaisdell FW: The use of fresh blood in the treatment of critically injured patients. J Trauma 15:670–677, 1975
4. Isbister JP: Haemotherapy for acute haemorrhage. Anaesth Intensive Care 12:217–228, 1984
5. Schmidt PJ: Whole blood transfusion (letter). Transfusion 24:368–369, 1984
6. Counts RB, Haisch C, Simon TL et al: Hemostasis in massively transfused trauma patients. Ann Surg 190:91–99, 1979
7. Robertson HD, Polk HC, Jr: Blood transfusions in elective operations: comparison of whole blood versus packed red cells. Ann Surg 181:778–783, 1975
8. Hollinger FB, Mosley JW, Szmuness W et al: Non-A, non-B hepatitis following blood transfusion: risk factors associated with donor characteristics. p. 361–376. In Szmuness W, Alter HJ, Maynard JE (eds): Viral Hepatitis. Franklin Institute Press, Philadelphia, 1981
9. Shackford SR, Virgilio RW, Peters RM: Whole blood versus packed-cell transfusions. a physiologic comparison. Ann Surg 193:337–340, 1981
10. Miller RD, Robbins TO, Tong MJ, Barton SL: Coagulation defects associated with massive blood transfusions. Ann Surg 174:794–801, 1971
11. Coté CJ, Liu LMP, Szyfelbein SK et al: Changes in serial platelet counts following massive blood transfusion in pediatric patients. Anesthesiology 62:197–201, 1985
12. Lim RC, Jr., Olcott C, IV, Robinson AJ, Blaisdell FW: Platelet response and coagulation changes following massive blood replacement. J Trauma 13:577–582, 1973
13. Murphy S, Gardner FH: Platelet preservation. Effect of storage temperature on maintenance of platelet viability—deleterious effect of refrigerated storage. N Engl J Med 280:1094–1098, 1969
14. Murphy S, Gardner FH: Platelet storage at 22°C; metabolic, morphologic, and functional studies. J Clin Invest 50:370–377, 1971
15. Handin RI, Valeri CR: Hemostatic effectiveness of platelets stored at 22°C. N Engl J Med 285:538–543, 1971
16. Valeri CR: Hemostatic effectiveness of liquid-preserved and previously frozen human platelets. N Engl J Med 290:353–358, 1974
17. Slichter SJ, Harker LA: Preparation and storage of platelet concentrates. II. Storage variables influencing platelet viability and function. Br J Haematol 34:403–419, 1976
18. Penner JA: Blood component therapy for patients with coagulation disorders. p. 501–526. In Petz LD, Swisher SN (eds): Clinical Practice of Blood Transfusion. Churchill Livingstone, New York, 1981
19. Tomasulo PA: Platelet transfusions for nonmalignant diseases. pp. 527–549. In Petz LD, Swisher SN (eds): Clinical Practice of Blood Transfusion. Churchill Livingstone, New York, 1981
20. Tomasulo PA, Lenes BA: Platelet transfusion therapy. p. 63–89. Hemostatic In Menitove JE, McCarthy LJ (eds): He-

mostatic Disorders and the Blood Bank. American Association of Blood Banks, Arlington, VA, 1984

21. Howard JE, Perkins HA: The natural history of alloimmunization to platelets. Transfusion 18:496–503, 1978

22. McFarland JG, Aster RH: Clinical significance of platelet-specific antigens. p. 55–69. In McCarthy LJ, Menitove JE (eds): Immunologic Aspects of Platelet Transfusion. American Association of Blood Banks, Arlington, VA, 1985

23. Howland WS, Schweizer O, Gould P: A comparison of intraoperative measurements of coagulation. Anesth Analg 53:657–663, 1974

24. Zuckerman L, Cohen E, Vagher JP et al: Comparison of thrombelastography with common coagulation tests. Thromb Haemost 46:752–756, 1981

25. Kang YG, Martin DJ, Marquez J et al: Intraoperative changes in blood coagulation and thrombelastographic monitoring in liver transplantation. Anesth Analg 64:888–896, 1985

26. Guyton AC, Lindsey AW: Effect of elevated left atrial pressure and decreased plasma protein concentration on the development of pulmonary edema. Circ Res 7:649–657, 1959

27. Levine OR, Mellins RB, Senior RM, Fishman AP: The application of Starling's law of capillary exchange to the lungs. J Clin Invest 46:934–944, 1967

28. Holcroft JW, Trunkey DD: Extravascular lung water following hemorrhagic shock in the baboon: comparison between resuscitation with Ringer's lactate and Plasmanate. Ann Surg 180:408–417, 1974

29. Shoemaker WC, Hauser CJ: Critique of crystalloid versus colloid therapy in shock and shock lung. Crit Care Med 7:117–124, 1979

30. Stein L, Beraud J-J, Cavanilles J et al: Pulmonary edema during fluid infusion in the absence of heart failure. JAMA 229:65–68, 1974

31. Hillman KM: Resuscitation in diabetic ketoacidosis. Crit Care Med 11:53–54, 1983

32. Skillman JJ, Restall DS, Salzman EW: Randomized trial of albumin vs. electrolyte solutions during abdominal aortic operations. Surgery 78:291–303, 1975

33. Jelenko, C, III, Williams JB, Wheeler ML et al: Studies in shock and resuscitation, I: Use of a hypertonic, albumin-containing, fluid demand regimen (HALFD) in resuscitation. Crit Care Med 7:157–167, 1979

34. Boutros AR, Ruess R, Olson L et al: Comparison of hemodynamic, pulmonary, and renal effects of use of three types of fluids after major surgical procedures on the abdominal aorta. Crit Care Med 7:9–13, 1979

35. Virgilio RW, Rice CL, Smith DE et al: Crystalloid vs. colloid resuscitation: is one better? A randomized clinical study. Surgery 85:129–139, 1979

36. Lowe RJ, Moss GS, Jilek J, Levine HD: Crystalloid vs colloid in the etiology of pulmonary failure after trauma: a randomized trial in man. Surgery 81:676–683, 1977

37. Metildi LA, Shackford SR, Virgilio RW, Peters RM: Crystalloid versus colloid in fluid resuscitation of patients with severe pulmonary insufficiency. Surg Gynecol Obstet 158:207–212, 1984

38. Shires GT, III, Peitzman AB, Albert SA et al: Response of extravascular lung water to intraoperative fluids. Ann Surg 197:515–519, 1983

39. Goodwin CW, Dorethy J, Lam V, Pruitt BA, Jr: Randomized trial of efficacy of crystalloid and colloid resuscitation on hemodynamic response and lung water following thermal injury. Ann Surg 197:520–531, 1983

40. Myhre BA: Fatalities from blood transfusion. JAMA 244:1333–1335, 1980

41. Pineda AA, Brzica SM, Jr., Taswell HF: Hemolytic transfusion reaction. Recent experience in a large blood bank. Mayo Clin Proc 53:378–390, 1978

42. Kahn RC, Jascott D, Carlon GC et al: Massive blood replacement: correlation of ionized calcium, citrate, and hydrogen ion concentration. Anesth Analg 58:274–278, 1979

43. Denlinger JK, Nahrwold ML, Gibbs PS, Lecky JH: Hypocalcaemia during rapid

blood transfusion in anaesthetized man. Br J Anaesth 48:995–1000, 1976

44. Drop LJ, Laver MB: Low plasma ionized calcium and response to calcium therapy in critically ill man. Anesthesiology 43:300–306, 1975

45. Borland LM, Roule M, Cook DR: Anesthesia for pediatric orthotopic liver transplantation. Anesth Analg 64:117–124, 1985

46. Boyan CP: Cold or warmed blood for massive transfusions. Ann Surg 160:282–286, 1964

47. Pepe PE, Potkin RT, Reus DH et al: Clinical predictors of the adult respiratory distress syndrome. Am J Surg 144:124–130, 1982

48. Collins JA, Gordon WC, Jr., Hudson TL et al: Inapparent hypoxemia in casualties with wounded limbs: pulmonary fat embolism? Ann Surg 167:511–520, 1968

49. Collins JA, James PM, Bredenberg CE et al: The relationship between transfusion and hypoxemia in combat casualties. Ann Surg 188:513–520, 1978

50. Durtschi MB, Haisch CE, Reynolds L et al: Effect of micropore filtration on pulmonary function after massive transfusion. Am J Surg 138:8–14, 1979

51. Reul GJ, Jr., Greenberg SD, Lefrak EA et al: Prevention of post-traumatic pulmonary insufficiency. Fine screen filtration of blood. Arch Surg 106:386–394, 1973

52. Barrett J, Tahir AH, Litwin MS: Increased pulmonary arteriovenous shunting in humans following blood transfusion. Relation to screen filtration pressure of transfused blood and prevention by Dacron wool (Swank) filtration. Arch Surg 113:947–950, 1978

53. Snyder EL, Underwood PS, Spivack M et al: An *in vivo* evaluation of microaggregate blood filtration during total hip replacement. Ann Surg 190:75–79, 1979

54. Mason KG, Hall LE, Lamoy RE, Wright CB: Evaluation of blood filters: dynamics of platelets and platelet aggregates. Surgery 77:235–240, 1975

55. Cullen DJ, Ferrara L: Comparative evaluation of blood filters: a study *in vitro*. Anesthesiology 41:568–575, 1974

56. Marshall BE, Wurzel HA, Neufeld GR, Klineberg PL: Effects of Intersept® micropore filtration of blood on microaggregates and other constituents. Anesthesiology 44:525–534, 1976

57. Silverstein MD, Mulley AG, Dienstag JL: Should donor blood be screened for elevated alanine aminotransferase levels? A cost-effectiveness analysis. JAMA 252:2839–2845, 1984

58. Bove JR: Fresh frozen plasma: too few indications—too much use (editorial). Anesth Analg 64:849–850, 1985

59. Braunstein AH, Oberman HA: Transfusion of plasma components. Transfusion 24:281–286, 1984

60. Oberman HA: Uses and abuses of fresh frozen plasma. p. 109–124. In Garratty A (ed): Current Concepts in Transfusion Therapy. American Association of Blood Banks, Arlington, VA, 1985

61. Corpe RF, Liang J: Autogenous blood transfusions in surgery. Abdom Surg J 8:45–50, 1966

62. Technical Manual of the American Association of Blood Banks. 9th Ed. American Association of Blood Banks, Washington, DC, 1985

63. Gilcher RO, Belcher L: Predeposit programs. p. 11–22. In Sandler SG, Silvergleid AJ (eds): Autologous Transfusion. American Association of Blood Banks, Arlington, VA, 1983

64. Sandler SG: Overview. p. 1–9. In Sandler SG, Silvergleid AJ (eds): Autologous Transfusion. American Association of Blood Banks, Arlington, VA, 1983

65. Hamstra RD, Block MH: Erythropoiesis in response to blood loss in man. J Appl Physiol 27:503–507, 1969

66. Zuck TF: Donor response to predeposit autologous transfusion phlebotomy. p. 51–67. In Dawson RB (ed): Autologous Transfusion, a Technical Workshop. American Association of Blood Banks, Washington, DC, 1976

67. Brzica SM, Jr., Pineda AA, Taswell HF: Autologous blood transfusion. Mayo Clin Proc 51:723–737, 1976

68. Bell W: The hematology of autotransfusion. Surgery 84:695–699, 1978

69. Popovsky MA, Devine PA, Taswell HF:

Intraoperative autologous transfusion. Mayo Clin Proc 60:125–134, 1985

70. Swisher SN, Petz LD: Autologous transfusion and blood salvage. p. 345–356 In Petz LD, Swisher SN (eds): Clinical Practice of Blood Transfusion. Churchill Livingstone, New York, 1981

71. Fleming AW: Intraoperative salvage. p. 41–56. In Sandler SG, Silvergleid AJ (eds): Autologous Transfusion. American Association of Blood Banks, Arlington, VA, 1983

72. Mattox KL: Comparison of techniques of autotransfusion. Surgery 84:700–702, 1978

73. Saarela E: Autotransfusion; a review. Ann Clin Res, 13: suppl. 33, 48–56, 1981

74. Wilson JD, Utz DC, Taswell HF: Autotransfusion during transurethral resection of the prostate: technique and preliminary clinical evaluation. Mayo Clin Proc 44:374–386, 1969

75. Wilson JD, Taswell HF, Utz DC: Autotransfusion: urologic applications and the development of a modified irrigating fluid. J Urol 105:873–877, 1971

76. Brener BJ, Raines JK, Darling RC: Intraoperative autotransfusion in abdominal aortic resections. Arch Surg 107:78–84, 1973

77. Wall W, Heimbecker RO, McKenzie FN et al: Intraoperative autotransfusion in major elective vascular operations: a clinical assessment. Surgery 79:82–88, 1976

78. Brewster DC, Ambrosino JJ, Darling RC et al: Intraoperative autotransfusion in major vascular surgery. Am J Surg 137:507–513, 1979

79. Thomas Gl, Jones TW, Stavney LS et al: Experiences with autotransfusion during abdominal aortic aneurysm resection. Am J Surg 139:628–633, 1980

80. Cordell AR, Lavender SW: An appraisal of blood salvage techniques in vascular and cardiac operations. Ann Thorac Surg 31:421–425, 1981

81. Ottesen S, Frøysaker T: Use of Haemonetics Cell Saver for autotransfusion in cardiovascular surgery. Scand J Thorac Cardiovasc Surg 16:263–268, 1982

82. Warnock DF, Davison JK, Brewster DC et al: Modification of the Haemonetics Cell Saver for optional high flow rate autotransfusion. Am J Surg 143:765–768, 1982

83. O'Hara PJ, Hertzer NR, Santilli PH, Beven EG: Intraoperative autotransfusion during abdominal aortic reconstruction. Am J Surg 145:215–220, 1983

84. Cali RF, O'Hara PJ, Hertzer NR et al: The influence of autotransfusion on homologous blood requirements during aortic reconstruction. Cleve Clin Q 51:143–148, 1984

85. Stanton PE, Jr., Shannon J, Rosenthal D et al: Intraoperative autologous transfusion during major aortic reconstructive procedures. South Med J 80:315–319, 1987

86. Hallett JW, Jr., Popovsky M, Ilstrup D: Minimizing blood transfusions during abdominal aortic surgery: recent advances in rapid autotransfusion. J Vasc Surg 5:601–606, 1987

87. Chapler CK, Cain SM: The physiologic reserve in oxygen carrying capacity: studies in experimental hemodilution. Can J Physiol Pharmacol 64:7–12, 1986

88. Fan F-C, Chen RYZ, Schuessler GB, Chien S: Effects of hematocrit variations on regional hemodynamics and oxygen transport in the dog. Am J Physiol 238:H545–H552, 1980

89. Lipowsky HH, Firrell JC: Microvascular hemodynamics during systemic hemodilution and hemoconcentration. Am J Physiol 250:H908–H922, 1986

90. Murray JF, Escobar E, Rapaport E: Effects of blood viscosity on hemodynamic responses in acute normovolemic anemia. Am J Physiol 216:638–642, 1969

91. Chapler CK, Cain SM: Blood flow and O_2 uptake in dog hindlimb with anemia, norepinephrine, and propranolol. J Appl Physiol 51:565–570, 1981

92. Glick G, Plauth WH, Jr., Braunwald E: Role of the autonomic nervous system in the circulatory response to acutely induced anemia in unanesthetized dogs. J Clin Invest 43:2112–2124, 1964

93. Messmer K, Kreimeir U, Intaglietta M: Present state of intentional hemodilution. Eur Surg Res 18:254–263, 1986

94. Krämer AH, Hertzer NR, Beven EG: Intraoperative hemodilution during elective vascular reconstruction. Surg Gynecol Obstet 149:831–836, 1979

95. Cutler BS: Avoidance of homologous transfusion in aortic operations: the role of autotransfusion, hemodilution, and surgical technique. Surgery 95:717–723, 1984

96. Jan K-M, Chien S: Effect of hematocrit variations on coronary hemodynamics and oxygen utilization. Am J Physiol 233:H106–H113, 1977

97. Holtz J, Bassenge E, von Restorff W, Mayer E: Transmural differences in myocardial blood flow and in coronary dilatory capacity in hemodiluted conscious dogs. Basic Res Cardiol 71:36–46, 1976

98. Most AS, Ruocco NA, Jr., Gewirtz H: Effect of a reduction in blood viscosity on maximal myocardial oxygen delivery distal to a moderate coronary stenosis. Circulation 74:1085–1092, 1986

99. Crystal GJ, Salem MR: Myocardial oxygen consumption and segmental shortening during selective coronary hemodilution in dogs. Anesth Analg 67:500–508, 1988

100. Van Der Linden P, Baron JF, Philip I et al: Normovolemic hemodilution in anesthetized patients with coronary artery disease: effects on hemodynamic and LV function (abstract). Anesthesiology 67:A135, 1987

101. Laks H, Handin RI, Martin V, Pilon RN: The effects of normovolemic hemodilution on coagulation and blood utilization in major surgery. Surg Res 20:225–230, 1976

102. Rosberg B: Blood coagulation during and after normovolemic hemodilution in elective surgery. Ann Clin Res, 13: suppl. 33, 84–88, 1981

31

The Bleeding Patient

Charise T. Petrovitch

NORMAL HEMOSTASIS

Anesthetists transfuse over half of the blood administered in the United States, giving them a primary role in diagnosing and managing patients with bleeding disorders.[1,2] Although normal hemostasis—the arrest of bleeding—consists of a complex sequence of events, a grasp of major concepts rather than great detail is fortunately sufficient to care for most bleeding problems that arise within the scope of anesthesia care.

Normal hemostasis involves balancing two processes, coagulation and fibrinolysis. Each process is complex and involves enzymatic activators and inhibitors. The proper interaction of both processes produces a dynamic equilibrium that maintains the fluid state of the blood. A defect or imbalance in either process can lead to excessive clotting or prolonged bleeding.

Under normal circumstances, a fibrin clot is formed at the site of vascular injury. Then, excess fibrin is lysed to allow blood to flow after the injury has healed. The endpoint of coagulation is formation of fibrin; the endpoint of fibrinolysis is removal of fibrin. In this way, the hemostatic mechanism confines circulating blood to the vascular bed, arrests bleeding from the site of vascular injury, and restores patency of the vascular bed. Attainment of these goals requires proper interaction of normal vasculature, normal platelets, normal blood coagulation, and normal fibrinolysis.

Primary Hemostasis

The initial response to vascular injury is called "primary hemostasis," a process that must be distinguished from coagulation. This process does not involve coagulation proteins. Specifically, injury to a blood vessel is followed by local vasoconstriction and tissue swelling; these actions reduce bleeding and shunt blood away from the site of injury (Fig. 31-1, step 1).[3] Platelets clump together and adhere to the injured vessel wall to form a platelet plug. This platelet plug initially seals the vascular defect and temporarily arrests bleeding.

The function of the vasculature and of platelets is actually more complex than just summarized. Blood vessels have an obvious role—to contain the blood, which circulates throughout the body—but they serve three crucial and different functions with regard to hemostasis: (1) the intima of blood vessels is non-thrombogenic, preventing clotting under normal circumstances, (2) in response to vas-

465

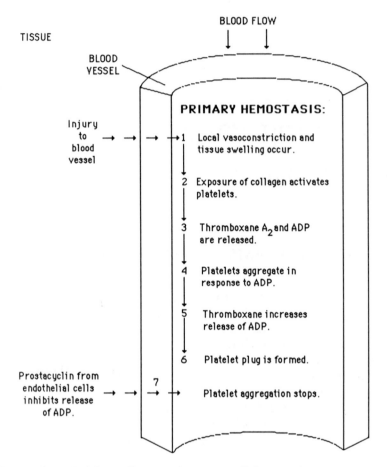

Fig. 31-1. Steps 1 through 7 depict "primary hemostasis," the initial response to vascular injury. Primary hemostasis is the first of three major stages of normal hemostasis, the arrest of bleeding (see text for complete explanation). ADP = adenosine diphosphate.

cular injury, they initiate primary hemostasis, and (3) they activate the fibrinolytic system following clot formation to restore normal blood flow.

The intima of blood vessels is lined with a monolayer of endothelial cells. This lining is nonthrombogenic due to the secretion of prostacyclin, which is a prostaglandin. Prostacyclin inhibits platelet aggregation and acts as a powerful vasodilator. These actions prevent platelet plug formation and maintain normal blood flow.

Just as the endothelium protects the vessel from platelet adhesion, loss of the endothelial surface promotes it. Circulat-

ing platelets exposed to collagen in the subendothelial layers of the intima adhere to the vessel wall at the site of injury. This platelet adherence to collagen induces a change in the platelets, causing them to be "activated platelets" (Fig. 31-1, step 2).[1,2] They change from a disk-like shape to a spheroid with the extrusion of many pseudopods. They also expose a new lipoprotein surface known as platelet factor 3 (PF3). The exposure of this phospholipid surface is crucial because subsequent interactions of some coagulation factors require the presence of a phospholipid surface.

Activated platelets release several intrinsic substances, including adenosine diphosphate (ADP) and thromboxane A2, (TxA2) (Fig. 31-1, step 3).[4,5] ADP causes platelets to aggregate (Fig. 31-1, step 4). Thromboxane A2, which is also a prostaglandin and a potent vasoconstrictor, increases release of ADP and causes further platelet aggregation (Fig. 31-1, step 5). In this way, prostacyclin secreted by normal endothelial cells and thromboxane secreted by activated platelets have opposing actions. Prostacyclin limits ADP release and consequent platelet aggregation on normal vasculature; thromboxane increases ADP release and platelet plug formation at the site of injury (Fig. 31-1, step 6, 7).

Platelet adhesion to subendothelial layers of blood vessels is aided by several substances, one of which is called von Willebrand factor (VWF). von Willebrand factor is thought to be secreted by both activated platelets and by endothelial cells. It circulates in the plasma and serves as an "intercellular glue" attaching platelets to subendothelial connective tissue proteins, particularly collagen. Similarly, fibrinogen aids platelet aggregation, acting like a glue to hold platelets together.

In summary, the denuded endothelium exposes collagen, which induces circulating platelets to adhere to the connective tissue; platelets become activated, change shape, release their contents and aggregate into a platelet plug. Primary hemostasis, which takes place within seconds of vessel injury, arrests bleeding temporarily and provides a surface (PF3) upon which blood coagulation may occur.

Coagulation

Coagulation involves many proteins (clotting factors), calcium, and phospholipid. They interact with each other to form a tough fibrin meshwork or clot, which reinforces the friable platelet plug to stop bleeding until tissue repair can occur.

The coagulation process has been made more difficult to understand because of the many different names given to the original 12 coagulation factors. To resolve this problem, their nomenclature has been standardized by assigning each factor a Roman numeral that corresponds to the order of their discovery. Most of the factors are referred to by their number, except for fibrinogen (I), prothrombin (II), calcium (IV), and tissue thromboplastin (III). Some of the numbered factors do not exist, such as factor VI; it was found to actually be activated factor V. Additionally, there are several new factors that have no numbers, such as prekallikrein and high molecular weight kinogen.

The process of blood coagulation occurs as a series of complex reactions in which one clotting factor activates another in chain reaction fashion to form the fibrin clot (Fig. 31-2). Most of the clotting factors circulate in an inactive form called a procoagulant molecule or a proenzyme. During the process of coagulation, a portion of this protein molecule is cleaved off and the remaining protein becomes an active clotting factor or cleavage enzyme. This "activated clotting factor" (designated by a small "a" after the Roman numeral of the factor) cleaves off a portion of the next clotting factor. In succession, one factor "activates" another until fibrinogen (factor I) is cleaved to form fibrin.

Some factors (V and VIII) serve as "cofactors" in the clotting cascade and do not become cleavage enzymes. They circulate in active form, but are very labile. These cofactors must be present in reactions that take place on a phospholipid surface. The cofactor binds together with one of the activated clotting factors to the phospholipid surface in the presence of calcium. This paired binding creates certain spacial relationships that are neces-

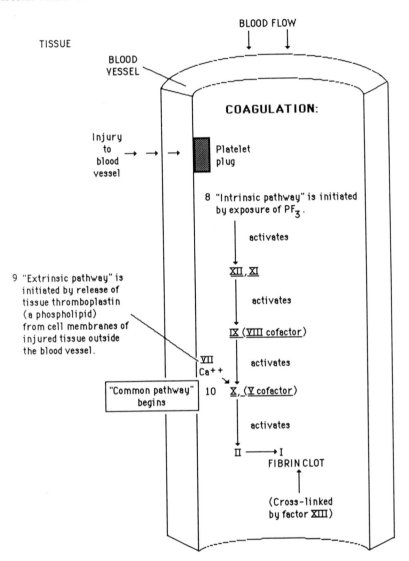

Fig. 31-2. Steps 8 ("intrinsic pathway"), 9 ("extrinsic pathway"), and 10 ("common pathway") are the processes constituting coagulation, the second major stage of normal hemostasis (see text for complete explanation). PF3 = platelet factor 3, also known as "platelet phospholipid." Roman numerals apply to clotting factors.

sary for the activation of the next clotting factor. These reactions therefore involve five components: the cofactor, the activated clotting factor, calcium, a phospholipid surface, and the clotting factor that is to be activated.

Four of the clotting factors (II, VII, IX, & X) require vitamin K for their proper

synthesis. Vitamin K enzymatically adds a carboxyl group to each of these factors, which enables them to bind via a calcium bridge to phospholipid surfaces. In the absence of vitamin K, these proteins are produced in normal amounts by the liver, but are not functional because they cannot bind to phospholipid. It is this group of clotting factors that is decreased when a patient receives coumadin therapy, because the coumadin competes with vitamin K for binding sites on the hepatocyte. Of these four vitamin K dependent factors, factor VII has the shortest half-life. It is the first protein to disappear from the circulation when a patient is placed on coumadin.

Since most of the coagulation proteins are synthesized by the liver, their normal structure and function are dependent upon normal hepatic activity. Only one factor, coagulant factor VIII, is thought to have some extrahepatic origin. Factor VIII circulates as a huge plasma protein with a molecular weight in excess of one million and is really a complex of two components. The major portion of this protein, VIIIR:Ag, is the "von Willebrand factor," which is involved with primary hemostasis. The von Willebrand factor (VIIIR:Ag) serves as a carrier protein for the smaller moiety, VIII:C, which is associated with factor VIII clotting activity. The factor VIII antigen or von Willebrand portion is produced in endothelial cells and megakaryocytes. The source of the low molecular weight portion of the factor VIII molecule (that portion responsible for the factor VIII coagulant activity) is still unknown. It may be that this portion is synthesized in the liver.

Several clotting factors require binding to a phospholipid surface for their proper interaction. This prerequisite serves to localize and limit clot formation to these membrane surfaces. Two phospholipid surfaces normally exist. Platelets activated during primary hemostasis expose a phospholipid surface called platelet factor 3 (PF3). Because it exists within the boundaries of the blood vessel, the clotting process that follows on that surface is called the "intrinsic pathway" of coagulation (Fig. 31-2, step 8). A similar phospholipid, tissue thromboplastin (also known as tissue phospholipid), is released from cell surface membranes of injured tissues located outside the blood vessel. Therefore, the process associated with this substance is called the "extrinsic pathway" of coagulation (Fig. 31-2, step 9). Both clotting sequences lead to the formation of factor Xa. At this point, the two pathways merge into the "common pathway" of coagulation that ultimately produces fibrin (Fig. 31-2, step 10).[6]

The intrinsic coagulation sequence is usually initiated within the blood vessel, when factor XII comes into contact with injured endothelium. Apparently, when the factor binds to a negatively charged surface, this binding alters and exposes the active enzyme site of the factor creating activated factor XII (XIIa). Factor XII may also be activated by contact with antigen-antibody complexes, complement, endotoxin, glass, and uric acid crystals.

Factor XIIa activates two major substrates, factor XI and prekallikrein, generating XIa and kallikrein. High molecular weight kinogen (HMWK), serves as a cofactor for the activation of each proenzyme in these two reactions. Kallikrein, formed by activated XIIa, activates more factor XII to XIIa. This forms a positive feedback loop between the two factors; the synthesis of one factor leads to generation of the other.

After the activation of XI (XIa), the intrinsic pathway proceeds with the conversion of factor IX to IXa. Factor IXa then binds via calcium to a phospholipid surface (PF3). In the presence of factor VIII, a cofactor, activated IX (IXa) converts X to Xa. The formation of activated factor X (Xa) is the first key reaction in the coagulation cascade and is the point at which the intrinsic and extrinsic pathways merge (Fig. 31-2, step 10).

Factor X is also activated via the extrinsic system (Fig. 31-2, step (9). This pathway is initiated by tissue thromboplastin, a phospholipid released from cell membranes of damaged tissue outside the vascular tree. Tissue phospholipid binds factor VII in the presence of calcium ions. This complex converts factor X to Xa. It is thought that much of factor VII circulates in the blood in activated form but is unable to activate factor X without tissue thromboplastin.

With the formation of Xa by the intrinsic and extrinsic systems, the common pathway begins. The second key reaction in the coagulation sequence is the formation of thrombin. Like the formation of factor Xa, this reaction is comprised of a five-component system. Factor Xa must be bound with its cofactor, factor V, via calcium onto the platelet phospholipid surface. Activated factor X (Xa) then cleaves prothrombin (factor II) to form thrombin (IIa).

The final key step, fibrin formation, occurs by the action of thrombin on fibrinogen. Thrombin bound to platelet factor 3, splits off two small peptides on each side of the fibrinogen molecule to produce the fibrin monomer. These fibrin monomers then aggregate end to end and side by side to form a fibrin polymer. This fibrin clot is known as fibrin S (soluble) and is held together only by hydrogen bonds. The fibrin clot is stabilized when covalent peptide bonds are formed between the fibrin monomers. This conversion from hydrogen bonds to peptide bonds is accomplished by factor XIII (fibrin stabilizing factor), which is activated by thrombin and calcium ions. The action of factor XIII crosslinks these fibrin monomers to form the stable fibrin clot (insoluble).

In all likelihood, the coagulation process has several triggers besides factor XII. Patients with a deficiency of either factor XII, prekallikrein, or high molecular weight kinogen (HMWK), clot without difficulty and do not have a bleeding tendency. As a rule, patients with factor XI deficiency have no bleeding symptoms, or only very mild ones.

The concept of the intrinsic and extrinsic pathways as two distinct systems leading to the activation of factor X is probably oversimplified but is useful from a diagnostic standpoint. There are probably many interactions between the two pathways. It is thought that factor VIIa can also activate factor IX.

Thrombin is the master coagulation enzyme, playing many roles. When present in low concentrations, it stimulates the intrinsic pathway of coagulation by increasing the activity of factors V and VIII. When thrombin is present in high concentration, it inhibits their action. Thrombin has a role in primary hemostasis. It stimulates platelets to release ADP, which causes them to aggregate. It also stimulates endothelial cells to produce prostacyclin, which stimulates vessel relaxation.

As coagulation proceeds, fibrin is laid down upon the growing platelet mass. A final step involves retraction of the platelet actin and myosin fibers, which leads to consolidation of the clot.

Fibrinolysis

Once a clot forms and bleeding stops, the clot is normally replaced by fibrous tissue or liquefied by fibrinolysis, the third major stage of normal hemostasis. As in coagulation, fibrinolysis also occurs through an intrinsic and an extrinsic pathway. The intrinsic pathway is initiated within the blood vessel, by activated factor XIIa (Fig. 31-3, step 16). The extrinsic pathway is initiated by tissue activators outside the vessel (tissue plasminogen activator) (Fig. 31-3, step 15). In both pathways, plasminogen (synthesized in the liver) is converted to plasmin, which degrades and lyses fibrin.

Although plasmin acts mostly on fibrin,

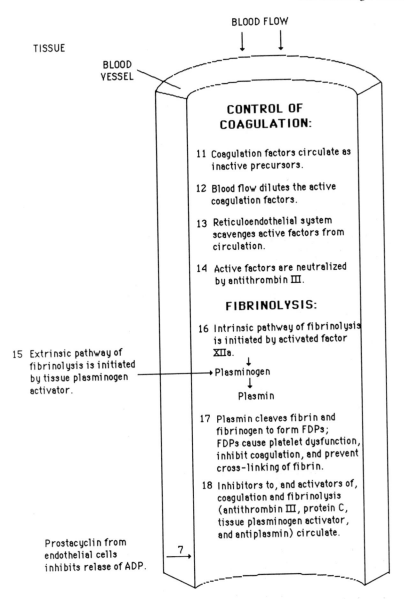

Fig. 31-3. The control of coagulation (steps 11 through 14) and the process of fibrinolysis (steps 15 through 17) are shown. Fibrinolysis is the last of the three major stages of normal hemostasis (see text for complete explanation). FDPs = fibrin degradation products.

it also cleaves fibrinogen and other clotting factors to produce fibrin degradation products (FDPs) or fibrin split products (FSPs). The structure of FDPs varies according to whether plasmin is cleaving fibrinogen, fibrin that is cross-linked, or fibrin that is not cross-linked. As clots are liquefied by plasmin, the FDPs are removed from blood by the liver, kidney and reticuloendothelial system. They normally have halflives of about 9 hours. If their production exceeds their clearance, the FDPs accumulate. High concentrations of FDPs inhibit coagulation, prevent cross-linking of fibrin, and disrupt normal platelet function[7,8] (Fig. 31-3, step 17).

Under normal circumstances, fibrinolytic activity is balanced perfectly by thrombotic activity: the hemostatic mechanism stops active bleeding; fibrinolysis removes excess fibrin; and normal blood flow returns in the healed blood vessel.

MECHANISMS REGULATING HEMOSTASIS AND FIBRINOLYSIS

The clotting and fibrinolytic systems must be regulated precisely to prevent widespread thrombosis or excessive bleeding. Several mechanisms protect this delicate balance.

Control of Primary Hemostasis

Two prostaglandins, thromboxane A_2 and prostacyclin, control primary hemostasis. These two compounds have opposing actions and different sites of synthesis. Platelets activated by contact with collagen in the subendothelial layers of an injured blood vessel release thromboxane A_2 (Fig. 31-1, step 3). Thromboxane A_2 increases release of ADP and causes further platelet aggregation at the site of injury. However, extension of the aggregating mass of activated platelets beyond the site of injury causes normal endothelium to produce prostacyclin (Fig. 31-1, step 7). Prostacyclin decreases release of ADP and slows platelet aggregation and plug formation. In this way, primary hemostasis is limited to the site of injury.

Prostaglandin control of primary hemostasis has clinical significance. Drugs containing aspirin inhibit synthesis of thromboxane A_2 and the consequent release of ADP and aggregation of platelets. The effect of aspirin on these platelets is irreversible and causes a defect in primary hemostasis that prolongs bleeding time for several days, until new platelets are synthesized. Transfusion of two units of normal platelets corrects this defect. The new platelets release enough ADP to cause aggregation of both new and aspirin-impaired platelets.[9,10]

Foreign materials, such as vascular grafts or cardiopulmonary bypass tubing, inhibit the normal prostaglandin control of primary hemostasis. Unlike normal endothelium, foreign materials do not produce prostacyclin. Platelet aggregation can proceed uninhibited, well beyond the site of injury, to initiate clot formation and graft thrombosis.

The real significance of prostaglandin control of primary hemostasis is that limiting platelet aggregation localizes clot formation. Some of the clotting factors require a phospholipid surface for their interaction. This surface is provided by activated platelets. By controlling the extent of platelet aggregation with prostacyclin, clot formation is limited to the site of injury.

Control of Coagulation

Coagulation is regulated in several ways. Most of the coagulation factors circulate in inactive (precursor) forms. Several factors require a phospholipid surface (platelet factor 3) or tissue thromboplastin for their proper interaction. Once activated, the factors are diluted by rapid blood flow and are removed from the circulation by the reticuloendothelial system[3] (Fig. 31-3, steps 12 and 13).

A naturally occurring inhibitor of coagulation, antithrombin III (AT 3), binds to thrombin and other clotting factors, forming inactive complexes and preventing normal coagulation. In the presence of heparin, AT 3 binds more avidly (100 times more rapidly) to thrombin. In fact, without AT 3, heparin has little anticoagulant effect. Deficiencies of AT 3 result in excessive coagulation. This type of deficiency can occur in disseminated intravascular coagulation (DIC), and occasionally in women taking birth control pills. Transfusion of fresh frozen plasma (which contains AT 3) permits patients with low or absent levels of AT 3 to undergo anticoagulation with heparin.

Further control of coagulation is provided by a negative feedback loop in the coagulation cascade. Higher concentrations of thrombin destroy the activity of factors V and VIII:C and thus decrease the rate of its own synthesis. Conversely, low concentrations of thrombin stimulate the activity of those factors.

CAUSES OF PATHOLOGIC BLEEDING

Bleeding disorders are most easily categorized according to which component of the hemostatic system is affected: the blood vessels, platelets, clotting factors, or the fibrinolytic system. The defect may also result from the production or presence of inhibitors. These defects are further categorized as being qualitative or quantitative in nature and as being inherited or acquired.

Vascular Disorders

Vascular bleeding may result from a structural defect in the vessel wall or from an altered ability of the blood vessel to interact with platelets and coagulation proteins. These vascular disorders are sometimes hereditary, but more often are caused by immune or inflammatory processes that damage the blood vessel.

The most common hereditary vascular abnormality that leads to bleeding is called hereditary hemorrhagic telangiectasia (Osler-Weber-Rendu disease). Telangiectases appear in the skin and mucous membranes. (Telangiectases are red spots caused by blood in abnormally dilated vessels that blanch on pressure). In this disorder, a defect in the subendothelial connective tissue results in multiple dilatations of capillaries and arterioles. The thinning of the blood vessel walls leads to subsequent rupture and bleeding.

Other inherited vascular defects are rare but include disorders of collagen synthesis. Collagen, which is in the subendothelium of blood vessels, is important both for structural support and for platelet adhesion. Defects of collagen synthesis lead to fragile blood vessels and impaired hemostasis. The most well known of the collagen "inborn errors of metabolism" is Ehlers-Danlos syndrome. Another example of a connective tissue disorder is osteogenesis imperfecta, a disease that leads to extreme vascular fragility.

The more commonly acquired vascular defects are purpura simplex (simple easy brusing), senile purpura, purpura associated with infections and drugs, scurvy, and the purpura of rheumatoid arthritis and amyloid disease.

Purpura simplex is a common disorder of young healthy women. The "simple easy bruising" is seen mostly on the legs or trunk and is due to fragile blood vessels in the skin. It has only cosmetic significance as does senile purpura. In this disorder elderly patients bruise on their forearms and hands where the skin is inelastic and thin with marked collagen loss.

Purpura caused by infection may be the result of vascular damage or microthrombi. Several drugs are associated with purpura production that clears when the drug is discontinued. Long-term corticosteroid therapy is thought to produce bruising or multiple petechial hemorrhages due to a vascular defect. These patients lose subcutaneous tissue that normally surrounds their blood vessels. This makes the blood vessels more subject to trauma.

In general, vascular defects do not cause significant hemorrhage with the exception of hereditary hemorrhagic telangiectasia. They are usually only associated with easy bruising and spontaneous bleeding from small vessels.

Platelet Deficiency or Dysfunction

Platelet disorders may be either quantitative or qualitative in nature. Thrombocytopenia may result from impaired platelet production or from the sequestration, destruction, or consumption of platelets. For example, production of platelets can decrease if bone marrow is infiltrated with tumor or is destroyed by radiation or drugs. Hypersplenism may cause sequestration of platelets. Platelet antibodies formed after multiple transfusions may destroy platelets (see Ch. 30). The idiopathic immune destruction of platelets is called idiopathic thrombocytopenic purpura (ITP). Acute ITP usually occurs in children or young adults and develops after recovery from a viral infection. The patients apparently develop a platelet autoantibody that is responsible for the destruction of the platelets. In chronic thrombocytopenic purpura, effective treatment usually consists of corticosteroid therapy or splenectomy because the spleen removes the platelets that are coated with the antibody. Transient platelet antibodies may be induced by infections or drugs. This is thought to be the mechanism of heparin-induced thrombocytopenia. The thrombocyto-

penia seen in autoimmune diseases, such as systemic lupus erythematosus, autoimmune hemolytic anemia, or rheumatoid arthritis, is also of an immune origin with antigen-antibody complexes that damage the platelets and lead to their destruction. Thrombocytopenia frequently complicates septicemia and is thought to be immune complex induced. The concentration of platelets may be decreased by massive transfusion with platelet-poor blood or crystalloid (see Ch. 30), and platelets may be consumed during DIC.

Many functional platelet disorders exist. In congenital platelet dysfunction, the count is normal or slightly reduced, but bleeding time is prolonged. Platelets may have an abnormal form and usually respond abnormally to platelet aggregation tests. Most of these hereditary platelet disorders are very rare. Both platelet dysfunction and a factor defect occur in von Willebrand's disease, a congenital hemorrhagic diathesis. In this syndrome, the VWF portion of the factor VIII complex is deficient and leads to defects in platelet adhesion to collagen. Bleeding also occurs because VWF serves as a carrier protein for factor VIII:C, the coagulant portion of the complex. With deficiencies of VIII:VWF, factor VIII:C levels are also reduced, producing clotting abnormalities and bleeding.

Acquired qualitative platelet defects are much more common and often caused by medication. Anti-inflammatory agents (aspirin, indomethacin, phenylbutazone, and prostaglandin synthesis inhibitors such as ibuprofen), antidepressants (amitriptyline), and other drugs (phenothiazines, ethanol, dipyridamole, dextran, propranolol, and diphenhydramine) cause varying degrees of platelet dysfunction. The defect caused by aspirin is the most potent and remains for the lifetime of exposed platelets (7 to 10 days). Transfusion of two units of platelets will allow platelets impaired by aspirin to function.[9,10]

The platelet dysfunction occurring in uremia is thought to be caused by accumulation in serum of compounds like guanidinosuccinic acid. These substances prolong bleeding time by inhibiting platelet adhesiveness; many, if not all, of these substances are small enough to be filtered by dialysis.[11]

Qualitative platelet defects are associated with cirrhotic liver disease, systemic lupus erythematosus, and alcohol consumption. Fibrin degradation products produced during DIC inhibit platelet function and impair primary hemostasis.

Factor Deficiencies

Clotting abnormalities may be categorized according to whether they are inherited or acquired. Hereditary factor deficiencies normally pertain to a single factor; acquired deficiencies usually involve several factors.

Hereditary deficiencies of all of the factors have been described. With the exception of hemophilia A and B (factors VIII and IX respectively) and von Willebrand's disease, congenital factor deficiencies are extremely rare. These factor deficiencies may be the result of inadequate synthesis or due to the synthesis of factors that are inactive.

Unlike hemophilia A and B and von Willebrand's disease, not all factor deficiencies produce significant clinical bleeding. Inadequate fibrinogen, factors V, VII, and X, all predispose to mild to moderate bleeding. Factor XI deficiency causes bleeding only after trauma or surgery. Deficiency of factors XII, prekallikrein, and high-molecular weight kinogen present no bleeding problems, although there may be a marked laboratory defect. Factor XIII deficiency causes delayed bleeding after trauma or surgery, but all screening coagulation tests are normal.

Hemophilia A and B and von Willebrand's disease are the most common and most important hereditary factor disorders. There is a wide clinical spectrum within each disease. For hemophilia A, activity levels of less than 1 percent of normal are associated with severe bleeding, levels of 1 to 5 percent with moderate bleeding symptoms, and levels between 5 and 20 percent with mild bleeding. Because of these wide clinical variations, not all hemophiliacs are diagnosed in childhood. Patients with hemophilia who present for elective surgery should have their hematologist involved in their perioperative management. In an emergency, the deficient factor must be replaced, using the appropriate factor concentrate or cryoprecipitate for factor VIII. Determination of factor levels before and after infusion is useful for judging the adequacy of, and need for, continued therapy.

Acquired clotting factor disorders are far more common in clinical practice. Because the liver synthesizes most of the clotting factors (except factor VIII), liver disease produces a multifactorial bleeding disorder. If vitamin K is not present for any reason, the vitamin K dependent factors (II, VII, IX, X) will be produced by the liver, but will be inactive. This results in a multifactorial defect. Vitamin K deficiency may result from antibiotic destruction of the intestinal flora that produce the active vitamin, from malabsorption syndromes, from biliary obstruction, and from malnutrition. Anticoagulation with coumadin affects the vitamin K factors because coumadin competes with vitamin K for a specific binding protein on hepatocytes. It therefore produces a "vitamin K deficiency" state; the net effect of coumadin depends on the availability of vitamin K and the plasma level of this compound.

Clotting factor deficiencies occur with DIC because the factors are consumed at a rate that outstrips production. Patients who receive multiple transfusions with stored blood or who receive large volumes of crystalloids develop clotting factor deficiencies on a dilutional basis. Stored blood is deficient in the labile factors, factors V and VIII.

Presence of Inhibitors of Coagulation

The possible presence of endogenous or exogenous inhibitors of coagulation or fibrinolysis should be considered in the patient with a bleeding disorder. Fibrin degradation products (present with DIC) and heparin are the most common examples. Naturally occurring inhibitors of coagulation include antithrombin III and protein C. However, some pathologic inhibitors develop in different disease states and produce clinical bleeding. Patients with hemophilia who have received multiple transfusions sometimes develop circulating antibodies that inactivate any transfused factor VIII:C. Patients with systemic lupus erythematosus are known to also develop circulating antibodies that inhibit coagulation.

Heparin therapy promotes the inhibition of coagulation by AT 3. This effect can be reversed rapidly with administration of protamine, which binds to heparin and prevents the complexing of heparin with AT 3. "Heparin rebound" is a poorly understood phenomenon that sometimes occurs after presumed reversal of heparin with protamine. Such patients should be reevaluated for residual heparin effect. In addition, administration of heparin can lead to thrombocytopenia.

Disseminated intravascular coagulation is associated with many conditions—sepsis, liver disease, hemolytic transfusion reaction, shock, acidosis, cardiac arrest, and others. Ironically, the cause of DIC-induced bleeding is excessive clot formation. That is, coagulation occurs throughout the microcirculation, exhaust-

ing the supply of clotting factors. The fibrinolytic system becomes active, producing FDPs that inhibit clotting and disrupt normal platelet dysfunction. As platelets are consumed, signs of vascular-platelet defects and factor deficiencies appear. In particular, bleeding occurs from the gastrointestinal tract and other mucous membranes, and blood often appears in the urine. Bleeding also occurs from cutdown and operative sites. Coagulation abnormalities include vascular fragility, platelet deficiency and dysfunction, factor deficiencies, and the presence of inhibitors of coagulation. Compounding the problem is an active fibrinolytic system that is trying to lyse the fibrin clots that do form.[3,12]

CLINICAL APPROACH TO BLEEDING: PREOPERATIVE CONSIDERATIONS

The History

The patient's history is important in the diagnosis of a bleeding disorder; screening laboratory tests are not a substitute. Patients may have experienced many challenges to their hemostatic mechanism that are more significant than routine laboratory testing. Some bleeding disorders, such as scurvy, do not alter screening coagulation tests. Other disorders, such as factor XII deficiency, prolong the laboratory tests, but do not cause clinical bleeding. If a patient's history suggests the presence of a bleeding disorder, laboratory testing is appropriate; routine screening is unnecessary.

Many disease processes are associated with abnormal bleeding, such as peptic ulcers and hemorrhoids. It is the task of the physician to determine whether a patient's history of bleeding is due to local causes or due to a generalized hemostatic defect.

It is extremely helpful if the patient has previously undergone a major surgical procedure, since this is a good test of the hemostatic mechanism. The patient's response to circumcision, tonsillectomy, tooth extraction, or trauma is also valuable.

If the patient describes unusual bruising or bleeding, an attempt should be made to differentiate clinically between a platelet or vascular disorder and a clotting disorder. The pattern, onset, and duration of bleeding usually suggest the more likely diagnosis.

Abnormalities in primary hemostasis (platelet or vascular defects) result in bruising, petechiae, and "mucous membrane bleeding," such as nosebleeds, menorrhagia, or gastrointestinal bleeding. After trauma or surgery, bleeding is immediate and perhaps prolonged but often controllable by application of direct pressure. To elicit a history characteristic of this type of hemostatic defect, the anesthetist can ask whether the patient bruises easily, gets frequent nosebleeds, or has seen blood in the urine. The patient can also be asked whether the gums usually bleed during brushing of teeth and whether prolonged bleeding has occurred after surgery or dental extractions. The presence of petechiae certainly suggests a platelet or vascular disorder, whereas easy bruising may occur in elderly patients, in some normal women, and in many clotting disorders.

Clotting factor defects often manifest as soft tissue bleeding or hemarthrosis. Patients may report that after surgery or trauma, bleeding stops initially (owing to formation of a platelet plug) but resumes within several hours. Because single-factor deficiencies are usually hereditary, the age of onset of a bleeding problem and the family history are important. Most acquired clotting disorders involve multiple-factor deficiencies and have their onset in adulthood.

Even if the patient has no history or evidence of bleeding problems, the physician should evaluate the patient for medical conditions associated with hemostatic defects. Such conditions can be categorized by the hemostatic defect they produce: (1) vascular problems, (2) platelet disorders, (3) factor deficiencies, and (4) the presence of inhibitors of coagulation.

Laboratory Tests

Patients suspected of having a hemostatic defect by history normally then undergo coagulation tests. No single test is sufficient to diagnose a bleeding disorder. Although the clinical picture may suggest a particular diagnosis, it is difficult to differentiate among the various causes of abnormal bleeding on clinical grounds alone.

The initial coagulation tests often include a platelet count and determination of prothrombin time (PT), partial thromboplastin time (PTT), thrombin time (TT), and fibrinogen levels. Determination of bleeding time is desirable but unpleasant for the patient and does not need to be done routinely. This test should be reserved for patients whose platelet counts are normal but who are suspected of having abnormal platelet function. A microscopic smear of peripheral blood and a test to detect the presence of FDPs yield helpful information but are usually not included in the initial set of coagulation tests.

Drawn blood should be collected in three tubes. One tube should contain ethylenediaminetetraacetic acid (EDTA); one, citrate; and one, nothing. Blood mixed with EDTA is suitable for the blood smear, platelet count, and determination of hemoglobin and hematocrit, if desired. The PT, PTT, and TT clotting studies and determination of fibrinogen levels are performed on blood mixed with citrate, which chelates calcium and prevents clotting. The specimen in the tube without an additive coagulates and provides the whole-blood coagulation time. If a transfusion reaction is suspected, this sample can be examined for the presence of free hemoglobin.

The results of the coagulation studies must be evaluated together to deduce the probable source of the bleeding defect. For this reason, it is best to classify the tests according to the part of the hemostatic system examined.

Tests for Primary Hemostasis

A *platelet count* of less than 100,000/mm³ often prolongs bleeding time. A platelet count inadequate for coagulation is the most common cause of serious bleeding. When the platelet count is 10,000 to 100,000/mm³, an inverse relationship exists between the number of platelets and bleeding time.[3,13]

A normal *bleeding time* requires an adequate number of platelets and normal platelet function. Determination of bleeding time is indicated if a functional platelet defect is suspected and platelet count is normal. Bleeding time is determined by placing a blood pressure cuff on the upper arm, inflating the cuff to 40 mmHg, and making an incision 1 mm deep by 9 mm long on the flexor aspect of the forearm. Normally, when this area is blotted every 30 seconds, serum will not appear after 4.5 minutes (the accepted normal range is 3 to 9 minutes). Bleeding time may be prolonged in the presence of thrombocytopenia, qualitative platelet defects, von Willebrand's disease, and vascular defects.[13]

Coagulation Testing

When coagulation pathways are tested, the endpoint is always formation of the fibrin clot. Because the intrinsic and extrinsic pathways occur on different phospholipid surfaces, each pathway can be tested by adding a specific phospholipid to the patient's blood.

Tests for the Intrinsic and Common Pathways of Coagulation

Three tests examine the intrinsic and common pathways. *Partial thromboplastin time* is determined by adding platelet phospholipid or a substitute, cephalin, to the patient's blood and noting the time to formation of a fibrin clot. When the PTT test is modified by surface-activating factors XII and XI before addition of platelet phospholipid, the result is a test for *"activated" partial thromboplastin time*. Normal values are less than 35 seconds. In the third test, *activated clotting time* is determined by adding diatomaceous earth for surface activation of factors XII and XI. This test relies on the patient's blood providing platelet phospholipid. Normal values are in the range of 90–120 seconds.

The clotting times for all of these tests will be prolonged if there is a deficiency, abnormality, or inhibitor of one or more of the factors involved in the intrinsic and common pathways (i.e., factors XII, XI, IX, VIII, X, V, II, and I). Prolonged times commonly occur with heparin therapy, inadequate fibrinogen levels (as occur in DIC), or factor dilution after massive transfusion.

A Test for the Extrinsic Pathway

In the test for *prothrombin time*, tissue phospholipid is added to the patient's blood, and the time to formation of a fibrin clot is noted. PT will be prolonged by deficiencies, abnormalities, or inhibitors of one or more of the factors involved in the extrinsic or common pathway (i.e., factors VII, X, V, II, or I).

PT is used to monitor the effect of the anticoagulant coumadin, as factor VII is the first coagulation protein to be depleted with this therapy. PT is also a sensitive test for liver disease or vitamin K deficiency. Although patients with these conditions often lack many factors, factor VII is the first to be depleted, thereby prolonging PT. Further depletion of other factors by vitamin K deficiency also prolongs PTT.[14]

Tests for the Final Common Pathway

Three tests evaluate the final common hemostatic pathway. In the determination of *thrombin time*, thrombin is added to the patient's blood, and the time to formation of a fibrin clot is noted. This test detects abnormalities in the conversion of fibrinogen to fibrin. TT will be prolonged if the level of fibrinogen is inadequate (as occurs with DIC) or if inhibitors of thrombin (which converts fibrinogen to fibrin) are present, such as heparin or FDPs. TT is the most sensitive indicator of the presence of heparin.

Fibrinogen levels are also an indicator of the status of the final common pathway. Normal levels range from 150 to 300 mg/dl, and levels lower than 100 mg/dl may be inadequate to produce a clot. Although fibrinogen may be depleted with severe liver disease, this condition most commonly occurs in DIC states.

When thrombin time is prolonged, the test for *reptilase time* can distinguish an effect of heparin from a defect caused by the presence of FDPs and low levels of fibrinogen. This is possible because heparin causes avid complexing of thrombin with AT 3 but does not affect the enzyme reptilase. Therefore, regardless of the presence or absence of heparin, reptilase will still cleave fibrinogen to form fibrin. Additionally, reptilase time is prolonged by the presence of FDPs. Thus, if both TT and reptilase time are prolonged, the cause must be low fibrinogen levels or the presence of FDPs. If TT is prolonged but reptilase time is normal, prolongation of TT is caused by heparin.

A Test for Fibrinolysis

The amount of *fibrin degradation products* in the circulation is determined by mixing plasma with antibodies against FDPs. Serial dilutions of antibodies are used until no clumping occurs. Elevated FDP levels indicate that the rate of production of FDPs exceeds the normal mechanisms for their removal. This occurrence is a sign of accelerated clot lysis (fibrinolytic system). The presence of FDPs does not differentiate primary fibrinolysis (which is caused by massive release of plasminogen activator, as may occur during prostate surgery) from secondary fibrinolysis (which is initiated by DIC).

The combination of prolonged thrombin time and decreased fibrinogen levels is highly suggestive of DIC.

Measurement of Clot Formation

The thromboelastograph measures the speed of clot formation and the firmness of the clot. Measurement of five basic variables produces a characteristic tracing that differentiates between thrombocytopenia, factor deficiency, and excessive fibrinolysis. The thromboelastograph is often used during liver transplantation because of the need for massive blood transfusion.[2,15]

Analysis of the results of the clotting profile should identify the pathway involved by the hemostatic defect and may indicate the need for further tests or the assistance of a hematologist.

Preoperative Treatment

Vascular Bleeding

Vascular bleeding caused by infection or inflammation is often difficult to treat. The underlying disease must be addressed to decrease the tendency to bleed. Most vascular causes of bleeding require surgical intervention.

Platelet Deficiencies or Dysfunction

Treatment of platelet deficiencies or dysfunction depends on the cause of thrombocytopenia or platelet defect. If platelets are being destroyed rapidly and the mechanism for their destruction remains, transfusion will be of little value. Therapies such as splenectomy or administration of steroids may be indicated. Examination of bone marrow can distinguish impaired production of platelets from platelet destruction. If abnormal production is the cause of thrombocytopenia, platelet transfusions should dramatically improve hemostasis. Dialysis improves platelet dysfunction caused by renal failure, and removal of FDPs would improve platelet function in DIC. Aspirin-containing drugs are a common cause of platelet dysfunction, which is easily treated by transfusing platelets or by withdrawing the drug for 7 to 10 days.

Factor Deficiencies

Single-factor deficiencies (usually hereditary) require replacement therapy before surgery. The patient's hematologist should be involved in the preparation of such patients for surgery.

More commonly, patients present with multiple-factor acquired deficiencies as a result of liver disease, vitamin K deficiency, coumadin therapy, or DIC. Inadequate hepatic synthesis of clotting factors caused by liver disease cannot be corrected rapidly; transfusion of fresh frozen plasma will best restore the deficient factors. For the patient receiving coumadin therapy, PT will return to near normal if the daily dose is discontinued 36 to 48 hours before surgery. Vitamin K therapy can correct an abnormal PT within 8 to 12 hours. If the patient must

undergo emergency surgery, two to four units of fresh frozen plasma may be given to replenish the vitamin K-dependent factors. Preoperative bleeding in patients with DIC can also be caused by the presence of inhibitors of coagulation.

Inhibitors of Coagulation

Heparin therapy is reversed rapidly by administering protamine. This compound binds to heparin and prevents the complexing of heparin to AT 3. Inhibiting the action of AT 3 in turn promotes coagulation. However, the potential side effects of protamine make it preferable to discontinue heparin and wait 8 hours before surgery, if possible. This period permits metabolism of heparin.

Correction of bleeding caused by DIC depends on treatment of the underlying cause of this syndrome. Although the patient may benefit from administration of platelet concentrates and fresh frozen plasma, the production of FDPs and the consumption of factors must be stopped. Then normal mechanisms will clear the circulation of these inhibitors (FDPs), and normal coagulation can proceed. Severe DIC merits the advice of a hematologist.

Two other issues regarding preoperative hemostatic interventions deserve mention but are not sufficiently evaluated in the literature to allow definitive statements about their perioperative implications. The first issue involves the patient given a fibrinolytic agent such as streptokinase or tissue plasminogen activator (TPA) who then requires emergency surgery. Both streptokinase and TPA are used to relieve acute vascular occlusions in extremities and in renal or visceral vessels.[16] Insufficient data have accumulated to prescribe ideal preoperative preparation and intraoperative management of hemostasis in such patients. Postponing surgery for three half-lives of the drug (increases in plasmin activity in blood can be assayed for at least 4 to 8 hours) may not be possible, and observing the operative field for meticulous attention to hemostasis may not suffice.[17] To correct fibrinogen deficiency in such patients, I have administered fibrinogen before surgery and ε-aminocaproic acid (EACA) at the time of heparin administration. I delayed giving EACA until heparin administration to minimize the risk of thrombosis.

The second issue relates to routine use of desmopressin to decrease bleeding and transfusion requirements. Such therapy began as a treatment for platelet dysfunction in von Willebrand's disease but has since expanded to routine use in healthy patients undergoing cardiovascular surgery. This increased use occurred because desmopressin was found to decrease bleeding and transfusion requirements.[18] Whether the side effects of desmopressin exceed the benefits remains to be determined and will probably influence the likelihood that therapy with desmopressin becomes routine.

INTRAOPERATIVE BLEEDING

Although diagnosing intraoperative bleeding is a much shorter process than diagnosing preoperative bleeding, the former is more dynamic, and often more than one cause of bleeding exists.

Most intraoperative bleeding is surgical in nature. Therefore, when diffuse bleeding occurs during surgery, a surgical cause should first be suspected, as vascular disruption will certainly require surgical correction. Nevertheless, surgery-related intraoperative bleeding is often diagnosed only by the exclusion of other causes. For example, a surgical source is likely if the patient continues to bleed but laboratory tests of coagulation

are normal. Also, surgical bleeding is usually localized, whereas bleeding caused by a coagulation defect is not. Additionally, the appearance of clots in pooled blood usually indicates that bleeding is related to a surgical defect and not to a coagulation defect.

If bleeding does not appear to be related to surgery, the possibility of a hemostatic defect should be considered. Intraoperative coagulopathies are usually caused by acquired hemostatic defects; congenital hemostatic defects are unlikely to manifest during surgery without a prior history of bleeding. Coagulopathy would most probably result from multiple transfusions, a transfusion reaction, or from ongoing DIC.

Acquired Defects Causing Intraoperative Bleeding

Acquired defects are few and somewhat predictable. They are caused by (1) residual heparin effect, (2) dilutional thrombocytopenia, (3) dilution of factors V and VIII, (4) preexisting liver disease or anticoagulant therapy, (5) DIC, and (6) transfusion reaction.

Residual Heparin Effect
Continued intraoperative bleeding in patients given heparin and protamine reversal of heparin may be attributable to residual heparin effect. Because patients vary in their response to this anticoagulant, standard dose regimens do not always produce uniform effects. A popular way to monitor the effect of heparin is to measure activated clotting time.[19] After a baseline value has been established, an initial dose of heparin is given. In a few minutes, another value is obtained, and the ability of that quantity of heparin to prolong activated clotting time is determined. Repeating this sequence allows

one to generate a dose-response curve.[20,21]

Heparin is administered systemically or locally in vascular procedures when occlusion of the aorta is expected to exceed 10 minutes or when the adequacy of peripheral collateral flow has not been determined. Such patients are usually given doses that do not cause full anticoagulation (i.e., 4,000 to 5,000 units of heparin per 70 kg of body weight). This dose of heparin increases activated clotting time to approximately 260 seconds within 15 minutes. In these instances, the effect of the anticoagulant is not reversed. Heparin prevents thrombosis but may complicate the differential diagnosis of intraoperative bleeding.

Patients deficient in AT 3 are resistant to heparin. Administering fresh frozen plasma restores AT 3 levels and permits anticoagulation with heparin.

Reversal dosages of protamine may be calculated empirically. First, activated clotting time is determined. Then, 1.3 mg of protamine per kg is given for each 100 units of heparin remaining in the patient, as calculated from the activated clotting time. Protamine administration can be associated with some undesirable side effects, including systemic hypotension, pulmonary hypertension, and, in excess, with coagulopathy.[22–24] Heparin-induced anticoagulation can be distinguished from protamine overdosage by determining TT. That is, TT is normal with excess protamine but prolonged with residual heparin effect.

Chronic administration of heparin causes mild thrombocytopenia in 5 to 30 percent of patients and severe thrombocytopenia in 1 to 2 percent. Severe thrombocytopenia is believed to result from production of platelet antibodies.[25,26]

Dilutional Thrombocytopenia
Massive transfusions (usually more than 10 units of blood for a 70-kg patient) commonly result in defects in primary hemostasis because of thrombocytopenia and platelet dysfunction. The platelet count decreases when more than 80 percent of the patient's original blood volume has been replaced within a short period of time. This results because platelets lose viability in stored blood; their hemostatic effectiveness decays within 48 to 72 hours. Current recommendations are that platelets be given routinely after blood loss exceeding one and one-half times the patient's estimated blood volume (see Ch. 30).[2]

Dilution of Factors V and VIII
Stored blood is also deficient in labile clotting factors V and VIII. Massive transfusion dilutes these two factors and decreases their level in the circulation. However, in the absence of DIC, factor deficiencies are rarely a cause of intraoperative coagulopathy, as only 30 percent of factor VIII and only 20 percent of factor V are needed for adequate hemostasis. The current recommendation is that coagulation factors, in the form of fresh frozen plasma, or fresh plasma that accompanies platelet transfusions, should be given after blood loss exceeding two times the estimated blood volume.[2]

Disseminated Intravascular Coagulation
The surgical patient can have or acquire conditions associated with the occurrence of DIC during surgery. Such conditions include sepsis, tissue injury, burns, transfusion reaction, and shock.

In DIC, the normal mechanisms that localize clot formation are disrupted. Because clotting factors require a phospholipid surface on which to interact, coagulation is usually limited to the site of injury. DIC occurs in conditions that cause phospholipids to be circulated diffusely. The presence of immune complexes or bacteria in the blood will cause platelets to aggregate and expose platelet phospholipid (platelet factor 3) throughout the circulation. This condition can occur with sepsis. Tissue thromboplastin (tissue phospholipid) is released into the circulation with massive crush injuries, and hemolyzed cells release phospholipid after a transfusion reaction. Diffuse clotting also is initiated when large surfaces of denuded vascular endothelium are present. Platelet aggregation exposes platelet factor 3, and DIC ensues. This denuded vascular surface is common in patients with vasculitis or burns.

Disseminated intravascular coagulation is likely to develop in patients undergoing vascular surgery if shock has occurred, if the operation has been technically difficult, or if vascular occlusion time has been prolonged. This condition occurs because the tendency for clotting increases when blood flow decreases. That is, low blood flow allows platelets to aggregate on irregular arterial surfaces or on vascular graft material and to initiate the clotting sequence. In contrast, normal cardiac output and good microcirculatory blood flow counteract the tendency toward diffuse coagulation. Clotting factors are diluted by rapid blood flow, and the reticuloendothelial system clears activated factors from the circulation. Fibrinolysis begins concurrently with clot formation. When the natural mechanisms that prevent diffuse clotting are overwhelmed, the fibrinolytic system becomes critical in determining whether the patient will bleed or clot. If FDPs are produced at a rate greater than their clearance, or if their clearance is inhibited (as occurs when blood flow to the liver is interrupted), the balance is lost and the patient with DIC bleeds.

Vascular surgery patients may undergo shock or low-flow states (because of poor cardiac output or hypovolemia). They may also require massive transfusions (which deplete platelets and factors V and VIII) or have tissue damage (which releases tissue thromboplastins). Finally, they may be septic, or develop an anaphylactoid reaction to the material of which their vascular graft is made.[27] All of these conditions can lead to DIC.

Although early diagnosis of DIC may be difficult, DIC should be suspected in the bleeding patient who has not received multiple transfusions, has no history of liver disease, and has not been given heparin. Early in the development of DIC, the platelet count will decrease before PT or PTT increases. Fibrinogen levels, which normally increase during surgical stress, may be normal or reduced. In fact, until clotting factors are markedly depleted, laboratory test results on coagulation may be almost normal. The thromboelastogram may be helpful in such circumstances.[2]

When DIC is well established, laboratory tests will reveal the following: thrombocytopenia (platelet count of less than $150,000/mm^3$), hypofibrinogenemia (fibrinogen levels of less than 160 mg/100 ml of plasma), prolonged PT (greater than 15 seconds), prolonged activated PTT, clot lysis within 2 hours, and the presence of FDPs.

Treatment of DIC obviously involves treating the underlying cause that led to uncontrolled coagulation. This may require the restoration of normal circulation, a good cardiac output, and establishment of normal acid-base balance. The source of platelet activation or release of tissue thromboplastin must be controlled. This may require the treatment of sepsis or immunologic disorders.

The second step of treatment involves replacing deficient blood products, consumed by coagulation. If diffuse platelet activation has occurred, the patient may be thrombocytopenic and require platelet transfusion. Administration of fresh frozen plasma will replace fibrinogen and factors V and VIII consumed by DIC.

Cryoprecipitate may also be used as a source of fibrinogen and factor VIII. The goal is to maintain a platelet count greater than 100,000, a normal activated partial thromboplastin time, and a fibronogen level greater than 200 mg/dl.

Administration of ε-aminocaproic acid, which blocks fibrinolysis, is never indicated in DIC. Fibrinolysis (secondary to coagulation) is a defense mechanism that reduces the effects of diffuse coagulation. On the other hand, heparin is sometimes indicated in DIC; however, a hematologist can help in confirming the need for this controversial therapy.

Overview of Intraoperative and Postoperative Bleeding

Clearly, intraoperative bleeding is more dynamic in nature than preoperative bleeding and often results from multiple sources. Diagnosing these sources may be a difficult process. For one thing, coagulopathies may be obscured by surgical bleeding, or trauma. The patient may need massive transfusion and may be undergoing DIC from shock, sepsis or extensive tissue damage. If cardiac bypass is necessary, heparin will be given. Although protamine can neutralize the effect of heparin, it will not prevent the action of FDPs (from DIC), that is, inhibition of coagulation. In addition, excess protamine causes yet another coagulopathy.

Treatment of this complex situation depends on correction of surgical lesions, replacement of platelets and clotting factors, and removal of any inhibitors to coagulation that are present. Arresting DIC may require restoration of normal circulation, good cardiac output, and normal acid-base balance. Only after FDPs have been cleared from the circulation will normal hemostasis return.

After completion of surgery, continued bleeding is most likely attributable to the same conditions causing intraoperative bleeding, with the exception of the unusual phenomenon of "heparin rebound." This syndrome occurs within 4 or 5 hours of surgery. Some of the heparin administered is believed to be sequestered from the normal circulation. The circulating heparin is neutralized by protamine; then, hours later, the sequestered heparin enters the circulation. The patient begins to bleed as anticoagulation takes place. Treatment requires administration of more protamine.

SUMMARY

The approach to the bleeding patient varies according to the time frame involved. Abnormal preoperative bleeding should be considered in terms of platelet or vascular defects if bruising, petechiae, or mucosal bleeding occurs; or in terms of probable coagulation disorders caused by factor deficiencies if soft tissue bleeding is evident from history. This latter coagulopathy is further classified according to whether the lesion is congenital and due to a single-factor deficiency or whether it is an acquired defect involving multiple-factor deficiencies.

Preoperative laboratory tests evaluated with the patient's history can usually produce an accurate diagnosis and appropriate therapy. Platelet abnormalities may be treated with platelet transfusions unless some mechanism is present that is destroying platelets. Factor deficiencies require transfusion of the appropriate factor concentrate or fresh frozen plasma. A final source of bleeding is the presence of inhibitors (endogenous or exogenous) of coagulation. These include heparin, coumadin, and FDPs, which are produced during DIC. Heparin-induced anticoagulation is reversed with protamine;

coumadin-induced factor deficiencies can be replaced with vitamin K therapy or administration of fresh frozen plasma. To reverse the bleeding tendency with advanced DIC and the production of FDPs, one needs to correct the cause of DIC; normal reticuloendothelial (largely hepatic) mechanisms will then remove the FDPs from the circulation. The patients may be given platelets and fresh frozen plasma in the interim, before the inciting cause of DIC has been eliminated.

Intraoperative bleeding is usually surgical in nature. However, massive transfusion of the patient can dilute the concentration of both platelets and factors, with consequent defects in hemostasis and in coagulation. Disseminated intravascular coagulation is a source of intraoperative bleeding that should be suspected in many clinical conditions, particularly those associated with sepsis or low-flow states. Signs of diffuse clotting and diffuse bleeding may be present.

The mechanism of intraoperative bleeding may not be totally clear, as several sources of bleeding can exist simultaneously. After initiating tests of coagulation, one can replace platelets and clotting factors, consider the presence of inhibitors (endogenous and exogenous) to coagulation, and ensure good circulation and proper acid-base balance. If bleeding continues after surgery and coagulation studies are normal, reoperation can be considered and a hematologist consulted before the situation becomes critical.

REFERENCES

1. Miller RD, Brzica SM, Jr: Blood, blood components, colloids and autotransfusion therapy. p. 1329–1367. In Miller RD (ed): Anesthesia. Vol 2. 2nd. Ed. Churchill Livingstone, New York, 1986

2. Freiberger JJ, Lumb PD: How to manage intraoperative bleeding. Prob Anesth 1:161–172, 1977

3. Fischbach DP, Fogdall RP (eds): Coagulation: The Essentials. Williams & Wilkins, Baltimore, 1981

4. Barrer MJ, Ellison N: Platelet function. Anesthesiology 46:202–211, 1977

5. Weiss HJ: Platelet physiology and abnormalities of platelet function (first of two parts). N Engl J Med 293:531–541, 1975

6. Roath S, Francis JL: Normal blood coagulation, fibrinolysis, and natural inhibitors of coagulation. Int Anesthesiol Clin 23(2):23–35, 1985

7. Kwaan HC: Disseminated intravascular coagulation. Med Clin North Am 56:177–191, 1972

8. Bolton FG: Disseminated intravascular coagulation. Int Anesthesiol Clin 23(2):89–101, 1985

9. Uppington J: Anesthetic management of patients with coagulation disorders. Int Anesthesiol Clin 23(2):125–140, 1985

10. Giddings JC, Evans BK: Drugs affecting blood coagulation and hemostasis. Int Anesthesiol Clin 23(2):103–123, 1985

11. Slater NGP: Acquired bleeding disorders. Int Anesthesiol Clin 23(2):73–87, 1985

12. Ellison N: Diagnosis and management of bleeding disorders. Anesthesiology 47:171–180, 1977

13. Harker LA, Slichter SJ: The bleeding time as a screening test for evaluation of platelet function. N Engl J Med 287:155–159, 1972

14. Moir DJ: Investigation of bleeding disorders. Int Anesthesiol Clin 23(2):37–47, 1985

15. Kang Y, Lewis JH, Navalgund A et al: Epsilon-aminocaproic acid for treatment of fibrinolysis during liver transplantation. Anesthesiology 66:766–773, 1987

16. Boley SJ, Borden EB: Acute mesenteric vascular disease. p. 659–671. In Wilson SE, Veith FJ, Hobson RW, II, Williams RA (eds): Vascular Surgery. Principles and Practice. McGraw-Hill, New York, 1987

17. Lee KF, Mandell J, Rankin JS et al: Im-

mediate versus delayed coronary grafting after streptokinase treatment. Postoperative blood loss and clinical results. J Thorac Cardiovasc Surg 95:216–222, 1988

18. Czer LSC, Bateman TM, Gray RJ et al: Treatment of severe platelet dysfunction and hemorrhage after cardiopulmonary bypass: reduction in blood product usage with desmopressin. J Am Coll Cardiol 9:1139–1147, 1987

19. Cohen JA: Activated coagulation time method for control of heparin is reliable during cardiopulmonary bypass. Anesthesiology 60:121–124, 1984

20. Kamath BSK, Fozard JR: Control of heparinisation during cardiopulmonary bypass. Experience with activated clotting time method. Anaesthesia 35:250–256, 1980

21. Akl BF, Vargas GM, Neal J et al: Clinical experience with the activated clotting time for the control of heparin and protamine therapy during cardiopulmonary bypass. J Thorac Cardiovasc Surgery 79:97–102, 1980

22. Lowenstein E, Johnston WE, Lappas DG et al: Catastrophic pulmonary vasoconstriction associated with protamine reversal of heparin. Anesthesiology 59:470–473, 1983

23. Campbell FW, Goldstein MF, Atkins PC: Management of the patient with protamine hypersensitivity for cardiac surgery. Anesthesiology 61:761–764, 1984

24. Horrow JC: Protamine: a review of its toxicity. Anesth Analg 64:348–361, 1985

25. Vender JS, Matthew EB, Silverman IM et al: Heparin-associated thrombocytopenia: alternative managements. Anesth Analg 65:520–522, 1986

26. Smith JP, Walls JT, Muscato MS et al: Extracorporeal circulation in a patient with heparin-induced thrombocytopenia. Anesthesiology 62:363–365, 1985

27. Roizen MF, Rodgers GM, Valone FH et al: Anaphylactoid reactions to vascular graft material presenting with vasodilatation and subsequent disseminated intravascular coagulation. Anesthesiology 71:1989 (in press).

Index